Success in Practical/ Vocational Nursing

From Student to Leader

EDITION
11

Success in Practical/ Vocational Nursing

From Student to Leader

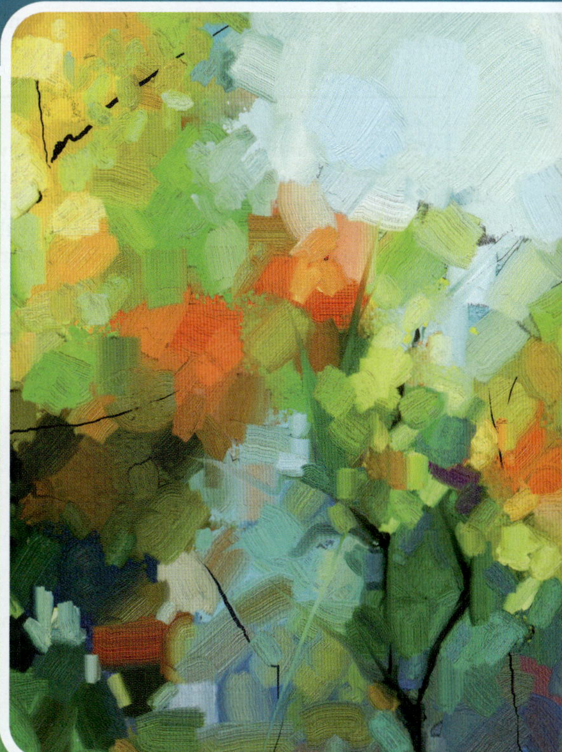

Janyce L. Collier, MSN, MBA, RN, CNE
Formerly, Director
Franklin County Career and Technology Center Practical Nursing Program
Nursing Education Consultant
Chambersburg, Pennsylvania

Ginger L. Peterson, DNP, RN, CNE
Assistant Professor
Department of Nursing, LPN-to-BSN Program
Wilson College
Chambersburg, Pennsylvania

ELSEVIER

Elsevier
3251 Riverport Lane
St. Louis, Missouri 63043

SUCCESS IN PRACTICAL/VOCATIONAL NURSING: FROM STUDENT TO LEADER, ELEVENTH EDITION

ISBN: 978-0-44328-191-4

Content Strategist: Brandi Graham
Content Development Manager: Lisa Newton
Content Development Specialist: Deborah Poulson
Publishing Services Manager: Deepthi Unni
Project Manager: Ashok Ravi
Design Direction: Renee Duenow

Printed in India at Replika Press Pvt. Ltd.
Plot No. 310-311, EPIP, HSIIDC, Kundli Industrial Park,
Sonipat, Haryana – 131028.

Last digit is the print number: 9 8 7 6 5 4 3 2 1

We dedicate the 11th edition of this textbook to
the past and present practical nursing students and nurse educators
who have the passion and the perseverance to attend to the health care needs
of all clients, families, and the community.

We are in constant awe of the motivation of practical nursing students
as they overcome the many obstacles to becoming a nurse.
Additionally, we have the utmost respect for the practical nursing educators
who dedicate their professional passion for nursing to support and mentor students
to successes in the beginning of their nursing career pathway.

Janyce L. Collier
Ginger L. Peterson

Contributor

Pamela Hoffeditz, BSN, MSN, CNE
Nurse Educator
Practical Nursing Program
Franklin County Career and Technology Center
Chambersburg, Pennsylvania

Spiritual Needs, Spiritual Caring, and Religious Differences

Reviewer

Cherie R. Rebar, PhD, DNP, MBA, RN, CNE, CNEcl, CLNC, COI, FAADN
Professor of Nursing
Department of Nursing
Galen College of Nursing
Louisville, Kentucky

LPN/LVN Threads

Standard LPN/LVN Threads series features incorporated into *Success in Practical/Vocational Nursing: From Student to Leader*, 11th edition, make it easy for students to move from one book to the next in the fast-paced and demanding LPN/LVN curriculum. The following features are included in the LPN/LVN Threads:

- A **reading-level evaluation** is performed on all LPN texts to increase the consistency among chapters and ensure that the text is easy to understand.
- **Full-color design, cover, photos**, and **illustrations** are visually appealing and pedagogically useful.
- **Learning Outcomes** (numbered) begin each chapter, provide a framework for content, and are important in providing the structure for the TEACH Lesson Plans for the textbook.
- **Key Terms** are listed at the beginning of each chapter. Key terms appear in color in the chapter with full definitions in the **Glossary**. The goal is to help the student reader with limited proficiency in English develop a greater command of terminology.
- A wide variety of **special features** relate to critical thinking, leadership and management, and more.
- Refer to the Preface for descriptions and examples of features from the pages of this textbook.
- **NCLEX-PN® Review Questions** and **Critical Thinking Scenarios** presented at the end of chapters give students opportunities to practice critical thinking and clinical decision-making skills with realistic student/patient scenarios.
- **Key Points** at the end of each chapter correlate to the learning outcomes and serve as a useful chapter review.
- A full suite of **Instructor Resources**, including TEACH Lesson Plans, PowerPoint Slides, Test Bank, and Image Collection, is included on the Evolve site.

Preface

The 11th Edition of *Success in Practical/Vocational Nursing: From Student to Leader* was revised to expand on the National Council of State Boards of Nursing (NCSBN) changes to the Next Generation NCLEX (NGN) first introduced in 2023. Additional NGN questions have been added to all of the chapters. Additionally, you will notice that Chapter 11 discusses culture and spirituality holistically.

If you are new to this textbook, Dr. Patricia Knecht made significant changes to the ninth edition to facilitate faculty and student interactions that promote critical thinking, robust discussion, and deep understanding of the material beyond content knowledge. The material in the textbook is meant to assist students in their lifelong learning journey and leadership development.

We wish you the best in becoming a licensed practical nurse/licensed vocational nurse (LPN/LVN) and with whatever comes next for you in your career. If you would like to share any comments or suggestions, we welcome you to contact us in care of the customer service department at Elsevier (support.elsevier.com).

Best!
Janyce L. Collier and Ginger L. Peterson

TEACHING AND LEARNING PACKAGE

We provide a rich, abundant collection of supplemental resources for both instructors and students.

FOR THE INSTRUCTOR

The comprehensive Evolve Resources provide a wealth of material to meet your teaching needs. Instructors will have access to all of the student resources, as well as the following:

- A Test Bank contains NCLEX-PN® Examination–style questions that include multiple-choice and alternate-format-item questions.
- PowerPoint presentations that include approximately 400 slides.
- TEACH Lesson Plans are based on textbook chapter objectives. These lesson plans provide a road map to link and integrate all parts of the educational package and can be modified or combined to meet your scheduling and teaching needs.

FOR THE STUDENT

- Evolve Student Learning Resources include NCLEX-PN® Examination–style interactive review questions that test your knowledge and help you prepare for licensure.
- Helpful phrases for communicating in English and Spanish are also provided.
- Additional ancillary material is included to supplement the content of the chapters.

READING AND REVIEW TOOLS

- **Objectives** introduce the chapter topics.
- **Key Terms** are considered essential to understanding chapter content and are defined within the chapter. Key terms are in color the first time they appear in the narrative and are briefly defined in the text, with complete definitions in the Glossary.
- Each chapter ends with a *Get Ready for the NCLEX-PN®* Examination section that includes (1) **Key Points** that reiterate the chapter objectives and serve as a useful review of concepts, (2) a list of **Additional Resources,** (3) a set of **Review Questions for the NCLEX-PN® Examination and Next Generation (NGN) NCLEX-PN®** with answers located in the back of the book, and (4) Scenarios with answers located on the Evolve site.
- References cite evidence-based information and can be found in the back of the text.
- Suggested Readings provide resources for enhancing knowledge and are located on the Evolve site.

CHAPTER FEATURES

Collaborative Care boxes are presented in four ways to introduce the reader to leadership and management in nursing:

- Management Tools provide practical instructions and resources and have the reader apply learned concepts to specific situations.
- Management Hints provide tips for handling management situations.
- Leadership Activities provide students with exercises to practice their leadership skills. Instructions and needed resources are provided.
- Leadership Hints give helpful hints to follow and remember when in a leadership situation.

Critical Thinking boxes encourage problem solving for both academic and personal situations.

Empowerment boxes have questions that contribute to more autonomous, self-directed, positive outcomes in academic and practice settings.

Keep in Mind boxes introduce the reader to the underlying theme of the chapter.

Professional Pointers give readers advice on nursing best practices in the professional arena.

"Try This" boxes challenge students to imagine, visualize, and think outside the box.

Acknowledgments

To the previous author of this textbook—Patty. Thank you, Patty, for your many years of leadership and advocacy in practical nursing education, and for your ongoing support in nursing education at large. Your passion, spirit, work ethic, scholarship, collegiality, and energy are unmatched and validated by all who know and work with you. As the authors of this textbook, we appreciate and cherish our years of friendship with you. You are truly a mentor to us all!

Contents

Personal Resources of an Adult Learner: Becoming a Practical/Vocational Nursing Student

1

Objectives

On completing this chapter, you will be able to do the following:

1. Identify the type of learner that best describes you.
2. Describe common characteristics and experiences shared by different types of adult learners.
3. Describe the role of empowerment in successful learning.
4. Describe various dangers adult learners need to avoid to be successful.
5. Recall special challenges for the practical/vocational nursing student.
6. Discuss your rights as an adult learner.
7. Describe various responsibilities of learners and their implications.
8. Create a personal plan, inclusive of your unique resources, aimed at successfully completing a practical/vocational nursing program within the designated time frame.

Key Terms

active learning	**generational personality**	**referral**
constructive evaluation	**informal education**	**returning adult learner**
facilitator	**learner**	**self-directed learner**
First Amendment	**paradigm**	**self-evaluation**
formal education	**performance evaluation**	**teaching**
generalization	**positive mental attitude**	**traditional adult learner**

Trinh, Akeno, Katie, and Jamal have just finished their orientation for the Success in Practical Nursing Program. As they exit the building, they overhear two other students, Darius and Olivia, recent high school graduates, talking about the age, cultural, and educational differences of the class. Darius states, "Those older students asked way too many questions and could barely fill out the information online. I just wanted to get out of there." Akeno approaches Darius and states, "Hi, Darius, I am one of those older people. I will try to be careful with my many questions, but I love how diverse the class is—I was afraid I was going to be the only older student. It will be interesting to see how we all learn together. I look forward to learning with you." Shrugging his shoulders, Darius walks to his car. "Well," Trinh states, "being a realist, let's hope for the best. It seems like understanding yourself and each other is critical to your personal and the program's success. All of us being different can be a strength, if we understand each other and keep communication open. Let's hope for low drama and keep it positive."

As you read the chapter, think about these students' comments. What knowledge will you develop to help you better understand yourself and others? Learning as a team is powerful. Remember, nursing is a team sport. Your educational journey with your team is beginning.

THE ADULT LEARNER AND RESOURCE MANAGEMENT "JUST IN TIME"

As an adult learner, resource management is a key to success. A successful person/student can identify key resources, knows where to find them, and knows when and how to use them effectively. Unfortunately, we often neglect to engage our resources in a timely fashion. We have all heard the expression "too little, too late." The chapters in Unit 1 are designed to assist you in creating a strong plan to engage your resources "just in time," ensuring success. Understanding your role as an adult learner, including your unique personal attributes, is one of your most valued resources. Self-discovery as an adult learner is a key first step to success. Let's start by understanding the different types of adult learners.

The adult learner (one who acquires knowledge and skills) comes in all ages, and it is possible to have **learners** from five generations in your nursing class. Depending on birth year, generational groups can be characterized. Time frames and names for the five generations vary among authors, but each generation is separated by approximately 20 years (Box 1.1).

Box 1.1 The Five Generations

- Traditionalist (Matures, The Silent Generation) born between 1925 and 1945
- Baby Boomers (Boomers) born between 1946 and 1964
- Generation X (Gen X) born between 1965 and 1980
- Generation Y (Millennials/Net Generation) born between 1981 and 2000
- Generation Z born between 2001 and 2020

Data from Halfer D, Saver C: *Bridging the generation gaps.* Nursing Spectrum/Nurse Week, Falls Church VA, 2008; Riggs CJ: Multiple generations in the nursing workplace: part I. *J Contin Educ Nurs* 44(3):105–106, 2013; Patel D: *8 ways Generation Z will differ from millennials in the workplace.* Forbes, 2017. Available at https://www.forbes.com/sites/deeppatel/2017/09/21/8-ways-generation-z-will-differ-from-millennials-in-the-workplace/#7d7a19576e5e; https://www.purdueglobal.edu/education-partnerships/generational-workforce-differences-infographic. Purdue Global, 2025.

Try This

The Five Generations

Using Box 1.1, identify your generation.

People born around the same time generally develop a **generational personality** of how they think and what they value. This personality is shaped by a common history of cultural events, images, and experiences. Income, religion, education, and geography also influence your generational personality. Understanding your generational perspective and the views of different generations will improve your communication and collaboration with your classmates, faculty, mentors, and colleagues.

Your goal is to be aware of each generation's shared experiences. Avoid stereotyping individuals of a specific generation. A stereotype is a false assumption. It is an expectation that all individuals within a specific group will act exactly the same because they are members of that group. Stereotypes ignore the individual differences that occur within a specific group, for example, a generational group. See Box 1.2 for characteristics of each generation.

Box 1.2 Characteristics of the Five Generations

TRADITIONALIST (THE SILENT GENERATION)

- Depending on birth year, generational personalities may be shaped by the Great Depression, World War II, and/or the Korean War.
- Are more conservative, prefer formal titles, are more formal with intrapersonal interactions, seek conformity.
- Consider work an obligation. Prefer one-to-one meetings and formal memos. Do not like ambiguity or change, prefer to learn in formal, structured ways, oriented to the past but are adaptable.
- Digital immigrants. May be reluctant to use advanced technology and need more time and hands-on to learn modern technology devices and protocols.

BABY BOOMERS

- Depending on birth year, generational personalities may be shaped by Watergate, the Vietnam War, the space race, civil rights, women's liberation, and the assassinations of John and Robert Kennedy and Martin Luther King.
- Dedicated, highly motivated and hard working, idealistic.
- Prefer learning in a relaxed, organized, and respectful atmosphere, like group discussions.
- Digital immigrants and have varying technology skills.

GENERATION X (GEN X)

- Depending on birth year, generational personality may be shaped by the Challenger explosion, the end of the Cold War, MTV, AIDS, Google, Amazon, and dual-career households.
- Accept diversity, less judgmental, pragmatic (practical), flexible, self-reliant (had Boomer parents), multitask well, used to change, informal, conservative/traditional.
- View work as a challenge and opportunity to make changes in the world. Intolerant of "busywork," like small chunks of information, prefer self-study.
- Digital immigrants and are technically literate.

GENERATION Y (MILLENNIALS)

- Depending on birth year, generational personality may be shaped by Columbine, 9/11, the Clinton scandal, and the Afghanistan and Iraq wars.
- Dynamic, confident, straightforward, opinionated, optimistic, sociable, embrace change, multitask, like group discussion, and are high-achieving rule followers.
- View work as a means to an end and have a sense of entrepreneurialism.
- More liberal, tolerant of people different from them, for example in terms of race and sexual orientation.
- Digital natives (Net Generation); grew up using cell phones and computers.

GENERATION Z (IGEN, CENTENNIALS)

- Generation Zers are influenced by the Great Recession.
- Generational personality is influenced using technology and always being highly connected.
- Prefer using smartphones and would rather text than talk; however, prefer face-to-face meetings at work.
- Instinctual relationship with technology.
- Seek security, independence, and welcome competition.
- Willing to work hard but expect compensation.
- Digital natives.

Data from Halfer D, Saver C: *Bridging the generation gaps.* Nursing Spectrum/Nurse Week, Falls Church, 2008; Billings D, Halstead J: *Teaching in nursing: a guide for faculty*, St Louis 2019, Elsevier/Saunders; Mehallow C: Generational conflict in nursing: how to relate to colleagues across generations. Available at http://career-advice.monster.com/in-the-office/workplace-issues/generational-conflict-in-nursing/article.aspx; Riggs CJ: Multiple generations in the nursing workplace: part I. *J Contin Educ Nurs* 44(3):105–106, 2013; Patel D: *8 ways Generation Z will differ from millennials in the workplace.* Forbes. Available at https://www.forbes.com/sites/deeppatel/2017/09/21/8-ways-generation-z-will-differ-from-millennials-in-the-workplace/#7d7a19576e5e; Stewart JS, Oliver EG, Cravens KS, Oishi S: Managing millennials: embracing generational differences, *Harv Bus Rev* 60:45–54, 2017.

Try This

Your Generational Personality

Using Box 1.2, Characteristics of the Five Generations, identify the characteristics of your generation that do/do not apply to you. Discuss with a classmate or family member generational characteristics that cause you to be judgmental. Seek to understand why this characteristic is viewed as important to the respective generational group.

The **traditional adult learner** comes to an educational program directly from high school or as a transfer student (i.e., from another program of study). They are in transition from late adolescence to young adulthood. In addition to their own developmental tasks, these students are being propelled into situations of responsibility for others. Traditional adult learners grew up in a digital, wireless world and are known as the Generation Zers (iGen or Centennials). This group was born in 1994 or after.

The **returning adult learner** or nontraditional learner has been out of school for several years. Many of these learners have not taken any courses since high school. Returning adult learners can include Generation Y (Millennials), Generation Xers, Baby Boomers, and Matures. Returning adult students are experiencing many different life transitions and have diverse reasons for enrolling in nursing school. Perhaps an employer shut down a business or a layoff occurred, resulting in a need for job training. In addition, a change in marital status, children leaving the household, a change in the health of a spouse, or an impending retirement might have created a need for a stable income source, including health insurance benefits. Lastly, recent retirement may also have provided the time to pursue personal passions.

Despite these diverse reasons, a common theme prevails across generations, simply stated as, "I always wanted to be a nurse." Because of valued life and work experiences, returning adult learners have built a strong foundation for the personal commitment and transitions needed in nursing school and practical/vocational nursing. Complex lives, inclusive of competing demands from grown children and aging parents, can contribute to the stress of nursing school.

A subset of the returning adult learners are those adult learners with prior education beyond high school. This learner shares some of the characteristics of both traditional and returning adult learners. However, this adult learner might have experience in on-the-job training; a certificate program, technical school, or college; or have an undergraduate or graduate degree in a discipline other than nursing. Depending on the level of academic success and degree of program completion, this learner may have a strong academic skill set. However, in some cases, this adult learner has had limited success in the academic world and may question their abilities. It is common that adult learners who have been unsuccessful in many other types of postsecondary programs can excel in a practical/vocational nursing program when academic and social support services are readily available and easily accessible. Reasons for choosing to enroll in the practical/vocational nursing program include the following:

- Desire to change careers
- Desire to become a nurse
- Desire to develop new or advanced job skills
- Desire to achieve a financially sustainable career
- Desire to pursue a career with strong projected job growth/opportunities

Regardless of the reason for enrolling in a 9- to 12-month practical/vocational nursing program, most learners find this program meets their needs in both time and cost. The diversity of the learners is a benefit to practical/vocational nursing programs. Nursing in general, and practical/vocational nursing in particular, is challenged to build a diverse nursing workforce to meet the needs of our changing demographics in the United States. Learning together with students from diverse backgrounds contributes positively to building a culturally competent skill set and workforce. Listening carefully to your peers will increase your understanding of others.

Critical Thinking

Which Type of Adult Learner Am I?

Which type of adult learner are you? Survey your classmates. Determine which ones consider themselves to be traditional or returning adult learners. Identify different strengths that you can share with each other.

FORMAL AND INFORMAL LEARNING EXPERIENCES

Generalizations are broad, sweeping statements and can be made about each type of learner. However, the characteristics of each type of adult learner are not found in every individual.

- Traditional adult learners are accustomed to **formal education**. The practical/vocational nursing program in a vocational-technical school, community college, or private school is an example of a program of formal education.
- Returning adult learners, however, have been learning. More likely, they have been experiencing informal education, unless recently attending or graduating from college. Examples of informal educational experiences include learning new technology for personal and business use, developing time management and organizational skills while managing an office or household, or leading or participating in a community event. These experiences are invaluable when learning in a formal education setting.

Try This

Informal Educational Experiences

List at least five informal educational experiences you have had since high school.
1.
2.
3.
4.
5.

How will these informal educational experiences positively impact your personal and classmates' success in nursing school?

GEARED FOR SUCCESS

All adult learners have strengths that assist in succeeding in the practical/vocational nursing program.

Traditional adult learners are likely to be:

- At their prime physically, often with high energy levels, and may have fewer out-of-school responsibilities to distract them from their studies
- Experts at educational routine and given the opportunity to develop reading, writing, studying, and test-taking skills
- Digital natives who have always had cell phones and computers in their lives. They know how to register for classes, take tests online, and use electronic apps. When they need information, they "Google," and when they want to contact a friend, they send a text or instant message. Social media and gaming are everyday communication tools.

Returning adult learners are likely to:

- Feel they have energy drain caused by their varying personal responsibilities
- Have had responsibilities and life experiences that help them relate well to new learning, make sense out of it, and get the point quickly
- Be digital immigrants who have had to learn to live in a digital world. Some find it easy to adapt, but others may find it more difficult. When these learners need information, they consider going to the library, seeking paper resources, and enlisting children and younger friends to assist with technology. Communication with friends and family can vary greatly, from using their landline, cell phone, or e-mail. They are continually learning how to improve communication via social media.
- Be **self-directed** learners who have set goals for themselves. Many have made economic and personal sacrifices to return to school.

Depending on their previous level of academic success, they may have developed a strong academic skill set or may have struggled and never really achieved academic success.

Critical Thinking

Reasons I Can Succeed

Identify and list three attributes you possess that will help you succeed in the practical/vocational nursing program.
1.
2.
3.

POTENTIAL HIDDEN DANGERS TO AVOID

All adult learners are focused on success at enrollment. However, each group also has some liabilities, things that could stand in the way of success. Identifying these hidden dangers is a key strategy required to develop a successful plan.

HIDDEN DANGER SHARED BY ALL ADULT LEARNERS

One of the greatest liabilities shared by all adult learners is the fear of failure. Fear of anything is a very strong motivator, but in a negative sense. Fear of failure in school is a feeling that usually develops as a result of past negative experiences with learning situations. Perhaps you did not do well in some high school or college classes. Maybe you did not study, studied the wrong way, or allowed yourself to be put down by teachers or professors in the past. Instead of becoming stronger, you retreated, thereby losing confidence in yourself. Regardless of the cause, you may look at school in a negative, threatening way.

Your past is history. You have a clean slate ahead of you! Many adult learners with the same history and fears as you have succeeded in educational programs. You are an adult in an adult educational experience. Begin to picture in your mind the rewards of succeeding in the practical/vocational nursing program. Forget the failures and setbacks you may have suffered in high school and other educational experiences. Replace your fear of failure with the desire for success. Keep your thoughts positive, and practice these positive thoughts continuously. Watch the content and tone of your thoughts and words. Negative thoughts and words can play like a song in your head.

As surely as you learned this negative script, you can learn a positive script. However, it does take time. Replace your "I cannot" and "I never could" with "I want to," "I can," "I will," and "I am going to." Avoid dwelling on the past and look to the future. Go all the way with PMA: **positive mental attitude**. If you consistently expect to succeed, and combine this expectation with hard work in your studies, you *will* succeed. Did you know that your brain believes anything you tell it? If it learned to believe you could fail, it can also learn to believe you can succeed. Start today to engage in positive self-talk. Positive music lyrics can also help. Listen to lyrics such as "Fight Song" by Rachel Platten when you feel discouraged.

Surround yourself with positive peers. Sometimes, students who may not have succeeded in other nursing programs or a previous nursing course may be your classmates. Active listening to this group of peers can be positive and assist you in avoiding common student pitfalls. However, remember that reasons for lack of academic success are varied, personal, and confidential. If negativism prevails, politely avoid these conversations. New beginnings are good for all!

Try This

Positive Mental Attitude

Every night, write down one or two positive events of the day related to your school performance/growth. Revisit this list weekly on Sunday evening, reflecting on your accomplishments, and identify one strength you can share with your classmates this coming week.

DANGERS FOR THE TRADITIONAL ADULT LEARNER

Many explanations can be given for the liabilities listed below for traditional adult learners. Some traditional adult learners may still be developing an awareness of who they are and what life is all about. Some may lack a sense of direction or have no clear goals or life plans. Some may lack inner motivation to be a practical/vocational nurse. These learners can succeed by taking responsibility for making decisions about priorities and personal use of time to help them meet their personal goals. The following examples of dangers for traditional adult learners are examples of generalizations. They may or may not apply to the traditional adult learners you know.

Grade Expectations

A grade of C on a test or for a nursing course surprises some traditional adult students initially because the same high school studying routine may have gotten "A" grades in the past. Some traditional adult students may need to improve their time management skills or motivation when it comes to studying. Study time required to master content in a practical/vocational nursing program is personal to each student. Minimal study effort will typically not lead to success in the practical/vocational nursing program. More focus may be essential to achieve success.

Social Activities

Social activities and work may compete with school and study time. In a 24/7/365 wired/wireless world, learners are accessible at all times to friends and family through communication devices. Learning to "turn it off" is essential. Set limits by sharing class and clinical schedules with family and friends, and restrict being contacted for emergencies only during those times. Develop awareness of distractions when online, and recognize when valuable time slips away. Be cognizant of the need for some downtime daily, even if only for 15 minutes. The need to clear your mind and reenergize is critical to your success.

Employment

The amount of time occupied by employment outside of school hours may be another interference. Ask yourself, "How much of the time that I am employed outside of school is necessary for food, shelter, and other realistic expenses?" Planning your finances, including costs of education, is essential to ensure that your focus in school can be on your studies and self-care to stay healthy throughout your enrollment. Some learners may need to work full time to keep health care benefits for themselves and their families. Some learners have resources, either support persons or savings, which will require only part-time work hours or not at all. Contact your school's financial aid office to determine what grants, loans, or work study programs may be available.

DANGERS FOR THE RETURNING ADULT LEARNER

Physical Changes

Returning adult learners may lack confidence in or recognize that they do not have a strong academic skill set. Their reading, writing, test-taking, and study skills may be rusty. Technology skills may pose even more of a challenge. In the normal aging process, physical changes can affect learning. Energy levels may decrease and impact endurance for extended study time. Vision and hearing, at their peak in the adolescent years, decline gradually through the adult years. Older adults may need more illumination when reading or performing clinical skills. Eye strain can contribute negatively to energy level. Hearing in the classroom, skills lab, and in clinical settings may be a challenge. Seek solutions early. Assistive devices are available to address these issues.

Social and Family Responsibilities

Success as a student requires the ability to juggle relationships and responsibilities effectively. The role as student will compete with established roles such as family member, employee, friend, and any other community roles.

Because of these roles, more demands are placed on returning adult learners. Although many people will be excited for you, others may not want you to change the status quo. Some family members may not support the student's choice to continue their formal education. Spouses/significant others may object to changing roles and accepting extra relationship or family demands. Needing others to help care for children and aging parents may make the student develop a continual feeling of inadequacy. Common comments include "I feel like I am not doing anything well" and "No one is happy, particularly me." It is not unusual for students to express feelings of guilt.

Recognize and acknowledge this inevitable struggle. Identify resources and support people to assist. Do not hesitate to reach out to confirm and resolve your feelings of frustration, guilt, and inadequacies before the stress level mounts. Managing time is important. Realistic goal setting is essential. Self-care must be a priority, as 4 hours of sleep nightly will not be a viable long-term plan for success.

All humans, when faced with obstacles, have thoughts of giving up at some point. The strategies in this book will assist you in recognizing that your feelings are normal, help you anticipate some of the usual roadblocks, and identify and implement quick solutions to keep you on the road to success. A solid realistic plan is the key.

EMPOWERMENT

Empowerment is a term you may hear in the news/social media and general conversation. Many definitions exist. According to Merriam-Webster (2025), *empowerment* is "the granting of the power, right, or authority to perform various acts or duties." Empowerment is important to the role of the nurse. You will need to feel empowered by others and empower others on your nursing team (i.e., assistive personnel [AP]). Chapter 17 will explain empowerment in your work as a nurse in more detail.

> **? Critical Thinking**
>
> **Personal Needs for Improvement**
>
> Identify and list three things that could stand in your way of success in the practical/vocational nursing program.
>
> 1.
> 2.
> 3.

SPECIAL CHALLENGES FOR PRACTICAL/VOCATIONAL NURSING STUDENTS

No matter what type of adult learner you are, some learners have special challenges to success in practical/vocational nursing. Learners with a spouse/significant other at home may be extremely busy with school and family affairs. Learners with aging parents may be involved with their needs for assistance. Single parents may feel overwhelmed when the learner role is assumed in addition to their other roles. It may be good for learners with spouses/significant others to imagine what it would be like to be a learner without these individuals to offer support.

Practical/vocational nursing students who speak English as their first language sometimes indicate the difficulty of coursework and the amount of time it takes to complete assignments. It may be insightful for these learners to imagine being responsible for the same amount of coursework when English is their second language. Learners who speak English as a second or additional language need to strive continually to understand content presented in a language that is different from their native tongue. Reading assignments need to be translated by these students to their native language to be understood. Taking a test requires extra effort, as these students may need to translate test directions and items to their native language for understanding before answering an item. This is comparable with presenting English-speaking learners with textbooks and tests written in Spanish or Russian with the need to translate both to English.

These learners described are typical of the demographic of a practical/vocational nursing student. It is important to remember there were approximately 657,800 licensed practical/vocational nurses (LPN/LVN) jobs in 2023 in the United States (BLS, 2024). Thus facing the preceding challenges is common, and many graduates have achieved success despite the great odds that needed to be overcome. They are a testimonial that success is within your reach, even if you are faced with these special challenges.

STRENGTHS OF ALL ADULT LEARNERS

All adult learners possess unique strengths. These strengths often are the opposite of the dangers discussed above. Most importantly, adult learners need to recognize they would not be accepted into a practical/vocational nursing program unless they were able to demonstrate the essential academic skills necessary for success. Couple this with passion, self-confidence, perseverance, physical health, and a good plan (inclusive of identified academic and social supports), and you are ready to soar to success. Focus on the four "*P*"s to create your personal plan for success (Fig. 1.1). The four "*P*"s are Power, Passion, Perseverance, and

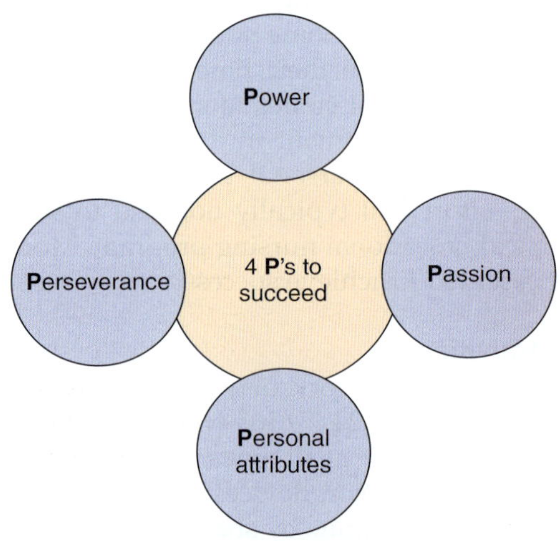

Fig. 1.1 The four "*P*"s of success.

Personal Attributes. *Power* is essential; belief in yourself and your ability to be successful is inherent to success. *Passion* fuels your inner drive when the barriers seem insurmountable. *Perseverance* ensures that you stay on track when exhaustion hits and all seems astray. Lastly, self-reflection to identify your personal attributes is essential to a realistic and successful plan. *Personal attributes* include finances, time, social supports, and academic skill set. An unrealistic evaluation of personal attributes, despite power, passion, and perseverance, can lead to an unsuccessful outcome, resulting in a course or program failure.

Empowerment

Begin to think about the term empowerment. Who has empowered you? Whose words make you feel stronger, more peaceful, and ultimately increase your confidence, leading to greater success and well-being? Why does this impact you positively and make you feel better? Do you see anyone at your school with similar qualities who may be your source of empowerment, increasing your chance to succeed? Seek them out to establish a relationship early in the program. Write down two to three key reasons that this person empowers you. Think about why this impacts your success. How can you use this same approach to empower others?

LEARNERS HAVE RIGHTS

As an American citizen, start thinking about some fundamental rights you have been granted through the US Constitution that will affect you as a learner. The **First Amendment** gives you freedom of expression as long as what you want to express does not disrupt class or infringe on the rights of your peers. When your instructor asks you to join in a discussion, do not be afraid to do so. Instructors want your input in a class session. They have no intention of holding your comments against you.

The Fourteenth Amendment assures you due process. Due process means that if you are charged with a violation of policies or rules, you will be presented with evidence of your misconduct and will be entitled to state your position. So relax. The institution in which you are enrolled cannot terminate you on a whim, nor does it want to. It exists to help you succeed.

A more detailed account of these two rights can probably be found in your school's student handbook. If you do not have a copy of the student handbook, download an online copy or obtain one from the student services department. An important learner's right is the right to have an organized curriculum and a responsible instructor who is prepared to teach it. You have the right to know the requirements of each course and how you will be graded for each course. Although your tuition and fees do not pay for all the services you receive through your school, you are the most important person in the educational system. You are the customer! You do not interfere with the instructor's or any staff's work; you are the focus of it.

RESPONSIBILITIES OF LEARNERS

The first responsibility of learners is to learn. The authors of this book want you to test your knowledge regarding the process of learning before you read any further. Read the following four statements and decide whether they are true or false. As the chapter continues, these statements will be discussed. You will be expected to check the accuracy of your responses. Remember, your answers are for your eyes only.

Critical Thinking

Responsibilities of Learners

Read the following four statements and indicate whether each is true or false.

1. The instructor has the responsibility for my learning.
2. If I fail, it is the responsibility of the instructor.
3. If I succeed, the credit for my success should go to the instructor.
4. My instructor has the responsibility to pass on to me all the information I will need to know in my career as a practical/vocational nurse.

TEACHING VERSUS LEARNING

Years ago, something wonderful happened in the area of adult education. Teachers were educated about the difference between **teaching** and learning. Greater emphasis was placed on the role of the learner. Changing emphasis from teaching to learning is called a **paradigm** (a way of thinking) shift. Learners need to be aware of the exciting world of learning and the roles of teaching and learning. Then you will know what is expected of you as an adult learner.

Passive Learners

Did your past educational experiences involve sitting in classes in which the teacher did most of the talking and you just took notes? Did you view the teacher as someone who possessed knowledge and somehow was going to pass it on to you? And, if you did not pass, did you say "The teacher flunked me"? When you think about it, these situations are characterized by the adjectives *dependent* and *passive*.

The last time you were dependent from necessity was when you were an infant. Even then you were far from passive. When you observe a 6-month-old infant, the spirit of inquiry is evident as they gaze up and watch a fan, look in the mirror and see their reflection, and listen intently as the sounds change on the television. We all inherently have a spirit of inquiry that resides within us. When you became a toddler, you became very independent and began to learn about the world in earnest. You very actively pursued your learning, that is, the acquiring of new knowledge and skills. And you did it with gusto! Now you are an adult learner. How unfair of an instructor to expect you to become dependent and passive in your learning. This is especially true because studies have proven that people learn best when they are actively involved in their own learning and have an interdependent relationship with the instructor.

Instructors—Facilitators of Learning

You have already learned that it is the instructor's responsibility to set up a curriculum. Your state's board of nursing dictates the core content of the curriculum in a school of nursing. It is then up to the faculty of your school to decide how that content will be included in the nursing program. Some practical/vocational programs might use the general structure of the National Council Licensure Examination for Licensed Practical Nurses (NCLEX-PN®) examination in developing a curriculum.

Instructors act as **facilitators** of your learning. They are responsible for creating an environment in which learning can take place. They arrange a variety of activities and experiences that trigger your spirit of inquiry. In addition, they provide access to academic resources to seek knowledge, discuss, debate, and make conclusions. A critical part of facilitation involves being available when you encounter questions and problems you cannot solve. Instructors also have the responsibility to evaluate learning. They do so by testing and observing learners.

As a student, you have the right and the responsibility to talk to an instructor when you have a concern about your relationship with him or her. Under rules of assertiveness, always go to the source. Follow the chain of command to resolve your concerns. The same rule applies if you have a problem with a classmate. Approach the classmate, not another student.

Active Learning

To *learn* is to acquire knowledge and skills. The verb *acquire* means to obtain or gain by your own effort. As a learner in a practical/vocational nursing program, you need to be your own agent of knowledge and skill acquisition. You have the personal responsibility to acquire the knowledge and skills needed to be a practical/vocational nurse. **Active learning** is not a passive activity. As a learner, you must open yourself up, reach out, and stretch to gain knowledge and skills. To be successful, you must be personally involved in your learning. It is impossible for instructors to pour knowledge and skills into your head. You need to become self-directed and curious in your learning. You need to use critical-thinking skills to help you comprehend what you read in texts and journals, what you see on multimedia in the classroom and online resources, and what you hear in class discussions. Instructors will not hover over you and guide your every step. Instructors are there to facilitate your learning and be a mentor and coach.

Do not expect the instructor to assume a skill for you, be your medical dictionary, or reteach Chapter 2 in *Anatomy and Physiology* because you did not have time to study. Instead, expect your instructor to observe you while you are trying to work through a difficult skill. The instructor will make suggestions and demonstrate a point or two to help you along. If you are having trouble, expect your instructor to help you put a definition of a medical term in your own words. Expect the instructor to answer specific questions you may have about Chapter 2 in *Anatomy and Physiology*. These are the roles of teacher and learner and examples of their interdependency.

If you are to learn and succeed in practical/vocational nursing, you need to become actively involved in your own learning. Studies of adult learning clearly indicate that the basic ability to learn remains essentially unimpaired throughout the lifespan. Now review the answers to your true/false questions from the Critical Thinking exercise earlier in the chapter. Are there any answers you want to change before looking at the key?

1. *False.* You have the responsibility for your own learning. You must become actively involved in the learning process.
2. *False.* If you fail, it is your own fault. Adult educational programs are geared for success. You are geared for success. Although you could list many reasons why you might not succeed, the teacher failing you is not one of them. Learners sometimes allow themselves to fail.
3. *False.* When you succeed (and you are perfectly capable of doing so), only you can take credit for the success. You were the person who assumed responsibility for your own learning. You became actively involved in the learning process.
4. *False.* Instructors have had much experience in nursing. They do not know all the experiences you will have in your career as a practical/vocational nurse. Even if they did, there would be no time or way to transfer this knowledge to you. Instructors help learners learn how to learn. This is important in an ever-changing field such as nursing. Your instructors will encourage you to develop critical-thinking and problem-solving skills, which will enable you to develop clinical judgement to handle new situations as they arise in your nursing career.

If you had no wrong answers, you should be an expert on learning. Now put your expertise to work for you. If you had one or more wrong answers, the author suggests you reread the "Teaching Versus Learning" section in this chapter. Chapters 2, 5, and 19 will help you become an active learner and a critical thinker and be successful in the practical/vocational nursing program, on NCLEX-PN®, and as a candidate for an LPN/LVN nursing position.

ROLE OF EVALUATION

The second responsibility of learners is to receive and participate in evaluation. Evaluation plays an important role in your education in the practical/vocational nursing program and throughout your career. You have set a goal to become a practical/vocational nurse. As the year goes on, your instructors will evaluate you in several different ways to determine whether or not you are progressing in the achievement of that goal. When you graduate, you will be evaluated periodically while on the job, sometimes as a means of determining whether or not you are to receive a salary increase or a job promotion. At other times you will be evaluated to see if you are functioning well enough to keep your job.

Evaluation in the practical/vocational nursing program occurs in several areas: written tests, presentations, and evidenced-based papers and projects that measure your knowledge of theory and understanding of that knowledge; simulations; and **performance evaluations** that measure your ability to apply your knowledge in the clinical area. Performance evaluations occur in the clinical simulation lab and a diverse array of clinical settings. Evaluation in these areas is a learning experience in itself. Following evaluations, students should assess their strengths and weaknesses and create a plan to improve their knowledge and performance accordingly.

Theory Tests

Learners and instructors review test results very differently. Learners focus on the number of items answered correctly. They concentrate on what they did right so they can apply the process of getting the right answer to future tests and apply this information in the clinical area. In addition, learners often only focus on the test grade. In a nursing program, identifying knowledge that you have not conquered is essential to your eventual success on the NCLEX-PN® exam. Instructors usually focus on the specific items the learner(s) answered incorrectly, which indicates critical knowledge the learner does not have. Understanding why each answer choice was incorrect is an important learning experience.

Upon receiving a test grade, if available, review the questions answered incorrectly and determine why you missed the question. Then arrange time with your instructor to review the test. Grades do count! You must earn the minimum grade established by your nursing program. Consider this: If you achieved 80% on a test, it means you did not answer 20% of the questions correctly. Now place yourself in the client's slippers. If my nurse got 20% of the test questions wrong, can my nurse care for me safely? Also, this 20% of information not learned may impact your ability to successfully pass the NCLEX-PN® on the first attempt. For these reasons, look at tests as learning experiences. Study the rationales for your correct and incorrect answers. Review all your tests with the goal of understanding why the correct answers are correct and the incorrect answers are wrong.

Clinical Performance Evaluations

The most meaningful evaluations you receive during the year are the clinical performance evaluations based on your performance in clinical lab simulations and diverse clinical areas. Understanding this form of evaluation and your responsibilities with it give you an important opportunity for personal and career growth. Clinical performance evaluations also provide an example of how you will evaluate others in your expanded role.

In the clinical area, instructors observe you as you care for clients. They are observing for positive behaviors that indicate you are learning, applying your knowledge, and progressing toward your goal to become an LPN/LVN. Instructors are also observing for behaviors that will keep you from reaching your goal and consequently will be discouraged. Your instructor will update you daily on your progress, either verbally or in a written format. At the end of a clinical rotation, a written performance evaluation will be reviewed with you during a conference with the clinical instructor.

Look at performance evaluations positively as a two-sided coin. On one side, as part of their job, instructors have the responsibility of evaluating your performance. As a learner, you have the responsibility of being aware of your clinical behaviors. You are responsible for **self-evaluation**. Students, at the time of graduation, should know their strong nursing actions and behaviors and those that need improvement.

The ability to be aware of one's behaviors begins the first day in the practical/vocational nursing program. Learners must consistently work at viewing themselves objectively. A learner does not automatically have this ability, and one of the instructors' roles is to support you in this self-evaluation. For example, when learning how to make a bed, ask yourself, "Does the finished product meet the standard as listed step by step on the skill procedure?" Do not wait for the instructor to identify areas of success or areas needing improvement. Peer learning and continual evaluation is a great strategy to implement in both the simulation lab and the clinical area. View your peers as a resource with the unique strengths and resources they bring to the learning experience. For example, have a peer critique your lab procedure before the clinical skills evaluation by the instructor. Recording (if available) can be a powerful tool in the simulation lab. Direct observation of skill performance encourages immediate feedback to improve identified weak areas and correct errors.

Professional Pointer

Objective awareness of one's own behaviors is an important skill to have as an employee.

Think back to when you received comments from your teachers and parents about your behavior in grade school and high school. How did you feel when you received these comments? Many people grow up with negative feelings about these episodes of criticism and even the word itself. Criticism means evaluation. Some people view it as a put-down.

The phrase "constructive criticism" may evoke negative feelings. The phrase "**constructive evaluation**" is frequently used instead. This choice of words may help you look at evaluation of your behaviors in a positive way. Distinguish what is being evaluated. You must separate your behaviors or actions from yourself, the person.

Constructive evaluation directed toward your behaviors has no bearing on your value as a person. Look at your behaviors as either being positive, and helping you reach your goal, or as needing improvement. Behaviors that need improvement should be modified so you can reach your goal of being a practical/vocational nurse.

As you progress in the nursing program, you will learn about a systematic way of conducting client care called the "nursing process" (see Chapter 12). An important part of the nursing process is evaluation of client goals while giving client care. If your actions are not helping clients reach their goals, they need to be modified. Knowledge of the nursing process will help you develop the ability to look at your actions and evaluate them. Comments from instructors help your self-awareness.

To start learning self-evaluation, look at yourself in everyday life. Ask yourself how you look through the eyes of others:

- Would you like to be your own spouse?
- Would you enjoy having yourself as a learner?
- Would you like to be your own mother or father?
- Would you trust and like to be your own nurse?

If you would not like to be any of these people, identify the reasons why.

Another good exercise is to make two lists: a list of your assets or strong points, and a list of your liabilities or areas that need improvement. When asked to evaluate themselves, learners traditionally rate themselves more negatively. They tend to neglect their strong points. Identifying strong points is not proud or vain behavior. It is dealing with yourself honestly and openly. After you have identified assets and liabilities, review your assets periodically. Make an effort to grow these strong points while modifying your liabilities. Work on one liability at a time. You will see your assets list grow and your liabilities list shrink.

A good place to start self-evaluation in nursing is in the skills lab of your basic nursing course. Observe the results of your actions. Are you using a drape during procedures to maintain the client's privacy and avoid chilling? Are you aware of the effect of the tone of your voice on your instructors and peers?

Evaluation is a reality in any career. Getting into the practice of self-evaluation early in your program of study will help you develop a skill you will use daily in your career and personal life.

> **? Critical Thinking**
>
> **Self-Evaluation**
>
> List one of your strong areas you identified as a new practical/vocational nursing learner. (Review your answers to "Critical Thinking: Reasons I Can Succeed" earlier in the chapter.)
>
> ____
>
> List one area needing improvement that you have identified as a practical/vocational nursing student. (Review your answers to "Critical Thinking: Personal Needs for Improvement" earlier in the chapter.)
>
> ____

> **? Critical Thinking**
>
> **Plan to Eliminate My Areas That Need Improvement**
>
> Discuss with an instructor, peer, or significant other the areas you identified as needing improvement. Request verification and identification of any other areas you have not identified. Avoid the temptation to become defensive and list why these areas exist. Instead, focus on developing a plan to eliminate at least one of your areas that need improvement. How can you convert this area into a strength?
>
> ____
>
> ____
>
> ____

THE VALUE OF A REFERRAL

If you are evaluated by your instructor as having areas that need improvement, the instructor might refer you to a counselor at school. Examples of areas that require a **referral** are a grade below passing in a major test and frequent absences from class. Counselors at technical colleges and community colleges are academic counselors who have expertise in helping students identify reasons for academic problem areas. A referral to a counselor is an attempt to help you succeed. These counselors can help students set up a plan of action to remedy the problem.

Unfortunately, some students resist going to the counselor because they think it is a waste of time. An external counseling system may also exist. Be proactive. In most schools, you can initiate the need for assistance before the instructor referral. If you are struggling with academic or clinical performance, seek out help early and often. In addition, remember that counselors can also assist with a variety of personal crises. These could be extreme situations, such as the death of a loved one or an abusive situation, or they could be less urgent but still important, such as struggling with time management or communication skills.

Critical Thinking

Referral to a Counselor

Identify how you access counselors at your school.

What could be one reason for thinking that an appointment with the counselor is valuable?

Consider one potential area where you may need to access a counselor while enrolled in school.

OTHER RESPONSIBILITIES OF LEARNERS

In addition to assuming responsibility for your own learning, becoming actively involved in the learning process, and receiving and participating in evaluation, it is necessary to be aware of other responsibilities you have as a learner. Ultimately, these responsibilities are preparing you for employment, so see your role not only as a student, but as a future LPN/LVN.

1. Be aware and agree to abide by the rules and policies of your school and the practical/vocational nursing program.
2. When a problem develops, follow the recognized channels of communication both at school and in the clinical area. The rule is: Go to the source. Avoid "saving up" gripes. Instead, pursue them as they come up. Deal with them in an assertive manner (see Chapter 9).
3. Come prepared for classes and clinical experiences. You expect teachers to be prepared, and they expect the same of you. Arriving unprepared for classes wastes the time of the instructor, your peers, and yourself. When unprepared for clinical experiences, you are violating an important safety factor in client care. When scheduled for a clinical assignment, your state board of nursing expects you to function as an LPN/LVN would function under your state's Nurse Practice Act, under the supervision of your instructor.
4. As a self-directed learner, seek out learning experiences at school and in the clinical area. Set your goals higher than the minimum. In postconference, learn from your peers and their experiences and knowledge. Learn from one another.
5. Seek out resources beyond the required readings. Examples of these resources can be the learning resource center, information from past classes, electronic resources at the clinical sites, and the Internet.
6. Assume responsibility for your own thoughts, communication, and behavior. Avoid giving in to pressure from your peers. BYOB: be your own boss, as appropriate.
7. Be present and on time for classes and clinical experiences. Follow school and program policies for reporting absences. Frequent absences and late arrivals, despite a passing grade average, could result in disciplinary action up to and including dismissal from the program. In addition, developing a strong commitment to be dependable and accountable will contribute to job success and advancement in the future.
8. Be an active, self-directed learner. Know what you know, what you do not know, and where to find the evidence needed.
9. Treat those with whom you come into daily contact with respect—peers, instructors, leaders, clinical staff, health care providers, and certainly clients and their families. Be mindful of their rights as individuals.
10. The clinical area can be very stressful for the student, instructor, staff member, and client. You must remain professional at all times. Learn the fine line between assertive and aggressive. Observe others for their response to challenging situations, and self-evaluate often.
11. Seek out your instructor when you are having difficulties in class or the clinical area. Often instructors can tell when students are having problems. More important are the times when they cannot tell and only the student knows a problem exists. Do not be afraid to approach your instructors. They are there to help you.
12. Keep a record of your grades as a course proceeds. At the beginning of a course, the instructor and/or your course syllabus will explain the method of calculating your final grade. You are responsible for knowing your average grade at all times.

Get Ready for the Next-Generation NCLEX® Examination

Key Points

- Adult learners develop diversity in age, resulting in differing ways of thinking and valuing.
- The adults in your class could be Matures (The Silent Generation), Baby Boomers, Generation Xers, Generation Ys (Millennials), or Generation Z.
- Adult learners can be classified as traditional adult learners and nontraditional (or returning adult) learners.
- Each category of adult learner possesses characteristics that may help the learner succeed in the practical/vocational nursing program.
- Each group of adult learners also possesses characteristics that may prevent success.
- Learners have control over solutions for liabilities that may occur in learning situations or personal circumstances. Implement the solutions early. Seek assistance when the solutions are not evident.
- Although learners have rights, they also have responsibilities. Important responsibilities include actively participating in the learning process and in the evaluation of their learning and growth.

Additional Learning Resources

Go to your Evolve website (http://evolve.elsevier.com/Carroll/success/) for the following FREE learning resources:

- Answers to Critical Thinking Scenarios
- Additional learning activities
- Additional Review Questions for the NCLEX-PN® exam
- Helpful phrases for communicating in Spanish and more!

Clinical Judgment Questions

1. A student enrolled in a practical/vocational nursing program. Select the appropriate behavior for the student practical nurse/vocational nurse (SPN/VN).

a. To accept responsibility for personal success, including grades, in the nursing program
b. To be as passive a learner as you can possibly be, both in classes and in the clinical area
c. To learn everything from the nursing instructors that is needed to function as a LPN/LVN
d. To blame the nursing instructor for any failures that occur in class or the clinical area

2. A practical/vocational nursing learner has been referred to the counselor because of a failing grade on the final exam in a course. Which of the following learner responses indicates the understanding of the purpose of the referral?

a. "The instructor does not like me and wants me to quit the program."
b. "This is a warning that I will be asked to withdraw from the program."
c. "The purpose of a referral is to help me identify problems to avoid failure."
d. "A psychologist will evaluate me for psychological problems that may be interfering with success."

3. A SPN/VN has just received the end-of-course clinical evaluation. Which of the following attitudes is most appropriate regarding the role of clinical evaluation of students?

a. Instructors and SPN/VN have the responsibility to identify positive behaviors and those that need improvement.
b. It is the job of the instructor only to identify positive clinical behaviors and behaviors that need improvement.
c. When SPN/VN identify positive behaviors, it indicates that they are proud and overly confident individuals.
d. When behaviors that need improvement are identified, clinical evaluation may destroy self-esteem in the SPN/VN.

4. Four practical SPN/VN were absent the day tests were returned and reviewed in a nursing course. Which of the following students has a plan that will benefit the student in future testing and clinical situations?

a. The student who on the next class day will ask the instructor for the grade on the test for personal records
b. The student who on the next clinical day asks the instructor to schedule time to go over test items that were correct
c. The student who thinks that because the test is over, it is unnecessary to review test items because the grade is final
d. The student who asks the instructor for an appointment to review all the test items so the reasons for wrong answers can be identified

5. Which of the following students is *not* demonstrating behavior for success in the practical/vocational nursing program? (*Select all that apply.*)

a. A recent high school graduate who expects the instructor to teach her everything she needs to know
b. A student who is a mother of four and spends time in the library each afternoon reviewing class notes
c. A student who has not been in school for 20 years and seeks out the instructor when content is not understood
d. A student with college experience who works part time and joins a group that crams before each examination
e. A student who speaks English as a second language and studies every night in preparation for class and clinical

6. A 37-year-old student just started the practical nursing program at the local technical college. The class is composed of students in their late teens, twenties, thirties, fifties, and one retired individual. From the following list of generalized characteristics, select those that describe this student's generational age. (*Select all that apply.*)

a. Accepts diversity in the members of their class
b. Is more formal when approaching classmates
c. Works long hours to get the job done
d. Does not readily use the computer lab
e. Is self-reliant when learning nursing skills

Critical Thinking Scenario

Anya, 36 years old, has been accepted to the practical nursing program. Initial excitement is followed by concern. Anya begins to think: "Can I really do this? I have three kids, am a single parent, and haven't had any classes since high school! And high school was a bad dream for me. I never got along with my teachers. And how am I going to be able to afford school both in time and money? I work full time now and have a hard time making ends meet in time and money. And I heard you have evaluations of what you do when taking care of clients. I don't like people being critical of me." Identify at least three different areas Anya should evaluate before enrollment. What can you suggest to Anya to include in a success plan to help with her concerns?

Academic Resources (Study Skills and Test Strategies)

2

Objectives

On completing this chapter, you will be able to do the following:

1. Describe key biological and psychological components of learning.
2. Discuss learning preferences and learning preference thinking.
3. Describe categories of multiple intelligences and how they are used.
4. Describe the learning process.
5. Describe how to overcome barriers to learning. Apply techniques in learning situation that will enhance your comprehension (understanding) of information needed for critical thinking as a licensed practical nurse/licensed vocational nurse (LPN/LVN).
6. Describe strategies for learning new information.
7. Describe strategies for effective reading comprehension.
8. Discuss strategies for retaining new information.
9. Discuss strategies for successful test taking
10. Describe resources commonly available to a student through their school's learning resource center (LRC).
11. Identify other learning resources that can fully prepare you to SUCCEED, including course syllabus, or outline, tutoring, simulation labs, and study groups

Key Terms

active listener
app
artificial intelligence (AI)
blended course
bucket theory
call number
case scenario
comprehension
computer-aided instruction
computer simulation
cooperative learning
copyright laws
course outlines
discussion buddy
distance learning
distracters
electronic devices
electronic simulation
external distractions
interlibrary loan services
internal distractions
Internet
key
key concepts
learning management system
learning resource center
lecture-discussion strategy
mnemonic devices
mobile devices
nursing skills/simulation lab
online catalog
options
passive listener
peer-reviewed
periodical index
periodicals
podcast
reference materials
simulation
stacks
static simulation
passive listener
study group
study skills lab
syllabus
tutoring
understanding
virtual clinical excursions

Keep in Mind

Success is dependent on a strong self-analysis. Knowing who you are, what your academic strengths are, and how to find/use available academic resources will help you SUCCEED!

During lunch, five students, Olivia, Katie, Jamal, Akeno, and Darius, sit together and discuss the morning's class about academic success. Olivia states, "I am kind of scared. That pile of books and list of assignments due next week is overwhelming. There were times the instructor was going so fast that I could hardly keep up." Akeno continues, "I agree. I was grateful when the instructor outlined on the whiteboard a chart with the schedule of our clinical, class, and lab days, although I could tell some people were bored with this detail. It was very confusing until I saw it on the board. It helped me organize my week." Katie chimes in, "I felt the same way and realized that I need to see things in writing. Just hearing the information is often confusing to me." Jamal states, "I can see how everyone learns differently. There are many resources. I think we will need to carefully identify what works best for each of us and not assume a peer's successful study strategies will definitely be our best option. They may work, but not if we are a different type of learner. For example, I want to join a study group but know that I am a solitary learner. So I will need to choose carefully and balance the study group with solo study. I am excited but a bit nervous. Oh, it's 11:56. Let's go. I don't want to be late for class."

An in-depth academic self-analysis before starting your education is critical. This analysis already began when you completed the required nurse school entrance test. Although several types of tests are used for nursing school entrance, most measure key areas of academic aptitude. A good starting point to a self-analysis, examining test results can assist you to focus your efforts. Reviewing your test results, were you strong in reading comprehension, English, language usage, math, science, or making deductions? For example, if your overall math score was below average (below the fiftieth percentile), what specific math concepts do you need to review? If you did not take a nurse entrance test, examine your performance on prerequisite courses (if required) for areas needing further development.

In addition to this analysis, you will also want to ask yourself several other questions:

- What is your learning preference?
- Do you have effective study skills?
- What are academic resources? Are they available to you, and how do you use them?

Let's start by identifying your learning preference.

> **Keep in Mind**
>
> Identify your learning preference(s): Discuss how your learning preference can impact your learning, comprehending, retaining, and applying information in the care of clients. Remember: Everyone's learning preference is unique.

Everyone learns differently. Some student practical nurses/student vocational nurses (SPNs/SVNs) take voluminous notes. Some just listen. Others learn best by hands-on activities and group instruction. In contrast, some are solitary learners and prefer to learn independently on the computer. Listen to student conversations about studying to get clues on different preferences of learning. Examples include "I like absolute silence," "I like my music blaring," "I study best in the wee hours of the morning," "I like to munch when I study," "I make up rhymes to help me remember," "I read on a treadmill," and so on. All students can be equally successful. There are many theories about what affects learning preference. It is possible for students to have more than one learning preference.

> **Try This**
>
> Take a few minutes to list your "favorites" when studying. Discuss these "favorites" with a peer. How are they similar? How are they different?

Brain dominance impacts the way you think. Your thinking preference impacts the way you learn. Your learning preference is the way you receive information most efficiently and effectively.

BRAIN DOMINANCE

The battle of biology (hardwiring) versus socialization (how you are raised) in brain development is finally backed by scientific evidence. Originally, biology alone was credited for male/female differences in areas such as learning and behavior. For a number of years, until the late 1980s, the importance of socialization became the focus. It was thought that a person became what they are based on specific socialization. Looking back, it has not worked out this way, and persons have suffered because of this singular emphasis.

RIGHT AND LEFT SIDES OF THE CEREBRUM

We often hear people talk about being "right brained" or "left brained." In reality no one is completely "right or left brained." We achieve our best when both sides of our brain work together, as partners. For example, the left side of the brain is verbal and fluent, and without the help of the right side to add tone and inflection, it would make our speech robot-like. In school, the left side of the brain helps break down information so we can master it. The right side gives a total picture of our learning (Fig. 2.1). However, specific parts of the brain impact different attributes. For a brief overview, visit https://www.thoughtco.com/left-brain-right-brain-1857174.

RIGHT BRAIN–DOMINANT INDIVIDUALS

Primarily **right brain–dominant** individuals tend to be intuitive, imaginative, and impulsive. They prefer to start out with a broad idea and then pursue supporting information. They apply creativity to problem solving and learn best by:

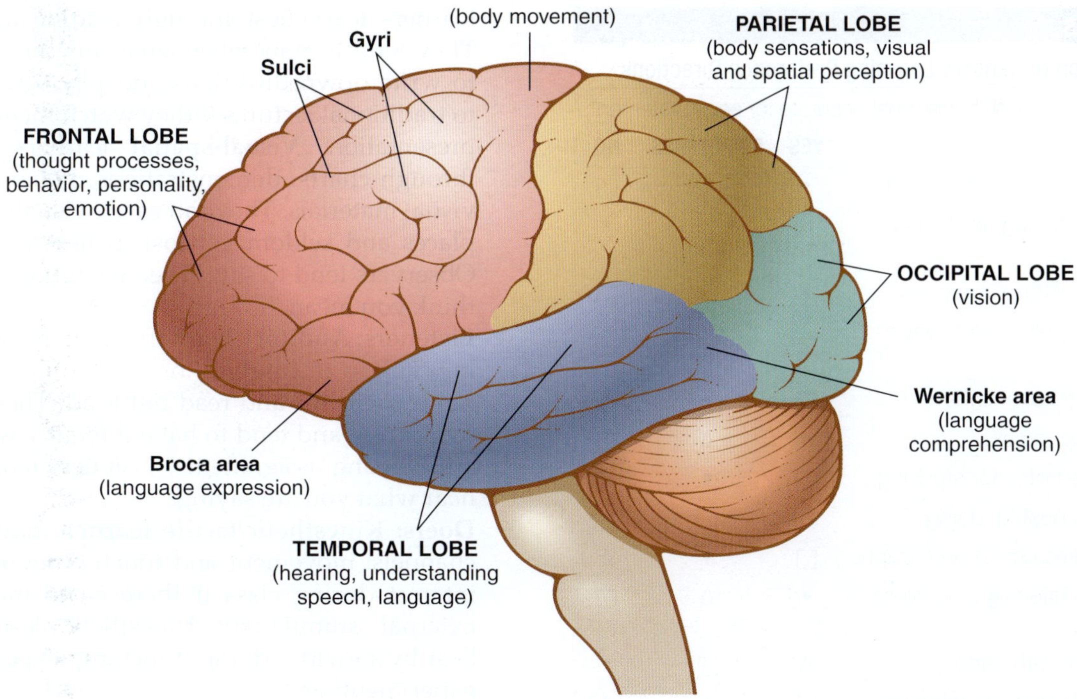

Fig. 2.1 Left and right hemispheres of the cerebrum. (From Chabner DE: *The language of medicine*, ed 11, 2017, St Louis: Elsevier.)

- Seeing and doing in an informal, busy, somewhat unstructured environment.
- Participating in simulations, group discussions, panels, and activity-based learning. This group will embrace the "flipped classroom."

LEFT BRAIN–DOMINANT INDIVIDUALS

Left brain–dominant learners tend to be analytical, rational, and objective. They apply logic to problem solving and learn best by:

- Putting together many facts to arrive at an understanding.
- Having traditional lectures, demonstrations, and assigned readings.

THINKING PREFERENCE

Usually one side of the brain is dominant and affects the way you process information. The two most common preferences are linear and global.

Linear thinkers (also known as left brain dominant):

- Prefer a very structured approach to learning. They are most comfortable doing things in order. For example, when going to their first day of the nursing program, linear thinkers will have checked ahead of time the route they will take, which door to go in, where the room is located, the time they are expected to arrive, and what supplies they are expected to bring.
- They will review the information carefully *before* leaving home and often prepare a list.

Global thinkers (also known as right brain dominant):

- Are more comfortable going to the nursing program their first day by accessing information and relating it to their overall goals.
- They are likely to get into their vehicle and drive, without any preplanning, on that first day.

LEARNING PREFERENCES

Learning takes place in different ways. It is important not to label anyone, including yourself. Everyone is capable of learning with any learning style preference and use another preference to reinforce learning.

PERCEPTUAL LEARNING PREFERENCES

Perceptual learning preference refers to our three main sensory receivers:

- Visual (learn primarily with their eyes)
- Auditory (learn primarily by listening)
- Kinesthetic/tactual (learn primarily by hands-on tasks).

The majority of individuals in Western countries prefer the visual learning preference. The next most natural is auditory, and the least common is the movement (kinesthetic) and tactile (touch) preference. Many practical nursing programs, particularly clock hour–based programs, have more "hands-on" training than a traditional prelicensure registered nursing (RN) program. This may attract students who have a visual or kinesthetic learning preference.

Try This

Self-Evaluation of Sensory Learning Preference Directions

Underline the symbol that is most accurate for each statement

	YES	SOMETIMES	NO
Prefers to talk rather than read	•	Δ	□
Likes to touch, hug, and shake hands	Δ	□	•
Likes to brainstorm in groups	•	Δ	□
Uses finger spelling as a way to learn words	Δ	□	•
Prefers written directions	□	•	Δ
Sings or talks to self	•	Δ	□
Likes to take notes for studying	□	•	Δ
Remembers best by doing	Δ	□	•
Likes or makes charts and graphs	□	•	Δ
Learns from listening to lectures and tapes	•	Δ	□
Likes to work with hands	Δ	□	•
Might say, "I don't see what you mean"	□	•	Δ
Good at jigsaw puzzles and mazes	□	•	Δ
Has a good listening skill	•	Δ	□
Presses pencil down hard when writing	Δ	□	•
Learns words by repeating out loud	□	•	Δ
When traveling, prefers to have oral directions	•	Δ	□
Plays with objects during the learning period	Δ	□	•

Count all of the symbols. The highest number indicates the sensory reading preference.

□, Visual; •, auditory; Δ, kinesthetic/tactile.
Adapted from the Barsch Learning Style Inventory, Penn State Learning Style Inventory, and the University of Georgia Education Technology Center Learning Style Inventory.

Critical Thinking

Summarizing Your Learning Preferences

After you have completed the Self-Evaluation of Sensory Learning Styles exercise, make two columns on a piece of paper. Label the columns "A" and "B." Write the statements you answered as "Yes" or "No" in column "A," and write the statements you answered as "Sometimes" in column "B." You have identified your sensory learning preference. The "Perceptual Learning Style Preference" section tells you how the information can be helpful to studying.

PERCEPTUAL LEARNING PREFERENCE THINKING

People think differently. They think in the system corresponding to the sense of vision, hearing, or kinesthetic/tactile.

- **Observers: Visual learners** have two subchannels: visual linguistic and visual spatial. **Visual-linguistic** learners learn best through reading and writing. They tend to remember what they read. They like to write down directions and pay better attention to traditional lectures if they watch them on a video presentation. **Visual-spatial** learners learn best through charts, demonstrations, videos, and other visual materials. They can easily visualize faces and places and seldom get lost in new surroundings. Observers tend to say, "I see what you mean" or "I think you mean."
- **Listeners: Auditory learners** think in terms of hearing, talk to themselves, or hear sounds. They may move their lips and read out loud. They learn best by hearing and tend to have difficulty with reading and writing assignments. Listeners tend to say, "I hear what you are saying."
- **Doers: Kinesthetic/tactile learners** have two subchannels: movement and touch. They tend to lose interest during class if there is no movement or external stimulation. Kinesthetic learners learn best by moving, doing, touching, experiencing, or experimenting.

Being identified as a specific type of learner does not mean that a learner thinks exclusively in any one of these overall systems. What it means is that most people think more in one system than another. There are ways to enhance learning by supporting the overall system. No learning preference is better than another. It is usually easier to feel connected to someone who shares a similar learning preference: "We think in the same language."

Critical Thinking

Think about instructors you have had from past education to the present. Which instructor was your favorite? What was their teaching preference? Did it match your learning preference?

Professional Pointer

A learning preference is just that. Think about resources available to reinforce information using your learning preference. For example, if you are a kinesthetic "hands-on" learner and your teacher lectures most of the class, you may need to visit the lab or use a screen-based simulation tool to fully understand the concept presented in class.

Visual Learner Preference

If you are a visual learner, you learn best by watching a demonstration first. Make this preference work for you by using the following techniques:

- Sit in the front seat of a face-to-face class.
- Stay focused on the teacher's facial expression and body language.
- Take notes in class, and highlight color code, and use mind maps to process and learn content.
- Rewrite notes in your own words as a form of studying (e.g., write notes or draw pictures in the margin of your book or as a note on the screen).

- Use index cards for review or memorization.
- Review video clips.
- Look for reference books that contain pictures, graphs, or charts, or draw your own.
- Request demonstrations and observational experiences before practicing a new skill.
- Try to "picture" a procedure rather than just memorizing steps.

Auditory Learner

If you are an auditory learner, you learn best by hearing. Make this preference work for you by using the following techniques:

- Listen carefully if the instructor outlines what you will be learning, emphasizes what is important to remember, and summarizes what has been covered during class.
- Read aloud or mouth the words. Concentrate on hearing the words, especially when reading test questions.
- When attending a lecture, listen to the words instead of taking notes during class. Record the presentation and discussion if the instructor and students grant permission. Play the recording back several times. Playing the recording in the car on your way home from school, while doing routine tasks, or just before sleeping can be beneficial to learning.
- Find a "study buddy" or group with whom to discuss class content. Compare notes and verbalize the information to aid in learning the material.
- Request permission to make a recording or give oral reports (instead of written reports) for credit.
- Make up silly rhymes or songs (mnemonic clues) to remember key points.
- Request a verbal explanation of illustrations, graphs, and diagrams. Record the explanation, if permissible. Your cell phone can be a quick resource to record the interaction.
- Listen to podcasts.

Kinesthetic/Tactual Learner

If you are a kinesthetic learner, you learn best by touching, moving, or hands-on tasks. Traditional lectures, in which one is required to sit, read, or listen for long periods of time, may be difficult for you. Processing both visual and auditory input may be a challenge.

Using your muscles by gesturing can help improve memory of information by matching a gesture to information that needs to be remembered. When the gestures and word are associated in your mind, performing this gesture can retrieve the word. Physical motion can jog memory and promote recall. You should see the motions students go through during an examination. Make this preference work for you by using the following techniques:

- Handle the equipment before you practice a nursing procedure.
- Move while reading or reciting facts (e.g., rocking, pacing, or using a stationary bike).
- Change study positions often. During traditional lectures, you may want to sit in back so you can stand up and take notes without distracting others.
- Use background music of your choice when studying away from school.
- Take short breaks and do something active during that time.
- Offer to do a project as a way of enhancing a required classroom presentation. For example, if you have been asked to explain how oxygen gets out of a capillary and carbon dioxide gets in, develop a project to use as the basis for your explanation.
- Use arrows to show relationships when taking notes. Use flash cards, games, mnemonic clues, and other game-like activities to reinforce content of long reading assignments.
- Highlight key concepts; make diagrams and doodles.

Try This

Enhance Your Learning

List two suggestions that you think will help enhance your learning and commit to implementing them within the next week. Ask a peer to verify if you achieve this goal.

MULTIPLE INTELLIGENCES

Gardner (1999) described what he termed "multiple intelligences" as being more accurate than the single measure of the intelligence quotient (IQ) with which most people are familiar. The seven distinct intelligences include the following:

1. Linguistic
2. Logical/mathematical
3. Visual/spatial
4. Musical
5. Bodily/kinesthetic
6. Interpersonal
7. Intrapersonal

This knowledge provides additional information that will further enhance your learning.

LINGUISTIC LEARNER (THE WORD PLAYER)

If you are a **linguistic learner**, you learn best by saying, hearing, and seeing words. You like to read, write, and tell stories. You are good at memorizing names, places, dates, and trivia. Make this preference work for you by using the following techniques:

- Take notes when you read this text and reduce the number of words you have included in the notes. Your love of words and vocabulary may cause you to become distracted from the key points. Use these notes as your study source.

- Review all written work before handing in the assignment. Delete extra words and phrases that are not directly related to the topic.

LOGICAL/MATHEMATICAL LEARNER (THE QUESTIONER)

If you are a **logical learner** as well, you learn best by using an organized method that involves categorizing, classifying, and working with abstract patterns and relationships. You are good at reasoning, math, and problem solving. Make this preference work for you by using the following techniques:
- Take the time to organize a method of study that fits you personally.
- Redo your notes to fit your study method, categorizing the material under titles and themes.

VISUAL/SPATIAL LEARNER (THE VISUALIZER)

If you are a **visual/spatial learner**, you learn best by visualizing, dreaming, working with colors and pictures, and studying diagrams, boxes, and special lists in the textbook/e-book. You are good at imagining things, sensing changes, puzzles, and charts. Make this learning preference work for you by using the following techniques:
- Make your own diagrams, boxes, or lists when they are not available in the text/e-book.
- Redo your notes using key concepts only.
- Box key information in the text. Highlight in your e-book.

MUSICAL LEARNER (THE MUSIC LOVER)

If you are a **musical learner**, you learn best by humming, singing, or playing an instrument. You are good at remembering melodies, rhythms, and keeping time. Make this preference work for you by using the following techniques:
- Play your favorite music, or hum while studying. Remind yourself which music relates to the content you are studying.
- Play an instrument while reviewing information in your head.
- Create songs to remember key information.

BODILY/KINESTHETIC LEARNER (THE MOVER)

If you are a **bodily/kinesthetic learner**, you learn best by touching, moving, and processing knowledge through bodily sensations. You are good at physical activities and crafts. Make this preference work for you by using the following techniques:
- Move around when studying. If you work out on a treadmill or stationary bike, it becomes a good time to read or review notes. You can also listen to podcasts or video clips.
- Dance or act out concepts you are studying to experience the sensations involved.

INTERPERSONAL LEARNER (THE SOCIALIZER)

If you are an **interpersonal learner**, you learn best by sharing, comparing, cooperating, and interviewing. You are good at understanding people, leading others, organizing, communicating, and mediating. Make this preference work for you by using the following techniques:
- Organize and/or participate in a study group.
- Compare your understanding of material with that of other students.
- Practice mock simulations in the lab with a peer.

INTRAPERSONAL LEARNER (THE INDIVIDUAL)

If you are an **intrapersonal learner**, you learn best by working alone, self-paced instruction, and having your own space. You are good at pursuing interests and goals, following instincts, understanding yourself, and being original. Make this learning preference work for you by using the following techniques:
- Work on individualized projects.
- Contribute to team projects as needed. Align team projects with individualized projects.
- Trust your instincts in regard to study needs (Gardner and Hatch, 1990).

Be aware of the type of learner you are, but do not limit yourself to those preferences. Try out suggestions listed under other preferences. Some of them will further enhance your learning.

Critical Thinking

Implementing Suggestions

Make a realistic plan involving learning preferences that you think will work for you. Include observable, desired outcomes; a plan of action; and dates by which you will accomplish this plan. Remember that the dates are just educated guesses based on intimate knowledge of how you function. Be sure you note how you will determine progress toward a behavioral change. Use a format that works for you: columns, clustering, doodling, pictures, and so on.

Professional Pointer

Identify your client's learning preference and use it as a basis to support teaching started by the RN or health care provider.

HOW WE LEARN

Scientists are not exactly sure how the brain can rewire itself with each new stimulation, experience, or behavior and cause learning. However, the science of neuroplasty is unraveling the mystery. The Cleveland Clinic (2023) discusses the power of neuroplasty in the brain adapting throughout life. One idea is that a stimulus occurs and is processed in different areas of the brain. Neural pathways (traces) become more efficient when a learning exercise, such as reviewing notes, is repeated. This is done through myelination (coating) of the neurons. Stimulation occurs when you learn something new such as receiving a new assignment or clinical experience. The mental or motor stimulation lights up the brain in several areas, producing greater beneficial energy.

The brain gets its energy for learning primarily from blood, about 8 gallons per hour. Remember to stay hydrated; drinking water is essential. A glass of water with each meal and between each meal will keep most adults hydrated under normal environmental conditions. Other factors that impede long-term memory include lack of sleep, multitasking, distraction, and physical health. Sleep is essential to learning. Routinely skipping sleep to study may result in a negative outcome.

MAPPING (CONCEPT MAP)

Brain researchers have suggested an alternative to the linear method of note making. It encourages using the *right side* of the brain, with its emphasis on images. Color and drawings are processed by the right side of the brain and are important components of **mapping**. Information presented in a linear manner, as in traditional note-taking, is not as easily understood as information presented by key concepts. The use of key concepts is the primary way in which the brain processes information. The brain takes these key concepts and integrates them in relationships. So if the brain does not work in lines or lists, the method of note-making called mapping can enhance your ability to understand, review, and recall this information. Mapping is a method in which information is organized graphically so it is seen in a visual pattern of relationships. Mapping is most meaningful to the person who draws the map. Box 2.1 gives hints for note-making, using the mapping method. Fig. 2.2 is an example of a summary using **clustering**, a basic form of mapping that helps simplify topics. Clustering is especially helpful for *visual* learners.

Some nursing programs have found mapping helpful in developing critical-thinking skills by having learners use this format to develop nursing care plans as concept maps, instead of the traditional column format. There are many web-based sites that will support creation of a concept map on your computer. Lucidchart is one example that has free access (www.lucidchart.com)

Box 2.1 Hints for Note-Making: Mapping Method

Start with your notepaper in a horizontal position.

- Start with a small circle in the middle of the paper.
- Put the main topic of activity in the circle.
- Add branches off the circle for important ideas and subtopics. Arrange these branches like the spokes of a wheel. Use a different-colored pen for each of the branches. Draw more branches off branches as needed for each topic. Draw a picture to go with each key topic or idea. Artistic ability does not count here. What is important is that the picture gives meaning to you!
- Visit the website www.mindmup.com to create a concept map on your computer.

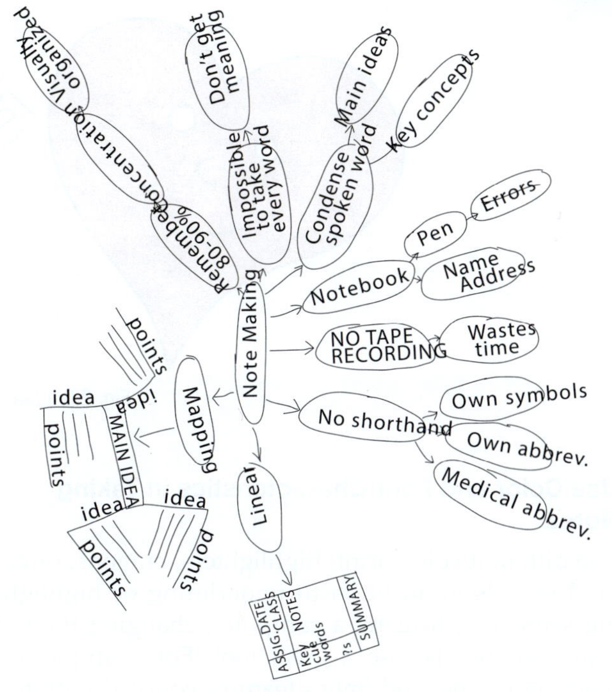

Fig. 2.2 Clustering.

VISUAL STRATEGIES TO ENHANCE UNDERSTANDING

Your academic world is bombarded with words, sentences, and paragraphs. One of the most beneficial techniques to comprehend (understand) and remember all new information is to balance this verbal mixture with visual strategies. Each of the following visual strategies will help you understand and ultimately remember information better. They deal with the right side of the brain. You will be tapping a resource that possibly you have not used often if your left brain is dominant. These strategies include creating pictures and drawings that capture the key information.

Draw Idea Sketches

These drawings will probably be comprehensible only to you. The emphasis of **idea sketches** is not on the quality of the drawing but on the process you must go through to take a verbal concept and represent it graphically, without words. To go through this process, you must understand the verbal concept. You can even set it up as a cartoon. Use stick figures and describe the concept verbally. Fig. 2.3 is an idea sketch illustrating the function of the drug Lanoxin (digoxin), which is used to slow and strengthen the heartbeat.

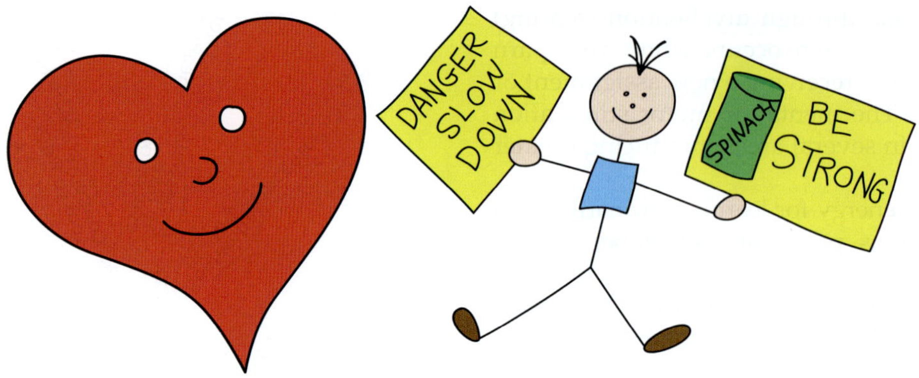

Fig. 2.3 Idea sketch: Lanoxin (digoxin).

Use Color and Font Characteristics in Taking Notes

Use different color print, highlighters, crayons, or colored pencils in addition to underlining or highlighting sentences. If using a computer, changing the font characteristics is also a great tool. For example: use bold, underline, and italics features coupled with font color and highlight options to assist in categorizing information, thus enhancing your understanding and retention. These strategies help your brain organize and retrieve information more effectively.

Make Your Own Diagram as You Read

If you commit to memory by using words only, you are using only half of your brain's resources, those of the left side. If you also produce a sketch of that idea or view a sketch on a website, you will have brought the right side of your brain into use. Using both sides of the brain enhances your success.

Engage in Mental Imagery

Engaging in **mental imagery** will help you remember material because it demands that you understand the information. When you use mental imagery, you become the idea that you are having difficulty understanding. The right side of your brain generates pictures of the idea, and the left side supplies the script to explain what is going on in the pictures (and always in your own words). Box 2.2 provides a mental image developed by a practical nursing student to provide a simple understanding of the function of insulin, a hypoglycemic agent that increases glucose transport across muscles and fat cell membranes. Notice how *the* use of senses of hearing and feeling and also body movement help achieve understanding. This is a good example of the use of a metaphor to tie it to something when trying to learn. Have someone read the story and try to visualize the scenario. Then recite the image to yourself, closing your eyes and visualizing it.

Mental imagery can be fun. If you are a social learner, this could be a fun activity with peers, at the end of a long week. A difficult concept such as tonicity of fluids or fetal circulation can become easy to remember.

Box 2.2 Mental Images Depicting the Function of Insulin: I Am Insulin—A Job Description

I am insulin, and I am shaped like a canoe. In fact, I am a green canoe. My job is to make sugar or glucose in the blood available to most of the cells of the body for energy. I like my job. I like things that are sweet, but not too sweet, so normal blood sugar is just my thing. Sometimes after the person who owns the pancreas (where I am stored in my canoe rack) eats a meal, a whistle blows, and I know this is a signal to launch myself into the bloodstream. As I ride the currents of blood, I rock gently back and forth, and the sugar in my bloodstream jumps right in to be a passenger in the canoe. Blood sugar likes me. I think it is because I am green, but I might be wrong. When I am pretty full, but not full enough to swamp, I pass through the blood vessels, paddle through the sea of tissue fluid (it smells salty) around the cells, and pass through the cell membrane. Then I deposit the sugar by making these molecules jump out of the green canoe and into the fluid inside the cell. I feel pretty important in my job. Without me, the blood sugar molecules would be unable to pass through the cell membranes. Because of this, I am given the official job title of hypoglycemic agent. I lower the level of sugar in the blood.

Excuse me! There goes the whistle.

? Critical Thinking

Increasing Understanding of Concepts

Choose a concept you are having trouble understanding in one of your nursing classes or text/e-book readings (i.e., trace a drop of blood), and try to increase understanding by using the following:

1. Draw an idea sketch.
2. Use mental imagery.
3. Locate an online resource.

Which strategy was most useful for the concept you chose?

BARRIERS TO LEARNING

UNDEPENDABLE MEMORY AND LEARNING SYSTEM

All students can experience barriers to learning. The discussion that follows is focused on strategies to assist students who are diagnosed or are possibly undiagnosed with attention deficit hyperactivity disorder (ADHD). Although the strategies discussed focus on this diagnosis, they can be helpful to all students, particularly when students experience high levels of stress (e.g., a new nursing student).

Average and above-average individuals with potential talent may embrace failure messages, low self-esteem, and loss of hope. These individuals may live with untreated **adult ADHD**. A few of the characteristics are an undependable memory and learning system and problems with self-regulation and self-motivation. The individual may have problems with procrastination, distractibility, organization, prioritization, and impulsive decision-making. Because of previous poor performance at school or work, they may have been labeled as "lazy" or "stupid." Students diagnosed and treated with ADHD often become high achievers, experiencing academic success for the first time in their life.

Possible Behaviors

- Procrastination
- Indecision, difficulty recalling and organizing details required for a task
- Poor time management, losing track of time
- Avoiding tasks or jobs that required sustained effort
- Difficulty initiating tasks
- Difficulty completing and following through on tasks
- Difficulty multitasking
- Easily bored
- Impatient
- Easily irritated
- Impulsive
- Endless energy

Adults with ADHD may have experienced a lot of pain caused by repeated failure resulting in embarrassment, self-blame, and a loss of hope. Intelligence is not affected in ADHD. Excellent information is available at the National Resource Center (NRC) on ADHD (https://chadd.org/), funded by the Centers for Disease Control and Prevention (CDC) (CDC.gov). This is the nation's clearinghouse for the latest evidence-based information on ADHD. As a nursing student you will gain a deep understanding of the importance of reputable evidence. The CDC is a trusted government resource providing evidence and latest news regarding many health issues. Chapter 3 will address in detail community resources available to enhance your success.

Suggestions for the Student With Attention Deficit Hyperactivity Disorder (These Can Help All Learners!)

- Educate yourself about ADHD. Understanding the disorder is a useful tool in learning to manage symptoms.
- Get a coach; both a classmate and a friend/family member are ideal. A coach assists you in staying organized, encourages you, and reminds you to get back to work while supporting you. Humor can be helpful.
- Create a list of tasks to be accomplished, organizing tasks into manageable sections with deadlines. Prioritize your lists so the most important assignments are accomplished first.
- Procrastination is a major issue. Be alert to the possibility, and discipline yourself to avoid procrastination. Do not deviate from deadlines unless a crisis occurs.
- Color coding: The adult with ADHD is often visually oriented. Color helps focus attention and also makes what you are looking at memorable. Use color in your text/e-book as you read to bring out important points. Highlight as you read and take notes on your computer.
- Pay attention to the different learning preferences you read about in this chapter and try out the preferences that appeal to you. The student with ADHD may need to multitask to study successfully (e.g., listening to a study tape while jogging). Because physical activity is generally a part of ADHD, you may discover that reading or reviewing notes works best for you when you are on a stationary bike, treadmill, or other apparatus that moves. Having music may help drown out distracting noises when studying.
- Be alert to what time of day works best for you for studying. Decorate your personal study environment to inspire you. Invent your own way of studying. Do what works for you even if other students study differently.
- Note what is important and jot down ideas. Daydreaming is an important part of ADHD, and noting ideas may be a way of staying on task while studying and attending class.
- When studying, give yourself a mini time-out before you switch to a different subject. Transition is often difficult for the student with ADHD, and a little break will help.
- Find ways to recharge your batteries without guilt.

> **Try This**
>
> Most students can benefit from some of the strategies noted above. List two that you will implement.
>
> 1.
>
> 2.

MORE BARRIERS TO LEARNING

Barriers may or may not be of your own making. Regardless of the reason for their existence, they belong to you now. It is up to you to identify if barriers exist and if they affect your learning. It is also up to you to seek help in dealing with the barriers, if needed. Your level of reading and math academic readiness, despite entrance test screening, can be a barrier. See Chapter 3 for specific details.

Try This

Personal Learning Preference Related to Academic Readiness

Review your individual nursing entrance test scores in comparison with the national average (50th percentile point on the test). Seek guidance from your faculty or advisor to understand the impact.

Critical Thinking

Personal Learning Preference Related to Academic Readiness

Identify strategies discussed that can assist you in improving your reading, writing, or other related skills. Be specific. Based on your weak areas, list two implementations related to your learning preference to improve in these areas.

1.
2.

INABILITY TO UNDERSTAND (COMPREHEND) CONTENT

Almost everyone in the United States can read and recognize words, but not everyone understands the meaning of the words they read. Years ago, a renowned reading researcher, Dr. Jeanne Chall (1958), identified predictable stages of reading development, which are still valid today. They are as follows:

- Before a child starts grade school, the foundation for reading and learning has been established. By being read to, a child learns what books are for and how they are used. In addition, the alphabet is introduced.
- In grades 1 and 2, a child learns to translate written letters and symbols into sounds and words.
- In grades 3 and 4, the school-age child develops speed and accuracy in reading (fluency). The child has not yet learned to comprehend what is being read.
- In grades 4 through 8, the school-age child masters vocabulary and learns how to pick out the main parts when reading. This is the beginning of reading for content.
- In high school, students learn to weigh evidence in messages they are reading and evaluate and make judgments about what they read. These behaviors demonstrate the ability to read for content and understand what is being read.
- By the end of high school, adolescents have reached a stage in which they are able to manage their own learning process, choosing what to read, and knowing how to use what they have learned in areas of interest.

Many people in the United States have not reached the level of comprehending what they read. Memorization is not comprehension. Although some memorization is necessary, the SPN/SVN must be able to analyze information critically and make deductions and conclusions about client care. This is a role of a licensed person. Reading skills are important to your success.

PUTTING IT ALL TOGETHER

Quality education encourages you to explore and apply alternative thinking, multiple answers, and creative thoughts. You can become a self-directed learner using the following techniques:

- Practice thinking critically (see Chapter 5).
- Identify your major and specific learning preferences. Studying becomes easier.
- Understand basic right brain and left brain functions and how they work together. It helps you appreciate your capacity for learning.
- Do your part to prevent dehydration when studying and participating in classes. Water is a major ingredient of blood, which motivates the brain. Nutrition and sleep are also important.
- Maintain a positive attitude as you continue to learn and apply what you are learning.
- Set realistic goals and evaluate the results to see whether or not these goals were met.
- It is an obstacle to learning to believe it can take place without effort.
- Remember that established preferences of learning may not be working for you. Learning preferences can be changed or modified as needed. It is also worth it to try suggestions from other preferences to see if the suggestions enhance your learning.
- Tie in new learning to previous lessons and experiences. This gives the material meaning and makes it easier to remember.
- Seek help when it is needed. See Chapter 3 for additional community resources. Do not hesitate to contact these sources and get help early! Once you have failed a test, it becomes difficult to meet the minimum grade to pass the course. Be proactive!
- Identify your reading level and make sure you reach your potential.
- Seek to understand the clinical task versus simply performing the steps. Practice with a partner while they are quizzing you, modeling the instructor's expected behavior.
- Question what you do not understand and question the source of information when you have reason to believe it is incorrect. Always be professional in your approach. Cite evidence when questioning the source.
- Remember that whatever your learning preference is, the best way to remember is to write it down.

- According to a Chinese proverb, "the weakest link lasts longer than the strongest memory."

Empowerment

If you are having difficulty learning and feel no one "hears" you, try the following:

Leave your emotions behind and use the evidence to explain specifically how you studied (based on learning preferences) and why you are frustrated with the grade you achieved. Listen to the recommendations provided by your faculty or peer.

Study skills are critical to success in a practical/vocational LPN/LVN program. They are learned skills and become habit once practiced well. It is never too late to improve your study skills!

Knowledge is power! You can do it!

Many educational institutions offer courses in how to study before learners enter a program and have departments that offer study skills services after a learner has enrolled. There are many Internet sites that provide information about study skills. Visit the Education Corner as an example (https://www.educationcorner.com/study-skills/).

Despite these resources, lack of study skills, including test-taking skills, is a major factor for failure or withdrawing from a nursing program. Learners who need these services are not always aware that they need them or try to develop them "too late." Often students do not focus on improving study skills until they have received several failing grades.

Learners cannot assume they have the study skills necessary to succeed in the LPN/LVN program because they have attended high school or college. It is possible for students to have been successful in college in a different area of study (i.e., fine arts, music, history) and struggle to succeed in a nursing program. It takes time and effort to comprehend, store, and recall the knowledge and skills needed for critical thinking in a nursing career.

GENERAL HINTS FOR LEARNERS

CONCENTRATION

Concentration is the ability to keep your mind completely on the task at hand. The major enemy of concentration is distraction. Many distractions in a learner's life compete with the need to focus on school assignments. These distractions can be summarized as two types: **external distractions**, which are those that come from outside you; and **internal distractions**, which are those that come from inside you. Remember your learning preference and strive for a study environment that meets your unique needs.

External Distractions

External distractions occur in your physical and social environments. An obvious distraction is hunger and thirst. Satisfy these needs before settling in to study. Keep nutritious snacks and water close by for break time.

Personal study area. Your physical environment can be a potential enemy of concentration. Here are some tips to avoid distractions:

- Identify the type of environment that allows you to get the most out of your study time. Your grades will be the criteria by which you can judge whether your environment is helping or hurting. Everyone's environment is unique. Some students like total quiet, whereas others need music to drown out other distractors.
- A specific study area, conducive to learning, should be identified in your living space and organized with the necessary tools and equipment to benefit your learning. When you enter the space, your mind knows it is time to study, and so does your family!
- Alternating areas where one studies can improve retention of information. The learning resource center (LRC) can be used between classes and after school. At some schools, study rooms can be reserved.
- Have on hand the tools you will need, including course outline (syllabus), computer, Internet access, highlighters and colored pencils, print or e-book, and notes or reference materials

Lighting. Eyestrain can occur if lighting allows glare, shadows, or flicker to exist in your study area.

- E-readers may require additional external lighting.
- Reading lamps should have bulbs with natural white light and a light grid to reduce glare.
- Use ceiling lights, if available, to reduce shadows, in addition to your table lamp.
- A table lamp with a properly seated bulb needs to be shaded to reduce flicker.
- Your writing surface needs to be a light color to reflect light and reduce glare.
- When reading, if you experience symptoms of eyestrain, such as headaches, dizziness, tiredness, or blurred vision, and you have tried to eliminate glare, shadows, and flicker, it may be time to have an eye examination to rule out the need for corrective lenses.
- Some learners discover they need glasses only after they enroll in an educational program that demands much reading, such as the LPN/LVN program.
- If you wear contacts, limit the amount of time for reading before switching to your glasses. If experiencing dry eyes from significant amounts of reading, especially on a computer screen, take occasional breaks and seek medical guidance early to avoid any eye complications.

Background noise

- Television, music, podcasts, conversation, and other noises can be distracting background noise to some learners, but others find that they study best with these noises.

- Establish new habits if these noises are interfering with your concentration and test grades.
- Be sure your family and friends understand why you need to implement these changes.

Internet and social networking. Being online offers a vast amount of resources for all your classes.

- It is easy to get distracted by the Internet and social media sites.
- If you use search engines, e-books, and social networking services such as X (formerly Twitter), TikTok, and so many more for personal and recreational purposes, you need to learn how to use the Internet and social media professionally (see Chapter 18).
- Monitor your time when online for educational, personal, or professional reasons because hours can slip by before you know it.
- Using the Internet to find evidence to enhance understanding is a great strategy. However, time can slip away. For example, you may realize 3 hours have passed, you have only completed 25% of the assignment, and the assignment is due in 1 hour. Be careful of this trap!

Your peers and friends. Peers could be a possible external distraction. The energy devoted to any of the following behaviors can seriously deplete the energy needed to achieve success in the practical/vocational nursing program and can create unneeded stress and frustration. Answer "Yes" or "No" to the following questions about your peers in the LPN/LVN program.

1. Are the people you associate with encouraging your progress in the practical/vocational nursing program?
2. Do you and your peers support and encourage one another?
3. Do you seek out students who have negative attitudes? If so, do the conversations reflect negativity?
4. Do the people you associate with belittle, complain, and tear down the instructor, the course, the school, and/or various students in your group?
5. Does your anxiety level increase when you carpool with certain students on test days?
6. Do your peers, who are not enrolled in school pressure you to join them and take time away from study/sleep time?
7. Can you identify a peer who is motivating to you?

Try This

Personal Distractions

List any external physical distractions that are affecting your concentration.

What can you do to eliminate these distractions?

Internal Distractions

You can have the study space, lighting, noise level, equipment, and peers for studying but still not be able to keep your mind on the task at hand. The culprit may be distractions arising from inside you. Examples of internal distractions and suggestions for overcoming them are discussed below.

Complaints of mental fatigue. Some learners confuse boredom with fatigue.

- Avoid studying one subject for so long that you get bored with it.
- Keep self-energized physically with proper nutrition, sleep, and exercise.
- Take scheduled short breaks and come back to new material to get your mental "second wind."
- Intermix concepts you like to study versus areas you dread.
- Intermix reading, writing, and interactive assignments.

Daydreaming. Daydreaming can be a creative adventure or wasted time.

- Every time you find your mind wandering from the topic at hand, try putting a checkmark on a piece of paper kept at your side. This may remind you that you are drifting off and need to get back to work.
- Students who use this technique find that the number of checkmarks decreases dramatically over time.

LISTENING/VIEWING

The Active and Passive Listener/Viewer

Whether you are involved in a mini-lecture or a group discussion, viewing videos, websites, or watching an instructor or resource presentation as part of your course assignments, you will miss a lot if your mind wanders. Listening/viewing is more than the mechanical process of hearing or seeing. There are two kinds of listeners/viewers. Which type are you?

The **passive listener/viewer** receives sounds or sees words with little recognition or personal involvement.

- Passive listeners/viewers may be doodling, staring out the window, staring at the instructor, aimlessly trying to copy everything, all the while thinking about personal problems, family needs, or work issues.

The **active listener/viewer** is always thinking, not just hearing or seeing words.

- Active listeners/viewers listen and look with full attention, are open-minded and curious, and ask themselves questions about content.
- The active listener/viewer, who really listens to hear and thoughtfully looks to see, is searching for relevant information, strives to understand it, applies it to other knowledge, and is always trying to figure out how content fits into the big picture, as you will do in clinical assignments.
- Active listeners/viewers realize that listening and seeing are important means of gathering information, and they work at developing these skills.
- Active listeners/viewers identify and define words that are unfamiliar and seek out other resources to

Box 2.3 Hints for Active Listening/Viewing in Classes

- Be well rested for class or activity.
- Complete assignments, extra readings, and exercises before class or activity.
- Focus on what is happening with the lesson. Listen and/or look for key information, central ideas, examples, and study hints.
- Capture key points of the PowerPoint presentations.
- Ask questions before, during, and after class.
- Make eye contact with the speaker.
- Listen when other students are speaking.
- Seek help when a difficult concept is not understood.

increase their understanding of the content while reading.

- The active listener/viewer searches for ways in which the words can be put to practical use or drawn in a picture to give meaning. Box 2.3 gives you hints on how to become an active listener/viewer.

Empowerment

Active Versus Passive Listener/Viewer

Identify and list behaviors that indicate you are an active or passive listener/viewer.

My active listening/viewing behaviors:

____

My passive listening/viewing behaviors:

____

Discuss your comments with a peer. How can you increase your active listener/viewer skills to positively impact your school outcomes (i.e., grades, evaluations)?

Note-*Making* Versus Note-*Taking*

An important part of listening/viewing is remembering what you have heard or seen. Some students say that taking notes interferes with their listening/viewing skills. They are correct if they are in the business of taking notes. Research by Hermann Ebbinghaus in 1885 identified the forgetting curve. This research has stood the test of time and is still widely referenced. The forgetting curve shows that retention drops from an immediate 90% to 100% to less than 40% in the first few days. This retention can be impacted by many external factors (i.e., difficulty level of content, stress level, delivery method). Luckily, you can improve those percentages to as much as 80% to 90%. Whether using your tablet or paper and pen, one of the secrets is to engage in note-*making* whenever you are listening/viewing. Because instructors derive test questions from mini-lectures, discussions, activities, videos, web links, instructor presentations, and texts, that 80% to 90% of a specific learning activity could translate into a comparable test score. Note-*making* will help you pay attention, concentrate, and organize your ideas.

Note-making hints

- Never try to capture every spoken or written word. This is note-*taking*, and it is impossible.
- Actively listen/look for the main ideas. Capture them in a way that reflects your personal learning preference or preferences. You are recording ideas or **key concepts** that you will later add to, correct, and study. Your goal is to understand the information, *not* memorize it.
- Engage in note-making, condensing what is said or seen in a text-like manner.
- Develop personal symbols, abbreviations, and/or shorthand of sorts to help capture the main ideas, yet retain readability without having to completely rewrite the notes.
- With practice, notes will improve. Your goal is a set of notes you can use for review and test preparation.
- Outlining is a structured form of note-making that starts with major points and indents supporting points. Numbers or letters can be used to outline but are not necessary. Indentations will do. Box 2.4 contains excellent hints for note-making.
- Some students think that just making notes will help them retain the material. However, active and frequent review of your notes is an important step in retention of material for later recall.

HOW TO UNDERSTAND (COMPREHEND) INFORMATION

READING ASSIGNMENTS

"I read the material four times and got a D. My friend read the material once and got an A. It isn't fair." The learner who is speaking is correct. It takes a lot of time to read material four times for a test. The missing ingredient is the lack of **understanding (comprehension)** of information that is read.

Box 2.4 Hints for Note-Making

- When using a tablet or pen and paper, include the date and general topic of class/activity at the top of the page and any assignments that are given.
- Place specific topics of the class to the left of the page.
- Indent points as they are presented to explain/discuss the topic.
- Leave spaces between topics to add information to clarify the topic as needed.
- After class, in the left margin of a paper page, record any questions to clarify your understanding of the content.
- At the bottom of the page, summarize the content of the notes on that page, *in your own words*. This summary forces you to think about the ideas in your notes. You are critically thinking about the information, not passively copying it to be memorized later.

- To think critically in nursing, you must have information.
- To acquire information, you must be able to read with understanding.
- Reading with understanding makes possible retention of the information.
- Retention ensures recall.

Earning only a D by merely reading words is a poor return on your time investment. Did you ever walk/drive somewhere without remembering how you got there? That is the same as reading the text four times or getting to the end of a page and not knowing what you read. These readers have zoned out and have mindless reading. As they read, their minds are somewhere else. They may be hungry, thirsty, tired, need to go to the restroom, or are thinking about other things. Their comprehension of the information is low to absent, and test scores will suffer.

Because you are responsible for large amounts of reading in the practical/vocational nursing program, the ability to read with understanding is a necessary skill. Most of us are able to read printed words on a page. However, the reading demanded of a learner and future employee requires understanding of the meaning of the words. Reading to learn and understand involves a rate of speed and degree of understanding that are effective.

You probably had to take a reading test as part of your pre-entrance tests for the LPN/LVN program. Generally these tests are brief. If you scored low, you were referred for help with this skill. Perhaps you were one of those who achieved an acceptable score on these short reading tests but could use some hints on how to increase your reading efficiency. Evaluate your reading habits by answering "Yes" or "No" to the questions in the following Try This exercise.

Try This

Reading Habit Evaluation

Circle the reading habits that apply to you.

1. Do you ever reread a sentence before you come to the end?
2. Do you ever have trouble figuring out the main point of an author?
3. Do you stop reading every time you come across a word you cannot define and look up the word immediately?
4. Do you read novels, popular magazines, newspapers, and textbooks at the same speed?
5. Do you ever have trouble remembering what you read?
6. Do you have trouble understanding what you read?
7. Do you ever think of other things while you read?
8. Do you read every word of a sentence individually?
9. Do you focus on details when you read?
10. Do you tire quickly when reading?
11. Do you skip uncommon words when you read?

If you answered "Yes" to any of the previous questions, you could benefit from help with your reading. A visit to your school's study skill center or a consultation with your instructor for assistance with reading can help improve your skill in reading more efficiently and effectively.

Reading Effectively

- Read in phrases, a few words at a time, rather than word by word. Although the brain can view only one word at a time, it understands only when words are in phrases. For better understanding, you should read as you speak (i.e., in phrases).
- Put expression into your reading. You do not speak in a monotone, so why read that way? Musical learners can benefit by singing what they read.
- Be aware of your reading assignments that are technical or scientific in nature, and vary your reading speed accordingly. The more recreational your reading material (e.g., novel or magazine), the faster you can read. For more technical or scientific material, you must slow down. Regardless of your learning preference, when the going gets tough in a paragraph of assigned reading, reading the difficult material out loud may help clear up more challenging information.
- Highlight unfamiliar words as you read. When you are finished reading, copy the words on an index card and look them up in the appropriate dictionary. Most of the unfamiliar words you come across will be medical terms, which can be found in a medical dictionary. At first you will think these words are Greek, and you are right. Many of them are derived from the Greek language, the rest from Latin. You may need to look up the unknown words immediately while reading. If so, be sure to reread the content.
- Write the definition on the other side of the card. Break down the word with vertical slashes into its prefix (the word beginning), root (core word), and suffix (word ending) so you can begin making associations with other words that have the same prefix, root, or suffix. If your medical dictionary does not include this information with each word, the information can be found in medical terminology texts or software. Listen to the word, especially if you are an auditory learner or if English is not your first language.
- Nursing involves learning a new language. Regardless of learning preference, to help recall the meaning of the word, consider drawing a picture to represent the definitions of these words. Create a song to remember difficult information. Use index cards to frequently review on errands or standing in a grocery line. Create flash cards on your computer, use cards shared by others (i.e., cram.com or quizlet.com), and retrieve these cards on your smartphone or tablet. Caution: if reviewing cards made by others, check first to see if they are accurate. Learning can occur whenever you have a few minutes to spare.

- Highlight key phrases in your text/computer resources/class notes and write notes in the margins. Highlighting will keep you active and result in the identification of key concepts.
- Consider recording words that you needed to define and your notes. Listen to the recordings when you are commuting, performing household chores, or walking between classes. It is best to record your own notes, emphasizing key points to understand.
- Be sure to use resources provided by your instructor on the learning management system (LMS) (i.e., Moodle, Blackboard, Canvas). Determine mandatory versus optional assignments and resources. It is easy to become overwhelmed with all the resources available in today's digital learning environment.

Remember, an important part of any textbook is the index at the back of the book. This index will help you locate information quickly. The glossary (alphabetical listing of boldfaced terms in this text) at the back of the book will provide the definition of these words. Glossaries also usually exist in the textbook's web-based support materials or in e-books. In addition, pay close attention to the charts, figures and tables, and recommended websites included to enhance your learning.

? Critical Thinking

Improving Reading Habits

Write your plan to increase your reading comprehension. Note how you will determine progress.

Include in your plan school and community resources.

REMEMBERING AND FORGETTING

We all can recall things from the past, indicating that our brains have the ability to store information. But how many times have you said, "I forgot" or "I cannot remember"? Possible causes of forgetting include a negative attitude toward the subject, which interferes with the motivation to remember. Perhaps the most common reason why students cannot remember is that they never understood, stored, and comprehended the information in the first place. Perhaps they did not listen/view actively, or they just read words without comprehending.

Do not fool yourself when studying. Always close your book and describe "the top five" critical concepts regarding the area studied. Explaining health-related concepts to a peer or significant other who does not work in health care can be very helpful in determining if you understand the concept. Their questions and confusion will prompt you to review your resources and try to explain again.

FROM TEMPORARY TO PERMANENT MEMORY BY WAY OF A NEURAL TRACE

Once you understand information, you need to store that information so you can recall it when needed in the clinical experience (and on tests!). To store information in your long-term memory, a neural trace or record of the information must be created. It takes 4 to 5 seconds for information to move from the temporary (or short-term) memory to the permanent (or long-term) memory. To form a long-term memory of information, you must strive to understand that information and give meaning to it. In doing so, you will give your brain the chance to create a neural trace. Presto! You have formed a memory of that information. Short but frequent study periods with concentration will help you understand information and store it in your long-term memory. Then it is ready for recall. In addition, teaching a peer or family member can be helpful to improve your memory recall.

Remember that a positive mental attitude is a factor in learning, allowing you to understand and remember. Remind yourself that all the prerequisite and basic courses in your nursing program are essential. They are the building blocks for the remaining courses in the LPN/LVN program. The following techniques help increase understanding of your studies by allowing neural traces to be recorded in your brain. (See the PQRST Method of Textbook Study in this text for further study systems.)

- Scan the reading material first, noting headings, bold words, charts, and tables.
- Next, read the entire selection. Seek out key concepts, basic principles, and key ideas. Be selective and sift out unnecessary details. The activity of being selective helps you lay down neural traces. Emphasize accuracy, not speed. You want correct information to make a clear neural trace. It is difficult to unlearn wrong information and replace it with correct information. You cannot memorize everything. If you could, you would not have an understanding of anything. The student who focuses on memorization has difficulty in applying course information and solving problems in the clinical experience.
- Short study periods followed by short rest periods are better than long study marathons. This type of study will reenergize you and allow neural learning to continue during rest periods. It seems that cramming for examinations is treated like a rite of passage among some students. Brain research has shown that short but frequent study periods help you store information in long-term memory. This will make the information available for testing and for application in the clinical area.
- Regardless of your learning preference, use as many body senses and body movement as possible when trying to learn new information. Recite the information out loud as you read, using your own words. If you can explain it, you understand it. Hearing you say the information out loud allows neural traces to be recorded.
- Write down the information in your own words. This muscle action will help you clarify ideas and

improve thinking. *Do not copy word by word from a book.* Mueller and Oppenheimer's (2014, 2018) study provides evidence that typing notes on a laptop can be less beneficial than writing notes for some learners. Assess what works best for you and stick to it!

The techniques of using body senses and body movement are elements of tactual learning and help lay down a neural trace. Try them, and see if they work for you. Adopt the suggestions that help you understand the material in your classes to increase your long-term memory.

MEMORY AIDS

Mnemonic devices are examples of memory aids. Some examples include the following:

- *Rhymes*
  Thirty days hath September.
  I before *e* except after *c*.
  In fourteen hundred and ninety-two.
- *Acronyms*
  Every good boy does fine (to remember the line notes of the treble clef in music)
  There are also devices in nursing that can help you remember information. For example:
- *CMTSP* (for assessment of the nerve and blood supply to an extremity)
  C 5 color
  M 5 motion
  T 5 temperature
  S 5 sensation
  P 5 pulse
- *PERRLA* (for assessment of the pupils)
  P 5 pupils
  E 5 equal in size
  R 5 round
  R 5 regular in shape
  L 5 react to light
  A 5 accommodation (pupils constrict)

Memorizing these acronyms can help the LPN/LVN student remember groups of information. They do not take the place of or help you understand the information. The Internet, including YouTube, has many examples created by other students.

SUCCESSFUL TEST TAKING

According to the National Council of State Boards of Nursing, Inc., "the practice of practical/vocational nursing requires application of knowledge, skills, abilities, and clinical judgment; therefore the majority of items are written at the application or higher levels of cognitive ability (NCLEX-PN® Test Plan, 2023). Therefore you can anticipate that your theory tests in the LPN/LVN program will be asking these types of questions to prepare you for the licensure exam, but more specifically for clinical practice. Application and analysis questions require you to know the information and then apply it to a clinical scenario.

Test-taking skills are divided into three general areas: preparing for the test, taking the test, and reviewing/analyzing the test results.

PREPARING FOR THE TEST

- Preparation for test taking begins the first day of class by striving to understand information to do well on the test and meet lesson, course, and clinical outcomes.
- Clarify content to be covered on the test and the type of test—types of questions, number of questions, time allotted, computer or paper format. The test will be measuring your understanding of the lesson/unit/course outcomes.
- Clarify the types of questions that will be asked on the tests. For example, will the test be multiple choice, short answer, and/or NextGen (NGN)-type questions. Specific hints for taking multiple-choice, fill-in-the-blank, multiple-response, and prioritizing questions are included later in this chapter.
- To store information in your long-term memory, review class information often.
- In study groups, write practice questions you believe might be on the test and share them to formulate accurate answers. Discuss the rationale for (why) other answers are incorrect. Understanding why answers are wrong enhances deeper understanding of the subject matter.
- Cramming (last-minute studying of material for a test) sometimes results in short-term memory of material that might help you pass a test. However, because you did not engage in repetitions spaced over days, storage in long-term memory will not occur, and application of the material to the clinical area will be difficult. In addition, you may score poorly on the course final comprehensive exam, NCLEX-PN® preparation examinations, and ultimately the NCLEX-PN®.
- *Do not reread the textbook.* You completed your reading with understanding. Because you have studied the material periodically since the last test and used study skill techniques, all you need to do is focus on your highlights, margin writings/onscreen notes, and index cards to check your understanding and retention of the information. Only reread sections of the text where you need to enhance your understanding of the concept.
- The night before the test, go to bed at your usual time. Eat, hydrate well, and use relaxation techniques before the test.
- Be sure you have thoroughly completed assignments that will be reviewed by the instructor as a "ticket to test."

TAKING THE TEST

- Stay positive: Avoid discussions in the days prior that make you nervous by saying things like "You didn't study *that*, did you?" or "You mean you *didn't* study that?"

- Be sure to arrive at least 15 to 30 minutes early for the test, allowing time for minor delays.
- Carefully read and follow the school's testing policy. If you are taking a computerized test, be sure to have any necessary ID/log-in numbers, and make sure your personal computer battery is fully charged.
- If taking a test on a paper test form that will be machine corrected, be sure to complete accurately any information specific to the test, such as a test form (i.e., A or B).
- Keep a positive mental attitude. Visualize yourself being successful. Take slow, deep breaths to reduce tension.
- Avoid spending large amounts of time on difficult questions and avoid getting upset about them. Both of these activities waste time and do not earn points. Go on to the next question and return to the skipped item later (if allowed). However, be aware that on the NCLEX-PN®, you will not be able to skip items and then go back to them. For the NCLEX-PN®, you need to answer each item as it comes up on the test.
- Take the full time for the test. If you finish early, return to answer the questions you skipped. Review your answers.
- CAUTION: It is not encouraged to change your answers. Usually your first reaction in selecting an answer is correct. Retake the question without looking at your previous answer selected. Compare your answers if more than one answer was chosen and decide which is the best possible answer. If a math exam, recalculate questions that caused you difficulty. Compare your steps and confirm that your final answers are the same. Do not look at your previous answer or work until you have recalculated and arrived at a final answer.
- Make sure you have not missed an item or group of items.
- If is the exam is a paper multiple-choice with an answer sheet, make sure your answers match up with the proper slot on the answer sheet.
- If you are using a separate answer sheet that will be machine corrected, be sure you erase your first answer completely if you change answers.
- Should you change an answer? Although research has shown that test scores are generally improved by changing answers, generally we have seen learners decrease their test scores by the same action. If you have given the item further thought and feel it should be changed, change it. Test by test, keep tabs on your test scores to see whether changing answers is improving your final score; if not, then modify your behavior accordingly.

REVIEWING YOUR TESTS

Tests are a learning tool. When the examination is corrected and returned to you:

- Read the items you missed. Why are they wrong? Did you make a careless mistake? Did you know the material? Can you correct the item without looking in your textbook or notes? If not, look up the answer.
- Read the items you answered correctly. What did you do right to get credit for these items? Do you understand why the other answers were wrong, or did you "luck out"?
- Decide which of your study skills and test-taking techniques are and are not working to your benefit. Modify your test-taking strategies accordingly.
- After reviewing your tests, you may realize that you need to study more, study differently, and/or read the test questions more analytically to succeed.
- Discussing content you did not know immediately after a test can assist in providing a deeper understanding and increase long-term retention needed for the final exam, clinical practice, and NCLEX-PN® the Next Generation.

Some students who have organized their notes and their time, and who systematically reviewed and understood the material, have nevertheless done poorly on tests. A reason for this could be that they did not follow the directions on the test. How well do you follow directions? Take out a blank sheet of paper and do the How Well Do You Follow Directions exercise in the Try This box.

How did you do? If you did not follow the directions, do you feel tricked? You were not. The directions were clear, and you did not follow them. Listen meticulously to oral directions and read the written directions completely before each test. IF you did follow the directions, keep up the good work! If directions are ever unclear, ask the instructor before proceeding. Clarify the time limit of the examination. Now you are ready to begin. The hints in the following sections will come in handy for test taking.

Try This

How Well Do You Follow Directions?

Directions: Read the following directions carefully. You will have 1 minute to do the exercise after reading the directions. Be sure to write legibly. When you have finished, check your answers against the directions before handing in the paper. Be sure to read the entire exercise before beginning.

1. On a sheet of paper, print your name in the upper left-hand corner, last name first.
2. Under your name, write the last four digits of your social security number.
3. In the upper right-hand corner, write the name and number of the course for which you are taking this exercise.
4. In the lower left-hand corner of the paper, write today's date.
5. In the lower right-hand corner, write your instructor's name, last name first.
6. Fold your paper in half lengthwise.
7. Number the left half of your paper 1 to 6, skipping three lines between each number.
8. Number the right half of your paper 7 to 12, skipping three lines between each number.
9. Now that you have read all the steps in this exercise, do only number 1 of the exercise and hand your paper to the instructor.

REDUCING ANXIETY BEFORE TESTING

It may be presumed that if a person does not do well on tests, odds are that he or she is less intelligent than the average student, has poor study habits, has weak test-taking skills, or is distracted by personal issues. Less intelligence does not apply, or you would not have been admitted into the nursing program. Poor study habits do not apply if you established good study habits, organized your study time as suggested in this chapter, and made use of your personal learning preference to comprehend course content. If poor study habits are an issue, you would be aware of poor test grades and should seek help.

Normal anxiety is healthy and your friend. This type of anxiety actually makes you sharper and more alert during a test. Only when anxiety overwhelms you does it become your enemy. Accept the energy resulting from normal anxiety as supportive. Total personal comfort is not the key. Normal anxiety places you between too much relaxation and too much tension, perfect for testing.

Make the days before testing work for you through positive thinking. Reflect on your thoughts. Are you in the habit of seeing yourself failing or just squeaking by? Everyone daydreams and sets the stage for their reality. Daydreaming is a natural way to practice being confident and successful. Visualization may be helpful. For additional ways to relieve anxiety, see the suggestions in Chapter 1.

Spend the evening before the test studying as needed, but also focus on one activity that is normally relaxing/refreshing. Get a good night's sleep by going to bed at your usual time. It is believed that sleep restores memories that were lost during a hectic day. Going to bed extra early and not falling asleep may result in a new worry. Follow through with your usual morning habits.

Try This

Relax!

Make a *tentative* plan for what you will do the evening before any test examination.

HINTS FOR SPECIFIC QUESTIONS

The types of tests you will be taking in the practical/vocational nursing program, including the NCLEX-PN® examination after graduation, are achievement tests. They measure how much you have learned. Following are some of the types of questions found on the NCLEX-PN®. The same types of questions will be used during testing in the LPN/LVN program. In the NCLEX-PN® since 2023, newer types of question formats have been introduced; see Chapter 19.

Multiple-Choice Questions

- Multiple-choice questions are called items. Each multiple-choice question includes a stem, three **distracters**, and a correct answer, referred to as the **key**.
- The stem is the first line of a multiple-choice question.
- It defines the situation for which the learner must pick out the correct answer. The stem is presented as a statement or a question.
- Four statements, called **options**, follow the stem. Three of the options are incorrect answers and are called distracters. One of the options is the correct answer and is called the **key**.
- Distracters are presented to test whether you have learned the material and can apply it.
- The format of the NCLEX-PN® examination since 2023 has changed; however, it is primarily multiple-choice questions, which measure application or higher levels of nursing knowledge. Box 2.5 gives general hints for taking multiple-choice tests.

Try This

Multiple-Choice Questions

Choose the appropriate option (the key) for the following multiple-choice statements. There is only one answer to each multiple-choice statement.

1. What is a multiple-choice question?
   a. Sentences for which one-word answers are required
   b. Questions or sentences with four options for answers
   c. Two vertical columns that must be matched item by item
   d. Statements that require a sentence on the answer sheet
2. When answering multiple-choice questions, which is *not* appropriate?
   a. Read all of the directions.
   b. Eliminate wrong options.
   c. Read each of the options.
   d. Ignore any negative words.

Answers to Multiple-Choice Questions

1. b. A question or sentence is given with four options. Only one option, the key, is correct. The rest of the options are distracters; that is, options that are there to test whether you really have learned the material and can apply it. Option 1 describes fill-in-the-blank items, option 3 describes matching tests, and option 4 describes short-answer items.
2. d. This multiple-choice item contains a negative word in the stem that can complicate things. Read the stem without the negative word to get some meaning out of it, and then read the options. One option should not fit in with the others. Now reread the original stem with the negative word and see whether or not the option you have already isolated fits in. Items with negative words in the stem are sometimes accused of being more of a reading test than a test of understanding of content. Although the test begins with directions, there may be additional directions before individual multiple-choice questions. These directions may ask you to select one best answer or select what is most important of four correct answers. *Do not stop reading when you think you have the correct answer*. There may be a better option yet to come. Options a, b, and c are true.

Box 2.5 Multiple-Choice Test Hints

- Read over all the options given before making any decision.
- Eliminate the options you know are definitely wrong.
- Remember the course subject matter for which you are being tested.
- Eliminate options that are not related to the subject.

Multiple-choice questions are not "multiple-guess" questions. Think through each response thoroughly before choosing your answer. Should you ever guess? To be able to make a decision about guessing, you must know whether you will be penalized for wrong answers. Even if you are penalized, figure out the odds. If you can eliminate one distracter for certain, you have a better chance of answering correctly. Can you eliminate two out of four distracters? Your chances are now even better. You make the decision. Remember, on the NCLEX-PN® you will have to answer every item as it appears on the computer screen. There is no penalty for guessing on the NCLEX-PN®.

Fill-in-the-Blank

These questions require you to calculate an item, for example, a medication dosage or intake and output. You may be asked to round the answer to the nearest whole number or the nearest tenth. Be sure to read directions carefully and include the unit of measure (i.e., mL).

Try This

Fill-in-the-Blank Questions

The LPN/LVN needs to chart intake for a client. The client drinks 8 oz of coffee, a slice of toast, and 8 oz of water. Record the intake in milliliters. (Fill-in-the-blank questions will be used in your courses with a clinical component.)

Answer

Intake is 480 mL. Thirty mL equals 1 oz.

Alternate Format: Multiple-Response—Select All That Apply

A question is presented and you need to select all the answer choices (responses) that apply. This could include a single response, more than one response, or all of the responses provided as answer choices. There are at least 5 options but no more than 10 options. In your program there may or may not be partial credit if correct items are not selected. For example, if there are five correct options and you select only four, you do not receive credit. The NCLEX-PN® does give partial credit.

Try This

Multiple-Response Questions

1. Indicate the strategies to improve reading comprehension. *(Select all that apply.)*
   a. Read text word by word.
   b. Highlight key information.
   c. Read quickly to complete the assignment.
   d. Avoid writing in book margins.
   e. Draw pictures to explain concepts.

   Answer

   b, e

Visit www.ncsbn.org Frequently Asked Questions (FAQs) to view other Alternative Item Formats include 1.

- Case Studies with 12 item question types.
  a. Matrix multiple-choice
  b. Matrix multiple-response
  c. Multiple Response: Select all that apply
  d. Multiple Response: Select N
  e. Multiple Response: Grouping
  f. Drag-and drop: Cloze
  g. Drag and drop: Rationale
  h. Drop-down: Cloze
  i. Drag and drop: Rationale
  j. Drop-down: Table
  k. Highlight: Text
  l. Highlight: Table 2
- Stand Alone items with a Bow-tie item or a trend item.
- Hot Spot and Ordered Response questions.

All item types may include multimedia such as charts, tables, graphics, sound, and video. In addition, the NCSBN is conducting ongoing research to determine whether clinical judgment and decision-making can be assessed through the use of innovative item types. The project is called Next Generation NCLEX® (NGN) project, and it will be used to help nurses think critically when caring for their clients. Monitor the NCSBN website (www.ncsbn.org) for ongoing updates. Not all of these items may be on your NCLEX-PN®, but there may be as many as seven different alternative item formats. No specific percentage or ratio is stated, and they will appear throughout the exam.

YOUR SCHOOL'S LEARNING RESOURCE CENTER

Beyond the study skill methods reviewed so far, many other academic resources are available to assist you. Identifying and using these academic resources will increase your likelihood of success. These academic resources are a critical component of your personal plan for success. As we discussed in Chapter 1, prioritization is important in time management. How you prioritize your use of academic resources will be important to your ability to SUCCEED!

Keep in Mind

Knowing where and how to access nursing information makes keeping up to date for client care and passing the NCLEX-PN® less stressful. In addition, it will protect your nursing license.

If you are a returning adult student, you know the **LRC** as the library. Today, many students may never physically access the library, but instead use a virtual library. Whether you visit the library in person or virtually, you will find today's library consists of books and countless electronic evidence-based resources. These diverse resources can support various academic levels and types of learning preferences.

DIFFERENT STUDENT SKILL LEVELS AND DIFFERENT RESOURCES OF THE LEARNING RESOURCE CENTER

All LRCs have *similar* print and digital resources or access to these resources. However, not all LRCs are *equal* in technology. As a result, some small schools may use their affiliating clinical site libraries and electronic medical resources to supplement their school resources. Some schools may partner with local colleges or universities for resource access. The students' ability to use the LRC and related resources is very varied (Box 2.6). If you are skilled in this area, be aware that some of your peers may not be as skilled in using the LRC and its general resources and technology. Given differences in LRCs across schools and differences in the student's skill level, the discussion that follows focuses on what tasks are needed to obtain nursing information for class and clinical experiences (Box 2.7).

- Box 2.6 includes a checklist of tasks you need to carry out to fully use the general print and digital resources and technology of your LRC for your student enrollment year and as a graduate.
- Box 2.7 includes a checklist of tasks you need to carry out to fully use the nursing resources and technology of your LRC for your student year and as a graduate.

Despite prior LRC experience, you need to identify and correct any deficiencies in regard to using nursing resources and technology in your school and clinical site's LRC. Knowing how to carry through the tasks will save you energy, time, and frustration.

Box 2.6 Checklist of Tasks Needed to Fully Use Learning Resource Center General Resources and Technology

Read and reflect on the following questions/statements. If you can answer the question, write "Yes" next to the item; if not, write "No." If no, follow up at your LRC to obtain the answers.

- Does the LRC staff provide tours and/or orientation to services in person or online?
- Are library staff available to provide support by phone, e-mail, and/or real-time online?
- How does my LRC classify all of its print and digital holdings (books, videos, periodicals, CD-ROMs, DVDs, etc.)?
- How can I find the call number of a specific item?
- Once I have the call number, how can I locate a specific item?
- Where do I check out a specific item for home use?
- Can I access resources in my LRC from my home computer?
- How do I check out AV equipment for home use?
- How can I access needed resources that are not in my LRC?
- How can I access reference materials? (These would include an English dictionary, medical and nursing dictionaries, encyclopedias, almanacs, yearbooks, atlases, handbooks, and other similar categories of books.)
- Can I access learning resources in other schools' LRCs?
- Where is the circulation desk?
- Where are the copying machines? Do I need a code?
- Are there computers for personal use? Do they have Internet access?
- Where can I study in the LRC?
- How can I reserve a room for group study?
- Where are pamphlets located?
- Is there a Wi-Fi hotspot for a personal laptop, smartphone, iPod Touch, or iPad (or other tablet)?

Try This

Checklist: General and Nursing Resources and Technology

On index cards or an electronic device, list the general and nursing LRC tasks from Boxes 2.6 and 2.7 with which you are *not* familiar. Indicate on your personal timeline when you will accomplish these skills.

Box 2.7 Checklist of Tasks Needed to Fully Use Learning Resource Center Nursing Resources and Technology

Read and reflect on the following questions/statements. If you can answer the question, write "Yes" next to the item; if not, write "No." If no, follow up at your LRC to obtain the answers.

- How do I access current print and digital nursing journals and periodicals?
- How do I access back issues of print and digital nursing journals and periodicals?
- How can I obtain a copy of articles in back issues of nursing journals and periodicals?
- How can I obtain a print or digital copy of an article in a nursing journal or periodical if my LRC does not subscribe to the publication?
- Does my LRC have online databases for nursing and general information?
- Where are the nursing texts located in the stacks?
- What is the procedure for accessing nursing materials that have been put on reserve for nursing classes?
- Are mobile devices available for use in the clinical area? If so, what nursing information is available for use with these devices? Are there any free or low-cost apps recommended?
- Are handheld computers available for class/clinical use?
- Can I use a tablet to meet my computer needs at school?
- Are earphones supplied?

WHERE TO START

Investigate your LRC. You need to know the physical layout of the LRC and general hours of operation. Is a tour available in person or online? Touring the LRC can save you many wasted hours and much frustration later in the school year. Ask the librarian the best way for you to find the answers to items on your checklists with which you are unfamiliar. The LRC staff are available to answer questions. The LRC staff are experts in their field and can help you immensely.

General Information About Resources of the Library

Librarian. The librarian is a college-educated specialist who knows what the library has to offer in the area of information and where that information can be found. Look at the librarian as a professional educator about information for learning and as a person who is always ready to assist you. They are experts in identifying evidence-based resources.

Circulation desk. The circulation desk is the area where library materials that can be checked out are processed. If materials that can be checked out are reserved by your instructor, they will probably be found here. Today, students often access materials electronically.

Online catalog. You can obtain a lot of information about your LRC by yourself once you understand the cataloging system. Most LRCs' card catalogs are online (computerized) catalogs. All print and digital materials found in your LRC are indexed in this computerized system. In addition to books, cataloged materials also include audiovisual (AV) materials (audio recordings, videos, CD-ROMs, DVDs, etc.). You can search for desired materials by subject, title, or author. The LRC may also have access to free or purchased access to digital databases. If the LRC does not have the material you are searching for, but another LRC on the online system does, this information might also be included.

In many systems, students are able to access the **online catalog** and digital resources from home via computer, username, and password. This system of cataloging saves students valuable time and energy. Keep your username and password easily accessible to decrease frustration.

LOCATING IN-HOUSE RESOURCES

Libraries may choose to use either of the two systems to classify in-house materials so they are easy to locate: the Dewey Decimal system and the Library of Congress classification system. Regardless of the system your library uses, the **call number** shown on the author, title, or subject screens is the same number as that on the material itself. Copy, in order, all the letters and numbers in the call number.

The Stacks

Armed with the call number, you can proceed to the **stacks**, the place where the majority of materials that can be checked out are located. The books are placed in call number order according to academic disciplines. When you do find the material you are looking for, note that materials covering the same subject are shelved in the same area. You might find additional useful material on the same shelf.

Reference Materials

Reference materials include dictionaries and other similar categories of books, including medical and nursing dictionaries, almanacs, yearbooks, atlases, encyclopedias, and handbooks. Most of these resources can be found online. You will find up-to-date information on any subject. Print reference books generally do not circulate. Information from print reference materials may be copied on a copy machine if the book cannot be checked out. Online information can be printed. Be cautious to print only what is necessary. It is likely that you are allocated a certain number of copies per semester or program. Additional charges may apply after you exceed the semester or program allotment.

Interlibrary Loan Services

Interlibrary loan services allow your LRC to borrow materials you need that are not in your library's holdings. Print books and AV materials are available through this service. A link for a digital full-text version of an article may be provided. If your LRC does not have the periodical in which an article you need is located, or an electronic subscription to the source, a photocopy of the article or a link, free of charge, might be obtained from a library that does have some form of the periodical.

Professional Journals/Periodicals

LPN/LVN students need to be aware of sources that will provide up-to-date, relevant, and accurate information on nursing topics. Professional journals/periodicals consist of articles containing news or material of current interest to a particular discipline. These are important, timely resources for a learner in a field that is changing as quickly as nursing and health care. Because professional journals are published weekly, monthly, and quarterly (i.e., periodically), they are also called **periodicals**. Because of the frequent publication dates, they complement a comprehensive textbook that is published every several years.

Given the quantity of articles, the titles and authors of various articles cannot possibly be included in the online catalog of the LRC. Instead, articles can be located using bound books called print periodical indexes and/or digital databases. Today, the digital database is the common source and often can be accessed from home via the Internet. Once the article is located, it can be downloaded immediately to your computer or sent by e-mail via interlibrary loan.

A unique Digital Object Identifier (DOI) also exists today to assist in locating electronic documents. The DOI can identify a specific professional journal, article, or even a table within an article. The DOI is found in reference lists. You can click on the DOI and link directly to the journal/article (i.e., doi:10.1000/182), eliminating the need to use a digital database. This saves time! Professional journals of interest to LPN/LVN include, but are not limited to, *The Journal of Practical Nursing*, a research journal published by the National Association for Practical Nurse Education and Service, Inc.; *Nursing Made Incredibly Easy; Nursing2025* (the year in the title changes as the year changes); and *The American Journal of Nursing*.

Try This

Professional Journals

Identify the location of the aforementioned nursing journals in your LRC. Determine which of them will help you keep up to date in nursing. Identify the location of other nursing periodicals.

Digital Periodical Databases/Print Periodical Indexes

Entries in **digital periodical databases/print periodical indexes** are listed by author, title, and subject. Read/view the help sections to ease your use of these resources. The following are two digital periodical databases/print periodical indexes that are of special value to practical/vocational nursing students. Your instructor may suggest others.

1. *Cumulative Index to Nursing and Allied Health Literature* (CINAHL). This comprehensive and authoritative periodical index contains current listings for nursing and allied health fields and for others interested in health care issues, including biomedicine, consumer health, and alternative medicine. More than 5000 nursing, allied health, and related journals are reviewed and indexed. There are online tutorials to assist in understanding how to use the index. Fig. 2.4 illustrates the information found in a typical entry in the CINAHL print edition. Most schools have purchased access to online CINAHL databases or have access via a clinical site. CINAHL will be your primary source for current, accurate, and relevant articles used for evidence-based client care.
2. *ProQuest*. This digital database collection covers all disciplines, providing access to dissertations and theses; three centuries of newspapers; more than 450,000 academic e-books; and a diverse collection of important scholarly professional journals and other content.

1– Patient Safety **2–** What Frontline Nurses Need to Know
3– McKeon, L. and Cardell, B. **4–** (tables/charts)
5– Nursing Made Incredibly Easy **6–** Jan./ Feb. 2011
7– 9(1) **8–** 44-53 **9–** (11 ref)

Key: 1. Subject. 2. Title of the article. 3. Authors of the article. 4. Additional information found in article. 5. Periodical in which the article appears. If the periodical is abbreviated, the periodical index in the front of the book will have a list of periodical abbreviations and the full name of the journal for which those abbreviations stand. 6. Date of publication. 7. Volume and number of periodical. 8. Page numbers of article. 9. Number of references used.

Fig. 2.4 Cumulative index to nursing and allied health literature.

Your LRC will have a periodical listing that includes professional journals and magazines and the dates of the issues that are found in your library.

Remember, if the article you need is in a journal or magazine that is not held in your library in some form, see the librarian. The librarian can locate the article online in another library and arrange for you to receive a link or photocopy by interlibrary loan. Understanding how to use a digital database is a necessary skill.

Try This

Locate the following article using the digital database CINAHL search using the author and title of the article, then search using the DOI. Which was quicker?

Beroz S, Sullivan N, Kramasz V, Morgan P: The multiple-patient simulation toolkit: purpose, process, and pilot, *Nurs Educ Perspect* 39(3):180–181, 2018, doi: https://doi.org/10.1097/01.NEP.0000000000000236

Copyright laws prohibit the instructor from copying an article for each of you. For this reason, the required reading articles may be available on a reserve basis in the LRC by photocopy or digitally by a link within an LMS. Copyright laws generally allow you to have one copy of an article (i.e., photocopy, print the reserve article, or download the article from the LMS). Because of copyright laws, use caution in redistributing the article electronically. This action may be prohibited.

Magazines and Newspapers

Include newspapers and popular magazines as sources of information on health-related topics. Magazine articles never replace professional journal reading, but they do provide information that your clients read. As one practical nursing student said, "I had better be up to date and understand what my clients are reading." Be aware of the author's expertise. Examine the author's demographic information and any funding received. This will help you identify possible author bias and evaluate the accuracy of the information on the topic.

RESPONSIBLE USE OF LEARNING STRATEGIES

Face-to-Face Class

Lectures/mini-lectures. Some of your teachers may have been taught using the "bucket theory" of education. The **bucket theory** suggests that merely by lecturing, a teacher can transfer knowledge from the teacher's mind to the mind of the student. This teaching method evolved from Aristotle's day. The teacher was considered the source and the vehicle of transmission of information, similar to a sage on the stage. Of course, the printing press, computers, and the Internet had yet to be invented!

Research has shown that students learn best from methods other than traditional lectures. Although traditional lecturing is an outmoded form of instruction, *brief lectures* (mini-lectures) can be valuable as a means of enhancing your assigned readings and clarifying information. A mini-lecture situation is a brief episode, taking only a portion of class time. Mini-lectures are intended to enhance your reading assignment, not replace it. A mini-lecture reflects the fact that the teacher spent time searching, reading, selecting, and organizing information for your benefit. The instructor has done all the work and has become smarter in the process. However, mini-lectures are passive learning experiences that do not actively involve you in the learning process. You need to remain especially alert and actively involved. The instructor may introduce various techniques (e.g., clickers) to keep you actively involved during mini-lectures as well as class in general.

Lecture-discussion. In the **lecture-discussion strategy**, the instructor shares several ideas with the class and then stops to let the class discuss the ideas. Sometimes the instructor may say that the next class will be nothing but discussion of the assignment. The instructor then acts as a discussion leader, or ideally a student may lead the discussion. An example of a learning strategy to help keep the discussion focused on course outcomes includes the following:

- Box 2.8: an example of a learning strategy used in mini-lectures called **discussion buddy**
- Box 2.9: hints for participating in discussions and related activities

Cooperative learning. Cooperative learning is a technique that emphasizes individual accountability for learning a specific academic task while working in small groups. The teacher is a facilitator. Cooperative learning encourages you to:

- be actively involved in your learning
- develop critical-thinking skills
- develop positive relationships with your peers
- develop the ability to work in a team situation, a skill an employer is looking for in an employee.

What goes on in the classroom is just as important as what goes on in a reading assignment. There is, however, one great difference between the two: *You can repeat a reading assignment, but you can never repeat a missed face-to-face or synchronous online class.* Here are some hints to help you learn from any face-to-face *or synchronous online* class situation:

- Before recording a class activity, clarify if this is allowed.
- Never skip a face-to-face *or synchronous online* class unless an emergency arises. Some students skip class to get another hour's sleep, use the time to prepare for another class or an examination, or get in their allowable number of absences. When an emergency does make it necessary for you to miss class, ask a peer to review his or her notes with you and tell you about the class. Recall what you learned about personal learning preferences. Contact the instructor to ask for suggestions on getting caught up with the class material; however, your syllabus will also inform you on the topics covered.
- Come to class prepared. Review the syllabus, complete the read assignment, and know key terms and concepts. You will be ready to participate in learning activities.
- Keep vigilant and listen for verbal and nonverbal cues to inform you of key points during mini-lectures (Box 2.10). Examples are raising the hands; a long, dramatic pause; raising or lowering the voice; and leaning toward the class or into the computer screen with a comment such as "this is important to know." Copy key points or instructions written on the whiteboard/smartboard. If review materials are provided, focus on these.

Box 2.9 Hints for a Discussion Class

- Be prepared to participate in the discussion by completing your assignment before class. This will allow you to be an active participant.
- Be sure you have made a list of questions about the assignment. Discussions are the perfect time to clear up questions.
- While other learners are speaking, listen to what they have to say. Some learners make the mistake of using other learners' speaking time to formulate their own comments.
- You may disagree with others during a discussion. Do so assertively and firmly. Provide evidence. Avoid yelling matches. It enriches your world to listen to another's point of view before responding.

Box 2.8 Learning Strategy: Discussion Buddy

- You may be assigned to a discussion buddy before class.
- The two of you will be given a discussion task.
- Focus carefully on the mini-lecture and other resources on the Course Management System so you will be able to formulate an answer to the discussion task.
- After the mini-lecture, discussion buddies share their answers with one another. A new answer is formulated from both your responses.
- The instructor will choose students at random to share their newly composed answers with the class.

Box 2.10 Verbal Cues for Key Ideas in Mini-lectures, Discussions, and Online Activities

"The most important difference is."
"The major principle in this situation is."
"To sum up."
"The main point is."
"Finally,."
"In conclusion,."
"Moreover,."
"To repeat."

- The instructor speaks at a much slower rate than you are capable of thinking. The fact that you can think faster than the instructor can speak allows you to relate this new information to information you have learned in the past and to formulate questions that need clarification or for content you do not understand. Ask these questions in class and/or write down your questions during lecture to discuss with the instructor after class. It is *your* responsibility to question what you do not understand.
- Review your notes as soon after class as possible. Some students find that rewriting and organizing notes helps reinforce learning. Either way, this will support the information being stored into long-term memory.
- Stay actively engaged in class. Avoid using class time to work on other projects, such as care plans or upcoming presentations. Be an active listener.

Distance learning. Some of the courses in your LPN/LVN program or parts of courses may be available through **distance learning** or online learning. In this learning strategy, the student and teacher are separated by physical distance. The course may be synchronous (real time) or asynchronous (accessed at different times). In a *synchronous* class, all of the students in the course and the instructor participate simultaneously by means of interactive website. This is similar to a face-to-face class. However, most common is an asynchronous format in which the students choose when they will attend class. In an *asynchronous* format, it is critical to adhere to due dates for posts and online discussions. A **blended course** (hybrid course) combines face-to-face instruction with online learning and is more common in an LPN/LVN program.

Have the equipment or access to equipment needed to complete course assignments. You are in charge of your schedule. As with any class, self-discipline and motivation are important tools for success. It is important to establish a weekly class and clinical schedule. The nature of the course requires you to have access to social media (i.e., LMS, e-mail, e-book, Google account, and/or X). Check these sites daily for messages from instructors and fellow students.

Study skills are a must. Distance-learning/online learning courses require much reading and self-discipline. The ability to understand information by means of the written word is important. Individual learning preferences can impact your perception of distance learning.

Distance learning/online learning has proven to be at least as effective as traditional methods of instruction. Positive features include the fact that students become more active in personal learning and have more involvement in and control over the learning process. Some students report feeling less of a social connection. It is possible to plan a meeting with peers on campus to fulfill this need.

TECHNOLOGY USE DURING LEARNING ACTIVITIES

Class time requires active listening and participation in learning activities. Avoid using class time for snoozing, talking to friends, or any of the activities listed in Box 2.11. Your time in the LPN/LVN program gives you the opportunity to sharpen (bring to an excellent level) professional behavior that is appropriate for your future profession as a LPN/LVN.

OTHER LEARNING RESOURCES

SYLLABUS AND COURSE OUTLINES

A **syllabus** is an up-to-date course document available by handout or online as part of an **LMS** at the beginning of a course. At a minimum, the syllabus includes a course description, course objectives/learning outcomes (this text will use the term outcomes instead of objectives; however, they are considered the same thing, just a different term), course requirements for a passing grade, required textbooks/resources, grading scale, instructor information (office location, instructor contact information, office hours, response times for e-mails, etc.), course policies, and testing policies. A course outline may refer to policies in a student handbook. Be sure to review this material.

Your school may have **course outlines** for each course. These outlines are a great help to an adult learner. They contain unit-by-unit course objectives/student learning

Box 2.11 Technology Courtesy for Learning Activities

- Check school policy for the use of cell phones, smartphones, iPod Touch, iPad, laptops, and so on.
- If cell phones are allowed, turn off the ringer and put it on vibrate.
- If it is necessary to return a call, leave the immediate area, quietly make your call, and quickly complete it.
- Avoid e-mailing, texting, tweeting, instant messaging, taking photos, recording, and playing games during class activities.
- Avoid surfing the Internet during class activities.
- Avoid listening to music on your iPod during class activities.
- Record classroom lecture, activities, discussions ONLY if you have the permission of the instructor and anyone in the classroom.

outcomes and content areas, which indicate what the learner must know to pass the course. Each student learning outcome begins with a verb. Watch the verb carefully because it tells you the level of understanding you must achieve to meet the objective. If an objective states you must *list* something, that task is quite different from having to *compare* and *contrast* the same information. Instructors develop their test questions from the course content and outcomes. The course outline will include a list of resources indicating where the information to answer the outcomes is found. Supplementary material in the form of worksheets, charts, activities, and additional reading may be included to support your learning. An LMS contains complete online course content and includes, for example, a syllabus, library links, learning modules, a calendar for quizzes, tests, and assignments, chat rooms, and other features. If the amount of material is overwhelming, schedule a meeting with your instructor to prioritize the resource materials. This task could be dependent on your learning preference. A tutor can also assist you.

STUDY GROUPS

Do you have a desire to achieve better grades? Do you need to study more effectively? Do you need a little support? Joining a **study group** is a great strategy! Students usually form their own study groups out of need. Studies have shown that despite each person's learning preference, *actively* participating in a study group can improve academic performance. *Actively* participating is the key! Sometimes students join a study group thinking that the group will help them pass the course, and they avoid active participation. Study groups work when students use them to become actively involved in their own learning. The group provides an outlet for discussion of material, which promotes retention. A diverse study group is generally most effective, as each person's unique background stimulates the discussion and every member participates. Active study group members usually develop questioning and reasoning skills on a higher level.

TUTORING

Tutoring is a very select study group. Tutoring can be provided one on one or in small groups. For best results, the student arranges tutoring through a special department by means of instructor referral or self-referral. This referral can be electronic. The purpose of tutoring is to help a student understand the material better and pass the course. You must actively identify your learning needs. Specifically defining the content you do not understand will maximize your tutoring experience. Students who need tutoring *sometimes* have learning disabilities. In these situations, because of an excellent attitude on the part of these students and their active participation in the tutoring process, tutoring can be very beneficial.

NURSING SKILLS/SIMULATION LAB

The **nursing skills/simulation lab** is a resource that will allow you to practice and develop your hands-on nursing skills and clinical decision-making skills. This lab contains the physical items needed to make the practice area as similar to the workplace as possible. *Skills must be practiced.* In addition, the rationale for skills must also be verbalized. Reading about skills, watching a video or YouTube clip, and watching other students practice are only the first steps in developing a physical skill. **Practice until you are proficient in each skill so you feel competent performing these tasks in the clinical area**. Remember that you recall approximately 10% of what you hear, 20% of what you see, 50% of what you read, and 90% of what you do. Ben Franklin summarizes how SPN/SVNs need to approach the skills component of their nursing program: "Tell me and I forget, teach me and I may remember, involve me and I learn."

You may be required to make appointments to give a return demonstration of skills. Practice with a peer before this return demonstration. When you make an appointment with the skills lab, you are entering into an agreement with the lab personnel. Your responsibility is to practice the skill until you can perform it in the time frame of your appointment. If you are unable to keep your appointment, inform the lab personnel. This will allow them to schedule other students into lab time for skills testing.

Simulation is a learning activity that uses imaginary client situations that mimic the reality of the clinical environment. The learner has the opportunity to think like a nurse and gather data; set priorities; and plan, implement, and evaluate care in a virtual (reproduced/replicated by a computer) client situation without risk to the client. Simulation encourages decision-making and critical thinking. Working as a team is often integrated into a simulation. It is ideal if students from different health programs can work collaboratively during a simulation. Simulations foster the development of critical thinking and clinical judgment.

Simulation can take many forms:

- **Case scenarios** can be delivered in a printed format or by computer. In each type, an imaginary client story will bring reality to theory in the form of a clinical situation. Both forms may be used when the client census is inadequate for client assignments, when a desired client situation is unavailable, or when enhanced learning of specific concepts is desirable. **Computer simulation** can be a learning situation from a computer or be web-based learning. The computer-patient simulation changes, as it would in the clinical area. This requires the student to evaluate the situation and plan new assessments (data collection) and interventions.
- **Static simulation** uses mannequins that are full-size body models or models of specific parts of the body made to be realistic. These mannequins are used

for practicing skills before reaching the clinical area and returning demonstrations of procedures, for example, urinary catheterization, insertion of intravenous lines, and application of colostomy bags. Moulage makeup can enhance the "real" look of the simulated medical emergency (i.e., blood, bruising).

- **Electronic simulation** uses mannequins that are high-tech, more costly simulation models that can be programmed to set up different client situations and allow practice of nursing procedures and data collection (assessment). For example, Simchart, modeled on an actual electronic health record (EHR) used in a health care institution, can be used with a client simulation.
- **Virtual clinical excursions** are computer programs that electronically (controlled by a computer) provide a virtual hospital floor and clients whose conditions are constantly changing. This allows the student to practice in a safe environment. The data available mimic the data accessed if in a real clinical setting, thereby facilitating clinical decision-making as appropriate for the LPN/LVN role.

STUDY SKILLS LAB

If your school has a **study skills lab**, it is available to help you with academic problem areas. Examples of areas in which help is available are study skills, time management, reading (including vocabulary and comprehension), listening skills, math skills, test-taking skills (especially situation tests), note making, writing, and any other academic problem you may have. You can go to the skills lab on your own or by referral from your instructor or counselor.

? Critical Thinking

No Time for Tutoring or the Skills Center

Some students who need tutoring or the study skills center state they do not have time to go for help. Be sure to create a plan that allows some accessibility during available tutor hours. At some time in the program, most students need to access the tutoring or the study skills center.

AUDIOVISUAL MATERIALS

In addition to mini-lectures, discussions/activities, textbooks, and articles, the instructor may have included videos, CDs, DVDs, PowerPoint (or other types of) presentations, **podcasts**, and other electronic resources as part of your assignment. AV materials are not considered extra or additional assignments. They are a significant part of all areas of learning. These learning resources give faith to the saying: "A picture is worth a thousand words." AV materials provide an additional sensory channel for learning, compared with reading. In some nursing courses, especially autotutorial skills courses, the AV medium is the course. The student progresses independently, attending periodic lecture-discussion classes and seeking out the instructor when questions arise. Approach the AV material as you do a class. Realize that you have the option of repeating all or part of the material when you do not understand it.

INTERNET

The Internet offers unlimited resources on many subjects. The Internet is the physical infrastructure that allows the electronic circulation of billions of sites of information to Internet-ready computer users. An Internet provider charges a monthly fee and is a computer user's link to the Internet. Provider services can be dedicated service lines (DSL) or broadband (high-speed Internet), meaning that you have instant access when your computer is turned on. Broadband service is critical to effectively retrieve information from the Internet in a timely manner. In addition to computers, many types of electronic devices exist today to support students (i.e., iPads, tablets, smartphones).

The World Wide Web (www) is the most effective means of providing access to the vast amount of information available on the Internet. Everything on the Internet has an address (called a URL) that helps in locating a specific site. Most addresses begin with www, followed by a dot. The next letters in the address are specific to the site you wish to access; for example, www.ncsbn indicates the site that provides information about the National Council of State Boards of Nursing (NCSBN). This is followed by three letters, called a domain name, which denote the site's source. For example, the complete address for the site for information about NCSBN is www.ncsbn.org. The following are common domain names and their meanings:

- com: for-profit sites
- gov: government sites
- edu: colleges and universities that grant 4-year degrees
- org: usually reserved for nonprofit organizations
- net: network organizations
- mil: military

Search engines are programs that can help students zero in on the exact information for which they are searching. Search engines periodically scan the web and index it. Therefore search engines are like the telephone book. Popular search engines include Google, Bing, Yahoo, Firefox, Ask, and AOL. There are more suggestions of Internet sites that can be used as learning resources and for client teaching resources on Evolve (Elsevier's online resources).

It is critical for the LPN/LVN to develop information literacy in finding health information for your clients and yourself. Although the Internet provides the means of obtaining that information, it is up to you to evaluate if that information is recent, accurate, reliable, and relevant. The HON code is a private and independent certification that helps identify reliable and trustworthy health information on the Internet. Wikipedia, known as a free online encyclopedia, is an example of a source that nursing students should *not* use to obtain evidence-based information for class or clinical. Wikipedia is written by volunteers, and the articles can be edited by anyone with site access. The quality, accuracy, and appropriateness of Wikipedia articles are not checked by scholars in the related field of study (**peer reviewed**).

Box 2.12 contains guidelines for gathering Internet information for your use or to share with clients. Let the user beware: Students can spend a lot of time on the Internet. To save time, take a few minutes to read the section that gives hints for using a specific site. Stay focused on your purpose. Avoid getting sidetracked.

Box 2.12 Guidelines for Gathering Internet Information

- The Internet is not regulated in any way. Anyone can publish anything they want on the Internet. When searching the Internet, you can find the most recent and accurate information, as well as the most inaccurate and out-of-date information.
- Let the user beware: People can spend a lot of time on the Internet. To save time, take a few minutes to read the section that gives hints for using a specific site. Stay focused on your purpose. Avoid getting sidetracked.
- Check the professional credentials and qualifications of the author of the information.
- Determine the organization, group, agency, and company that created the site. This will help you evaluate the credibility of the information. The domain name is helpful in evaluating credibility. For example, a site that has a ".gov" domain name may be more credible than a ".com" site that may be promoting a product.
- Check the date the information was created and last modified. This will ensure up-to-date material.
- What are the objectives of the author of the material? Does the author express opinions? Does the author have a personal bias?
- Seek the assistance of the librarian to effectively search key words.
- When conducting searches, supply key words to help the search tool narrow the document results to just the ones you want to see.
- When using key words for a search engine, use phrases or single words that are pertinent to your topic and describe it objectively.
- Use nouns only, and put the most important words that describe your topic first.
- When searching with a phrase (e.g., "study skills"), surround the phrase with quotation marks. This forces the database to search for words that are next to each other.
- Plus signs (+) or the word "AND" identify words that must appear in the search (e.g., nursing + practical).
- Minus signs (–) or the word "NOT" excludes words from the search (e.g., NCLEX-PN®, NOT NCLEX-RN®).

Try This

Peer Assistance With Computer/Internet

If you do not have computer/Internet experience, ask students in your class who are familiar with using computers for hints on using this technology and information resource. Consider taking a short instructional course offered by your school or local library. In addition, you can ask the Internet a question when you are unsure of how to do or find something. Many refer to this action as "Googling it."

MOBILE DEVICES

Because of Wi-Fi, your educational institution and/or clinical site may provide wireless access to the Internet. **Mobile devices** with **Internet** capabilities are useful for obtaining information for class and the clinical area. Before utilizing the following information, clarify the policy of your school and clinical area for using computers and mobile devices while on the clinical area.

- **You must separate your private and professional uses of mobile devices.** If your device is capable of taking photos or videos, do not use these functions with clients. Health Insurance Portability and Accountability Act (HIPAA) requirements (see Chapter 7) prohibit the use of **electronic devices** for these purposes. If you are a student, you could be suspended or dismissed from the program. If you are licensed, you could receive a sanction regarding your license if you take photos or videos of clients in the clinical area.
- Nursing-based software that contains drug information, laboratory values, disease processes, and a medical dictionary is available as a subscription to be downloaded on your mobile device.
- Reference e-books for downloading on your mobile device can be purchased.
- **Apps** can provide instant clinical reference materials at the point of care for medications, lab studies, and medical/surgical conditions. Some apps are free, but others charge a fee. Check the app store of your device.
- Check the appropriateness of selected software/apps with your instructor.
- Sites that provide information for mobile devices can be found on Evolve.
- Use of **artificial intelligence or AI** is a new dimension of the internet and can be accessed by going to various websites such as ChatGPT, Claude AI, Microsoft Copilot. The 11 Best Free ChatGPT Alternatives in 2025 – AI Tools Like ChatGPT https://docsbot.ai/article/the-11-best-free-chatgpt-alternatives). Use of this resource should be used with caution. It is always best to check with your instructor and school policy before using for studying or assignment completion.

COMPUTER-AIDED INSTRUCTION

Computer-aided instruction (CAI) has the following benefits:

- Allows learners to be actively involved in their learning.
- Encourages problem solving, a skill that employers expect of LPN/LVN.
- Provides immediate feedback by quickly evaluating answers and decision-making strategies.
- Provides an opportunity to develop the ability to follow directions.

CAI simplifies concepts and reinforces skills that have been presented previously. If you do not have computer skills, and CAI is used in your practical/vocational nursing program, you will be taught the skills necessary to use this type of teaching strategy. The process is simple even if you do not have any computer experience. The computer is essential in the clinical area to store and retrieve client information via the electronic medical record (EMR).

GUEST SPEAKERS

Nurses and other health professionals are sometimes invited to visit nursing classes as **guest speakers** or to make presentations via distance modalities (i.e., Skype, FaceTime, AdobeConnect, GotoMeeting, Podcast, Zoom). These speakers donate their time to present current information on their areas of expertise and updates on specific nursing topics. Often their employers have released them to visit nursing classes.

Get Ready for the Next-Generation NCLEX® Examination

Key Points

- Brain dominance impacts thinking preference, which in turn impacts the way you learn.
- Each side of the brain processes things differently. It is accepted that the left hemisphere is more verbal and processes in parts and sequences. The right hemisphere is nonverbal and sees a total picture. A connection between the right brain and music has been established.
- The two most common thinking preferences are linear (left brain dominant) and global (right brain dominant).
- Some people think in pictures (visual learners). Some hear sounds (auditory learners). Some experience a feeling in regard to what they are thinking about and learn best by doing (kinesthetic/tactile learners). Each learning preference can be enhanced, and it is possible to use more than one learning preference to reinforce learning.
- Multiple intelligences translate into learning preferences. Identifying whether you are a linguistic learner (likes words and new vocabulary), a logical learner (organized and consistent), a spatial learner (prefers boxes and diagrams to words), a musical learner (likes to hum, sing, or play a musical instrument), a bodily/kinesthetic learner (likes touching and moving), an interpersonal learner (likes sharing, comparing, and cooperating), or an intrapersonal learner (likes working alone, self-paced instruction) further enhances your learning ability.
- Your personal attitude toward learning also influences the learning process. Attitude is closely related to whether you are a reactive learner who expects to be taught or an active learner who takes charge of his or her own education.
- Clustering, a form of mapping, is a method of notemaking. Concept mapping is a common strategy in nursing education programs.
- Visual strategies such as drawing idea sketches, using color in whatever form of note-making works for you, maximizing font characteristics when using a computer for note-taking, diagramming information so it makes sense to you, and using mental imagery are all additional ways of study to assist in developing long-term memory of what you are studying.
- Most people in the United States can recognize words and read with fluency and accuracy. Because of being able to read with fluency and accuracy, there is an assumption that the person understands what they are reading. Studies show that many people in the United States have not progressed past the fourth-grade level in reading. In fact, newspapers and magazines are generally written at the fourth- to sixth-grade level.
- ADHD does not affect intelligence. There are numerous effective techniques to help the person diagnosed with ADHD succeed in school.
- Learning how to learn is important because study skills enable the SPN/SVN to understand (comprehend) and store in long-term memory the theory and skills required to be an LPN/LVN.
- When theory and skills are stored in long-term memory, they can be retrieved or recalled as the basis for critical thinking.
- Perhaps your most important skill for success in the LPN/LVN program is your reading/comprehension skill.
- There is no fast and easy way to learn information.
- Techniques that have been proven effective in increasing your level of concentration are creating personal study areas, evaluating the influence of peers, and decreasing daydreaming.
- Improving your listening/viewing skills requires you to be an active, rather than a passive, listener/viewer.
- Effective note-*making* may enhance your ability to understand information.
- The LRC is your most valuable resource for learning as a student and for keeping up to date as a graduate.
- In addition to textbooks, mini-lectures, lecture-discussions, and cooperative learning are specific course-learning strategies that are used by the SPN/SVN.
- Methods of delivering instruction, such as distance or online learning, can make learning more student oriented.
- Additional learning resources include articles from periodicals, the syllabus, course outlines, LMS, study groups, tutoring, AV materials, the Internet, CAI, web-based classes, and simulation.
- Staying current in practical/vocational nursing is made possible by using print or digital periodical indexes,

databases, the Internet, skills labs, nursing organizations, community resources, and guest speakers.
- It is necessary for SPN/SVN to distinguish between personal and professional use of social media.
- After learning the information you need to be an LPN/LVN, you must demonstrate that learning has taken place by your performance in the clinical area and on tests.
- Determining your learning preference and aligning key learning strategies and academic resources found in this chapter will help you obtain the information you need to SUCCEED in a practical/vocational nursing program and, ultimately, be a successful LPN/LVN.

Additional Learning Resources

Go to your Evolve website (http://evolve.elsevier.com/Carroll/success/) for the following FREE learning resources:

- Answers to Critical Thinking Scenarios
- Additional learning activities
- Additional Review Questions for the NCLEX-PN® examination
- Helpful phrases for communicating in Spanish and more!

Clinical Judgment and Next-Generation NCLEX® Examination-Style Questions

1. A student is enrolled in a practical/vocational nursing program. Which statement best describes how a *kinesthetic* student learner will prefer to learn a lab skill?

a. Watch a demonstration video and then practice the lab skill.
b. Listen to a demonstration podcast and then practice the lab skill.
c. Draw a visual image of the lab skill and then practice the lab skill.
d. Watch a demonstration interactive video while practicing the skill simultaneously.

2. A student is enrolled in a practical/vocational nursing program. Which statement best describes a student who primarily uses the left side of their brain?

a. When learning a new procedure, you pay more attention to what the total information is rather than focusing on the steps.
b. You break down information into smaller units and work to understand each step before proceeding to the next step.
c. You have a tendency to give up on reading because it feels like too much of an overload.
d. You would rather participate in a group demonstration to learn a concept.

3. Your instructor is involving all of the students in the teaching/learning process. You will work in groups of four, representative of each major learning preference. Which type of learning preference would align with the task of developing a concept map related to the information being studied?

a. A visual learner
b. An auditory learner
c. A tactual learner
d. A logical/mathematical learner

4. Which of the following student's statements indicate an effective reading/study method?

a. "When I read an unfamiliar word, I highlight it and look up the definition as soon as possible."
b. "I read each and every word separately so I am sure to understand the content."
c. "I realized the best student in the class tapes all classes and listens to them repeatedly. I am going to do the same thing to improve my grades."
d. "Time management is important to me. I skip the tables and boxes in the textbook so I can read more pages of the chapter."

5. A nursing instructor suggests that an SPN/SVN receive help with study skills at the school's Skills Center. Which student response *most* accurately indicates that the student understands the purpose of the Skills Center?

a. "I cannot afford the fee to attend study programs in the Skills Center at my school."
b. "In high school, only students with learning disabilities attended the Skills Center."
c. "It will take too much time out of my limited study time to go for help with studying."
d. "Even a few visits to the Skills Center can help me get more out of my study sessions."

6. Classes in an LPN/LVN program may be conducted in a lecture-discussion format. Which student behavior is most effective for this learning strategy?

a. When time is needed to study for a test in a different class, arrange for a peer to take notes for you in your absence.
b. Complete all assignments before going to class and prepare questions you have about parts of readings that are unclear.
c. If you disagree with a student during a class discussion, interrupt the student and clarify the information, preventing other students from becoming confused.
d. While the instructor is answering a student's question, review the notes and document any questions you need answered.

7. Understanding information that is read in the LPN/LVN program is necessary to save that information in long-term memory so it can be retrieved when needed for critical thinking. Which of the following students are using strategies that help in accomplishing this task? *(Select all that apply.)*

a. A student who previews a reading assignment and formulates questions from chapter titles that they answer while reading the assignment
b. A student who is having difficulty understanding a concept and creates a story in their own words while visualizing the story
c. A student who repeats what she reads in her own words after completing the assignment and again several times after the initial reading
d. A student who takes a verbal concept that he is having difficulty understanding and, without using words, draws a picture to explain the concept
e. A student who teaches a difficult concept to her significant other, assessing his understanding and answering his questions about the concept

8. Students are attending a medical/surgical class. Which of the following describes students who are demonstrating active listening behavior? *(Select all that apply.)*

a. A student who listens with full attention to whoever is speaking
b. A student who questions the content of the discussion
c. A student who thinks about the speaker's hairstyle
d. A student who tries to relate this discussion to her last clinical assignment with their peer during class
e. A student who is working on the related care plan that is due later in the day

9. A variety of learning resources and strategies are used in an LPN/LVN program. Which of the following students are using these resources and strategies to their advantage? *(Select all that apply.)*

a. A student who joined a study group that meets every day after school to review and discuss class notes
b. A student who frequently skips lectures to study for a test in another class and finish care plans to submit by deadline
c. A student who borrows notes from friends who reviewed AV materials instead of watching them
d. A student who signed up for a distance learning class to save more study time
e. A student whose primary preparation for scheduled tests includes completing 50 NCLEX style questions

Anya has just completed the fourth week of the practical/vocational nursing program. Frustrated with low grades, the following information is shared:

10. Carefully examined how a few successful students/graduates studied
11. Implemented similar strategies
12. Has been recopying class notes nightly
13. Is using flash cards to study
14. Discovered that recopying notes word for word is time consuming and not helpful to understand and recall the information

You determine that Anya is an *auditory learner*. Provide some advice to assist Anya.

Anya should consider which of the following alternative methods of studying, based on learning style will better support retention of information? Select all that apply.

15. re-read and highlight key points in the class notes
16. have someone read the material out loud
17. read aloud to self, concentrating on the words
18. make up "silly" rhymes or songs (mnemonic clues)
19. listen to the words of the instructor instead of taking notes (obtain permission of the instructor and students to record the instructor)
20. use background music when studying
21. change study positions frequently
22. take notes in class and color code
23. look for reference books that contain pictures or draw on your own

Critical Thinking Scenarios

Scenario 1

A new student who has been diagnosed with ADHD insists on being in the back of the classroom and walks around during class. Today's discussion is about different learning preferences and how to identify personal preference(s). When the instructor talks about undependable memory and learning preferences, the new student listens and realizes that parts of discussion describe the student's behaviors, including impulsive behaviors. The student reflects on many discussions with parents about jumping into things without first thinking it through. The new student is doubting the decision to enroll in this nursing program. How would you suggest the new student get started and get support?

Scenario 2

While on a class break, a peer nursing student states that time management skills are improving. However, the student can't make sense of class notes, earned a C in the first Fundamentals quiz, and flunked the second quiz. What advice can you give the peer student regarding study habits and reading assignments?

Scenario 3

Your classmate is present daily for class and shares that grades have shown slow but steady improvement. While changing classes, your classmate tells you there is no time to go to the LRC because of child care responsibilities. Give your classmate some suggestions for using the LRC.

3 Community Resources

Objectives

On completing this chapter, you will be able to do the following:

1. Discuss community resources that can contribute to your success in the practical nursing program.
2. Identify financial aid resources, nursing organizations, and online resources that will support your success as a student practical/vocational nurse (SPN/SVN).

Key Terms

community resources
Maslow's human needs theory
nursing organizations
social media
social networking

> **Keep in Mind**
>
> It is essential to meet your and your immediate family's basic needs, such as food, shelter, and safety, to achieve success in a practical/vocational nursing (LPN/LVN) program.

Trinh and Darius are sitting waiting for the bus after school. Trinh shares, "My mom was laid off from work. With three younger siblings living at home, I increased my work hours to 32 hours per week to help out. My grades are slipping and I overheard my mom telling her friend about her fear of the cold weather and inability to pay the oil bill. Maybe I should withdraw from school and help her out. I am not sure I can work many more hours and still be able to pass the course. My mom has always had a job. We really don't know what to do." Darius listens and responds, "I have been in tough spots with my family over the last several years. There are great community resources available. Mrs. Jones in the practical nursing program office can help you and your mom find resources. This is my second time enrolled; last time I did just as you described—increased my hours and ended up failing. It was not the right decision. I waited too long to ask for help—my ego would not let me. This time round, I am reaching out early if anything happens. I suggest you do the same. Let me know if I can help."

As you read this chapter, think of the resources that can assist Trinh in this scenario. Do you need similar resources or maybe different options? Diverse community resources can support you in achieving your goals. Keeping an open mind and seeking resources early can make a difference in completing the LPN/LVN Program.

Feeling true hunger, lacking sleep, feeling unsafe, or sensing a lack of belonging can impact your ability to learn. A famous psychology theorist, Abraham Maslow, in the late 1940s identified a hierarchy of needs common to all people. (See Chapter 13 for more details.) **Maslow's human needs theory** is portrayed as a five-step pyramid. The steps include physiological needs, safety, love/belonging, esteem, and self-actualization. Starting at the pyramid base, the first step, basic physiological needs (i.e., air, water, food, clothing, and shelter), is essential for human survival. As the needs are met in the lower level, the person focuses on the next higher level of needs, which is safety. The person can then proceed to focus on love and belonging, self-esteem (i.e., respect), and finally self-actualization.

To maximize your success in a LPN/LVN program, it is important to feel respected and have self-confidence. These attributes are represented in the pyramid as self-esteem. Difficulty meeting your physiological or safety needs can impact your ability to feel respected, be confident, and learn effectively. Being aware of these personal needs and finding resources as soon as possible to meet these needs will be key in keeping you focused on learning.

This chapter will to provide examples of possible local **community resources**. Your school's counseling center is a first great resource in identifying where these agencies exist and how you can contact them directly.

You are encouraged to seek assistance early and not wait until a situation is serious or possibly dangerous, negatively impacting your health and grades. Equally important, this knowledge can be used to teach your clients about community resources. Community resources have become significantly more important as health care continues to change. Our clients' hospital stays are very short, transitioning to same-day services, outpatient care, and ambulatory care settings. Knowing community resources will be essential to your role as a student and a licensed practical nurse/licensed vocational nurse (LPN/LVN) as you assist the client and the family unit as a whole entity.

TYPES OF COMMUNITY RESOURCES

There are diverse types of community resources, such as school, city, county, and state resources. Private resources may also exist. Frequently, religious organizations offer assistance and/or resources to individuals and families. Depending on the size of your school, your school community resources may include academic (i.e., writing center, mathematics center, office of career development, academic accommodations), financial aid, health services, housing, and social resources.

Empowerment

An orientation to your school resources is generally completed when you enter school. It is easy to forget what is available. Take a moment now to visit your school's website/student handbook. List some resources that may be helpful in the near future. Bookmark the links for easy access when needed. Remind your peers about resources if they express unmet needs. Use your resources to be a successful student.

Community resources can be different across cities, counties, states, and the nation. However, common types of assistance are available in most areas of the country. The following are major categories of community resources:

- Information and referral agencies
- Housing and shelter programs
- Financial and legal assistance programs
- Health and medical services
- Drug and alcohol and mental health treatment centers
- Food programs
- Transportation programs
- Employment/educational/training programs

INFORMATION AND REFERRAL AGENCIES

Information and referral agencies can serve as a first stop if you are unfamiliar with services in your county. Your school's counseling center may refer you to these agencies to determine the best resources to address your unique needs. These referral agencies provide free assistance in finding help. They may be able to guide you to resources based on income eligibility guidelines, usually those using state or federal government dollars, as a best fit and to save you time in researching. As a student, your time is precious. However, faith-based or philanthropy-funded resources may evaluate your immediate situation when qualifying you for a service. This can be helpful when you are a student, as your income has likely decreased dramatically. Despite your best-laid plans, the perfect storm may have hit (i.e., a car died, a child became very sick, water pipes burst). Consider calling 211, a special telephone number designated in the United States, usually available 24/7, which acts as an information/referral service to health, human, and service organizations in your local area (www.211.org). Finding the right resource is key.

HOUSING AND SHELTER PROGRAMS

Adequate housing is an essential element of survival for you and your family. In addition, adequate housing will support you in your study habits, as discussed in Chapter 2. There are a variety of shelters, including homeless, women's, family, and youth shelters. Rehab centers also may provide short-term housing. Examples include the YWCA, YMCA, Salvation Army, and various other faith-related missions. Many counties and states also have a homeless hotline that can be easily found online.

Housing programs can assist with rent, temporary housing, or even permanent housing. Many times, you may not even realize that you qualify for housing assistance due to a recent layoff, divorce, or other life event. Rental housing assistance programs generally consist of affordable rental housing, housing counseling, rapid rehousing assistance, foreclosure/eviction assistance, home buying assistance, home repair programs, and weatherization services. Habitat for Humanity has a unique approach, engaging the family with the community as they build the house. Contact your local housing authority to seek assistance.

FINANCIAL AND LEGAL ASSISTANCE PROGRAMS

Worry regarding finances and legal issues can be a compelling reason that some students do not successfully complete a LPN/LVN program. You may be aware of the county assistance office, also referred to as the *welfare office*. The type and amount of aid vary from state to state. The services provided through county assistance include financial assistance for food (Supplemental Nutrition Assistance Program, or SNAP, formerly called food stamps), child care, unemployment, and housing. Lesser-known services include assistance with utility bills, credit counseling, tax preparation, and legal services. There are usually multiple legal aid services available in your community. Given that you are on course to achieve a new financially sustaining career pathway, consider using financial planning and budgeting services. These services will teach you, while you are in school, about how to manage your bills and tuition needs; however, they will also assist you in future planning, including goal setting, debt reduction, credit repair, and savings/retirement programs. This truly is a great time to transform your life and create financial stability for the future. Tapping these resources during or close to completion of the program will empower you and your family for the future.

Civil legal service clinics and legal-related workshops are conducted regularly and are free of charge. Topics can include "How to have a criminal record (i.e., DUI) expunged" and "Child custody laws—What you need to know." Citizenship educational classes and support are also available to assist in this complicated process. These services may be funded by governmental entities or faith-based centers. Immediately contacting any of these services, when needed, is a great first step in decreasing your stress level.

HEALTH AND MEDICAL SERVICES

Various types of health and medical services are available in your community. The cost of these services is usually on a sliding scale depending on your household income. These services may help you complete your physical and immunization requirements to attend clinical sites. Multiple clinics are available that provide medical services. Maternal and child health consortiums, Planned Parenthood, and other women's services often exist independently to meet the unique needs of this population. Your local health care institutions, along with your public health department, offer a wealth of health and wellness classes and services to meet the community's needs, including your and your family's needs. Be sure to access them when needed.

Rehabilitation is available through drug and alcohol treatment centers and 12-step programs (i.e., Alcoholics Anonymous). Mental health crisis centers, as well as residential and day treatment centers, also exist to support community needs. Counseling services are often available through your Family Service county outreach office.

Maintaining dental hygiene can be cost prohibitive because many people are uninsured or underinsured. Fortunately, dental services may be available for adults and children through local clinics and dental or dental hygiene schools.

Health insurance is available through your specific state's Affordable Care Act Health Insurance Exchange and specific state-related children's insurance programs. Lastly, prescription expense assistance can be available through state, pharmaceutical-funded programs, and local clinics.

Empowerment

Access Health Services

Visit the website of your local hospital/health care system. Make a list of any services that they offer that may be helpful to you, your family, or your nursing practice. Determine if there is a charge, and plan/advise accordingly.

FOOD PROGRAMS

Countless food programs exist in our nation. They can be government, community, or faith-based funded. In recent years, there has been an increase in farm-raised produce that is harvested by volunteers and donated to food banks. This has assisted in improving the nutritional value offered by food banks and serving a nutritionally balanced meal. In addition to food banks, soup kitchens and other subsidized food events may exist in your local area. Hot meal programs may also be provided. Seniors and disabled individuals can have special programs that deliver meals to their doors (i.e., Meals on Wheels).

Try This

Identify a minimum of two food banks in your city/county. Determine the following:

- When are they open?
- Who is eligible?
- What foods are available?
- Is it client choice or prepackaged foods?
- Is there any assistance for individuals with dietary restrictions?

TRANSPORTATION PROGRAMS

Transportation can be a challenge for all students, particularly nursing students, because of the travel required to attend diverse clinical sites. Given the complexity of scheduling clinical sites, it is unlikely that your school will be able to adapt to your unique transportation barriers when scheduling your clinical rotation. Most nursing schools, unless it is in a completely urban area, will counsel students about the necessity of a car while enrolled. Knowledge of public bus and train service may assist you in some situations; however, having a car in good condition is often essential. Car repairs are costly and can often be the "straw that broke the camel's back" when a student is missing clinical because of lack of transportation.

Although these programs are limited, students should inquire regarding technical schools or auto shops that provide free repairs for people in financial need. An example of this type of program, Repair Angel, exists in the Philadelphia area. The auto shop owner covers the cost of the parts, and some of their technicians donate their time to fix the car. Local practical nursing students have benefited from this amazing outreach service. Other examples include Charity Motors, Car Donation Wizard, and access through Salvation Army or Habitat for Humanity.

Unique transportation programs exist for seniors and/or disabled people. In addition, some communities have volunteer transportation programs, often focused on a particular disease process, such as cancer. Although the hours that these services function may be limited, they may be instrumental to meet your family's needs while in school or to refer clients.

Critical Thinking

- A student's car breaks down. It is going to cost $500 to repair. You find them crying in the parking lot and deciding not to return to school. What should you do?
- You are discharging a client from a rehabilitation center. They live alone and have limited family support in the area. How will they access outpatient therapy 3 days per week?

EMPLOYMENT/EDUCATIONAL/TRAINING PROGRAMS

Employment and educational training opportunities are available through your city/county. Some of you may have used these services to attain your GED or prepare for the nursing program entrance test. If you need assistance with basic math, reading, or literacy skills, free programs exist in most areas of the country. If you need assistance, seek out the Adult Basic Education (ABE) or the adult literacy program in your county. You will receive free individual or small group training. Improving these basic skills will be integral to your academic success. See Chapter 2 for additional academic resources.

In your city/county there will be an employment center (i.e., Career Link). Many states have created a central resource center where many of the resources noted above are available and combined with access to employment and educational/training opportunities. Most importantly, there may be a possibility that training dollars through the Workforce Innovation and Opportunity Act (WIOA) and Trade Adjustment Assistance (TAA) funds are available to you to assist in paying your nursing tuition. If you are a dislocated worker or underemployed, you may be eligible for several thousand dollars in funding. When seeking access to these funds, inquire about the Workforce Innovation and Opportunity Act funding and training grants. Use these as key words to narrow your search. Your school's financial aid office should also be able to assist you.

The Office of Vocational Rehabilitation (OVR) is available to assist people with disabilities to achieve employment and independence. This office may be able to assist with adaptive equipment or low-interest loans to assist a student. An example of a student who may seek out this service would be someone with a hearing disability who is in need of an expensive amplified stethoscope. OVR may be able to provide the evaluation and funding for this service.

There are many different types of employment services available. Although job-seeking skills are generally available through your school, additional services are available through these employment sites. Assistance with interview preparation, résumé creation, and possibly even clothing for an interview are a few of the services to benefit you. Lastly, job locator/placement services will be a great resource upon successful completion of your LPN/LVN program or when you are looking for a suitable part-time job while enrolled in the program.

Try This

Find a Community Agency

Identify an actual or potential need for a community resource as described above. Locate this community resource on the Internet and determine if you are eligible for their assistance.

Critical Thinking

You see a peer who is crying in the parking lot as you exit school. You recognize the person from class and offer assistance. The person explains that their husband locked her out of the house and she stayed in their car last night. Tonight it is going to be cold. What advice will you share with this peer of yours?

BEYOND COMMUNITY RESOURCES

The Internet provides an opportunity for you to identify resources well beyond your school or local community to contribute to your success. Various nursing organizations, social media sites, scholarship opportunities, and academic and clinical resources are available on the Internet.

FEDERAL FINANCIAL AID RESOURCES

Your school has a financial aid office that can assist you to find federal, state, and nongovernmental funds to help pay for tuition, books, resources, and in some cases, living expenses. Contact the financial aid office to find out how to apply for funding and determine financial need. Most students qualify for federal student loans by completing a Free Application for Federal Student Aid, or FAFSA (see https://studentaid.gov for more information). Based on your income/assets and other details, some students with greater financial needs may qualify for a variety of federal programs to include PELL grants, Perkins grants, and other programs.

NURSING ORGANIZATIONS

Nursing organizations identify or offer speakers, seminars, and workshops on up-to-the-minute nursing topics and related health care topics. These programs are frequently made available to students, thereby enhancing their content knowledge and creating for them a new network of colleagues.

There are two long-established licensed practical/licensed vocational nursing membership organizations in the United States: the National Association for Practical Nurse Education and Service, Inc. (NAPNES, www.napnes.org) and the National Association of Licensed Practical Nurses (NALPN, www.nalpn.org). Both of these organizations are dedicated to promoting competence and advancing the profession of LPN/LVNs. They provide continuing education, networking opportunities, and information regarding topics important to LPN/LVNs. Visit the respective website for specific information.

SOCIAL MEDIA (ELECTRONIC MEDIA) AND SOCIAL NETWORKING

LinkedIn is a preferred professional network. In addition, nurses are using Facebook, YouTube, Instagram, WhatsApp, and TikTok, the most commonly used **social media** platforms for communicating with family and friends, to communicate and collaborate with nursing organizations, and keep up to date with colleagues.

Professional organizations also use these networks to allow nonattendees to follow conventions, seminars, and so on. The interactivity of these sites allows one to consume as well as contribute information. It is critical to realize that social media and networking must be used with caution so as to develop an awareness of the professional versus personal use of these sites. The 2011 National Council of State Board Examiners (NCSBN) white paper, "A Nurse's Guide to the Use of Social Media," states that 46 Boards of Nursing (BON) were surveyed by the National Council, and 33 boards reported receiving complaints about nurses who violated client confidentiality/privacy by posting client information on **social networking** sites. Sanctions ranged from a letter of concern, mandatory continuing education, to suspension of license. The NCSBN has updated an extensive brochure. It emphasizes to nurses to "be mindful of employer policies, relevant state and federal laws, and professional standards" to see benefits and consequences of using social networking."

- NCSBN provides a free download or hard copy of the brochure *A Nurse's Guide to the Use of Social Media*, 2024. It is available at https://www.ncsbn.org/brochures-and-posters/nurses-guide-to-the-use-of-socialmedia along with other resources at www.ncsbn.org.
  Key points follow:
- Violation of client privacy is a violation of the Health Insurance Portability and Accountability Act (HIPAA) and can result in a fine for your employer and sanctions for you from your State Board of Nursing.
- Violation of client confidentiality is also a violation of your professional code of ethics (see Chapter 6).
- Whether or not you engage in social media is a personal choice. If you choose to participate, carefully check the privacy policy of the site. Thoughtfully develop a profile and carefully set your privacy settings. Remember that caution is needed even when using privacy settings.
- Avoid putting on the Internet *anything* you would not put on television or the front page of a newspaper. Prospective employers may "Google" you. Be especially scrutinizing of pictures posted by you and your friends.
- LinkedIn is the world's largest professional networking platform, impacting social media professional connections. This is a site for posting résumés, education, work history, accomplishments, and professional memberships. The goal is to connect or reconnect with colleagues/classmates, creating a network to assist in advancing your career. If you include your current employer, remember that you are then a representative of that agency. The power of LinkedIn lies in making a second connection when job seeking. You leverage someone you know (your LinkedIn connection) to introduce you via e-mail to their supervisor/administrator (their LinkedIn connection). This is especially helpful when job seeking.
- The American Nurses Association (ANA) has identified Social Networking Principles to guide your professional participation in social networking (https://www.nursingworld.org/social/). Connecting with groups on social media provides an opportunity to chat with students throughout the country and in various levels of nursing education and experience. Facebook provides various opportunities for nursing students including:
- NurseGroups.com
- AllNurses.com

Watch your time manangement represents a social media community exceeding 1,000,000 members and provides an opportunity for nursing students/nurses to connect with other students and nurses. A specific "student" site allows students the opportunity to discuss, debate, share best practices, and find camaraderie amid the perils of nursing school. Watch your time management while on the many website resources, and not just because of the fees. It is easy for several precious hours to slip away, leaving minimal time to study and prepare for the next day's class/clinical. Balance occurs when there is a great plan in place.

Remember the four "*P*"s needed to create a plan to SUCCEED: Power, Passion, Perseverance, and Personal Attributes. These Internet sites can fuel all four "*P*"s but can also limit your power, built through knowledge, if they conflict with study time. Use your social media savvy wisely. Create a plan and stick to it, changing it only when absolutely necessary!

Professional Pointer

Presentation of self on social media requires professional behavior. Try to search for yourself on the internet and critically evaluate all sources.

Try This

Social Media Policies

Investigate social media policies developed by your school, clinical areas, State Board of Nursing, and the National Council of State Boards of Nursing.

INTERNET ACADEMIC RESOURCES

Although many of the Internet-based academic/clinical resources are geared toward registered nurse (RN) students, SPN/SVN can also benefit. For example, Practical Clinical Skills (www.practicalclinicalskills.com) is a website that provides free clinical simulation aids that help you in tasks such as assessing blood pressure and simulating heart, lung, and bowel sounds. This resource, although focused on RN students, provides an excellent resource that helps practical/vocational students to develop skills for real-life applications. Sites, such as Off The Charts (http://ajnoffthecharts.com), a blog by the *American Journal of Nursing*, also provide additional reference sources for students.

Get Ready for the Next-Generation NCLEX® Examination

Key Points

- Maslow's human needs theory, portrayed as a pyramid, has five steps, with the most basic needs existing at the bottom of the pyramid. The five steps include physiological needs, safety, love/belonging, esteem, and self-actualization.
- According to Maslow, if you are hungry, thirsty, fear for your safety, fear for lack of food for your children, or feel unsafe, you need to address and resolve these issues the best you can. If not, your learning can be affected.
- Community resources are a significant focus in health care reform. Our clients' hospital stays are very short and often nonexistent. Most care occurs in a community setting. Community resources will be integral to your role as a student and as an LPN, assisting not only the client but also treating the family unit as a whole entity.
- Diverse community resources exist in your school community and community at large (i.e., city, county, state, nation).
- The following major categories of community resources exist: Information and Referral Agencies; the Housing and Shelter Program; Financial and Legal Assistance Programs; Health and Medical Services; Drug and Alcohol and Mental Health Treatment Centers; Food Programs; Transportation Programs; and Employment/Educational/Training Programs.
- All students may benefit by accessing a community resource while enrolled in a LPN/LVN program. Securing assistance before a crisis occurs is the goal.
- The OVR is available to assist people with disabilities to achieve employment and independence.
- There are two long-established practical/vocational nursing membership organizations in the United States: NAPNES and NALPN.
- Professional social media networks consist of varied groups including LinkedIn, Facebook, and Twitter. These sites are commonly used social media networks to communicate and collaborate with nursing organizations and keep up to date with colleagues.
- Social media and networking must be used with caution. Develop an awareness of the professional versus personal use of these sites.

Additional Learning Resources

Go to your Evolve website (http://evolve.elsevier.com/Carroll/success/) for the following FREE learning resources:

- Answers to Critical Thinking Scenarios
- Additional learning activities
- Additional Review Questions for the NCLEX-PN® exam
- Helpful phrases for communicating in Spanish and more!

Clinical Judgment Questions

1. **Maslow's human needs theory stresses the importance of humans meeting basic physiological needs and safety needs. If these basic needs are not met, what may a student be unable to do?**
   a. Feel respected and have self-confidence
   b. Have a casual discussion
   c. Access a digital database
   d. Identify a community resource
2. **A student is struggling with basic math concepts in their pharmacology class. Which of the following may be a good community resource to access?**
   a. Office of Vocational Rehabilitation
   b. Adult Basic Education (ABE) Program
   c. NALPN
   d. Repair Angel
3. **A SPN/SVN, who is very active on social media, took pictures of students engaged in a catheterization simulation during a clinical lab simulation and posted them on her Facebook page. Did this create a social media issue related to professionalism?**
   a. Yes, she will probably be counseled or possibly suspended from nursing school.
   b. Yes, the school will need to report this student to the local police.
   c. No, it is in the spirit of team building that she posted the pictures.
   d. No, because it is a private site. However, it would be best in the future to ask her classmates before posting the pictures.
4. **Which of the following SPN/SVNs would be well served from seeking out a student assistance program or community resource? *(Select all that apply.)***
   a. A student whose wife just lost her job.
   b. A student whose husband came home drunk the last three evenings.
   c. A student who has a long history of credit card debt accumulation and now has poor credit.
   d. A student who achieved a B on the first pharmacology test.
   e. A student who just won a $1000 tuition scholarship.
5. **Community agencies may be able to assist with the following: *(Select all that apply.)***
   a. Short-term rental housing
   b. Tax preparation
   c. Time management
   d. Anger management
   e. Citizenship

Critical Thinking Scenarios

Anya, continued.
Anya is now in the third month of the practical nursing program and has been late for class four times and absent 4 days since school started. Anya is fearful dismissal from the program is a real possibility and is thinking it is best to stop going to classes and just disappear. Anya is currently passing all the courses but having car issues for the third time this week and doesn't have money to get it fixed. In addition, Anya's babysitter just gave 2 weeks' notice of unavailability for 3 months due to surgery. Anya feels like the odds are impossible. This was the only chance to go to school. Anya says, "I feel so defeated. I just want to run and hide." What suggestions would you give Anya?

How Practical/Vocational Nursing Evolved: 1836 to the Present

4

Objectives

On completing this chapter, you will be able to do the following:

1. Recall milestones in nursing history since 1836 and in modern practical nursing.
2. Discuss the contributions of Florence Nightingale.
3. Discuss early nurse training school in America before and during the Civil War.
4. Discuss advancement in formal training for practical/vocational nurses.
5. Summarize the evolution of practical/vocational nursing education and practice during the 20th century.
6. Discuss key events in practical/vocational nursing education and practice in the 21st century.
7. Present the rationale for your personal stand on entry into nursing practice.

Key Terms

Anna Goodrich
Anna Mae Hays
Clara Barton
Cadet Nurse Corps
Dorothea Lynde Dix
Florence Nightingale
Glenna Goodacres
Jane Delano
Lenah S. Higbee
Lillian Kinkela-Keil
Lillian Wald
Lystra Gretter
Mary Seacole
M. Adelaide Nutting
Mildred I. Clark
Notes on Nursing

Keep in Mind

The first nurses were practical nurses, and you are part of that proud heritage.

Today, formal educational programs are the norm for all nurses, including practical/vocational nurses. The length of the full-time program for the modern practical (or vocational) nurse is approximately 9 months to 1 year in most states. Part-time programs can last as long as 2 years.

EVOLUTION OF PRACTICAL/VOCATIONAL NURSES OVER TIME

MODERN PRACTICAL/VOCATIONAL NURSES

Nursing has experienced many changes throughout its history (Table 4.1), and the changes continue. Two major changes that have occurred in practical nursing are a gradual increase in the required formal knowledge base and a requirement for licensing to practice practical/vocational nursing. Unlike the historically untrained or poorly trained practical/vocational nurse, who had unlimited and unsupervised freedom to practice, the present licensed practical/vocation nurse (LPN/LVN) is now trained in an educational program consisting of theory, clinical simulation, and clinical hours. The practical/vocational nursing program prepares the student to successfully pass the National Council Licensure Examination for Practical Nurses (NCLEX-PN®) examination and meet minimum standards to practice safely as a graduate practical/vocational nurse. After licensing, the LPN/LVN is permitted to perform the role of the LPN/LVN as aligned with the respective state regulations. Most state regulations stipulate that LPN/LVNs work under the supervision of the registered nurse (RN) or health care provider.

FIRST SCHOOL OF NURSING (1836)

The first real school of nursing was founded by the Lutheran Order of Deaconesses under the supervision of a German pastor, Theodor Fleidner, in Kaiserswerth, Germany in 1836. The purpose of the program was to teach principles of nursing care to the Lutheran Order of Deaconesses. Many of the graduates of Kaiserswerth Deaconess Institute settled in other parts of the world and established similar programs. The school's most famous pupil was Englishwoman **Florence Nightingale**, the founder of modern nursing. She attended the school for 3 months and studied under Caroline Fliedner.

Table 4.1 Nursing Milestones

PERIOD IN HISTORY	EVENT
1836	First real school of nursing, in Kaiserswerth, Germany. Florence Nightingale attended for 3 months.
	Eighteen years later, after start of Crimean War, Nightingale nursed the wounded with 38 self-identified (untrained) nurses.
1860	Nightingale established a school of nursing in England. She wrote several books. The most famous was *Notes on Nursing*.
Civil War (1861–1865)	In the South: Most nursing done by infantrymen assigned to the task. Southern women volunteered services. In the North: Dorothea Lynde Dix, a teacher, was appointed Superintendent of Nurses and organized a corps of female nurses (untrained).
1864	Clara Barton, a teacher, collected supplies for soldiers. This led to her appointment as Superintendent of the Department of Nurses for the Army.
1881	Clara Barton established the first chapter of the American Red Cross in Danville, New York.
1892	First class for formal training of practical nursing: YWCA, Brooklyn, New York.
1893	Nightingale Pledge written by Canadian-born Lystra Gretter, principal of Farrand Training School in Detroit. Henry Street Settlement founded by Lillian Wald, a social worker who graduated from a nursing program. Practical nurses pioneered in this new public health movement. They went into homes and taught the basics of cleanliness and control of communicable diseases to families in New York slums.
1893	Ballard School for Practical Nursing opened in New York.
1907	Thompson School for Practical Nursing opened in Brattleboro, Vermont.
1914	Mississippi is the first state to pass a law to license practical nurses.
1917	Standardization of nursing requirements for practical nursing by National League of Nursing Education (now the National League for Nursing [NLN]).
World War I (1914–1918)	Shortage of practical nurses. Army School of Nursing established. Highlighted the need for more and better-prepared nurses. Smith Hughes Act of 1917 provided money for developing additional schools of practical nursing.
1920s	Acute shortage of practical nurses. Many did not return to nursing after the war.
1920–1940	Most practical nursing limited to public health agencies and visiting nurse associations.
1938	New York only state to have mandatory licensure.
World War II (1939–1945)	Shortage of RNs created need for LPNs. At home, practical nurses worked in clinics, health departments, industries, and hospitals. In the war, they ventured into hardship tours in Europe, North Africa, and the Pacific.
1940	The number of practical nurses peaked in 1940 at 159,009.
1941	NAPNES (National Association of Practical Nurse Education and Service), a nation's professional organization dedicated exclusively to practical nursing, was founded.
1943	Cadet Nurse Corps was founded; 2.5-year courses to become nurses.
1944	Comprehensive study of practical nursing by U.S. Department of Vocational Education. This was the first time that tasks of practical nursing were agreed on.
End of World War II	Nursing shortage saw movement of practical nurses into hospitals and gradually increasing responsibilities.
1949	NFLPN (National Federation of Licensed Practical Nurses) was founded to provide structure nationwide through which LPNs could promote better client care and act on behalf of LPNs. The NFLPN-organized Joint Committee on Practical Nurses and Auxiliary Workers in Nursing Services recommended use of the title "licensed practical nurse" and differentiated between tasks of registered nurses and LPNs.
Korean Conflict (1950–1953)	Nurses finally became part of the military.
1951	*Journal of Practical Nursing* published by NAPNES (now *Practical Nursing Today*).
1952	Approximately 60% of the nurse workforce was made up of practical nurses.
1955	All states had licensure laws for practical/vocational nurses.
1957	NLN established a Council of Practical Nursing Programs.
1960	By 1960, every state had a nurse licensure law.

Table 4.1 Nursing Milestones—cont'd

PERIOD IN HISTORY	EVENT
1961	NLN began offering accrediting services for practical nursing programs
Vietnam War (1961–1973)	Military nurses were assigned to Vietnamese hospitals, MASH units, as flight nurses, and hospital ships.
1965	ANA (American Nurses Association) first moves toward two distinct levels in nursing: professional and technical.
1971	NBNA (National Black Nurse's Association) is established.
1975	1315 state-approved PN programs. More than 45,000 PN graduates. After 1975, number of PN programs and graduates declined.
1979	NLN published first list of competencies for practical/vocational nursing programs.
1980s	Resurgence of ANA moves toward two distinct levels of nursing. This resulted in some states adopting two levels of nursing and then rescinding their decision because of the nursing shortage.
1984	Creation of ALPNA (American Licensed Practical Nurses Association).
1989	The American Medical Association (AMA) initiated and subsequently dropped the registered care technician (RCT) proposal.
1990s	Unlicensed personnel are used for client care. The number of hospital nursing jobs has decreased. The primary employment site has moved into the community.
1994	First computerized adaptive test (NCLEX-PN®) available to practical/vocational nursing graduates.
1995	Full-time nursing positions in hospitals decreased. Client/nurse ratios increased. Primary employment in community continues.
1996	Long-term care certification examinations for LPNs/LVNs by National Council of State Boards of Nursing with the National Association for Licensed Practical Nurse Education and Service.
2000	Increased demand for LPNs/LVNs in nursing homes and extended care; demand down in hospitals.
Afghanistan War 2001–2014	Military nurses help set up surgical teams, MASH units, air evacuation, combat support units in Afghan and Iraqi hospitals.
Iraq War 2003–2011	Military nurses provide care and leadership to maintain the health and support units in Iraq.
2007	Nursing programs are turning students away because of the shortage of instructors.
2010	Institute of Medicine (IOM) Releases the *Future of Nursing: Leading Chance, Advancing Health* report.
2013	Health Resources and Services Administration (HRSA) report, *The US Nursing Service Report Trends in Supply and Education* released indicate a shift from acute care to long-term and community-based care.
2014	National League for Nurses (NLN) Releases Vision statement, titled *Recognizing the Role of the Licensed Practical/Vocational Nurses in Advancing the Nation's Health*.
2017	National Nursing Workforce Summary (2017) Highlights that the LPN/LVN workforce is more ethnically diverse than the RN workforce.

LPN, Licensed practical nurse; *MASH*, mobile army surgical hospital; *NCLEX-PN®*, National Council Licensure Examination for Licensed Practical Nurses; *RN*, registered nurse.

FLORENCE NIGHTINGALE (1820–1910)

Florence Nightingale was born in Florence, Italy. Her parents named her after the city and called her Flo. Nightingale's parents were wealthy, influential, and accepted in society. Florence was presented at court and was expected to follow the social pattern of other women of her day. Women were considered intellectually inferior to men. Education for middle-class and upper-class women often consisted of lessons in etiquette, dancing, music, manners, embroidery, painting, and modern languages. Instead of being tutored by governesses or in a private school, Nightingale's father tutored her in modern and ancient languages, history, composition, philosophy, and mathematics, including statistics. He was a strict disciplinarian, but she was an eager student (LeVasseur, 1998).

Nightingale turned down a proposal of marriage from a man her sister later married. Early on, Nightingale knew she had a purpose in life to fulfill. She begged her parents to permit her to go into the nurses' training program in Kaiserswerth, Germany. Her parents were not pleased because nursing was seen as a job suitable only for lower-class women. As we know, Nightingale got her way. Upon graduation, she became superintendent for the Institution for the Care of Sick

Gentlewomen in Distressed Circumstances, now the Harley Street Nursing Home in London (Romanoff, 2006). She began to take steps to make the work of nurses who served the gentlewomen easier. Dumbwaiters were installed so the nurses did not have to carry heavy trays up and down stairs. Nightingale also developed a system of call bells that could be seen in hallways to identify which person was summoning. Because the institution discriminated against Catholic and Jewish people, she dropped religion as a requirement for admission. Some of the governing board members were not happy with her changes.

The following year, as Nightingale was planning to become superintendent of King's College Hospital in London, the Crimean War broke out. She sent a letter to the Secretary of War offering her services. She did not know that he had also sent a letter to her requesting her assistance.

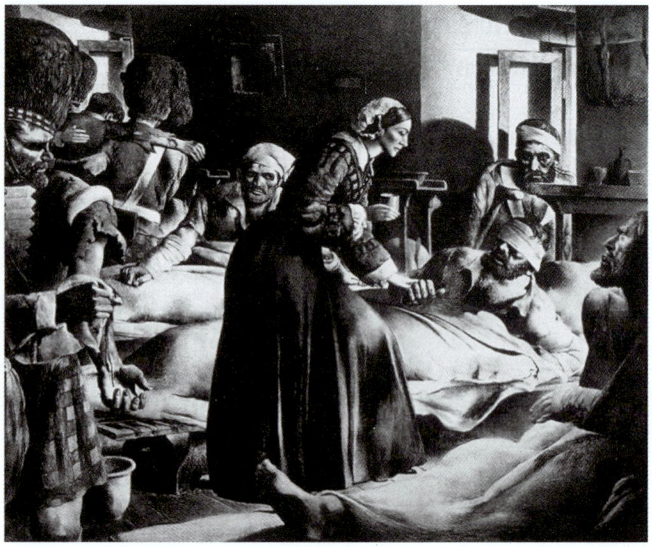

Fig. 4.1 Florence Nightingale ministering to soldiers at Scutari (lithograph). (Courtesy National Library of Medicine.)

CRIMEAN WAR (1853–1865)

Shortly after the start of the Crimean War in 1853 (in which Britain, France, Turkey, and Sardinia fought Russia for control of access to the Mediterranean from the Black Sea), information about the neglect and poor care of casualties began to reach England. A correspondent for the *London Times* newspaper wrote vivid accounts of the deplorable conditions and lack of medical and nursing care for the British troops. The Sisters of Mercy tended Russian troops, the Sisters of Charity tended the French, and the wounded of England were almost completely neglected. The correspondent's charges were so persistent that a commission was sent to investigate. As a result, the Secretary of War decided that England should also have a group of women nurses to tend the war casualties.

The Secretary of War contacted Florence Nightingale and explained the situation to her. Because she had both nursing and administrative experience, the secretary perceived her as the one nurse in England capable of organizing and supervising care in a foreign land.

Being appointed to the task of organizing and supervising nurses during the Crimean War gave Nightingale an unexpected opportunity for achievement. She left for Crimea, taking with her 38 self-proclaimed nurses of limited experience, 24 of whom were nuns. On arrival, they found overcrowded, filthy hospitals with no beds, no furniture, no eating utensils, no medical supplies, no blankets, no soap, no linens, and no lamps. Wounded soldiers lay on the filthy floor in their battle uniforms (Fig. 4.1). Soldiers were more likely to die from infected wounds than the wound itself. Nightingale took charge. Using the supplies she brought, and raising funds, she purchased supplies that health care providers could not obtain for the army. Nightingale hired people to clean up the "hospitals" and established laundries to wash linens and uniforms and prepare nutritious meals. She expected a great deal of herself and those who worked with her. It was not an easy task. A major prejudice that had to be overcome was that of medical officers, who considered the nurses intruders. The hours were long and difficult for Nightingale and her nurses. Many soldiers had family following them, and recreation rooms were set up for their use. She believed that the best nurses were those who had good character, who experienced a sense of calling, and who were well trained to meet the physical needs of clients. The barracks, a 4-mile labyrinth of cots meant for 1700 clients, packed in 3000 to 4000 clients. She did not want her nurses on the wards after dark and could often be seen after hours making additional rounds with her lamp to check on clients. The soldiers fondly referred to her as "Birdie." These extra efforts earned her the title, "The Lady with the Lamp," as immortalized in Longfellow's poem *Santa Filomena* (Box 4.1).

MARY SEACOLE; HONORED FOR HER WORK

Mary Seacole, a nurse from Jamaica, also played an important role in the history of nursing. She used her own money to build a lodging house in Crimea where she provided care for the soldiers. A memorial statue in London exists in her honor inscribed with words written in 1857 by *The Times'* Crimean War correspondent, Sir William Howard Russell: "I trust that England will not forget one who nursed her sick, who sought out her wounded to aid and succour them, and who performed the last offices for some of her illustrious dead" (BBC, 2016).

DEATH RATE DROPS; NIGHTINGALE DECORATED

After 6 months, it was obvious that the efforts of Nightingale and her nurses were paying off. The death rate among the wounded dropped from 420 deaths per 1000 casualties to 22 per 1000. She stayed throughout the war

Box 4.1 Santa Filomena

Whene'er a noble deed is wrought,
Whene'er is spoken a noble thought,
Our hearts, in glad surprise,
To higher levels rise.
The tidal wave of deeper souls
Into our inmost being rolls,
And lifts us unawares
Out of all meaner cares.
Honor to those whose words or deeds
Thus help us in our daily needs,
And by their overflow
Raise us from what is low!
Thus thought I, as by night I read
Of the great army of the dead.
The trenches cold and damp,
The starved and frozen camp—
The wounded from the frozen plain,
In dreary hospitals of pain—
The cheerless corridors,
The cold and stony floors,
Lo! in the house of misery,
A lady with a lamp I see
Pass through the glimmering gloom,
And flit from room to room.
And slow, as in a dream of bliss,
The speechless sufferer turns to kiss
Her shadow, as it falls
Upon the darkening walls.
As if a door in heaven should be,
Opened, and then closed suddenly,
The vision came and went—
The light shone and was spent.
On England's annals, through the long
Hereafter of her speech and song.
That light its rays shall cast
From portals of the past.
A lady with a lamp shall stand
In the great history of the land,
A noble type of good,
Heroic womanhood.
Not even shall be wanting here
The palm, the lily, and the spear.
The symbols that of yore
Saint Filomena bore.

—Henry Wadsworth Longfellow

and was the last to leave. Many of her nurses had become ill during the war and were sent home to recover. Nightingale became ill with Crimean fever, probably typhus, and almost died. When she returned home, Queen Victoria decorated her for her efforts in the war.

Critical Thinking

Medical Asepsis

Look up the term *medical asepsis*. Discuss with a peer how Florence Nightingale implemented many of the key aspects of medical asepsis to save the soldiers during the Crimean War. Does poor medical asepsis contribute to client's deaths today? If so, discuss where and how.

NIGHTINGALE ESTABLISHES FIRST SCHOOL OF NURSING IN ENGLAND

One of Nightingale's major goals was to establish a school of nursing in England. An overwhelming number of health care providers opposed such a school. Their opposition was that "because nurses occupied much the same positions as housemaids, they needed little instruction beyond poultice making, the enforcement of cleanliness, and attention to their clients' personal needs" (Kalish and Kalish, 1995). In 1860, Nightingale established the Nightingale Training School at St. Thomas Hospital in England. It was a 1-year program. She chose this site because of the hospital's reputation for progressive medical care. The school was independent from the hospital and financially independent as well. She believed nurses should work only in hospitals, not in private duty. Nightingale had strict admission standards that emphasized high moral character and intelligence. She was strict with her nursing students. The nurses were inaccessible in the evening as a way to reassure the middle-class parents that their daughters were safe from harassment. Upon graduation, she gave the nurses gifts of books and invited them to tea. When her graduates went to work in far-off places, she sent flowers to welcome them to their new home (Romanoff, 2006).

Nightingale's personal and nursing decisions reflected the influence of works by Plato and Hippocrates. Examples include her decision to remain single, her sense of mission, her concern with client environment, her focus on the whole client, and her belief in the need for keen observation and assisting nature to heal the client (LeVasseur, 1998). Nightingale wrote over 200 publications, the most famous of which is *Notes on Nursing*. Although she was reclusive, she was influential in matters of military and public health policy because she kept such precise notes, which included statistics. Nightingale's statistics, similar to evidence-based practice today, confirm her role as a visionary for the nursing profession.

Keep in Mind

Like Florence Nightingale, the director of your nursing program will need to attest to your moral character when he or she notifies the respective state board of nursing that you have met all the practical/vocational nursing program requirements. Moral character is an essential component of a licensed nurse. Self-reflect on this fact often, ensuring your moral character is and remains strong.

NIGHTINGALE'S CORE BELIEF ABOUT NURSING

The core of Nightingale's spirituality was a belief in perfection. To her, nursing was a sacred calling, a commitment to work for mankind, not a business. Other Victorian women like her shared the sense of the sacredness of time and belief that wasting time was a sin. Nursing became a way for Florence Nightingale to work toward the perfection of mankind and her personal salvation. She was against licensure. To her it was too much like nurses being in a union. She eliminated prejudice against a better class of women entering nursing and created a push toward the development of nursing as a respectable vocation.

Nightingale was intelligent, well educated, and skeptical. This combination made her the foremost critic of the meaning of nursing and the nursing role. She continued to be involved in health policy well into her eighties. She was the first woman to receive the Order of Merit from the King of England. In 1910, she died in her sleep of heart failure at age 90. The government offered to bury her at Westminster Abbey, but according to her wishes, she was buried in the family plot at East Wellow, Hampshire. The marker reads, "F.N. Born 12 May 1820. Died 13 August 1910."

In 1893, **Lystra Gretter**, the principal of Farrand Training School in Detroit, and a committee modified the Hippocratic Oath. They named it the *Nightingale Pledge* as a token of esteem for the founder of modern nursing. It continues to be recited in many schools during graduation, primarily because of the mistaken belief that Nightingale wrote it. It reads as follows:

> *I solemnly pledge myself before God and in the presence of this assembly, to pass my life in purity and to practice my profession faithfully. I will abstain from whatever is deleterious and mischievous, and will do all in my power to maintain and elevate the standard of my profession, and will hold in confidence all personal matters committed to my keeping and all family affairs coming to my knowledge in the practice of my calling. With loyalty will I endeavor to aid the health care provider in his work, and devote myself to the welfare of those committed to my care.* (Mosby's Medical Dictionary, 2009)

? Critical Thinking

Nightingale Pledge and Nursing

Review the Nightingale Pledge. Does it apply to the practical/vocational nurse in the 21st century? If you were to make changes, what would they be?

NIGHTINGALE MUSEUM ON THE SITE OF HER SCHOOL OF NURSING

In the spring of 1989, the Florence Nightingale Museum (https://florence-nighingale.co.uk) opened in London on the grounds of St. Thomas Hospital, the site of the Nightingale School of Nursing. The museum is a tribute to this nursing leader, despite the fact that she wrote in her journal, "I do not wish to be remembered when I am gone." Despite her great and courageous contributions to nursing, Florence Nightingale saw only her own faults and her failures.

EARLY NURSING TRAINING SCHOOLS IN AMERICA

PITTSBURGH INFIRMARY

Nurses in America were scarce and poorly trained. In 1849, Pastor Fliedner of Germany, who helped establish the first hospital and nursing school in Europe, came to America with four of his highly trained deaconesses. Although Pastor Fliedner was involved with establishing the first Protestant hospital in America, the deaconesses started the first formal training program for nurses in the United States. The hospital, known as the Pittsburgh Infirmary, still exists in Pennsylvania as the UPMC-Passavant Hospital. The training program was separate from the hospital with the intent to educate nurses.

As the nursing shortage continued, hospital-based schools of nursing emerged as a cost-effective (i.e., free) labor force for the hospitals. The living conditions and the long hours required a great deal of physical and emotional endurance of the students.

CIVIL WAR (1861–1865)

In the 1800s, women who worked in hospitals, particularly in the South, were victims of deep prejudice from men in general and especially from the medical profession. As one southern woman put it, "It seems strange that what the aristocratic women of Great Britain have done with honor is a disgrace for their sisters on this side of the Atlantic to do" (Kalish and Kalish, 1995).

Casualties were high on both sides during the Civil War. Many soldiers died right on the field, and others died because of a poorly trained medical corps. Southern women offered their services as volunteers, but most of the nursing was done by infantrymen assigned to do a task they did not want to do. It was many months before the Confederate government recognized southern women for their contributions.

In the North during the Civil War, women offered their services as nurses to the government. One hundred women were selected to take a short training course from health care providers in New York. **Dorothea Lynde Dix**, a teacher by profession, was appointed Superintendent of Nurses. Her task was to organize a corps of female nurses. She would recruit only women who were younger than age 30 and plain looking; they wore simple brown or black dresses and were forbidden to wear hoop skirts or jewelry. Women who did not meet these criteria nursed anyway but without official recognition or pay from the government. In addition, as a longtime advocate for better conditions for those who suffered from mental illness, Dix went on to establish the first hospital for the mentally ill.

Clara Barton

Clara Barton, a teacher by profession, was one of the first civilians in the Civil War to round up army supplies. She rented a warehouse, filled market baskets, and encouraged friends to send food, blankets, and other supplies for the soldiers. Her efforts resulted in her being appointed Superintendent of the Department of Nurses for the Army in 1864. Clara Barton's efforts frequently found her on the front lines, and she nearly lost her life on two occasions. After the war, President Andrew Johnson commissioned her to do what she wanted to do: find missing prisoners of war. Later, while visiting in Europe for health reasons, she met J. Henri Dunant, founder of the International Red Cross. He asked for her help in introducing the Red Cross to America. Through Barton's efforts, the first chapter of the American Red Cross was established in Danville, New York, in 1881.

? Critical Thinking

What is the relationship between the American Red Cross and nursing?

FORMAL TRAINING: PRACTICAL NURSING (1893–1984)

In 1893, the Ballard School under the auspices of the YWCA opened the first formal practical nurse program in Brooklyn, New York. The course lasted 3 months and focused on home health care for the chronically ill, invalids, children, and the elderly. It included cooking, nutrition, basic sciences, and basic nursing procedures. The graduates were referred to as attendant nurses. Other similar schools include the Thompson School for Practical Nursing, which opened in Brattleboro, Vermont, in 1907, and the Household Nursing Association School of Attendant Nursing, which opened in Boston in 1918. The Household School later changed its name to the Shepard-Gill School of Practical Nursing. The focus continued to be home nursing and light housekeeping duties. Hospital experience was not a part of the early programs. Before 1940, there were few controls, little education, practically no planning, and minimal supervision.

? Critical Thinking

As discussed above, the first formal practical nursing training focused on home health care of the chronically ill, invalids, children, and the elderly. Discuss with a peer how this aligns with practical/vocational nursing jobs found today.

NURSING IN THE HOME

Before World War I, most nursing done by practical nurses was home nursing, primarily because most people were cared for in the home. Even operations were performed in the home. There is some truth to how old Western movies portrayed surgery on the kitchen table. The nurse's 24-hour schedule included such procedures as cupping and applying leeches; preparing stupes for relief of abdominal distention, mustard plasters for relief of congestion, and poultices for drawing out pus from infections; and administering enemas, which were often nutritive enemas that contained eggnog with brandy or chicken broth. Intravenous infusions did not exist. Some practical nurses also assumed the then-accepted role of midwife. They taught new mothers the basics of cleanliness, diet, and child care (Fig. 4.2).

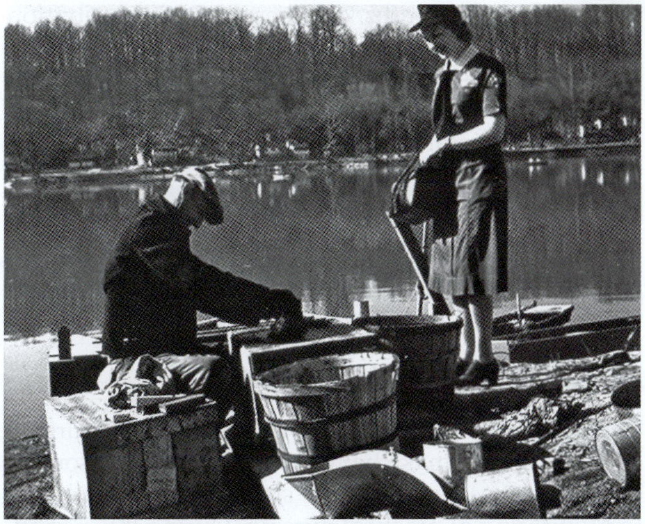

Fig. 4.2 Public health nursing follow-up visits. (Courtesy National Library of Medicine.)

FROM HOME TO PUBLIC HEALTH NURSING

By the end of the 19th century, there was renewed interest in charitable work and concern for the sick. Practical nursing began to expand from home nursing to public health nursing, care of clients in the slums, school nursing, industrial nursing, and well-baby care. Once again, practical nurses pioneered in this new public health movement.

One of the best-known centers in 1893 was the Henry Street Settlement in New York. **Lillian Wald**, a social worker, graduated from nursing school and intended to become a health care provider. Wald taught home nursing to immigrants and was so impressed by their need for medical care that she left medical school to begin a nursing service, the Henry Street Settlement. Practical nurses who were members of the Henry Street Settlement taught families in New York slums the basics of cleanliness and control of communicable diseases. There was a decrease in school absenteeism because the spread of childhood illness was reduced. School nurses visited schools and new mothers and their babies. They taught mothers the basics of preventing the summertime killer of infants: cholera infantum. It was estimated that their efforts resulted in the survival of 1200 more babies than average during the hot summer months. Another original contribution of the nurses was the development of Little Mother Leagues in the slums, in which all girls older than age 8 were taught how to take care of their younger siblings, including the infants.

? Critical Thinking

What programs exist in your local communities today aimed at decreasing the spread of communicable diseases?

TWENTIETH CENTURY (1901–2000)

The nursing profession evolved to meet the nursing shortage and to make better use of nursing personnel. By 1903, states began to take steps that ultimately led to monitoring of practical nursing. During this period, nursing organizations were developed. The National League of Nursing Education (now the NLN) took the most influential step. In 1917, the league developed a nationwide system of standardization of nursing requirements for practical nursing.

MISSISSIPPI: FIRST TO LICENSE PRACTICAL NURSES

In 1914, Mississippi was the first state to pass a law licensing practical nurses. This was an important event, because the public had no way of knowing who was providing nursing care. For centuries, self-proclaimed nurses were responsible for the majority of the nursing care given. Licensing, however, was not mandatory, and by 1938, New York was the only state to have mandatory licensure. Today, all states require mandatory licensure for nurses, including practical/vocational nurses.

WORLD WAR I NURSES (1914–1918)

The history of nursing is also the history of war and hard-fought women's rights. Women were considered fragile and delicate and kept at home to raise their babies and keep house. World War I made it necessary for women to work outside the home so men could go to war. Poster campaigns depicted the glamour of war to persuade young women to sign up as health care providers and nurses to help with the war effort. Women were encouraged to be tough, but they still struggled with those who did not want women working outside of the home. Nurses had been part of wars in the past but never as part of the military. World War I was the first war where nurses had professional training to serve. America declared war on Germany in 1917, and it was evident that there were not enough nurses to serve. **Jane Delano** of the American Red Cross began to recruit nurses and train and equip them for overseas duty. By 1918, about 20,000 nurses were assigned to go overseas, and many of them stayed overseas after the war to help with the postwar relief programs (Red Cross, 2019).

The US government insisted that only trained nurses could be sent to France with the Army. The reality was there were not enough nurses to meet both war and domestic needs. National nursing leaders **M. Adelaide Nutting, Anna Goodrich**, and Lillian Wald met and formed the National Emergency Committee on Nursing. As a result, the Vassar Training Camp was created to train college graduates in an intensive 3-month program to enter schools of nursing. Soon other universities began to offer similar nursing programs. In 1918, the Army School of Nursing was established at Walter Reed hospital in Washington, DC. It extended similar programs to other military hospitals throughout the United States.

World War I nurses were not allowed to serve at the advanced dressing stations on the front lines, although some nurses showed up there. They served primarily in hospitals organized for treating the wounded: field hospitals, which were sometimes just behind the front; clearing hospitals (known as evacuation hospitals) that were 10 miles back from the front; and base hospitals, where all the wounded were eventually sent. They dealt primarily with communicable diseases, wounds, infections, shock, hemorrhage, and poison gas inhalation, and they even performed minor surgeries. The work was long and exhausting, with deplorable conditions and few supplies. Young nurses were exposed to horrors, not the glamour that had been advertised on the posters.

At the peak of the war, 23,000 (some sources say 30,000) nurses were in service, and none held a military rank. Although governed by military discipline, they were neither officers nor enlisted personnel. Because of this, they had no authority to direct corpsmen or orderlies or to take on administrative duties. After the war, through an amendment to the National Defense Act, the Army Nurse Corps was given officer status. This did not increase their pay or allowance to that of their male counterparts.

There is no record of a nurse dying because of combat, but about 260 nurses died because of the influenza epidemic of 1918. Many women were recognized for their service with awards. Three nurses received the Distinguished Service Award, and four Navy nurses were awarded the Navy Cross. In her book *Nursing, the Finest Art*, Donahue (1985) states, "One of the four, **Lenah S. Higbee**, the second Superintendent of the Corps, from 1911 to 1923, had a destroyer named in her honor on January 1945. This was the first time a fighting ship was named after a woman in the military service."

World War I emphasized what nurses of that time were capable of accomplishing. It also highlighted the need for more and better-prepared nurses. Moving nursing into colleges and universities was a major step for nursing education. Admission standards for nursing schools were raised, and the expectations of graduates were increased.

It was the service of women in the military that positively impacted women's rights: the 19th Amendment, which was ratified in 1920. President Woodrow Wilson made a passionate plea to the Senate to pass the amendment. He emphasized that women were expected to work hard and make sacrifices without the privileges and rights enjoyed by men.

Canadian Nurses in World War I

Unlike American nurses in the military, the Canadian nurses were given the designation of lieutenants in the army and were stationed at nursing care wards. Canadian nurses worked around the clock to treat the wounded, who were brought in on stretchers or just dragged in because no stretchers were available. They had thousands of wounded to care for and try to prevent the onset of infections. Many lives were saved because of the nurses' diligence.

The shortage of beds in the military hospitals often made it necessary to put the wounded on the floor. These wounded men were the victims of the many hungry rats that overran the hospitals and were fearless and not afraid to bite the wounded soldiers. A Hall of Honor was built in Ottawa, Canada, to remember and honor the Canadian nurses who stood so strong in times of such difficulty.

SMITH HUGHES ACT OF 1917

The home front was facing a battle of its own in 1917 and 1918, with a major epidemic of pneumonia in 1917 and a worldwide epidemic of Spanish influenza in 1918. The mortality rate was high, especially in 1918. The Smith Hughes Act of 1917 provided money for developing additional schools of practical nursing. The first high school vocational/practical nursing program opened at the Minneapolis Girls Vocational High School in 1919. However, the new schools could not supply nurses quickly enough to meet the severe shortage in the United States.

NURSES RETURN HOME: ACUTE NURSING SHORTAGE FOLLOWS WORLD WAR I

After the war, many nurses did not continue nursing. Some stayed overseas to help with relief efforts. This led to an acute shortage of nurses in the 1920s. Many more hospitals opened schools of nursing, with the real purpose of providing staffing. Hospitals without schools were staffed heavily with untrained employees.

From 1920 to 1940, six states made laws licensing practical nurses, but only a small number of practical nursing schools existed in the United States. Much of the nurse's work continued to be in public health agencies and visiting nurse associations.

DEPRESSION OF THE 1930S

During the Great Depression in the 1930s, many nurses lost their jobs or worked in hospitals for room and board rather than a salary. When it became fairly obvious that America was becoming involved in World War II (WWII), nursing leaders began to prepare for the need for nurses at all levels. Not wanting to face the nursing shortage experienced during World War I, this effort became a monumental task because nursing had decreased in popularity as a vocation.

WORLD WAR II (1939–1945)

Although WWII began in 1939, the United States was unofficially involved by offering Lend Lease, which gave war materials to Allied countries in exchange for being allowed to use Allied bases. Initially noncombatants, American aircraft and warships escorted merchant ships and protected them against U-boat attacks. When Pearl Harbor was attacked, the United States declared war the following day. WWII involved about 50 countries and resulted in major changes throughout the world.

When Pearl Harbor was bombed on December 7, 1941, there were fewer than 12,000 nurses on duty in the Army Nurse Corps. Few of them had military experience and knowledge of Army protocol. Fifteen 4-week training programs were developed for new nurses. The programs stressed Army protocol; military customs and courtesies; field sanitation; defenses against air, chemical, and mechanized attacks; personnel administration; requisitions and correspondence; and property responsibility. More than 27,330 newly inducted nurses graduated from the 15 programs.

It became quickly obvious that there were not enough trained personnel to administer anesthesia. More than 200 nurses enrolled in the 6-month course on how to administer inhalant anesthesia, blood and blood derivatives, and oxygen therapy and how to recognize and treat shock. Nurses specializing in psychiatric care were in great need. One out of 12 clients in Army hospitals was admitted for psychiatric care. A 12-week course was developed by the surgeon general to teach nurses how to care for and medicate combatants with psychiatric disorders.

Approximately 59,000 American nurses served in the war. Army and Navy nurses served in both the European and Pacific theaters. They were closer to the front than in past wars. Nurses were assigned to field hospitals, evacuation hospitals, hospital ships, and as flight nurses on medical transport planes. Because of the care combatants received in field hospitals or during evacuation, fewer than 4% died from wounds or disease. The demand for nurses in the Army and Navy Nurse Corps helped create a nursing shortage at home. In 1943, Congress passed the Bolton Act, which became the basis for the **Cadet Nurse Corps**. The government subsidized schools that were willing to teach primary nursing skills in 2.5 years. More than 150,000 nurses graduated from these programs. The Cadet Nurse programs were discontinued in 1948, but the public considered these programs a great success.

When the war ended, the Army was still segregated and still had a quota system for black nurses.

Only 479 nurses of the 50,000 serving in the Army Nurse Corps were black nurses, and they were limited to taking care of black troops in black hospitals. The Army dropped its quota system in 1944 because of the negative public reaction. By the end of the war, black nurses had served in Africa, England, Burma, and the Southwest Pacific. Federal funding for the Cadet Nurse Corps made it possible for 2000 black students to enroll in the Cadet Nurse program.

Practical nurses played a significant role both at home and in WWII. At home, practical nurses worked in clinics, health departments, industries, and hospitals. At the battlefields, practical nurses and RNs could be found in both the European and Pacific theaters. Some officers were initially reluctant to have nurses assigned at combat zones. The dedication, organization, and professionalism proved their worth and won the respect of health care providers, corpsmen, clients, and military command. Nurses adjusted to long hours with little rest, loss of electricity, bombings, kamikaze attacks, frequent moves and setting up of field hospitals, internment in concentration camps, deaths of clients and other nurses, wounds and diseases, and dealing with members of numerous cultures. It was noted that nurses adjusted to difficult and dangerous situations with a minimum of complaints.

Nurses received 1619 medals, citations, and commendations during the war, 16 of them posthumously to nurses who died as a result of enemy fire. After the war, nurses were eligible for the G.I. Bill of Rights, which entitled them to continue their education funded by the government.

PRACTICAL NURSING RESPONSIBILITIES INCREASE AFTER WORLD WAR II

The end of WWII saw a continuing shortage of nurses. This shortage helped practical nurses play an important part in hospital nursing. Most hospitals gradually increased the responsibilities designated for the practical nurse. By the 1940s, there were nearly 50 approved practical nursing programs in the United States. The number of practical nurses in America peaked at 159,009 in 1940. By 1944, practical nursing was already experiencing a decline.

? Critical Thinking

How many practical nursing programs exist in your state today? How many LPNs/LVNs exist in the nation?

PRACTICAL NURSING DUTIES OUTLINED

In 1944, the US Department of Vocational Education made a comprehensive study of practical nursing. This marked the first time that tasks of practical nursing were agreed on. Extensive specific duties were outlined, with an emphasis on maintaining aseptic technique. The phrases "to judge," "to appraise," "to recognize," and "to determine" were often used to describe the scope of the practical nurse's job.

? Critical Thinking

Discuss with a peer whether these phrases used in 1944—"to judge," "to appraise," "to recognize," and "to determine"—describe the scope of the practical nurse's job today. What phrases would you suggest adding?

REGISTERED NURSE AND LICENSED PRACTICAL NURSE TASKS DIFFERENTIATED

Other important changes followed. In 1949, the Joint Committee on Practical Nurses and Auxiliary Workers in Nursing Services recommended use of the title "licensed practical nurse." Furthermore, the committee differentiated between the tasks of the RN and the LPN. They saw the LPN role to be under the supervision of the RN. The committee suggested that practical nurses organize to make decisions on their salary, working conditions, and employment standards.

Because of the work of the Joint Committee, many practical nursing programs were strengthened with regard to content. They focused, for the first time, on the preparation of practical nursing instructors. Up to this point, any graduate nurse was eligible to teach practical nursing. During the 1950s, the number of programs continued to increase, and programs were extended to 9-, 12-, and 18-month programs.

THE KOREAN CONFLICT (ALSO KNOWN AS UNITED NATIONS POLICE ACTION OR THE SECOND INDOCHINA WAR; 1950–1953)

Many in the military believed that women had no place in the armed forces. The term used was *demilitarization*, and it took place rapidly after WWII. Many women lost their jobs in industry. Multiple reasons were given for sending women back to the kitchen, but one reason not discussed openly was that men would have difficulty reporting to women officers. It took 3 years for the government to determine that women were an integral part of the military. General Eisenhower finally clarified the issue by strongly recommending that women become a part of the US military. Several senior officers who had worked with women during WWII had great praise for military women. This led to President Truman signing the Women's Armed Forces Act in 1948. By the time North Korea invaded South Korea, the number of women in the military was at an all-time low.

The United States entered the United Nations Police Action to support their ally South Korea when North Korea crossed the 39th parallel and invaded the Republic of South Korea. Because of the shortage of nurses in the military, nurses were recruited from civilian hospitals. According to records, 540 Army nurses served in Korea, and none died as a result of enemy action.

Of the 3081 active-duty Navy nurses and 1702 reserve Navy nurses, according to records, none were killed or wounded because of enemy action. The Navy nurses served on three troop ships in both US and overseas hospitals. Army nurses cared for wounded in Mobile Army Surgical Hospital (MASH) units, prisoner-of-war camps, makeshift shelters, and hospital trains. Nurses were known for serving in MASH units where their responsibility was beyond that of the usual nurse. The shortage of medical personnel pushed them into doing work past their scope of nursing and into advanced practice. One such task was that of first assistant in surgery, which has now become an accepted part of RN advanced practice (RNFA) nursing (Fig. 4.3).

Nurses also worked as flight nurses on evacuation aircraft. One of the women who served was **Lillian Kinkela-Keil**, a member of the Air Force Nurse Corps and one of the most decorated women in the US military. Captain Kinkela-Keil flew over 200 air evacuation missions during WWII, as well as 25 trans-Atlantic crossings, and she flew several hundred more missions as a flight nurse in Korea.

Captain Kinkela-Keil was the inspiration for the 1953 movie Flight Nurse *and served as technical advisor to the film. Her decorations include the European Theater of Operations with Four Battle Stars, the Air Medal with Three Oak Leaf Clusters, the Presidential Unit Citation with One Oak Leaf Cluster, the Korean Service Medal with Seven Battle Stars, the American Campaign Medal, the United Defense Medal, and the Presidential Citation, Republic of Korea. Captain Kinkel-Keil died in 2005 at age 88 (Wilson, 2011).*

The Korean War is called *the forgotten war*. The men and women who served were forgotten, as was the war itself. Finding records and information about the war is also difficult. Little factual information is available to the public.

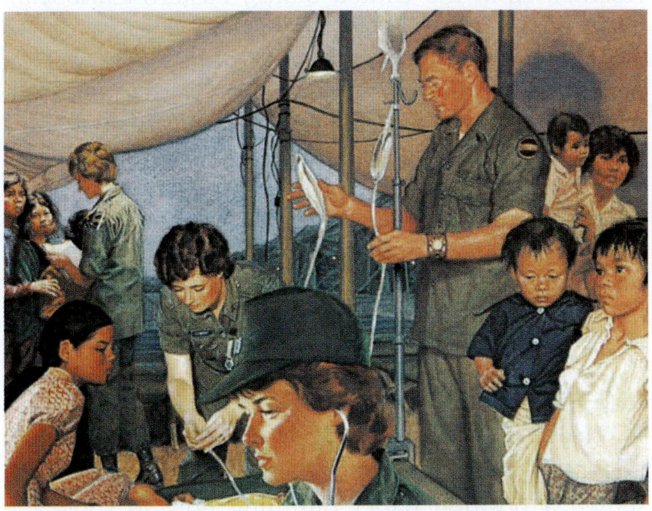

Fig. 4.3 The American Soldier, 1975. In the foreground, as concerned relatives look on, an Army nurse checks an injured Vietnamese citizen. The scene is typical of many long evenings in tents set up as emergency medical stations on Guam, the first stop for the refugees. (Courtesy US Army Center of Military History.)

REGISTERED NURSES REACT

By 1952, nearly 60% of the nursing workforce was made up of practical nurses. In many instances, RNs expressed bitterness because hospitals, clinics, and other agencies were hiring practical nurses for less money and assigning tasks to them beyond their educational level. RNs also expressed concern that the public was unable to differentiate between the levels of nurses. Both wore the same type of white uniforms, caps, and pins. Many practical nurses quickly stopped wearing the practical nursing insignia, which was meant to identify the practical nurse. LPN/LVNs performed tasks belonging to the RN one day and those belonging to nursing aides the next day. Many practical nurses felt trapped in such situations because of their need for employment.

TEXAS AND CALIFORNIA ADOPT NAME LICENSED VOCATIONAL NURSE (LVN)

In the early 1950s, both the Texas State Board of Vocational Nurse Examiners and the California Board of Vocational Nursing adopted the title "Licensed Vocational Nurse" as a result of state legislation. The title was based from the educational setting, as these nurses were educated in vocational schools.

PUBLIC LAW 911

In 1956, Public Law 911 provided for millions of dollars to expand and improve practical/vocational nursing programs. By 1975, there were 1337 programs, which graduated a total of 46,080 practical/vocational nurses. Approximately two-thirds of the LPN/LVNs were employed in hospitals, 17.3% in nursing homes, 7.5% in private duty, and 6.5% in health care providers' offices, clinics, and dental offices. Admission standards in most schools increased, as did the difficulty of the curriculum.

THE VIETNAM WAR (1961–1973)

The Vietnam War (1961–1973) was the second-longest war involving US military forces. According to the Vietnam's Memorial, nearly 10,000 women served. Most of these were newly trained nurses (DiFilippo, 2017). Nurses enlisted for various reasons including tuition forgiveness, free medical and dental care, opportunity to travel, and love for their country. All of the nurses volunteered and underwent a 6-week basic training course before being assigned to a 1-year assignment in Vietnam. Assignments were primarily in Vietnamese hospitals, MASH units, as flight nurses, and on board the hospital ships USS *Repose* and *Sanctuary*. Most of the nurses were in their early 20s and recent graduates with less than 6 months of clinical experience.

Living conditions varied from bug-infested tents to air-conditioned trailers to small, single-occupant rooms. Nurses in field hospitals wore white duty uniforms, and the rest of the medical personnel wore lightweight olive drab made of cotton poplin. It was difficult to keep uniforms clean, and nurses preferred to wear fatigues when available.

Nurses performed duties beyond what they had learned in nursing school. The 6-month basic training did not adequately prepare the nurses, physically or emotionally. Nurses worked 12-hour shifts, 6 days a week. Days off were often canceled out of necessity when massive casualties arrived. Combat injuries were different in this war. Artillery was specifically designed to inflict massive, multiple injuries. Napalm, white phosphorus, and "antipersonnel" bombs were used as well. Napalm and white phosphorus burned tissue right down to the bone. Nurses treated wounds they had never seen, did tasks beyond their nursing scope of practice, and dealt with illnesses such as typhoid, malaria, dengue fever, and bubonic plague. As in other wars, many of the admissions were for disease. In this war, it was malaria, viral hepatitis, skin diseases, venereal diseases, diarrheal diseases, and diseases of unknown origin. The rest were combat casualties. Assault rifles, rocket-propelled grenades, and booby traps were the major causes of wounds. Infection resulting from animal and human excreta in the paddy fields and waterways created additional problems in treatment. Nurses not only took care of the extreme physical wounds but also provided emotional support, playing the role of the soldiers' spouses and parents (DiFilippo, 2017).

As the war continued, service personnel were also being treated for drug addiction, especially heroin. Nurses had to deal with soldiers under the influence of illicit medications. Nurses were told to control their emotions when dealing with severely wounded and dying soldiers. According to the Vietnam Veteran's Memorial Foundation, the hospital mortality rate decreased in the Vietnam War compared to WWII due to various medical innovations and improvements in transportation.

In addition to practicing all the specialties, nurses also voluntarily gave medical assistance to Vietnamese civilians. This included basic care, immunizations, courses in child care, and sick calls at orphanages.

Mildred I. Clark, chief of the Army Nurse Corps from 1963 to 1967, and **Anna Mae Hays**, chief of the Army Nurse Corps from 1967 to 1971, led the Army Nurse Corps during the Vietnam War. On June 11, 1970, Colonel Hays also became a brigadier general, the first woman and the first nurse in American military to attain general officer rank (West, Army Nurse Corps Historian).

Women were treated as second-class citizens both in the military and when they came home. Nurses suffered from posttraumatic stress disorder (PTSD), experiencing feelings of isolation and anger. They had difficulty finding employment and suffered bouts of crying and depression. Vietnam veterans found it difficult to receive treatment, and both men and women were treated badly by many in the public.

The Vietnam Women's Memorial, designed and sculpted by **Glenna Goodacres**, is on the National Mall in Washington, DC. It is located at the south end of the Vietnam Veteran's Memorial and in the vicinity of the Three Servicemen memorial. The Goodacres monument shows three nurses in battle dress. One comforts a wounded or perhaps dying soldier, one is kneeling, and one is looking up in expectation.

? Critical Thinking

Preventing Posttraumatic Stress Disorder

If you were to join the military as a nurse and had to go into a war area, how would you prepare yourself to deal emotionally with the challenges you will face as a military nurse? What are work settings in the United States where you may experience PTSD?

NATIONAL BLACK NURSES ASSOCIATION

The National Black Nurses Association (NBNA) is a nonprofit entity, established in 1971. NBNA's mission is "to serve as the voice for Black nurses and diverse populations ensuring equal access to professional development, promoting educational opportunities and improving health" (NBNA, 2021). Many black nurses have contributed to the NBNA's legacy and organizational growth, beginning with the founder, Dr. Lauranne Sams, former Dean and Professor of Nursing, School of Nursing, Tuskegee University, Tuskegee, Alabama. NBNA represents 200,000 African American nurses representing a diverse group of nurses (RNs, LPNs/LVNs, nursing students, and retired nurses) focused on providing culturally competent health care to African Americans (NBNA, 2021). Members are represented from the United States, Eastern Caribbean, and Africa.

The organization's website (https://www.nbna.org) has in-depth information about its programs, policies, webinars, and conferences. The organization's most recent paper focuses on the COVID-19 pandemic with a focus on social justice and health equity when it convenes its annual National Black Nurses Day on Capitol Hill. In 2025, some of the key legislative priorities for discussion included tackling the global crisis in black maternal mortality and advocating for diversity in the nursing workforce.

AMERICAN NURSES ASSOCIATION MOVEMENT TOWARD TWO LEVELS OF NURSING

In 1965, the American Nurses Association (ANA) presented a position paper outlining how to solve the issues of the different levels of the nursing profession (Atkinson, 1966). They recommended that all RNs graduate from a 4-year collegiate program and all LPNs graduate from a 2-year technical program. Many hospital-based RN programs closed during that time. In the 1980s, a resurgence of the ANA 1965 movement toward establishing two levels of nursing temporarily gained momentum. This original movement was reinterpreted by many stakeholders, resulting in a surge of 2-year Associate's Degree (AD) in Nursing (RN) programs. However, some states did work toward adopting the ANA recommendations. Because a serious nursing shortage developed in the late 1980s, the ANA movement stalled in most states.

American Medical Association Moves to Ease Nursing Shortage

With the goal of easing the nursing shortage, in 1989, the American Medical Association (AMA) proposed a new health care worker: the registered care technologist (RCT). The RCT was to be trained in 1- and 2-year programs. Because this new level of health care worker correlated with existing personnel—the practical nurse and the AD nurse—the RCT proposal was not successful. This event is a gentle reminder for practical/vocational nurses to be strong, organized, and vigilant as a group. Changes in the health care system are occurring daily, as are opportunities for LPNs/LVNs. See Chapter 18 for a discussion regarding workforce trends.

Assistive Personnel

During the 1990s, assistive personnel (AP), originally called unlicensed assistive personnel (UAP), were hired to give client care. A major concern for LPN/LVNs and RNs was their legal responsibility for the care given by the unlicensed caregivers. Meanwhile, primary employment for nurses, especially for the LPNs/LVNs, moved out of hospitals and into the community.

First Computerized Testing: NCLEX-PN®

In 1994, the first computerized adaptive testing (NCLEX-PN® Examination) became available for the practical/vocational nursing school graduate. The computer format provided an individualized test for each graduate, based on the answer to the previous question. It excluded questions that were not within the nurse's scope of practice, according to their state's Nurse Practice Act.

Long-Term Care Certification

In 1996, long-term care certification became available to LPN/LVNs in some states. Since that time, other certifications have become available for LPN/LVNs in some states (see Chapter 18).

TWENTY-FIRST CENTURY (2001–PRESENT)

EVOLUTION OF NURSING LEVELS, TRAINING, AND EDUCATION

Nursing organizations continue to define the responsibilities of the different levels of nursing, However, there are still challenges. Nursing shortages created changes in nursing programs. Approximately 50 years ago, AD nursing programs were set up in technical schools and flourished. Today, approximately 23% of the current RN workforce hold an associate's degree as their highest nursing degree earned (Smiley et al., 2025). This is down from 36% in 2018. The goals of AD programs were to move nursing education out of hospital-based programs and to help ease the shortage by shortening the amount of time required to become an RN. However, the AD graduate, diploma graduate, and baccalaureate graduate all take the same licensing examination to become an RN. It was and continues to be confusing for those doing the hiring at a facility, because all RNs, regardless of their education, can legally assume the same responsibilities. Finances are always a major concern for health facilities. Years ago, when LPNs/LVNs earned much less than RNs, more LPN/LVNs were hired. When salary ranges were narrowed and the difference in salary became considerably less, more RNs were hired.

Nursing organizations continue to work on resolving the issue of nursing levels and present new recommendations and position papers. Nursing shortages continue especially with the COVID-19 pandemic of 2020. Changes in how health facilities are reimbursed for client care have had major impacts on client acuity, staffing ratios, overtime, client care loads, and client safety. The average age of the nurse workforce continues to increase.

In the last 15 years, fueled by the Institute of Medicine (2010) report *Future of Nursing: Leading Change, Advancing Health*, many stakeholders continue to discuss the levels of the nursing profession, an age-old debate that began in the 1960s. Given historical implications, such as the increase of AD in Nursing programs, the new discussion focuses on the need for Baccalaureate preparation as an entry point for RNs and a need for an increase in doctorally prepared nurses. In response, several states have introduced legislation to achieve these goals. In fact, BSN-prepared nurses increased from 39% in 2015 to 46% in 2024 (Smiley et al., 2025). However, the educational level of practical nurses has not been a focal point of the debate.

In 2014, the NLN released a vision statement, titled *Recognizing the Role of the Licensed Practical/Vocational Nurses in Advancing the Nation's Health*, supporting the critical role of LPN/LVNs in providing quality patient-centered, evidenced-based care to vulnerable groups across the health care continuum. In addition, the NLN also developed a guiding curriculum framework for practical/vocational nursing programs aligned with LPN/LVN workforce trends. This support is timely, as health care reform has created changing job roles for health care providers.

To build on the progress of the 2010 report mentioned earlier, *The Future of Nursing 2020-2030: Charting a Path to Achieve Health Equity* (National Academies of Sciences, Engineering, and Medicine, 2021) focuses on health equity, removing nurse practice barriers, social determinants of health, and diversifying the nursing workforce. The intention of this vision is to promote a culture of health for all. With this new vision the workforce has seen an increase in Black/African American RNs rose from 6% to 9%, and no change in male nurses, at a steady 10% proportionally.

IRAQ WAR (2003–2011) AND THE AFGHAN WAR (2001–2021)

The US involvement in the Afghanistan war (2001) was a result of the terrorist attacks on the United States on September 11, 2001. The war in Iraq (2003) began as a result of a belief that Iraq had weapons of mass destruction, which it did not. Very little has been written about nurses' experiences in Afghanistan and Iraq.

A total of 6326 nurses deployed between 2001 and 2015; to include 3296 nurses deployed to Afghanistan and 2683 nurses deployed to Iraq (Berry-Caban et al., 2018). At the onset these nurses quickly helped set up surgical teams and mobile hospitals to receive casualties. Issues arose regarding the lack of critical care nursing experience and the lack of experience using some equipment before deployment. Nurses were also assigned to air evacuation units, combat support units in Afghan and Iraqi hospitals, and hospitals for detainees. Living quarters varied from tents to primitive plywood shacks to container housing, depending on where they were sent. A layer of fine sand covered everything, showers were scarce, and feeling dirty all the time was common. Sanitation and sewer systems were minimal, and with the high temperatures, the smell of sewage was often in the air.

Some nurses described Afghanistan and Iraq as noisy, smelly places. It is not unusual to burn excreta and surgical waste. At the beginning of the war, little food was available, and most meals consisted of ready-to-eat fare, with water stored in containers that tasted like chlorine and was always warm because of the heat. This is a reason soldiers and medical people requested Kool-Aid and Crystal Light packets to add to the water (Desch and Doherty, 2010).

For nurses working in countries beyond our borders, being culturally sensitive when providing care to clients is an even greater issue. Clients' cultural preferences must be integrated into the plan of care. Nursing and medical care extends to America's wounded troops, civilians, National Army soldiers, and other coalition soldiers from around the world.

Although it is acceptable in Afghanistan for a male to be a nurse, male nurses cared for males only, and female nurses cared for female clients only. Families, when available, were involved in the care of hospitalized clients. Equipment and medicines were needed. Diarrheal illness was an issue in the civilian community, as was malaria, parasites, polio, and a protozoan illness caused by sand flies (especially in children playing in the sand).

Troops experienced severe injuries from mortar fire and roadside explosive devices, as well as gunfire. Gastrointestinal illness with nausea, vomiting, and diarrhea was an ongoing issue.

Although many nurses were not directly in harm's way, they were at risk for PTSD because of constant fear, exposure to trauma and loss, ethical dilemmas, and fatigue (Bolvin, 2010). Each individual undergoes an assessment when he or she returns to the United States. Sometimes symptoms do not appear until later, or the individuals' answers during an exit assessment may trigger concern and follow-up. They may be concerned about how they will be viewed when they are back home. It is not unusual for a nurse to grieve the person he or she was before going to Afghanistan or Iraq. Others appreciate professional growth and all that they learned to do and deal with, building their courage and self-confidence. What seems to stand out for many nurses is the sense of camaraderie and teamwork experienced between the nurses and the health care providers while overseas.

The United States continues to be involved in conflicts, and nurses continue to serve this great country and care for soldiers as the need arises throughout the world (Fig. 4.4).

The United States ended the conflict in September 2021. Nurses continue to serve this great country and care for soldiers and their families as the need arises within the United States and throughout the world.

Try This

If you know someone who has served in the Afghanistan or Iraq war, ask him or her about his/her feelings about nurses serving in the military.

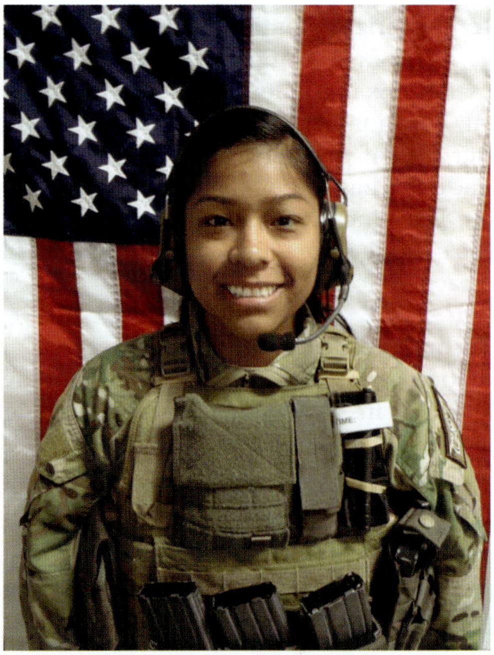

Fig. 4.4 Captain Jennifer Moreno. (From Cherry B, Jacob SR: *Contemporary nursing: issues, trends, and management*, ed 8, 2019, St. Louis: Elsevier.)

Box 4.2 Hospital Nursing 1887

In addition to caring for your 50 clients, each nurse will follow these regulations:

- Daily, sweep and mop the floors of your ward, dust the client's furniture and window sills. Maintain an even temperature in your ward by bringing in a scuttle of coal for the day's business.
- Light is important to observe the client's condition. Therefore each day fill kerosene lamps, clean chimneys, and trim wicks. Wash the lamp windows once a week.
- The nurse's notes are important in aiding the health care provider's work. Make your pens carefully; you may whittle nibs to your individual taste.
- Each nurse on day duty will report every day at 7 am and leave at 8 pm, except on the Sabbath, on which day you will be off from noon to 2 pm.
- Graduate nurses in good standing with the director of nurses will be given an evening off each week for courting purposes or two evenings a week if you go regularly to church.
- Each nurse should lay aside from each payday a goodly sum of her earnings for her benefits during her declining years so that she will not become a burden. For example, if you earn $30 a month, you should set aside $15.
- Any nurse who smokes, uses liquor in any form, gets her hair done at a beauty shop, or frequents dance halls will give the director of nurses a good reason to suspect her worth, intentions, and integrity.
- The nurse who performs her labors and serves her clients and health care providers without fault for 5 years will be given an increase of 5 cents a day, providing there are no hospital debts outstanding.

THE COVID-19 PANDEMIC (2020–2023)

In early 2020 people in Wuhan, China began to die from an unknown source. By March 11, 2020, the World Health Organization had declared a pandemic caused by a novel coronavirus currently named SARS-CoV-2. With the virus origin and source unknown, the transmission of the virus spread rapidly throughout the world, resulting in a shutdown of work, school, and everyday life activities (Dos Santos, 2020). Only essential workers could come to work—resulting in controversy about what was essential.

Nurses were involved from the start by caring for patients, with an incredible health care team effort, in the community and health care facilities. Especially fatal to the elderly and those with multiple morbidities, the deaths in long-term care facilities soared quickly in 2020. Hospitals, with few treatments available, were filled beyond maximum capacity, having to delay any nonurgent care. Research on vaccine development was sped up in a program called "Operation Warp Speed." As of December 2022 more than 80% of the US population has been given at least one dose of the vaccine, with lesser amounts in lower income countries. To take or not take the vaccine continues to be a very controversial topic and efficacy studies continue. (See http://www.ncbi.nlm.nih.gov.) The pandemic put a tremendous strain on the health care workforce, leading to a greater nursing shortage. As a student, you will learn much about the pandemic lessons learned regarding testing, mitigation efforts, and vaccination to keep you and your patients protected as much as possible.

NURSE LEADERS IN US GOVERNMENT

Increasing numbers of women serve in US Congress. As of January, 2025, there were 127 in the House of Representatives and 26 in the US Senate, and others have recently held senior management positions in diverse public entities. Of these three were nurses. As nurses have transformed from "doers" to "thinkers," their emergence in policy development is logical and beneficial to advancing the health of the nation. Their strategic positions can be a conduit for nurses to communicate their views regarding various issues that impact health care.

YOU HAVE COME A LONG WAY!

As a final note, it may be interesting to compare present practical/vocational nursing tasks with those that you would have been expected to perform in 1887. Practical/vocational nursing has indeed come a long way. The job description in Box 4.2 was given to floor nurses by a hospital in 1887 (author unknown).

Get Ready for the Next-Generation NCLEX® Examination

Key Points

- The nursing profession, including practical nursing, has experienced a history of transformation, emerging as a highly respected profession. Duties have changed according to the needs present at various times in history.
- Currently, practical/vocational nurses are taught both technical skills and critical thinking skills. This includes a focus on evidence-based (i.e., data-driven) decision-making, often described as critical thinking to evolve your clinical judgement during their educational program.
- According to some states' Nurse Practice Act, LPN/LVNs are allowed to perform more complex skills. LPN/LVNs work under the supervision and collaboratively with the RN and health care providers (i.e., health care provider, nurse practitioner).

- Historical figures in nursing include Florence Nightingale, founder of modern nursing; Clara Barton, founder of the American Red Cross; Lillian Wald, founder of public health nursing; Dorothea Lynde Dix, advocate for the mentally ill; and Mary Eliza Mahoney, first Black nurse to obtain a professional nursing license.
- Nurses have played a significant role in all wars and the COVID-19 pandemic, contributing positively to the development of the nursing profession.

Additional Learning Resources

Go to your Evolve website (http://evolve.elsevier.com/Carroll/success/) for the following FREE learning resources:

- Answers to Critical Thinking Scenarios
- Additional learning activities
- Additional Review Questions for the NCLEX-PN® examination
- Helpful phrases for communicating in Spanish and more!

Clinical Judgment Questions

1. **Florence Nightingale contributed greatly to the nursing profession. Which statement best describes Florence Nightingale's contribution to nursing?**
   - **a.** She established the first visiting nurse service for the poor in the Lower East Side slum section of New York.
   - **b.** She wrote the Nightingale Pledge in 1893 to set guidelines and inspire her nurses on graduation.
   - **c.** She discovered antibiotic use during the Crimean War.
   - **d.** She stressed environment, the need for careful observation, care of the whole person, and critical thinking.
2. **Periodically, various organizations have suggested eliminating practical/vocational programs. Which statement objectively provides a reason for continuing the LPN/LVN programs?**
   - **a.** LPNs/LVNs possess the same level of skill in client care as do RNs.
   - **b.** RN education is more focused on nursing theory, relying on LPNs to perform all tasks.
   - **c.** LPNs/LVNs are well prepared to provide evidenced-based care to vulnerable groups across the health continuum, collaborating with the RN as needed.
   - **d.** Health care providers prefer to work with LPNs/LVNs because they follow orders without question.
3. **Soldiers, in a war zone, receive care from a nurse. What are possible reasons why a nurse involved in the care of these soldiers may develop PTSD? *(Select all that apply.)***
   - **a.** Told to do tasks that are out of their scope of practice
   - **b.** Long hours with limited sleep
   - **c.** Faced with caring for clients with gruesome injuries
   - **d.** Lack of essential items required to give safe care
   - **e.** Adequate nutrition
4. **Florence Nightingale's beliefs formed the basis of medical asepsis, which continues to be a critical concept in health care delivery today. Which of the following beliefs were included? *(Select all that apply.)***
   - **a.** Brightly painted walls
   - **b.** Clean environment
   - **c.** Handwashing
   - **d.** Clean linens
   - **e.** Shades on windows

Critical Thinking and Clinical Judgment: A Lifelong Journey

5

Objectives

On completing this chapter, you will be able to do the following:

1. Describe why practical/vocational nurses should think critically and characteristics of thinking differently.
2. Explain why critical thinking is essential to decision-making as a practical/vocational nurse.
3. Discuss your personal need for help and how to find resources.

Key Terms

analysis
application
attitude
capability
clinical judgment
cognitive levels
comprehension
critical thinking
directed (or focused) thinking
knowledge
problem-oriented thinking

> **Keep in Mind**
>
> Become an active learner and critical thinker, and be successful in the practical/vocational nursing program, on the National Council Licensure Examination for Licensed Practical Nurses (NCLEX-PN®), and as a candidate for a job you will love as a licensed practical nurse/licensed vocational nurse (LPN/LVN).

As Kamy and Jamal are waiting for class to begin, you overhear them discussing the evolving role of the LPN/LVN from "doer" to "thinker." Kamy states, "Wow, it seems like the LPN/LVN has a much more challenging job today than they did 20 years ago. At first I thought, well I am a 'doer'; that is why I chose this career. But now I realize how important it is to be a 'doer' and a 'thinker.' Anyone can do but not everyone can use several pieces of evidence to think in a critical manner and arrive at the best decision for the client's plan of care. This is exciting. I feel like we really are a critical member of the health care team. This role seems very different than my role as a pharmacy technician." Hilary agrees and states, "I was thinking the same thing. My role as a nursing assistant is more heavily focused on 'doing.' Although a very important role, this 'critical thinking' really changes our job as an LPN/LVN. I am excited to learn about simulation and all the other ways to begin to think in a critical manner. Class is about to begin. Talk to you tomorrow." You reflect on this conversation as class begins.

OVERVIEW OF CRITICAL THINKING

REASONS TO THINK CRITICALLY

Now is the time to start thinking about how you think! The following are the Top 10 Reasons to Improve Thinking, adapted for practical/vocational nurses (LPN/LVN):[a]

10. Things are not what they used to be, or what they will be, in this changing health care system.
9. LPNs/LVNs care for clients, as a member of the health care team, who are stable, but may have multiple problems.
8. More clients and their families are involved in health care decisions.
7. LPNs/LVNs must be able to adjust from one health care setting to another.
6. Rapid change and information explosion requires LPNs/LVNs to develop new learning and workplace skills.
5. Clients, families, and insurance companies demand to see evidence of benefits, efficiency, and outcomes of care provided.

[a]Adapted with permission from Alfaro-Lefevre R: *Critical thinking and clinical judgement: a practical approach,* ed 7th, Philadelphia, (2019/2020), Elsevier.

4. Today's progress often creates new problems that cannot be solved by old ways of thinking (e.g., ethical and legal issues involved in end-of-life decisions, questions regarding stem cell research, determining who is entitled to receive expensive medical care when resources are limited).
3. Redesigning care delivery and education programs is useless if students and nurses do not have the thinking skills required to manage in today's health care environment.
2. Learning how to improve your thinking skills does not have to be difficult.
1. Your ability to focus your thinking on how to get the results you need can make the difference between whether you succeed or fail in the fast-paced health care system.

Years ago, nurses saw themselves as doers, not thinkers. Florence Nightingale, a pioneer in nursing, broke the mold to challenge nurses not to *just* follow instructions and carry out orders. It has taken significant time for nursing to change. However, over the past 30 years the acknowledged role of a thinking nurse has evolved. Changes in nursing practice is evidenced by the NCSBN Practice Analysis, completed every 3 years. Currently, the 2024 PN Practice Analysis: Linking the NCLEX-PN® Examination to Practice (NCSBN, 2025) is the most recent published. Access the NCSBN website at https://www.ncsbn.org/search.page?q=lpn+practice+analysis to check for updated documents.

As the expectation grew over time for critical thinking to be an essential skill for the LPN/LVN, now there is an even greater expectation of the nurse. The newer terminology is to develop clinical judgment. Clinical judgment is at the core of competent and safe client care (www.nalpn.org). According to Benner (2009), clinical judgment refers to ways nurses come to understand the problems, issues, or concerns of clients/client, to attend to salient information, and to respond in concerned and involved ways. According to Caputi (2022), students must learn a clinical judgment framework as the basis for thinking in nursing today. Older methods of evaluating student thinking that relied solely on students correctly answering questions with the assumption that if they answer correctly, they are able to use clinical judgment, is fatally flawed.

Professional Pointer

Critical thinking is a lifelong process (Alfaro-Lefevre, 2019).

DEFINITION OF APPLIED CRITICAL THINKING

What exactly is critical thinking, and how does it relate to the nursing decisions you will make at school and during your career? According to Marquez et al. (2023), critical thinking is defined as a mental process involving the perception, analysis, synthesis, and active and skillful evaluation of information collected through observation, experience and communication. Alfaro-Lefevre (2019) provides a definition of critical thinking and clinical judgment in nursing. **Critical thinking** in nursing, adapted for practical/vocational nursing, is defined as the following:[b]

- Entails purposeful, informed, outcome-focused (results-oriented) thinking that requires careful identification of the problems, issues, and risks involved (e.g., deciding whether a client needs one or more staff to move him from bed to chair in a manner that is safe for both client and staff).
- Is driven by client, family, and community needs. The LPN/LVN must be able to use knowledge to tailor approaches based on circumstances.
- Is based on the principles of the nursing process and on scientific methods; for example, making judgments based on evidence (facts) rather than guesswork. This is a major difference between LPNs/LVNs and assistive personnel (APs).
- Uses both logic and intuition, based on knowledge, skills, and experience of the LPN/LVN.
- Is guided by professional standards, such as those developed for the LPN/LVN by the National Association for Practical Nurse Education and Service (NAPNES) (www.napnes.org), the National Association of Licensed Practical Nurses (NALPN) (www.nalpn.org), and the practical/vocational nursing code of ethics.
- Calls for strategies that make the most of human potential (e.g., using individual strengths) and compensates for problems created by human nature (e.g., overcoming the powerful influence of personal beliefs, values, and prejudices).
- Is constantly reevaluating, self-correcting, and striving to improve (e.g., practicing skills, learning new skills, and attending classes and workshops).

Thinking is divided into unfocused thinking and **directed thinking**. At one time or another, most of us have used the following examples of thinking:

- **Unfocused thinking:** You engaged your brain out of habit without much conscious thought.
- **Habitual thinking:** We get up to go to the bathroom, shower, dress, and so on. This type of thinking involves any routine we do that is important but does not require us to think hard about how to do it (automatic pilot).
- **Random thoughts:** Multiple short scenes and thoughts come and go through the mind and have no particular purpose or goal (mental channel surfing).
- **Ruminative thinking:** The same situation or scene is replayed in the mind over and over, without reaching an outcome (instant replay).
- **All-or-none thinking:** The mind is made up, and no additional facts will be considered (black-and-white thinking with no grays in between).
- **Negative thinking:** The mind is stuck on negative thoughts and blocks worthwhile thinking (emotional sabotage).

[b]Adapted for practical/vocational nurses with permission from Alfaro-Lefevre R: Evidence-based critical thinking indicators, 2006. www.alfaroteachsmart.com/.

- **Directed (or focused) thinking:** Purposeful and outcome-oriented.
- **Problem-oriented thinking:** Focus on a particular problem to find a solution (e.g., planning your school, work, and home schedule). This could involve collecting information on school and work schedules and schedules of family members who rely on you. It might include delegating tasks, requesting help, making your goals known, and listening for input from those involved in the immediate situation. Once the schedule is developed, no further attention is given to the situation until another problem emerges (problem solving).
- **Critical thinking:** Critical thinking is an advanced way of thinking, a problem-solving method, and more. It is used to resolve problems and to find ways to improve a situation even when no problem exists. Critical thinking involves collecting and analyzing data to make a decision. It answers questions such as "How can we do this better?" and "How can we assist the client in achieving the highest-quality outcome; what resources are essential; and which can be eliminated to save costs?" "What is the actual problem?"

Try This

Survey of Your Current Level of Critical Thinking

Based on a scale of 0 to 10, with 0 as the lowest and 10 as the highest, rate each statement about thinking as it applies to you. Then list the items you rated starting with the lowest rated first.

___I identify the purpose of my thinking.
___My thinking is goal (or outcome) directed.
___I have an organized method of thinking.
___I question what I do not understand.
___I continually question: What does this mean? Is this useful? Is it fact?
___I question the reliability of sources and information available.
___I keep an open mind.
___My judgments are based on facts (evidence).

Empowerment

Make a Personal Plan for Success

1. Prioritize the critical-thinking items you need to work on from the previous learning exercise. Choose the items you think are most important to work on first.
2. Make a schedule and estimate the amount of time it will take to see progress. (We all need to work on critical thinking throughout our lives.)
3. Identify how you will determine what progress is being made.
4. Improving critical thinking skills can enhance self-confidence.

CRITICAL THINKING AND LICENSED PRACTICAL/ LICENSED VOCATIONAL NURSING

Critical thinking involves questioning with meaning. This type of thinking involves examining personal thinking and the thinking of others. Judgments are made on facts (evidence), not assumptions. The critical thinker avoids criticizing just for the sake of having his or her own way. Decisions are based on the right thing to do rather than emotions or a need to save face. New ideas and alternatives are offered in a constructive way. The thinker:

- considers other ideas and recognizes that there may be more than one right way to do something.
- realizes that a perfect solution may not be possible.
- realizes that collaboration is a key to effective critical thinking and decision-making.

Critical thinking is at its best when you have your brain purposefully engaged, for example, while you listen to a mini-lecture, view a video, listen to a podcast, participate in a discussion or study group, or are being tutored. A critical thinker is paying attention to what the speaker is saying.

- Do I understand it?
- What does it all mean?
- Where does it all fit in?
- Can I explain the key information in 3 to 5 minutes?

You are examining your thinking and the thinking of others. Critical thinking is based on science and scientific principles. The principles include the following:

- Collecting data in an organized way
- Verifying the data in an organized way
- Arranging the data in an organized way; this is often referred to as trending data
- Looking for gaps in information
- Analyzing the data
- Testing it out (Is the data purposeful and outcome/goal-oriented?)

These scientific principles align with the nursing process, as you will learn in Chapter 12. The critical thinker should routinely ask the following questions about the subject of the thinking task at hand (adapted from Alfaro-Lefevre, 2019):

1. What major outcomes (observable beneficial results) do you expect to achieve (e.g., when collaborating with the registered nurse [RN] to develop a care plan for a newly admitted client)?
2. What problems, issues, or risks must be addressed to achieve the major outcome (e.g., the hospital unit you are working on is short-staffed)?
3. What is the circumstance or context (e.g., the LPN/LVN is working in the client's home and assesses the environment to determine if equipment will need to be improvised)?
4. What knowledge is required (e.g., clinical areas where you had limited clinical experience, such as mental health)?
5. How much room is there for error (e.g., the client is positioned on his back as directed after surgery and begs to be on his side)?
6. How much time do we have (e.g., the client who was just admitted is bleeding profusely)?
7. What human and professional resources can help me/us (e.g., the client is acutely ill and refuses care because of lack of insurance or adequate personal funds)?

8. What perspectives must be considered (e.g., the client has refused to be examined because of religious beliefs)?
9. What is influencing my thinking (e.g., you are against abortion and do not want to take care of a client hospitalized because of self-induced abortion)?
10. What must we do to prevent, manage, or eliminate the problems, issues, and risks identified with question 2?

For each element, the thinker (in this case the LPN/LVN) must be able to reflect on the 10 key critical-thinking questions that shed light on the effectiveness of your thinking. In other words, is the thinking solving the problem or finding the answer you are seeking? Critical thinking is an essential part of nursing. The overall purpose of nursing is to assist people to maintain health, or regain the most maximum state of health possible as quickly as possible. Both purposes are to be achieved in a cost-effective manner and in a manner that fits within the client's culture and belief system. Nurses make decisions that affect both purposes. Nursing decisions must be accurate and based on evidence. The nursing process, evidence, and critical thinking coupled with assessment and recognition of the client's cultural diversity and other key demographics assist the LPN/LVN in making good decisions (Ignatavicius et al., 2018). As a nurse, your critical-thinking skill will vary according to your education and clinical experience. Box 5.1 lists suggestions to increase your critical thinking.

WHAT YOU NEED TO THINK CRITICALLY

For the LPN/LVN to think critically, it will be necessary to do the following:

1. Access information.
2. Comprehend (understand) information.
3. Store comprehended information in long-term memory. This includes having strategies to move information to long-term memory.
4. Determine what you know and what you do not know.
5. Recall the comprehended information when needed. (You will need to have the most important information in your head for client care on clinical.)
6. Know what to do when information is not in long-term memory. Where can you find the information needed?

As an LPN/LVN student, you will be exposed to a great deal of new knowledge during the year in the LPN/LVN program. You will gain knowledge, as stated in the course objectives. Your real test as an LPN/LVN will be your ability to access information, understand that information, recall it, and use it as the basis for critical thinking in the clinical area. Evidence needed to think critically is available in various sources, including the scientific literature and institution policy and procedure. Other members of the health care team can be a valuable source to assist in obtaining evidence for decision-making.

Box 5.1 Ways to Challenge Yourself to Think Critically

- Anticipate questions that the client or instructor might ask.
- Ask for clarification of what you do not understand.
- Ask yourself how you can improve the client's outcomes.
- Reword in your own words what you have read or been told (e.g., stating a nursing diagnosis as a nursing problem).
- Make comparisons with something similar to help you understand.
- Organize information in more than one way to see if you have missed anything important; this is to avoid being impressed when the "facts" fall into place but you have missed the obvious.
- Ask your instructor to check out your conclusions.
- Strive for objectivity. Keep an open mind and avoid drawing conclusions in advance.
- Review all your data again, especially after a period of time; trend the data as appropriate (e.g., how have the client's vital signs and symptoms changed over time) because they may look different, and you may reach a different conclusion.
- Get used to saying, "I don't know, but I will find out."
- Learn from your mistakes, fix them if you can, do not hide an error; someone's life may be at stake, and others can learn from your error.
- Think about what you are reading about while you are reading it; ask your instructor or peer to challenge you to think critically while you are on the clinical area.

FACTORS THAT INFLUENCE CRITICAL THINKING

Your current critical-thinking status is influenced by the following personal and situational factors:

- **Upbringing and culture**. Having family and teacher support and opportunities to learn to read well and understand the meaning of what you read; beginning to make simple, limited choices at an early age, which become more complex with consequences as you grow.
- **Motivation**. Whether you learned early to rely on others for motivation or decided you would learn in spite of the lack of external motivators, motivation determines in part the progress you have made in problem solving and critical thinking. You have the ability to think critically if you choose to do so. It is a preference on your part. Remember that the brain is like a muscle: The more you exercise it, the better it works.
- **Attitude influences thinking**. Critical thinkers are humble and recognize that they do not have all the answers and may be influenced by their beliefs and values. While in the process of client care, it makes a critical difference whether a problem is recognized,

missed, or ignored. Take time to collect some data on your **attitude** by completing the learning exercise in the Try This: Attitude Evaluation: My Attitude box.

Try This

Attitude Evaluation: My Attitude

Directions: On a scale of 0 to 10 (with 0 as the worst and 10 as the best), rate your attitude.

___I am aware of the limitations of my knowledge.
___I am aware that my dislikes, biases, and prejudices may influence my decisions.
___I try to be fair-minded.
___I am interested in understanding other people's thoughts and feelings.
___I check to find out if my statements are clear.
___I can be influenced by another person's conclusions, if based on facts.
___I question other people's sources of information.
___I acknowledge that what I have been thinking can be incorrect.
___I question the availability of additional alternatives.
___I listen to my intuition and compare it with my reasoning.
___I am aware that perfect solutions are not always available.
___I am willing to work as a team member.
___I try to anticipate problems before they occur.
___I am continually looking for ways to improve my thinking.

These items describe your strong attitudes for the development of critical thinking. The items are attitudes you need to improve to increase critical thinking.

Critical Thinking

Attitudes to Work On

Prioritize the attitudes you choose to work on first to help increase your critical thinking. How will you recognize improvement in each item you listed?

Try This

Bias

Personal bias can influence your critical thinking. In today's world, much of our bias occurs at the unconscious level but can influence our critical thinking. Psychologists at Harvard developed "Project Implicit" to measure unconscious bias. Go to https://implicit.harvard.edu/implicit/ to determine your unconscious bias. Categories include but are not limited to race, age, gender, and mental health.

ADDITIONAL FACTORS THAT INFLUENCE CRITICAL THINKING

Alfaro-Lefevre (2019) discusses the following personal factors that also influence critical thinking. These are summarized with some additional thoughts for LPNs/LVNs.

1. Effective reading
   a. Effective reading, as you have learned, is more than reading with speed.
   b. It means that you are able to identify the significance and potential application of what you are reading.
   c. An effective learning skill means that you are able to organize the data you have so you can access them efficiently.
   d. See Chapter 2 for suggestions to make studying and comprehending information work for you. Employers someone with more than random-access memory.
2. Maturity
   a. Maturity most often comes with age; however, age does not determine maturity.
   b. Maturity provides past opportunities to have worked through problems. It becomes easier to see problems through someone else's eyes.
   c. Do you work at understanding others before expecting them to understand you?
3. Problem solving and the nursing process
   a. Knowledge of problem solving and of the nursing process is based on many of the same principles as critical thinking.
   b. Do you use the problem-solving steps to work out problems now? Understanding and applying the problem-solving steps gives you a head start in thinking critically.
4. Communication skills
   a. Communicating effectively means being aware of the message you are sending verbally, in writing, and through body language. Are you willing to listen and consider ideas and views that are different from your own? Do you express yourself well in writing?
5. Self-confidence
   a. Self-confidence is often the personal characteristic that is the least available to a student.
   b. Without self-confidence, the student is wasting a lot of energy worrying that he or she will not "get it."
   c. No one can give you self-confidence. You develop self-confidence as you succeed in your endeavors. This is the meaning of the saying "Self-confidence is earned, not learned."
   d. Overconfidence can make people assume they are correct even before data are available to back up what they believe to be correct. Do you acknowledge the limits of your knowledge and skills? It is OK to admit that you do not know. The safe nurse seeks help to answer what is not known.
6. Moral development
   a. Moral development creates fair-mindedness, a strong sense of what is right, wrong, and just. Have you examined your values, and can you separate them from the values held by others? What are the core values/beliefs of your school or health care institution? Do your values align accordingly?

7. Capability in nursing
    a. **Capability** in nursing is essential. You must have nursing knowledge and skills to do the work of nursing and know how to access the resources.
    b. Nursing instructors have an enormous amount of factual information that they expect to introduce to their nursing students. The amount is often overwhelming to both the instructor and the student.
    c. Distinguishing what is absolutely necessary to know from what is nice to know is no easy task. The tendency is to hang on to what is fun to know and old information, just in case someone asks or it is in a test somewhere.
    d. With the knowledge explosion, it is not possible for instructors to infuse their students with all they need to know.
    e. Have the tools for locating and comprehending information, storing information in long-term memory, and recalling the comprehended information when needed. It is essential to evaluate whether or not a source of data (evidence) is reliable.
8. Collaboration
    a. A collaborative effort has been shown to promote critical-thinking skills. Interprofessional education occurs in many schools and clinical sites promoting this type of learning. Students can also facilitate this type of learning by presenting the instructor with a well-thought out collaborative plan (including observable, project outcomes/goals).
    b. Initially students become frustrated when they come to class and discover that lecturing is not the primary way of teaching. Working in teams, becoming immersed in clinical simulations and case studies can be much more beneficial to student learning. You are learning to apply what you read in the book. Challenging each other's ideas is a core component of critical thinking.
9. Anxiety
    a. When anxiety overwhelms, it effectively stops critical thinking.
    b. The same is true regarding a high level of fatigue. Adequate rest is essential to critical thinking.
10. Mentors and experience in nursing
    a. Work experience and the guidance of nursing mentors, starting with your instructor, will assist you in learning to identify priorities in nursing care.
    b. Depending on the work area, clients may be there to seek help for only a few hours or days (emergency or treatment) or for the rest of their life (nursing home).

CRITICAL THINKING, CLINICAL JUDGMENT, AND THE NCLEX-PN®

The NCLEX-PN®, the national licensing examination for LPNs/LVNs, includes test items that require various levels of thinking. These levels are called **cognitive levels**. The cognitive levels used on the NCLEX-PN® examination, based on Bloom's taxonomy, are knowledge, comprehension, application, and analysis. The following definitions will help you understand the meaning of the words *knowledge* (knowing), *comprehension* (understanding), *application*, and *analysis*.

1. **Knowledge** refers to the ability to recall and repeat information you have memorized. *Memorizing is not the same as understanding a concept*. Knowledge is the lowest level of learning. Defining a concept as stated in a dictionary is an example of knowledge level. Knowing a normal lab value is another example.
2. **Comprehension** refers to the ability to basically understand information, recall it, and identify examples of that information. To comprehend is to *grasp the meaning* of the material. Comprehension is the lowest level of understanding. An example of the comprehension level is the ability to repeat information in your own words. This indicates that you understand the information.
3. **Application** means being able to *use learned material in new situations*. For example, you apply what is learned in class to your clinical work. Application involves being able to prioritize or determine what is most important, what comes first. Application is a higher level of understanding. *You must be able to use knowledge to tailor approaches depending on circumstances*. Clinical simulation is used extensively today in nursing education, allowing students to apply theory information in a "safe" setting. Clinical simulation can also involve a higher level of cognition, called analysis. At this level, the student or group of students are challenged to collect data, analyze data, and make collaborative client care decisions based on evidence.
4. **Analysis** means to be able to *break down complex information into its basic parts* and relate those parts to the big picture. An example of analysis is the ability to *organize and prioritize* (what is most important, most urgent) two or more pieces of information in a client situation to *process a safe response*. Analysis is a higher level of application. Being able to identify the most important symptoms that a client with a specific problem presents, including the initial nursing response, is an example of analysis.

Your instructors will expect you to have competence in clinical and simulation experiences by comprehending, applying, and analyzing data as you continue to develop your critical-thinking skills. Nursing students with past college enrollment and/or degrees often state that the consistent requirement to apply and analyze past and newly learned information in the LPN/LVN program greatly differs from their college experience. They say the educational environment is much more challenging. Comprehension, application, and analysis and ultimately clinical judgment are what employers expect of an LPN/LVN on the job.

Critical thinking has been the theme of this chapter; however, it was mentioned earlier that there is a greater expectation that the nurse will develop strong clinical judgment skills over time. This skill set, based on the NCSBN Clinical Judgment Measurement Model, includes the ability to Recognize Cues, Analyze Cues, Prioritize Hypotheses Generate Solutions, Take Actions, and Evaluate Outcomes (NCSBN, 2019). See Chapter 19 for detailed information.

The chapter text review questions include items similar to the NCLEX-PN® examination. These multiple-choice, alternate format, and NextGen items will test you at the application and analysis or higher levels. A few will challenge your beginning clinical judgment skills. They will help you understand the cognitive levels, help you prepare for testing, and support your continued development of critical-thinking skills.

The NCLEX-PN® Measures Expected Practice

Just as practice changes in your role, the licensure exam must measure that you have the minimum competence to be eligible for a LPN/LVN license to practice. The NCSBN has evolved over the years to measure that minimum competence. The NCSBN revises its NCLEX-PN® test plan every 3 years after the practice analysis is complete. Examples of revisions include integrating the nursing process throughout the test plan (NCSBN, 1998) with questions at the cognitive level of knowledge, comprehension, and application; integration of critical thinking in 2001, with examination questions at application and analysis level. Critical thinking is an integral part of the nursing process, and analysis is an essential component of critical thinking.

In 2005, the NCSBN introduced *alternate format items*. These items may include multiple response, fill-in-the-blank (e.g., calculation, ordered response), and hotspot (e.g., the place on a diagram that answers the question). All format items may have charts, tables, or graphic images. Alternate format items are included at the end of the chapter with review questions. You have access to more NCLEX-PN®–type questions in Evolve. Your school may also utilize an NCLEX success product throughout the program. It is essential that you complete all assignments. This enhances your critical thinking and ability to succeed on NCLEX style questions.

As a nurse, you have to think critically and use clinical judgment to deliver safe, effective nursing at the entry level. A dramatic change occurred in 2023: the Next-Generation (NGN) NCLEX-PN® introduced a newer testing method to measure clinical judgment.

The 2023 NCLEX-PN® test plan (NCSBN, 2023) indicates that critical thinking and clinical judgment are needed to integrate increasingly complex knowledge, skills, technologies, and client care activities into evidence-based nursing practice. Thus the ability to critically think and develop clinical judgment is an essential role of the LPN/LVN. See www.ncsbn.org for NCLEX® timeline details.

Clinical judgment and decision-making in nursing practice has been an essential research focus because determining nurses are responsible for a significant proportion of the judgments and decisions made in health care. Newly licensed nurses are required to make progressively more complex decisions about clients (ncsbn.org). It was determined that the Next Generation NCLEX® item types and the NCSBN Clinical Judgment Measurement Model (NCJMM) represent a valid and reliable measurement of RN and PN minimum competence. This was based originally on earlier RN and LPN/LVN Practice Analyses (https://www.ncsbn.org/search.page?q=lpn+practice+analysis). In 2023, the new clinical judgment item types were incorporated into the licensure exam to measure entry level practice clinical judgment abilities. Keep in mind that through studying, information stored in your long-term memory and your ability to recall comprehended information when needed (discussed in Chapter 2) will make a difference in being prepared for highly variable clinical situations and for success on the NCLEX-PN® examination.

MAKING IT WORK FOR YOU

As a reminder, we all have special, although different, thinking abilities. The trick is to discover those abilities, embrace them, and make them work for you. You can choose whether or not to make the most of your abilities. However, not deciding is also a decision. There is a tendency to be impressed by those who begin to speak immediately on an issue as though they have all the facts, when in truth, their style of processing is external. Perhaps your way is to process internally and not speak out until you have all the words in place. The one who processes externally may ask the questions you wish you had asked. This difference is personality. Their verbalization can sound impressive and may intimidate the person who processes internally before speaking. Both types can be equally effective in their ability to think critically. Each way is different; a difference in personality is all it has to be unless you allow yourself to begin thinking negatively about your abilities.

WHERE TO GO FROM HERE

This chapter is written as a critical-thinking primer, and it is limited to need-to-know information. The questions and suggestions offered are those that are within the scope of the LPN/LVN and the nursing program. **Reflective (critical) thinking** will assist you in determining if you need outside assistance from your school's study skills center or the instructor in setting up realistic observable goals/outcomes. You may even decide that the awareness of personal and situational characteristics is enough to get you started on your own. The critical-thinking exercises provide you with a practical framework for increasing your critical-thinking ability.

Get Ready for the Next-Generation NCLEX® Examination

Key Points

- Thinking is divided into unfocused thinking and directed thinking.
- Critical thinking answers the question "How can we do this better?" or "What is the problem?"
- To think critically, it is necessary to access information, comprehend (understand) information, store comprehended information in long-term memory, and recall the comprehended information when needed.
- Comprehension, application, analysis, and ultimately clinical judgment are what employers will expect from LPNs/LVNs on the job.
- The cognitive levels used in the NCLEX-PN® examination are knowledge, comprehension, application, and analysis. Questions are written at the application or higher level of cognitive thinking.
- The ability to read with understanding is the cornerstone of critical thinking.
- Both personal and situational factors influence critical thinking.
- The decision is yours whether to use the abilities you already possess to enhance your critical-thinking ability.
- Clinical judgment and decision making skills are essential to ensure your client's safety.

Additional Learning Resources

Go to your Evolve website (http://evolve.elsevier.com/Carroll/success/) for the following FREE learning resources:

- Answers to Critical Thinking Scenarios
- Additional learning activities
- Additional Review Questions for the NCLEX-PN® examination
- Helpful phrases for communicating in Spanish and more!

Clinical Judgment Questions

1. **Students are discussing why critical thinking is a necessary component of nursing education. Which of the following statements indicate that the students understand the concept of critical thinking?**
   - **a.** Critical thinking ensures that all health care team members could speak the same language.
   - **b.** Critical thinking focuses on the new acute disease processes that are emerging in the 21st century.
   - **c.** Critical thinking assists the nurse in integrating knowledge (evidence) and skills and technology, resulting in data-driven decision-making.
   - **d.** Critical thinking aligns the nurse with other professionals and elevates the nursing profession.
2. **Students attended a class focused on Bloom's taxonomy. Which of the following indicates a solid understanding of this concept?**
   - **a.** Knowledge is the ability to understand and apply information to a situation.
   - **b.** Knowledge is the ability to explain information in your own words.
   - **c.** Application is the ability to break down information into its component parts.
   - **d.** Application is the ability to apply learned information in a new situation.
3. **Students are discussing the value of critical thinking in nursing. Which behavior best demonstrates the application of critical thinking?**
   - **a.** The nursing student decides to humor a new client who is short-tempered, do what is necessary, and give the client plenty of space the rest of the time.
   - **b.** The nursing student decides to increase a client's intake by sitting on the bed and feeding him, despite the fact he can feed himself independently.
   - **c.** The nursing student observes a client is crying. She tells the nursing student her baby died after birth. The nursing student states "That was 40 years ago. You have 15 healthy grandchildren now."
   - **d.** The student nurse is asked to hold a client in position for a spinal tap. The student nurse holds him firmly in position and speaks softly and reassuringly.
4. **A friend of yours is attending an RN program. They state, "Only RNs use critical thinking to assist with decision-making." Which of the following is the best response?**
   - **a.** The RN is not the only member of the health care team.
   - **b.** The LPN also learns to think in a critical manner, working collaboratively with the RN. A collaborative effort has been shown to promote critical-thinking skills.
   - **c.** Critical thinking is really only done by health care providers.
   - **d.** All members of the health care team, licensed and nonlicensed, are expected to engage in critical thinking as a key aspect of their job description.
5. **Practical nursing students are engaged in a critical thinking class. Which of the following statements support reasons for why the nurse must think in a critical manner? (*Select all that apply.*)**
   - **a.** The client often has multiple diagnoses requiring complex treatment modalities.
   - **b.** The way nursing has always been done is the best it can be for nurse and clients.
   - **c.** Rapid change and information explosion create a need for new learning and skills.
   - **d.** The interdisciplinary team collaborates to develop the best plan of care for the client.
   - **e.** Evidence is available from multiple resources.
   - **f.** The RN supervisors have more experience and education than I do, so their decisions and guidance do not need to be questioned.
   - **g.** Technology and equipment are always updating or new. Instructions are available online.

6. Faculty are observed assisting students to learn to think critically. Which statements most accurately describe the planning process? (*Select all that apply.*)

- **a.** When you feel strongly about a situation, you are usually correct.
- **b.** Remind yourself that you are not always correct in your analysis.
- **c.** Listen to another opinion even if it contradicts what you believe.
- **d.** Remember that a client can provide you with subjective information.
- **e.** Collaborate with other health care team members to discuss complex client diagnoses.

Critical Thinking Scenarios

Scenario 1

A practical/vocational nursing student is assigned to a client with the diagnosis of possible depression. The police brought the client to the hospital when a neighbor became alarmed by the client's attempt to cut both wrists. During the past 2 days since the client was hospitalized, the staff have seen no behaviors that alarm them. The client has participated completed activities of daily living (ADLs) independently without prompting. During staff checks, the client appears to be sleeping at night, eats modest portions of food at mealtimes, and greets staff with a smile and inquires about helping others.

Today, the client will go to court (which is held in the hospital) to determine if the decision to be committed for care will be made. The nurse will accompany the client. The nurse is troubled because the client asked the nurse to maintain secrecy regarding the client's "holding it together" to be discharged after court. Once the client goes home, the client states that "I will kill myself and this time my plan is foolproof." The nurse is torn about the promise of secrecy knowing the suicide plan.

As the nurse sits in court and listens to the client's story, what critical-thinking steps will help the nurse reach a decision of what to do?

1. Analyze the situation. Provide a rationale for what the nurse is thinking.
2. Identify all possible alternatives. What is the rationale for each of the alternatives?
3. Choose the best alternative and provide the rationale.

Scenario 2

The correctional institution in your community has just begun hiring LPNs. You interviewed and were offered the job. As a new LPN, you are excited about this opportunity; however, you became concerned when you found out that you are the only nurse in the prison on night shift.

1. Identify what data you will collect to assist you in determining your best next steps.
2. Analyze the situation.
3. Discuss your options with a peer.
4. How would you proceed?

6 Ethics Applied to Nursing: Personal Versus Professional Ethics

Objectives

On completing this chapter, you will be able to do the following:

1. Explain the differences between ethics, morals, and values.
2. Differentiate between ethical and legal responsibilities in nursing.
3. Describe the basis of nursing ethics and how those may influence one's personal ethics.
4. Identify ethical elements in a state/territory/country's Nurse Practice Act.
5. Differentiate between personal and professional ethics.
6. Differentiate nonmaleficence, beneficence, autonomy, fidelity, veracity, and justice as principles of ethics, including nursing implications.
7. Identify differences between beneficence and beneficent paternalism.
8. Discuss how the nurse promotes a client's right to autonomy through considering a client's privacy, as well as cultural, religious, and personal values.
9. Discuss the basis for making ethical decisions in health care, including the ethical responsibilities of nurses.

Key Terms

autonomy
beneficence
beneficent paternalism
ethics
fidelity
justice
morals
nonmaleficence
nursing ethics
personal ethics
privacy
values
veracity

Keep In Mind

Nurses are challenged daily to make decisions in situations that are complex; ethical dilemmas complicate many scenarios.

Two student practical nurses/student vocational nurses (SPNs/SVNs) share with their clinical instructor a concern regarding a conversation they overheard while caring for a resident at the nursing home earlier in the week. The resident's son, accompanied by their friend, had arrived to visit. The son was trying to convince their mother to sign a new will. The resident was asking questions, and the son stated, "Just sign right on the line, Mom. Everything will be okay. Trust me." The students stated that the resident seemed very uncomfortable but did sign the will. The students did not say anything to the staff because they thought they were respecting the resident's autonomy. Plus, they did not think it was their concern. However, after completing their reading for their ethics class today, they believe they may have made a mistake and should have reported this event. Their instructor indicates that this is an important issue and will notify the nursing home. The instructor thanks the students for reporting their concern and directs them to report any ethical issues immediately in the future.

As you read this chapter, think about all the ethical issues that a nurse can face daily.

The 21st century presents numerous ethical issues in health care, as reflected in agency policies and medical procedures that create life, prolong life, cure chronic diseases, ensure a peaceful death, and end life. Additional ethical issues will arise as scientific research continues to explore possibilities while people press their right *of* mak*ing* autonomous decisions. A few examples of current ethical issues in health care include in vitro fertilization, artificial insemination, surrogate motherhood, cloning processes, organ donation (including cadaver donations), child organ donors, procedures that use fetal tissues (stem cells) or organs from aborted fetuses, conception of a child to produce tissue for a sibling, abortion, experiments that destroy a human embryo, euthanasia, assisted suicide, advance directives (including living wills and durable power of attorney), and insertion and/or withdrawal of feeding tubes.

A clinical example of an ethical issue follows: A client has verbalized to a health care provider their wish to avoid further heroic *actions* as a means to stay alive. Two adult children arrive and insist that all means need to be taken to maintain life, but the third child, already at the bedside, does not agree. The client, unconscious at this point, lacks a living will and durable power of attorney. You may encounter similar scenarios as a student participating in a clinical assignment. These learning experiences are instrumental in providing time for self-discovery, self-reflection, and self-analysis. Understanding your own ethical values is an effective first step to providing unbiased ethical care to your clients.

? Critical Thinking

How does a nurse analyze their personal ethical beliefs?

ETHICS, MORALS, AND VALUES

Ethics is a system of ideal standards that determine actions as being right or wrong. Ethics is concerned with the meaning of words such as *right, wrong, good, bad, ought*, and *duty*. Ethics is concerned with the way people, either individually or as a group, decide the following:

- Which actions are *right* or *wrong*
- Which actions *ought* to be done
- Which actions are one's *right* to do
- Which actions are one's *duty* to do

? Critical Thinking

How does the nurse avoid imposing their personal ethical beliefs in the clinical setting?

Morals are similar to ethics as both are concerned with right or wrong behavior (conduct) and character. Moral beliefs can be different across cultures. For example, research shows that Koreans base their morals on how others think they should act. Americans base their morals on how individuals think they personally should act (Seo et al., 2021). Morals may be influenced by factors such as an individual's culture. **Values** involve the worth a person assigns to an idea or an action. Values are freely chosen and are affected by age, experience, and maturity. A child usually embraces family values during childhood. The teen years are a time of trying out family values while incorporating them or rejecting and replacing them with new values. Values continue to be modified throughout a person's lifetime while acquiring new knowledge and experience. Based on changes in values, one's code of ethics/morals can shift (e.g., organ transplants after learning about or caring for a client who receives a transplant).

? Critical Thinking

Your school and clinical sites are guided by a set of values and beliefs. How do your personal values and beliefs align with these respective values and beliefs?

NURSING ETHICS AND LEGAL ASPECTS OF NURSING

The law is thought to be a minimum ethic that is written and enforced. For licensed practical nurses/licensed vocational nurses (LPNs/LVNs), the Nurse Practice Act (NPA) in their state in which they are employed is the final authority on what LPNs/LVNs are legally obligated to do as a nurse regardless of where you are employed (see Chapter 7 for more about nursing and the law). It is essential for LPNs/LVNs to have a thorough knowledge of the NPA from their state.

Nursing ethics are similar to, but also different from, the legal aspects that regulate nursing practice. Table 6.1 presents a comparison of legal aspects and nursing ethics.

Table 6.1 Comparison of Legal Aspects and Nursing Ethics

	LEGAL ASPECTS	NURSING ETHICS
Definition	The state statutes that apply to licensed people and the situations in client care that could result in legal action	Set of rules of conduct (moral and practical) that guide decision-making
Focus	Rules and regulations Obligations under the law Safe care	Ideal behavior of a group of licensed people Morality Higher standards
Applies to	Member of a professional/career group	Member of a nursing group
Participation	Mandatory	Voluntary but expected
Source	Your state's Nurse Practice Act	NALPN and NAPNES codes, Florence Nightingale Pledge, PN Pledge

NALPN, National Association of Licensed Practical Nurses; *NAPNES*, National Association for Practical Nurse Education and Service; *PN*, practical nurse.

NURSING ETHICS

According to the *Miller-Keane Encyclopedia & Dictionary of Medicine, Nursing & Allied Health*, **nursing ethics** is described as "the values and ethical principles governing nursing practice, conduct, and relationships." Nursing ethics deals with the relationship of a nurse to the client, the client's family, associates and fellow nurses, and society at large. Nursing ethics attempts to look for underlying patterns or order in many ethical decisions and practices of nurses, individually or as a group. Codes provide a guideline for what the LPN/LVN ought to do. However, codes do not carry the weight of the law.

It is interesting to note how many ethical items are found in the law, such as in an NPA. When ethical items are included in a legal document, it places emphasis on the importance of these items. The law gives the LPN/LVN a source to fall back on to defend the choices in behavior made when caring for clients and families.

Because nursing education and the nursing profession promote the nursing process, critical thinking, and a focus on the total client (not just the physical disease or injured portion of the client), nursing ethics have advanced. The ethical principles in this chapter are about the application of nursing ethics to nursing decisions and action. SPNs/SVNs are encouraged to look at both sides of an ethical principle. Recognize that no principle applies in the same way to all clients; recognize the client's unique situation. No principle is absolute.

Critical thinking (see Chapter 5) plays a major role in sorting out ethical choices and legal responsibilities regarding the client. The client's knowledge of choices regarding care also affects their ethical decision-making.

NURSING CODE OF ETHICS AND THE NURSE PRACTICE ACT

Ethics are adopted by nursing groups in their codes of behavior. Both the National Association for Practical Nurse Education and Service (NAPNES; www.napnes.org) and the National Association of Licensed Practical Nurses (NALPN; www.nalpn.org) have ethical codes for LPNs/LVNs.

Try This

Ethical Issues and Your Nurse Practice Act

Discover how your state includes ethical issues (what you ought to do as an LPN/LVN) in the law, which is your Nurse Practice Act (what you must do as a licensed person).

- Search for the elements of these ethical codes in your Nurse Practice Act. Fill out the following worksheet.
- Summarize the ethical elements found in the Nurse Practice Act.

ETHICAL AREA	IS THIS ETHICAL AREA ADDRESSED IN YOUR STATE'S NURSE PRACTICE ACT?	IF "YES," CITE SECTION
1. Know and understand the scope of maximum utilization of the LPN/LVN, as specified by the Nurse Practice Act, and function within this scope.		
2. Safeguard the confidential information about the client, acquired from any source.		
3. Provide health care to all clients, regardless of race, creed, cultural background, disease, or lifestyle (e.g., single parent, sexual orientation).		
4. Refuse to give endorsement to the sale or promotion of commercial products or services.		
5. Uphold the highest standards in personal appearance, language, dress, and demeanor.		
6. Adhere to a community standard of justice, honesty, and good morals.		
7. Stay informed about issues affecting the practice of nursing and the delivery of health care, and, where appropriate, participate in government and policy decisions.		
8. Accept the responsibility for safe nursing practice by keeping mentally and physically fit and educationally prepared to practice.		
9. Strive to deliver the highest quality of care keeping current with best practices and the use of information technology.		
10. Accept the responsibility for membership in NALPN or the LPN/LVN organization of your choice and participate in its efforts to maintain the established standards of nursing practice and employment policies that lead to quality client care.		

PERSONAL CODE OF ETHICS OF NURSES

SPNs/SVNs and LPNs/LVNs have **personal ethics** that provide personal guidelines for living. A person ultimately chooses what their personal code of ethics includes. A nurse's personal code of ethics will influence their nursing ethics. Sometimes personal ethics conflict with the law (state's NPA). When this occurs, LPNs/LVNs have an obligation to follow the law.

If *LPNs/LVNs* object to a medical procedure on religious or moral grounds, *they should* discuss this concern during the interview process. This objection may be incompatible with the job description and the mission and beliefs of the institution. In this case, *the LPN/LVN is* not the right "fit" for the job. However, if an institution initiates a new procedure/service during *LPNs'/LVNs'* employment period that challenges *personal* religious or moral beliefs, *they should* discuss and submit in writing *their* objections. *They should* present the statement to *the* employer, including a possible solution to the issue. For example, *an LPN/LVN* may be ethically opposed to abortion. Abortion in the United States is permitted under certain circumstances. *An LPN/LVN* may ethically wish to refuse to assist with the abortion procedure.

Proactively creating a plan may prevent an ethical dilemma for *LPNs/LVNs*. However, *LPNs/LVNs* cannot refuse to give nursing care if needed. Abandonment is a legal matter, and maintaining *a* license may be at risk. The best strategy is to seek employment in a health agency that does not participate in procedures or nursing care of which *one* does not ethically approve.

Some nurses have tried to opt out of caring for clients who have an illness that may be related to a lifestyle of which they do not approve. A nurse needs to separate personal ethics from nursing ethics. *Nurses* are legally expected to care for a client regardless of their lifestyle. For example, when caring for a client with acquired immune deficiency syndrome (AIDS), *nurses should* use proper techniques during care as *they* would with any client with an infectious disease. You may not refuse to care for this client. Ethically and legally this client must receive the same level of care, with dignity and respect, that other clients do. Nursing is not about giving care selectively to those clients *the nurse* approves of and refusing care to others that have different beliefs or a different lifestyle.

? Critical Thinking

Personal Values

Write down your personal value system regarding health and illness. To get started, think about your family's value system. Be concerned with content, not form. What you write will be an ethical code in progress. You may want to add or subtract statements after you have completed this chapter. It will also be a code you can modify as your experience with clients increases.

PRINCIPLES OF ETHICS

As nurses in the 21st century, LVNs/LPNs recognize there is something unique that a nurse has to offer clients beyond the dependent role to health care providers. This realization places greater responsibility on SPNs/SVNs to learn all they can during the nursing program of study. For example, SPNs/SVNs can add knowledge of basic ethics to critical thinking as they assist the RN with the nursing process. The data SPNs/SVNs collect will have an added dimension of ethics. It will make a difference in developing a quality care plan that considers the client as a whole person and not just the part of his or her body that is sick.

At this level, SPNs/LVNs incorporate a basic understanding of how SPNs/SVNs and LPNs/LVNs practice nursing according to nursing codes. Learning about ethics is more than being able to recite the definition to pass a test; it means being able to help make ethical decisions when ethical dilemmas arise.

The following ethical principles are discussed in this chapter:

1. Nonmaleficence (do no harm)
2. Beneficence (do good)
3. Autonomy (free to choose)
4. Fidelity (be faithful)
5. Veracity (be truthful)
6. Justice (fair to all)

NONMALEFICENCE (DO NO HARM)

In the book *Leadership and Management According to Florence Nightingale*, Nightingale indicated that the first step of nursing should be to care for the sick without causing harm to them. Nightingale is referring to the ethical principle **nonmaleficence**, which comes from the Latin primum non nocere, meaning "first do no harm."

Nonmaleficence is the basis of many of the "rules" promoted by your instructors, such as the following:

- Six rights for giving medications.
- Use of ISBARR/SBAR (Introduction, Situation, Background, Assessment, Recommendation, Repeat/Situation, Background, Assessment, Recommendation) in collaboration with the RN for interdisciplinary communication (See Chapter 8 for details).
- Checking the temperature of bath or shower water.
- Checking the temperature of formula before feeding the infant or child.
- Returning the bed to its lowest position after completing a treatment or preparing to leave the room.
- Raising side rails after nursing care if it is in the plan of care.
- Providing care for your clients when their ethical principles conflict with yours.
- Performing only necessary procedures on clients, instead of unnecessary procedures just to gain additional experience.
- Protecting those who cannot protect themselves, for example, protecting clients who have a cognitive disability or who are unconscious, weak, or debilitated.

If the principle of nonmaleficence is taken to the extreme, however, SPNs/SVNs and LPNs/LVNs would not be able to perform many nursing duties. Few beneficial treatments are entirely without harm, including the following:

- Puncture the client's skin with a needle; there is some tissue damage, a risk of infection, and the possibility of an undesirable reaction to a solution if administered.
- Administration of medications can cause side effects: rare, serious, and mild.
- Insertion of a tube into a bodily opening (e.g., catheterization, irrigating a colostomy) could cause some trauma to surrounding tissue. There is the possibility of introducing infection and penetrating the tissue wall.
- Performance of a procedure can hurt a client physically (e.g., positioning a client properly after surgery, cleansing the mouth of an elderly client who has not had proper mouth care for a period, irrigating a pressure ulcer, moving a client with osteoporosis from bed to chair to toilet and back).
- Administration of a vaccine carries the risk of the client experiencing a side effect, but the overall effect for most people is the prevention of serious diseases.
- Administration of a solution through an intravenous (IV) line can cause harm. One thing to continually monitor is that the solution and additive, if any, are infusing as the health care provider ordered. A common additive is KCl (potassium chloride). KCl, within a narrow blood level range, is necessary for proper heart functioning. If too little or too much is administered, it can result in heart dysfunction, sometimes resulting in death. (Jack Kevorkian, a health care provider who participated in several assisted suicides, used KCl.) KCl can save lives, but it can also kill.
- Performing range of motion to an extremity after a stroke can elicit some discomfort because of stiff and slightly contracted muscles.

Each of the preceding procedures has the potential for doing good and doing harm. The question always is how to do the least amount of harm when doing something that is expected to result in good. The obvious answer is to never knowingly participate in any action that will deliberately harm a client. The client must also have agreed to the procedure verbally or in writing, depending on the procedure (clients have autonomy). This is the reason for practicing procedures in the nursing lab; preparing for nursing care; reviewing your nursing care plan with the instructor; and reviewing medication dosage, action, and side effects with the instructor before giving the medication to a client.

The following are negative examples of nursing actions that were meant to do no harm but resulted in injury:

- Putting down a client's side rail without first checking that the client's arm is not hanging between the rail and the bed. The client who immediately comes to mind is an 80-year-old client whose arm was fractured and who received several skin tears and bruises. The staff person who put the rail down was irritated because of "a bad night shift" and was hurrying to get off duty.
- Rapidly feeding large spoonfuls of food to a client who has a dry mouth as a side effect of medication. Because of the lack of liquid before beginning to eat, large spoonfuls of food, lack of adequate time to chew, and lack of additional liquid before the next bite, the client aspirated some of the food that accumulated in their mouth. The client survived but refused future attempts to eat when he or she saw the same nurse come in with their food tray.
- Applying an external (Texas) catheter (condom-like catheter applied to a male's penis) incorrectly, causing constriction of circulation resulting in gangrene of the penis. The client's penis required amputation.
- Leaving the bed in a high position and the client subsequently falls.

Try This

Procedures and Their Effects

Think about procedures with which you are familiar. Review the procedure. List two procedures that "do good" but also have the potential to do harm. State both the good and potential harmful effects of each procedure.

BENEFICENCE (DO GOOD)

Beneficence means to "do good" with nursing actions and is the basis of trust in nursing. It also involves preventing harm and removing harm. Nonmaleficence and beneficence are often difficult to separate and may go hand in hand. The following major nursing duties to the client are associated with beneficence:

1. Put the client's interests first, for example:
    - LPNs/LVNs do not go off duty until they hand over the care of clients to an equally skilled nursing staff to continue the nursing care. LPNs/LVNs are obligated to report to the nurse taking over the next shift what had transpired during the time they were responsible for nursing care.
    - When nurses give the wrong medication, they should report it as soon as they recognize the error. Their ethical concern is to "do good" and "prevent harm." Beneficence is a concern for the greater good than concern for self by reporting errors. In addition, an individual error may be related to a system error. Prompt reporting and investigation can minimize a similar event from occurring in the future. Unsafe staffing levels can be a root cause of many errors and need to be reported.
    - You go to work even though you are tempted to call in sick because you want to go out of town for the weekend.
2. Place the good of clients before the nurse's needs. This is where interpretation of duty gets more complex. Does this mean that duty to the client means

utmost sacrifice? No, it does not, but it does mean that a nurse may sacrifice something. Key points follow:

- Client needs are above organizational needs. LPNs/LVNs may have administrative responsibilities (perhaps as charge nurses) that must be completed by the end of the day, or they may have meetings they are expected to attend that day. If a client needs their skill and expertise, as in an emergency, their first duty is to the client.
- Prioritizing *doing good* to clients before the LPN's/LVN's needs does *not* mean that the LPN/LVN behaves as though no one in the world can assume the nursing care her or she can give to clients. LPNs/LVNs should not stay past their scheduled hours when there is someone ready to assume responsibility for nursing care. This also means that they do not call the client from home, accept calls at home from the client, or visit the client after hours. If an LPN/LVN is doing any of this, he or she has just entered an unhealthy codependent relationship with the client. These behaviors are usually prohibited by employers.
- Situations can be difficult. For example, a nurse receives an emergency phone call regarding a sick child and leaves abruptly. This would be viewed as client abandonment. A nurse must always ensure that the client receives adequate nursing care in their absence. Reporting off to the supervising RN and the colleague who is capable/competent of receiving the assignment is essential.

? Critical Thinking

Ethical Obligations

When a client is demanding, angry, or uncooperative and threatens to become violent, is the nurse obligated to put themselves in danger of serious harm? Are nurses ethically obligated to perform heroic acts of self-sacrifice?

Beneficent Paternalism

Beneficent paternalism continues to be confused with the ethic of beneficence. Beneficent paternalism is a disrespectful *attitude* toward the client and what the client can contribute to personal care and recovery. It is an "I know what's best for you" attitude that discounts the client's knowledge of self. The following are examples of beneficent paternalism:

- An LPN/LVN concludes that a client fits into a "specific category," discounting what the client wants the nurse to know. Many medication errors could have been avoided if nurses listened to clients when they stated, "That pill looks different to me." This error may occur in part because of beneficent paternalism. When assisting with collecting data, nurses should really *hear* what the client is trying to say.
- An LPN/LVN assists in developing the care plan without client input, reflecting the nurse's needs, not the client's needs. Later, the nurse complains that the client is noncompliant and will not cooperate with the plan of care. Nurse should ask themselves: "Did the client know what the alternatives were for treatment of this condition?" and "Did the client have the opportunity to offer input into the plan and agree to what the care plan would be?" It is difficult for clients to cooperate when they are not empowered.
- If the client asks a nurse's opinion for the choice, and the nurse responds with, "Well, if I were you, I would . . ." instead of saying, "The health care provider explained the alternatives for treatment and the possible side effects of each, and it is for you to decide what is best for you."

Beneficent paternalism is justified only in extreme circumstances and is most often a medical decision. An example would be a health care provider approaching the court to be allowed to do a potentially lifesaving procedure when parents have refused to sign an authorized treatment form for the child.

Paternalism and women's health. The issue of paternalism toward women in medical research and receiving health care is slowly changing through the efforts of women themselves and the advocacy of nurses. The term *paternalism* is derived from a Latin word that means "father" (i.e., father knows best). In the health care system, it can be interpreted as "the health care provider knows best because of their superior knowledge." Because the word is derived from the Latin word *pater*, some may believe that men know better than women.

Health care providers define what is considered ill health for women. Anything that is normally different from men is considered an illness and requires the health care provider's intervention. Because women are different from men biologically, medicine has defined what is normal for women as being abnormal. For example, menstruation, pregnancy, and menopause have been defined in the past as ill health instead of normal, healthy processes. Although this trend still can exist, great strides have been made in women's health care. Many factors have contributed, including the increase in female health care providers and empowerment of nurses and females, in general, in the United States.

Advocacy for women remains an important responsibility. Nurses should consider speaking up when they see decisions being made based on incomplete information (e.g., the health care provider or other health care worker not really listening to a female client). SPNs/SVNs will learn about assertiveness and personal responsibility in Chapter 9 of this book. An aggressive, rude approach does not gain someone anything except a bad reputation among peers and clients.

SPNs/SVNs should consider practicing assertiveness and remembering that change will occur slowly. Many female clients are already experiencing a change and assertively state their needs. Nurses who advocate for their female clients assist in this process of reducing a paternalistic attitude toward women, one client at a time, as the need arises, promoting justice.

? Critical Thinking

Do I Respond Differently to Male and Female Clients?

Keep track of the differences in your responses to male and female clients for 2 or 3 days. Record your response to the male or female client and what the client said.

When you think you have enough examples, review the data you have collected. Use critical thinking to determine what differences you noted in your response to male and female clients. Because this is for your eyes only, be candid. Are there any changes that you recommend for yourself? If so, write them down.

AUTONOMY (FREE TO CHOOSE)

Yoder-Wise (2019) describes **autonomy** as "the principal in which individuals are free to make personal choices about future happenings, while being accountable for those personal choices." We expect people to respect our rights, and we respect their rights as long as their rights do not interfere with someone else's rights. However, autonomy does not mean that clients can do whatever they want. Autonomy means the following:

- *Thinking* through all the facts
- *Deciding* based on an independent thinking process
- *Acting* based on a personal decision
- *Undertaking a decision voluntarily* without pressure, direct or subtle, from anyone else

For clients to make an autonomous decision, they must have all the facts without leaving out information to influence the decision in a particular way. For example, the nurse may unintentionally (sometimes intentionally) influence the client's decision by repeating what the health care provider has suggested as if it is best for the client ("The health care provider would not have suggested the treatment if he did not think it best for you").

There is also a fine line between autonomy and abandonment. Excessive control means interfering too much in a client's life. Not interfering enough results is neglect of the client. Here are some examples of autonomy:

- The right of the elderly to make decisions about their treatment
- A client's right to refuse treatment

More information is needed in both situations to determine if interference is recommended.

Role of Privacy in Autonomy

Privacy is both an ethical and a legal issue. Autonomy includes a client's right to privacy. This is the reason your instructor asks a client directly for permission to allow SPNs/SVNs to observe a particular treatment or to do a procedure. Similarly, the instructor checks with the client before assigning a student to give nursing care. In some cases, clients can sign consent upon admission to have students from all disciplines, participate in their care. The client has the right to refuse care from any practitioner, including the student nurse. Privacy includes the right to choose care based on personal beliefs, feelings, or attitudes, as well as the right to decide what is done to their body (accepting or rejecting treatment or exposure of the body). SPNs/SVNs will need to respect the client's decision. When giving care, such as giving a bath or inserting a urinary catheter, they should avoid exposing the client needlessly during the care. *This is an invasion of privacy.*

Role of Culture, Religion, and Personal Values in Autonomy

Culture or a religious belief system may be contrary to the accepted medical ethics. Examples of decisions based on culture and religion include the following:

- The client, a young woman, is diagnosed with breast cancer. Her husband has received a complete explanation from the health care provider about her illness, alternatives for each treatment, anticipated effects, possible side effects, and prognosis with each treatment. Her husband will not permit any treatment to take place (culture based).
- The client, a Jehovah's Witness, could benefit from a blood transfusion due to severe blood loss. The adult client has refused because blood transfusions are prohibited by their religion (religion based).
- If the client is an underage child, the parents may forbid the blood transfusion on religious grounds. The health care provider can decide to go to court to ask the court to overrule the parents' decision. An underage child is too young to understand all the facts to decide on informed consent. Parents can *authorize treatment* for what is appropriate for their children up to a certain age. In this case, the health care provider has decided that the value of beneficence is greater than the value of respect for the parents' autonomy. The court has greater authority and will decide if the health care provider can transfuse the child.
- A client in their late 60s is diagnosed with advanced prostate cancer. He has refused treatment, even though he understands that, although not curative, the surgery could result in less discomfort for a period and more time to live (personal value based).

FIDELITY (BE FAITHFUL)

Fidelity challenges each LPN/LVN to be faithful to the charge of acting in the client's best interest when the capacity to make free choice is no longer available to the client. This does not include rescuing behaviors and becoming paternalistic in making decisions for vulnerable clients (legal competency will be described in Chapter 7). LPNs/LVNs must *differentiate* between their feelings and choices regarding an issue and the feelings and wishes of the client. These points are foremost in decision-making. Charting the client's feelings and wishes as expressed, without personal interpretation, provides information for the health care provider when important decisions need to be considered. Examples of breaching fidelity include the following:

- Discussing a client in a public area such as the cafeteria, an elevator, at home, or when a nurse is out with friends. SPNs/SVNS should never mention a client by name or discuss any specific client characteristics or a detailed plan of care. These activities could allow individuals to conclude who the SPN/SVN is speaking about due to the unique characteristics shared. In doing so, fidelity and confidentiality (a legal term) would both be compromised, as would the client's dignity. The action says the client has limited worth in the eyes of the nurse and chips away at the client's dignity.
- Speaking disrespectfully about an obese client and complaining about how difficult it is to move them. SPNs/SVNs may consider what they would do if they overheard a nurse speaking this way. Why would they take this action? Is it an ethical response?

An SPN/SVN makes the decisions regarding what he or she should do when away from the immediate support and supervision of instructors. To ignore fidelity creates an ethical dilemma and a potential legal consequence. Dismissal from school or termination from a job could be the result.

VERACITY (BE TRUTHFUL)

Veracity is an important ethical principle involving truth. Nurses should report and document information accurately (ANA, 2024). It is unethical to report or document false information because it conflicts with the ethical principle of veracity. Another important aspect to remember about truth is that individuals are more accepting of instruction when they perceive the instructor as being honest. Likewise, clients accept education more easily when they perceive the nurse is expressing information accurately. Living a life of truthfulness or honesty allows a nurse to easily practice veracity on the job.

Veracity is not a clear concept at times. A dilemma could occur when telling the truth may not seem to benefit the client. For example, a client with dementia who believes their family member visits every day may become upset when being told that the family member has not visited for over a week. Although beneficial lies may appear to be desirable in certain circumstances, this could cause a conflict with one's belief in the obligation of truthfulness. It is important to carefully choose words appropriately. The nurse caring for the patient with dementia could say, "Let's see if your family member comes in today" to redirect the client's thinking.

JUSTICE (FAIR TO ALL)

Justice means that SPNs/SVNs and LPNs/LVNs must deliver fair and equal treatment to all clients, recognizing and avoiding personal bias. For example, each client with the same diagnosis should receive the same level of care. Being fair does not mean giving every client the same things. It means treating them all the same with high-quality care (i.e., with dignity and respect). As a nurse, you make daily decisions to provide the highest quality of care possible.

Personal bias can cloud our vision as nurses. Identifying hidden bias can assist the LPN/LVN in providing justice to all clients. For example, if clients in the hospital setting represent different levels of wealth, social status, culture, religion, and moral and value systems, yet all of them are acutely ill, is the LPN/LVN able to provide equal, yet client-centered care?

Consider the client who has Kaposi sarcoma, a defining component of AIDS. Do LPNs/LVNs classify AIDS as a life-threatening illness or as retribution for behaviors they consider immoral? If personal ethics interfere with the actions of LPNs/LVNs, they may find themselves giving this client more time than needed and doing less than needed for other acutely ill clients or providing minimal care to the client and lavishing attention on those who "deserve the care."

Consider a young, single mother who has five children and just found out she is pregnant. How a nurse proceeds can be impacted by a personal bias, if the nurse personally feels the pregnancy should have been prevented. All clients must be treated equally. This is the nurse's ethical duty.

It is within the nurse's power to make decisions about daily issues related to justice of individuals. Be careful to hear hidden bias within oneself: "They are so young; so much living left to do" or "They had a full life already" or "They are an alcoholic; never took care of their kids" and so on. Identifying a bias will assist the LPN/LVN in providing "just" care. Visit the following website to identify hidden biases: https://implicit.harvard.edu/implicit/takeatest.html

> **? Critical Thinking**
>
> At the end of your next clinical day, take time to reflect on your reaction to clients and how it affected your client's care. Did the word *deserve* enter your thoughts, or did you provide justice for all? Listen to the health care team. Did you hear any comments that would make you question if the quality of justice was met? If so, what did you do?

LPNs/LVNs should report clients' comments regarding ethical matters to the RN. Final ethical decisions are not within the LPN/LVN scope of nursing practice. Recall also that ethics is what nurses *ought* to do; law is what nurses *must* do.

ETHICAL DECISIONS IN HEALTH CARE

ETHICS COMMITTEES

Because of complex ethical scenarios, health agencies such as hospitals, hospice units, and long-term care settings establish ethics committees. This multidisciplinary team, which often consists of nurses, health care providers, clergy, social worker, and other allied health members, assists with difficult ethical decisions. Usually, discussions relate to new or unusual ethical questions. The recommendations of the ethics committee are expected to be given serious consideration by all stakeholders. In a faith-based organization, the principles of faith can be anticipated to impact the decision-making of this committee. Keep in mind that clients are influenced by their culture-based and/or religion-based ethics. What people can and cannot do regarding health care has already been established by the culture of which they are a part. See Chapters 10 and 11 for a discussion of cultural and spiritual needs, spiritual care, and religious differences.

WESTERN SECULAR BELIEF SYSTEM

In the Western secular belief system, the emphasis is shifted from duties to the rights of the individual. This system has the following characteristics:

1. *Individual autonomy* means "self-rule." Individuals have the capacity to think and, based on these thoughts, make decisions freely whether to seek health care (the freedom to choose).
2. *Individual rights* mean the ability to assert one's rights. The extent to which a client can exert his or her rights is restricted (i.e., their rights cannot restrict the rights of others). For example, the client's right to refuse treatment can be at odds with the health professional's perceived duty to always act in a way that will benefit the client (do good and prevent harm). Individual rights have become a central theme of health care:
   a. Right to consent to care
   b. Right to choose between alternative treatments
   c. Right to consent or refuse treatment
   d. Women's rights over their own bodies

Numerous bills of rights have been written, and fierce debates have taken place at both state and national levels. The question of individual autonomy and individual rights is far from being settled. Recently, some laws based on individual autonomy and rights have been passed (e.g., Health Care Reform; death with dignity laws). However, attempts to rescind laws that have been passed continue. The question is: To what extent do one's moral decisions (rights) get in the way of another's moral autonomy?

? Critical Thinking

Personal Beliefs That May Affect Medical Decisions

What cultural or religious values do you hold that may affect personal health care decisions?

Discuss with your significant other, family, coworkers, and peers your response. Reflect on how your discussion varied. Next, project to the future: Given the diverse client populations you will encounter as a student and as an LPN/LVN, how often will you encounter personal beliefs that differ from your own? Think about how you will respect the client's autonomy in these situations.

ETHICAL RESPONSIBILITIES OF NURSES

As the nurse's role has evolved from simply following physician orders to critically thinking, it is logical that the number of ethical issues has also increased. Adding the nursing process and critical thinking to nursing education changed the nursing focus to the whole client. Although the interdependent roles of the health care team members remain, unique responsibilities were added to nurses. The following responsibilities, both ethical and legal, emerged:

1. *Client advocacy:* Client advocacy is a key role of all nurses. Clients are often in a vulnerable state when they need nursing care because of the symptoms of the illness and because of the complexity of health care delivery. As a result, their need for advocacy often increases.

   Knowledge is power. Thus informing the client of the plan of care is essential. This needs to be done at least every shift and more often if indicated by the client's condition. Information, as simple as explaining the steps of a procedure, will empower clients. LPNs/LVNs need to include a brief overview of the role of all the members of the health care team in the plan of care.

   At times, LPNs/LVNs may need to advocate ensuring the plan of care is not altered inappropriately because of an error or misjudgment. Advocacy is usually done in collaboration with the RN. LPNs/LVNs need to fully understand their advocacy role. In most states, the LPN's/LVN's role is to support teaching done by the RN, health care provider, or other members of the health care team. If clients have questions, and LPNs/LVNs are unsure about whether they should provide an answer, they can discuss the next steps with the RN.

   When the client makes a decision, it is important that LPNs/LVNs are supportive even though they may not agree with the decision. LPNs/LVNs should ensure that the client has enough knowledge and resources (evidence) to make an informed decision. If not, the LPN/LVN can seek out the resources needed and offer them to the client.

2. *Accountability:* The word *accountability* means that a nurse is answerable to themselves, to their assigned client and their family, to their supervisor, to the health care team, and to their manager who evaluates their work. Accountability to the educational instructor as an SPN/SVN is replaced by accountability to the employing agency as an LPN/LVN. The LPN/LVN is held accountable for all the nursing actions performed or are assigned to perform. The measure of accountability is the nursing standards of practice. What a prudent nurse with education and experience would do in a similar situation becomes the standard.
3. *Client safety reporting:* It is the responsibility of the nurse to report behaviors of peers, supervisors, or any team members that are potentially harmful to clients (e.g., impaired at work because of alcohol and/or other drug use, stealing client's medication, substituting water or normal saline for injectable narcotics, leaving unstable clients unattended in the shower, sleeping while on duty, and displaying verbal or physical abuse).
4. *System-based issues:* Identifying system-based issues is essential to providing safe high-quality care (e.g., if new procedures are implemented without appropriate education and training on all shifts, the LPN/LVN needs to notify administration and suggest a plan to ensure safe practice). The role of the LPN/LVN in promoting ethics in health care involves client advocacy, personal accountability, incident reporting, and process improvement.

Get Ready for the Next-Generation NCLEX® Examination

Key Points

- Ethics is concerned with the meaning of words such as *right, wrong, good, bad, ought*, and *duty*.
- Nursing ethics provides guidelines for making ethical decisions in nursing.
- LPNs/LVNs need to be aware of the contents of their state's Nurse Practice Act regarding ethical issues.
- Ethics is something an SPN/SVN *should/ought to* do. However, ethics themselves do not carry the weight of the law.
- The content of the law (state's Nurse Practice Act) is something the SPN/SVN must do.
- SPNs/SVNs and LPNs/LVNs must know the nursing code of ethics and not confuse it with their personal code of ethics.
- The nursing role is now viewed as a collaborative role, providing nursing care to the whole client and being a client advocate as a member of the health care team.
- Encounters with ethical dilemmas have increased as the LPN transitions from a "doer" to a "thinker."
- Cultural and religious backgrounds and personal values may influence ethical decisions of clients seeking health care.
- Nonmaleficence means "do no harm." Few treatments are entirely harmless.
- Beneficence means to "do good" with your nursing actions and is the basis of trust in nursing.
- Autonomy means respect for a client's right to choose, if the client's rights do not interfere with the rights of others.
- Fidelity means to be faithful or dutiful. It challenges SPNs/SVNs and LPNs/LVNs to be faithful to the charge of acting in the client's best interests, even when the capacity of free choice is not available to the client because of his or her condition.
- Veracity means to tell the truth or be honest. The SPN/SVN and the LPN/LVN must be accurate with their communication, whether in reporting to others or in their documentation.
- Justice means that the SPN/SVN and the LPN/LVN must give the same level of care to all clients, with dignity and respect.
- The LPN/LVN has an ethical objection to carefully evaluate a job role before employment and avoid employment where ethical issues will routinely occur (e.g., working at Planned Parenthood while having a pro-life personal belief system).
- Beneficent paternalism is justified only in extreme circumstances and is most often a medical decision.
- Paternalism in women's health care is decreasing. Nurses' advocacy for women helps promote this change, one client at a time.

Additional Learning Resources

Go to your Evolve website (http://evolve.elsevier.com/Carroll/success/) for the following FREE learning resources:

- Answers to Critical Thinking Scenarios
- Additional learning activities
- Additional Review Questions for the NCLEX-PN® examination
- Helpful phrases for communicating in Spanish and more!

Clinical Judgment Questions

1. **SPNs/SVNs are discussing the concept of ethics. What statement indicates the SPN's/SVN's best understanding of the concept of ethics?**
   a. "Ethics is an understanding of each person's legal right to access care."
   b. "Ethics is the worth assigned to an idea or an action, freely chosen, affected by maturity."
   c. "An understanding to the meanings of words, such as *right, wrong, good, bad, ought*, and *duty*, is important to ethical decision-making."
   d. "An understanding of the customs, habits, and behaviors in a society that are approved by that society describes the term ethics."

2. The nursing profession has evolved over time. What statement best describes how the nursing profession has evolved?

a. Nursing discovered its unique role in providing care for the whole client, not just the diseased part, using evidence to make decisions.
b. Nurses now view themselves as independent practitioners, able to meet all their clients' needs.
c. Due to the implementation of the nursing process and critical thinking in nursing schools, nurses now need to think independently to develop the best client plan of care.
d. Nurses discovered that nursing education and textbooks have changed but not the work on client care units.

3. A parent has refused a blood transfusion for their 2-year-old son, but the health care provider has asked the court to overrule their refusal. What is the nurse's best response?

a. "In your child's case, beneficent paternalism [explain the term] overrules respect for your autonomy."
b. "In this hospital, the health care provider knows best because of their superior knowledge."
c. "We have saved many children by ignoring parents' religious beliefs and doing what is best."
d. "The child is too young to understand and make their own choice in something this serious."

4. After seemingly successful treatment for depression and a serious suicide attempt, a client will be in court this morning to be reviewed for release. The client tells the SPN/SVN, "As soon as I get out, I am going to kill myself. Promise me you won't tell anyone." What is the best ethical action by the SPN/SVN?

a. The SPN/SVN promises not to tell anyone. Their personal ethic is to never break a promise when one is made.
b. Despite respect for the client's autonomy, ensuring a safe environment is essential. The SPN/SVN reports the client's comment to their supervisor.
c. The SPN/SVN believes in waiting to see what will happen and plans to do the same during the court hearing.
d. The SPN/SVN keeps the promise made to the client but checks on the client very frequently.

5. An SPN/SVN is discussing the steps necessary to make an autonomous decision. Which statements indicate that the SPN/SVN understands the steps of autonomous decision-making? (*Select all that apply.*)

a. Voluntary without pressure
b. Fair to all parties involved
c. The health care provider suggests his personal solution
d. The nurse provides evidence to assist the client in decision-making
e. Personal gain is achieved

6. SPNs/SVNs are discussing the difference between personal and professional ethics. The SPN/SVN indicates understanding of this concept by identifying which statements are true and which are false.

	TRUE STATEMENT	FALSE STATEMENT
a. Personal ethics means the same as beneficent paternalism.		
b. Professional ethics sometimes conflict with the law.		
c. Personal ethics provide guidelines for one's life.		
d. Professional ethics means you cannot abandon the client.		
e. Personal ethics can conflict with professional ethics.		

7. The nurse is caring for a 74-year-old client who is on a medical-surgical floor and has a known diagnosis of squamous cell carcinoma of the bladder for the past 6 months:

Nurses' Notes	
1100	Client is complaining of sharp abdominal pain, nausea, and difficulty urinating even though his bladder feels full. Vitals signs: T: 100.0 °F, P: 92, RR: 22, BP: 148/92. Pulse Ox reading: 96% on room air. Client refuses any further treatment this morning and states, "I had a good life; I am ready to die."

What part in the nurses' notes would cause the nurse to respect the client's autonomy?

a. The client is complaining of sharp abdominal pain
b. Vital signs
c. Difficulty urinating
d. The client refuses any further treatment

8. Continuing with the scenario in question 7, for each nursing action listed below, check the box to indicate which ethical principle applies. Each action may support more than one principle.

NURSING ACTION	(1) NONMALEFICENCE	(2) BENEFICENCE	(3) AUTONOMY	(4) FIDELITY	(5) VERACITY	(6) JUSTICE
a. Ensure the room temperature is appropriate per the client.						
b. Continue to monitor the client's status frequently.						
c. Close the door when giving a bath per client's request.						
d. Report changes to the RN using SBAR technique.						
e. Chart findings in the electronic health record.						

9. Continuing with the scenario in question 7, complete the following sentence by choosing from the list of options.

When providing care to the client, the nurse should provide ______, demonstrating a respect for______.	
honesty	emotions
nourishment	autonomy
safety	culture
privacy	economics

10. Continuing with the scenario in question 7, what actions should the nurse avoid?

NURSING ACTION	DEMONSTRATE	AVOID
a. Perform a minimal physical assessment		
b. Leave work on time after completing responsibilities		
c. Forget to report to the oncoming nurse the client's wishes		
d. Research an unfamiliar medication after giving medications		
e. Verify client's name and DOB before providing care		

11. What statement(s) by the client demonstrates that the nurse provided ethical care (select all that apply)?

a. "Thank you for giving me a bath. I feel so much better."
b. "Why did you leave the bathroom door open when I was in there?"
c. "Your smile is contagious. It lifts my spirits."
d. "I appreciate that you checked on me several times this evening."

Critical Thinking Scenarios

Scenario 1

You are currently at the long-term facility 3 days a week on a geriatric nursing clinical rotation. The nursing instructor has talked to the class about being aware of sounds when walking in the halls. You see a resident being pushed to the shower room in a wheelchair by one of the nursing aides. On the way back down the hall, you hear a sound from the shower room and decide to open the door to the shower room. Much to your surprise, you see the aide putting a washcloth into the resident's mouth. The muffled sound from the resident is barely audible. The nursing assistant states, "The resident was screaming and disturbing another resident in the next room who has pneumonia and is trying to rest. I am just doing this for a few minutes. She hates this part of the bath." What will you do?

Scenario 2

The instructor asked the staff LPN and the client for permission to have an SPN observe the insertion of a urinary catheter. Permission was granted (the SPN had already watched a catheter insertion and given a successful return demonstration in class).

The SPN watched the LPN open the "catheterization tray" and noted a couple of breaks in sterile technique. The LPN contaminated their gloves when cleansing the client's perineal area. The LPN then began to reach for the sterile catheter. What should the SPN do?

7 Nursing and the Law: What Are the Rules?

Objectives

On completing this chapter, you will be able to do the following:

1. Summarize ways the nursing profession regulates itself.
2. Describe the responsibilities of a state's board of nursing (or nursing regulatory board).
3. Describe the board disciplinary process and actions.
4. Explain the limits, including prohibited acts, of a licensed practical nurse/licensed vocational nurse (LPN/LVN) license within your state.
5. Compare and contrast the state regulations governing registered nurse (RN) practice versus LPN/LVN practice.
6. Discuss the use of evidence-based resources to assist LPNs/LVNs to deliver safe care and avoid a potential lawsuit.
7. Define the nursing standard of care.
8. Summarize various aspects of the law and legal process that impact the provision of nursing care.
9. Recall issues and considerations regarding Good Samaritan laws.
10. Describe negligence and its implications in nursing practice.
11. Explain the four elements needed to prove negligence.
12. Discuss the typical steps for bringing legal action.
13. Differentiate between student practical/ vocational nurses (SPNs/SVNs) and instructor liability in preventing a lawsuit.
14. Discuss the need for personal malpractice insurance even if provided by your employer.
15. Summarize key legal responsibilities of the nurse to the client.
16. Summarize various end-of-life issues that impact nursing.

Key Terms

accountability
advance directives
assault
authorized consent
basic client situation
battery
breach of duty
causation
civil action
common law
complex nursing situation
confidentiality
continued competence
criminal action
damages
Death with Dignity Act
defamation
delegated medical act
depositions
direct supervision
do not resuscitate (DNR)
durable medical power of attorney
duty
end-of-life principles
euthanasia
felony
general (implied) consent
general supervision
Good Samaritan Act
Health Insurance Portability and Accountability Act (HIPAA)
informed consent
institutional liability
intentional tort
interstate endorsement
law
liability
libel
living will
malpractice (professional negligence)
misdemeanor
multistate licensure (Nurse Licensure Compact)
negligence
Nurse Practice Act (NPA)
nursing standard of care
Patient Self-Determination Act (PSDA)
personal liability
physician-assisted suicide (PAS)
preponderance proximate cause
slander
statutory law
unintentional tort
vicarious liability

Keep in Mind

Ethics, workforce trends/demands, and law drive the practice of nursing. When there is a dispute, the Nurse Practice Act (NPA) in your state is the final authority. No one has the authority to expand your scope of practice, not even your employer.

The licensed practical nurse (LPN) is struggling with a clinical decision. The LPN was working on a team with a registered nurse (RN) another LPN, and two nursing assistants. The RN, working with the LPN, became acutely ill during the work shift. As a result, the RN left early to go home. The evening shift RN was to arrive before the offgoing RN left; however, the incoming RN was stuck in traffic and did not arrive as anticipated. The RN left and stated to the LPN, "Just keep things quiet until the RN arrives." Minutes after the RN left, the LPN realized that the RN had neglected to initiate an IV infusion on a client who was septic. The LPN had practiced in another state where IV therapy was within the scope of practice of the NPA. Although the LPN realized that IV therapy was prohibited by the NPA in this state, the LPN thought this was an extenuating circumstance and, knowing what to do, initiated the IV.

As you read this chapter, think about how the LPN's actions violated the NPA. What could be the result of these actions? Would you have proceeded differently?

As we just reviewed in Chapter 6, ethics in nursing deals with rules of conduct, what is right, and how to act in a particular situation. Ethical values are the *basis* of nursing law. **Law** has to do with regulations that control the practice of nursing. Your state's NPA, discussed below, is your *legal* guideline in nursing practice. The state is the final authority.

Knowledge of your state's NPA is critical to making safe nursing decisions and protect you against acts and decisions that could involve you in lawsuits and criminal prosecution, which are commonplace in health care today. Your goal is to implement strategies to minimize malpractice claims (lawsuits) and decrease your personal chance of being involved in a lawsuit. In-depth knowledge and understanding of your state's NPA and your **continued competency** as an LPN/licensed vocational nurse (LVN) will provide a solid foundation to reach this goal.

NURSE PRACTICE ACT

Every state and territory in the United State has their own **NPA**. This document defines nursing practice and establishes standards for nurses for that specific state/territory. The privilege of having a state nursing license requires you to know and understand your state's NPA. Ignoring or not knowing the NPA is never a valid defense against legal proceedings regarding your license. As an LPN/LVN you must limit your work to the area of nursing defined in the state's NPA.

BASIC TERMINOLOGY

Similarities in basic terminology in an NPA exist in many states. As you study the scope of practice for LPN/LVNs in your state, an understanding of the following terms is necessary:

- **Activities of daily living (ADL).** Basic self-care tasks that an individual performs on a daily basis. These include but are not limited to basic hygiene (body and mouth), grooming, dressing, eating, exercising, and toileting. The nursing staff assists clients and their families in meeting these needs.
- **Basic nursing care.** Nursing care that can be performed safely by the LPN/LVN, based on knowledge and skills gained during the educational program. Includes ADL and skilled nursing procedures. Modifications of care are unnecessary, and client response is predictable.
- **Basic client situation.** The client's clinical condition is predictable. Medical and nursing orders are not changing continuously. These orders do not contain complex modifications. The client's clinical condition requires only basic nursing care. The professional nurse assesses whether the situation is a **basic client situation**. A basic client situation can include a chronic stable client with the need for skilled nursing procedures. However, the client's condition is stable (e.g., a client with chronic obstructive disease [COPD] who has a tracheostomy but whose disease process is currently stable; as a result, the health care provider orders do not contain complex interventions).
- **Complex nursing situation.** The client's clinical condition is not predictable. Health care provider orders or nursing interventions are likely to involve continuous changes or complex modifications. Nursing care practice is beyond what LPN/LVN was taught in LPN/LVN school curriculum. The professional nurse assesses whether the situation is a complex nursing situation.
- **Delegated medical act.** During a **delegated medical act**, a provider's order is given to an RN, an LPN/LVN by a health care provider, dentist, or podiatrist.

  Delegated responsibility (nursing act). A nursing activity, skill, or procedure that is transferred from a licensed nurse to a delegatee. The delegatee is one who is delegated a nursing responsibility by either an advanced practice registered nurse (APRN), RN, or LPN/LVN (where state NPA allows), is competent to perform it, and verbally accepts the responsibility. A delegate may be an RN, LPN/LVN, or nursing assistive personnel (AP) (NCSBN and ANA, 2019).
- **Direct supervision.** With **direct supervision**, the supervisor is continuously present to coordinate, direct, or inspect nursing care. The supervisor is in the building.
- **General supervision.** Under **general supervision**, a supervisor regularly coordinates, directs, or inspects nursing care and is within reach either in the building or by telephone.
- **Professional nurse.** In many states, the professional nurse is defined as the RN.

CONTENT OF NURSE PRACTICE ACTS

The NPA, the nursing law of each state may include the following content, according to the NCSBN Model Act (2021):

- Title and Purpose
- Definitions

- Scope of Practice for RN, LPN/LVN, and APRN
- Board of Nursing Organization and Functions
- RN, LPN/LVN Licensure and Exemptions
- Prelicensure Education
- Discipline and Proceedings
- Violations and Penalties

Try This

Get Familiar With Your Scope of Practice in Your State's Nurse Practice Act

Find your state's NPA online (visit https://www.ncsbn.org/policy/npa.page for links to state/territory NPAs). As you read it, note the major categories listed above. What did you learn about the following topics?

1. Definition of LPN/LVN nursing and professional nursing (RN)
   a. Compare and contrast the definition of practical/vocational nursing) versus professional nursing (RN).
   b. What differences are important?
   c. How do these differences impact respective scope of practices? Seek assistance from your instructor to fully understand the differences, if needed.
2. Use of the titles licensed practical nurse and licensed vocational nurse
3. Specific functions of the LPN/LVN
4. Prohibited functions of the LPN/LVN
5. Elements of unprofessional conduct

NURSING ORGANIZATION PROFESSIONAL GUIDELINES

In 2014, the National League for Nursing released a vision statement, *A Vision for Recognition of the Role of the Licensed Practical/Licensed Vocational Nurses in Advancing the Nation's Health.* In 2003, the National Association for Practical Nurse Education and Service Inc. (NAPNES) issued a professional guideline for LPNs/LVNs, titled *The LPN/LVN Fulfills the Professional Responsibilities of the Practical/Vocational Nurse.* These examples of national nursing organizations do not carry the weight of law. These statements are useful as *guides* for behavior and recommendations regarding workforce trends and LPN/LVN job roles. They may be used in a court of law as a point of reference and determination of what is expected of LPN/LVNs. However, *the NPA in your state is always your final authority.*

STATE BOARD OF NURSING

All 50 states, the District of Columbia, and four US territories have governmental agencies, or nursing regulatory bodies, that are responsible for regulating nursing practice. Their primary mission is ensure safe nursing care and issue licenses to practice nursing (NCSBN, 2025).

FUNCTIONS OF THE BOARD

State boards of nursing (also called nurse regulatory boards) can have a combined distinct NPAs to address the LPN/LVN and RN scope of practice. The boards have committees or councils that decide what specific nursing activities are within the state's scope of LPN/LVN practice. An activity that is legal in one state may not be legal in another state. See Box 7.1 for common board of nursing functions (NCSBN, 2018, https://www.ncsbn.org/public-files/What_Every_Nurse_Needs_to_Know.pdf).

Box 7.1 Common State Board of Nursing Functions

- Enforcing the State Nurse Practice Act (NPA) and nurse licensure
  - Licensing, determining duration and renewal of licenses
  - Monitoring continuing education credit requirements, if required, for license renewal
  - Maintaining inactive license status lists
- Developing practice standards.
- Approving/accrediting schools of nursing
- Establishing standards for educational programs
- Developing policies, administrative rules, and regulations
- Setting fees
- Addressing violations of the NPA
  - Suspending and revoking licenses and dealing with the appeal process
  - Carrying out disciplinary action for violators
  - Developing programs for impaired nurses

State Boards of Nursing (SBON) offer a variety of documents/services/information, usually accessible via its website. Some examples of resources include:

- Board laws (NPA) and regulations, Nursing Licensure Compact (if a participating state)
- State Board Member list, board meeting agenda, and minutes
- Licensure information and forms—Application, renewal, verification, reactivation
- Continuing education requirements
- Nursing education programs—Board-approved lists, NCLEX Exam pass rates

DISCIPLINARY RESPONSIBILITY OF THE BOARD

Keep in mind that your state board of nursing has a mandate to protect the public. Disciplinary action is focused on client safety. Each state's NPA, perhaps using different language, lists reasons for disciplining a nurse for unprofessional conduct. According to the National Council of State Boards of Nursing (NCSBN) (Discipline, 2025), disciplinary cases are often grouped into the following categories: practice related, drug related, boundary violations, sexual misconduct, abuse, fraud, and positive criminal background checks (see Box 7.2) Yoder-Wise (2019) provides examples of unprofessional conduct:

Typical examples of unprofessional conduct include the following: boundary issues; practicing while impaired; violating client confidentiality; failure to supervise persons for whom nursing functions have been delegated; inaccurate recording; falsifying or

Box 7.2 Categories of State Board of Nursing Disciplinary Cases

1. **Negligence:** The nurse does not do what a reasonable, prudent nurse would do in a similar situation. Negligence includes serious risk to the health, safety, or physical or mental health of a client. (This may include client injury. Injury can be physical, emotional, or spiritual.)
2. **Violation of the Nurse Practice Act (NPA):** Some states' NPAs list specific violations (e.g., unprofessional conduct, such as becoming personally involved with a client).
3. **Incompetence**: Examples include failure to meet generally accepted standards of nursing practice, negligence, and a nurse's mental disability that would interfere with client safety.
4. **Unethical conduct:** Examples include a breach of nurse–client confidentiality; refusal to provide nursing care for someone because of race, creed, color, national origin, disease, or sexual orientation; violation of the ethical code for licensed practice nurses/licensed vocational nurses (LPNs/LVNs); and failure to maintain nursing competence.
5. **Alcohol and/or other substance abuse:** Alcohol and other drug abuse by a nurse (e.g., diversion of medications, such as controlled substances, for personal use) is a threat to client safety. Some nurses steal and sell diverted substances and equipment such as syringes and IV tubing, falsify client records, and deprive clients of their medication. The number of nurses disciplined for alcohol and/or other drug abuse is increasing. Various programs exist to assist professionals, such as the Impaired Professionals Program.

altering a client or health care provider record; and sexual misconduct.

Practice-related cases may seem difficult to determine accurately as a newly licensed nurse. For example, practice-related issues can include failure to assess changes in client's condition, failure to adhere to the five rights of safe medication administration, and failure to accurately document. In addition, lack of adequate knowledge regarding the LPN/LVN scope of practice can lead to the LPN being asked to perform actions that are beyond your state's NPA. It is critical to remember that you are responsible to know your NPA, specific to your licensure. It is also important to understand your agency's policy and procedures relative to the responsible person (i.e., LPN, RN, NP) for a procedure or action. A supervisor or manager could ask you to do something beyond your NPA simply because they are not fully aware of the NPA relative to LPN practice, and perhaps your agency does not have a specific policy that assists in determining the safe action. Be sure to speak up if you believe you are being asked to do something that is prohibited by your NPA. It is your LPN/LVN license at risk.

Board actions resultant to unprofessional conduct vary based on many factors inclusive of the type of

Box 7.3 Possible Disciplinary Board Actions Relative to Unprofessional Conduct

1. Fine or civil penalty
2. Referral to an alternative to discipline program for practice monitoring and recovery support
3. Public reprimand or censure for minor violation of Nurse Practice Act, often with no restrictions on license
4. Imposition of requirements for monitoring, remediation, education, or other provision tailored to the particular situation
5. Limitation or restriction of one or more aspects of practice (e.g., probation with certain restrictions, limiting role, setting, activities, hours worked)
6. Separation from practice for a period of time (suspension) or loss of license (revocation or voluntary surrender)
7. Remediation (various educational content or exercises)
8. Other state-specific remedies

From NCSBN, 2025. https://www.ncsbn.org/nursing-regulation/discipline/board-action.page.

unprofessional conduct. See Box 7.3 for a list of possible board actions (NCSBN, 2025) and https://www.ncsbn.org/nursing-regulation/discipline/board-action.page for more details.

DISCIPLINARY PROCESS AND ACTION

The disciplinary process is based on law and follows the rules of law. See Box 7.4 for the steps of a disciplinary process.

NURSING LICENSURE

Nursing licensure defines and protects the title of LPN or LVN. Some states (e.g., Minnesota) have amended their NPA to include the provision that only an LPN or RN may use the professional title "nurse." This prevents an unlicensed person in a health care setting from misrepresenting themselves and stating, "Hi, I am your nurse Mary today." This is illegal in states where the title of nurse is protected. It is definitely also unethical.

On completion of a state-approved practical/vocational nursing education program, a graduate is eligible to apply for the National Council Licensure Examination for Practical Nurses (NCLEX-PN®).

In some states, immediately upon completion of their practical nursing program, the graduate may apply for a temporary permit (TPP) to practice nursing as a graduate practical nurse/graduate vocational nurse (GPN/GVN). Today, this is a less common practice, and it is less necessary, as technology has improved the speed of scheduling the exam date and receiving prompt notification of the examination results. If the graduate has passed the exam, then a nursing license is issued promptly by the State Board.

If the graduate nurse fails the NCLEX-PN® examination, the temporary permit is revoked. The graduate is

Box 7.4 Disciplinary Steps

FILING A COMPLAINT TO THE STATE BOARD OF NURSING OF A LICENSED NURSE OR LICENSURE APPLICANT

Anyone can file a complaint. Report immediately if you feel that a nurse has provided incompetent, negligent, or unsafe care or unethical. Some examples:

- You note the nurse's appearance seems impaired by drugs or alcohol while working.
- The nurse is stealing from a patient or client, including medications.
- The nurse is abusing a patient physically, emotionally, verbally, or sexually.
- The nurse is involved in criminal conduct.

STATE BOARD OF NURSING—INITIAL REVIEW OF COMPLAINT

- Verify if and in which state the nurse is licensed.
- Verify whether the alleged act is a violation of the Nurse Practice Act (NPA).
- Verify if practice-related, drug-related, boundary violations, sexual misconduct, or abuse and fraud.
- Verify if there is a positive criminal background check.

INVESTIGATION

- Documents and information from complainants
- Response from licensee
- Site visits
- Witness interviews
- Gather evidence

BOARD PROCEEDINGS (OPPORTUNITY FOR THE NURSE TO RESPOND TO ALLEGATIONS)

- Settlement conference
- Formal administrative hearing
- Alternative to discipline (ATD) programs (i.e., substance use disorder, practice related, remediation)

BOARD ACTION

- Statute of limitation
- Emergency actions (i.e., suspension of license if the nurse's action is clear and convincing evidence that continued practice by the nurse would present a danger of immediate and serious harm to the public))
- Disciplinary action
- Reciprocal

REPORTING AND ENFORCEMENT

- NURSYS (National database for verifying license, discipline and action privileges for nurses) reporting
- Federal law requires that adverse actions (disciplinary actions) taken against a health care professional's license be reported to the National Practitioner Data Bank (NPBD)

Data from National Council of State Boards of Nursing, 2025. https://www.ncsbn.org/nursing-regulation/discipline/filing-a-complaint.page.

responsible for reporting the unsuccessful exam immediately to the employer. Until successful completion of the NCLEX-PN® examination, the temporary permit remains revoked and the graduate cannot work as a GPN/GVN. The graduate may retest at a later date for an additional fee. The number of allowable retests and length of time between each exam is dictated by each state's NPA and varies across the United States.

Issuance of an LPN/LVN license can be impacted by a previous criminal or child abuse history. In many states, each individual situation is reviewed on a case-by-case basis and recommendations to issue a license are made by the state board of nursing legal counsel. This also remains true throughout a nurses' career as their license is renewed. Drug and alcohol violations, fraud, theft, and other infractions can result in license suspension or revocation or denial of renewal. Your license is essential to your profession. Be sure to protect it accordingly.

WORKING IN OTHER STATES

States have arrangements for **interstate endorsements** for nurses who choose to work in other states. It is possible to work in another state without retaking the NCLEX-PN® examination. The nurse applying must meet that state's criteria for licensure by endorsement. Thus once you pass the NCLEX-PN® examination, you will not need to retake the exam if moving to another state.

Some states are involved in **multistate licensure**: a mutual recognition model for nursing regulation. The Nurse Licensure Compact allows LPNs/LVNs and RNs to have one multistate license. NCSBN adopted the Nurse Multistate Licensure Mutual Recognition Model in 1997. Utah was the first state to adopt the NCSBN Nurse Licensure Compact (NLC) language that took effect in 2000. The NLC allows a nurse to have one license in his or her state of residency and practice in other states, depending on each state's NPA and legislation (https://www.ncsbn.org/compacts.page). To become law, each state must pass the law as part of their state NPA. As of January 2025, 43 states are members of the NLC. Eligible nurses must legally reside in a NLC state to participate. You cannot experience the benefits (Box 7.5) of the Nurse Licensure Compact unless you declare a NLC state as your primary residence. Check the NPA of the state in which you will

Box 7.5 Benefits of the Nurse Licensure Compact

- Ease of work mobility, ability to practice in multiple states
- Ability to practice telenursing and provide nursing services during disasters in all Enhanced Nurse Licensure Compact states for if the nurse is eligible for a multistate license
- Increased cooperation and collaboration between states boards of nursing
- Public receives safe nursing care protected by licensure laws across state boundaries
- Increases access to care while maintaining public protection at the state level
- The nurse can save time money by having one license, instead of completing and paying application and renewal fees for each state

Modified from National Council of State Boards of Nursing, 2025. Nurse licensure compact. https://www.nursecompact.com/.

be working to find out if it is a compact state or if any other special considerations with border states exist. The most recent annual report of the Interstate Commission of Nurse Licensure Compact Administrators, as of 2025, can be reviewed in detail at https://www.ncsbn.org/publications/2024-nlc-annual-report.

Try This

Compact States and the Nurse Practice Act

Access online the NPA of a compact state. If approved to work in a compact state, the LPN/LVN must know the contents of the NPA of the compact state. Confirm the residency requirements to participate in the Nurse Licensure Compact. Visit https://www.nursecompact.com/ to review details of the Nurse Licensure Compact.

Keep in Mind

To experience the benefits of the Nurse Licensure Compact (NLC), you must have legal residence in an NLC State. If your state is not a member of the NLC, you can apply for licensure in a Nurse Licensure Compact state; however, you will receive a single state license, not a multistate license.

VERIFICATION OF LICENSURE

Most boards of nursing have instituted online verification of nursing licensure. The board provides public information about nurses with current licensure. The verification system enables current and potential employers to use an online database confirming a nurse's license number, registration expiration date, and whether any board action (disciplinary) has taken place. The service is available 24 hours a day, 7 days a week. Check your state's board of nursing site to find out if this service is available.

Employers are able to use this option to comply with requirements for written verification of a nurse's registration by the Joint Commission (TJC) and other accreditation agencies.

NURSING STANDARD OF CARE

The **nursing standard of care** is your guideline for good nursing care. The phrase "you are held to the nursing standard of care" has important legal implications. The standard is based on what an ordinary, prudent nurse with similar education and nursing experience would do in similar circumstances. Resources for the nursing standard of care are found in Box 7.6. Note that health care institution routine ("I know you studied how to do this in nursing school, but this is how we do it here") is not on the list. All clinical decisions made must be based on evidence.

Keep in Mind

Accurate documentation is an important part of nursing care. In the eyes of the law, if it was not documented, it was not done.

Box 7.6 Resources for the Nursing Standard of Care

- **Nurse Practice Act (NPA):** Identifies the minimum level of competency necessary for a person to function as a licensed practical nurse (LPN) or licensed vocational nurse (LVN) or registered nurse (RN) in a particular state.
- **Nursing licensure examination** (NCLEX-PN® examination): Tests for minimum competence.
- **Practical/vocational nursing education programs:** Based on guidelines provided by the board of nursing, these programs guarantee a minimum knowledge base and the clinical practice necessary to provide safe nursing care. Curricula, textbooks, and instructors are resources for information about the standard of care.
- **Written policies and procedures:** The agency that employs the individual provides a standard of nursing care that must be followed. Read the policies of the agency to find out whether or not verbal directions are supported by written policies. If a question about care comes up in court, a lawyer will use the agency's policy and procedure manual as one guide to expected behavior. Remember that policies and procedures do not overrule the state's NPA and educational preparation. However, institutional policies may be stricter than state law.
- **Custom:** An unwritten, usually acceptable way of giving nursing care. Expert witnesses, not coworkers, would be called to testify to "the acceptable way."
- **Law (precedent):** Decisions that have been arrived at in similar cases brought up before a court (judge-made law).
- Statements from the National Association for Practical Nurse Education and Service Inc. and the National Association of Licensed Practical Nurses.
- Nursing texts and journals.
- Administrative rules of the board of nursing.
- Key resources such as The Joint Commission's National Client Safety Goals. For details, visit https://www.jointcommission.org/standards/. See Chapter 16 for more details.

ASSISTIVE PERSONNEL

The use of AP, previously called unlicensed assistive personnel or UAPs, to provide client care has grown dramatically in recent years. It is expected that the trend will continue. Licensed nurses need to be aware of specific AP training and facility AP job descriptions to safely make assignments. A major concern for safe client care is the supervision of APs by the RN and the LPN/LVN charge nurse in long-term care. The concern is that because of the lack of licensed nurses in aa facility, duties might be delegated and/or assigned inappropriately to APs. RNs and LPNs/LVNs put their jobs and licenses in jeopardy if the care provided by APs does not meet the standards of safety and effectiveness. Training programs for unlicensed persons teach a variety of nursing tasks. It is not the in-depth education and clinical experience provided in LPN/LVN or RN programs. Licensed nurses are accountable to both their employers and their state nursing boards (see Chapter 17). Providing safe, high-quality care is always the focus. Working conditions that prohibit safe care need to be reported to employers, state boards of nursing, and accreditation agencies.

HOW THE LAW AFFECTS LICENSED PRACTICAL NURSES AND LICENSED VOCATIONAL NURSES

COMMON LAW VERSUS STATUTORY LAW

The legal system in both the United States and Canada originates from English common law. **Common law** is called *judge-made law* because it originates in the courts. Common law is one way of establishing standards of legal conduct and is useful in settling disputes. Once the judge has decided, this decision *sets the precedent* for a ruling on a case with similar facts in the future. Thus common law can change over time, based on precedent. **Informed consent** and a client's right to refuse treatment are examples of common law.

Statutory law is law developed by the legislative branch of the state and the US Congress of the federal government. The NPA, which governs the practice of nursing, is an example of a statutory law. State boards of nursing can make nursing laws as long as the items in their laws do not conflict with any federal statutes. Because the NPA is statutory law, governed by states, differences exist across the United States.

CRIMINAL VERSUS CIVIL ACTION

The two classifications of legal action are criminal action and civil action. A **criminal action** involves people and society as a whole. It involves relationships between individuals and the government. It is unlikely for nurses to be involved in criminal action. A criminal action is classified as follows:

- **Misdemeanor:** A **misdemeanor** is the least serious charge and can result in a fine or prison sentence of generally no more than 1 year. This criminal act might include taking $100.00 from a client for an emergency personal need.
- **Felony:** A **felony** is a serious offense with a penalty that usually ranges from more than 1 year in prison to death, for example, when the nurse injects a client with a lethal drug to hasten death or removes life support before the client has been pronounced dead by the health care provider.

Guilt on the part of the nurse needs to be established by producing proof *beyond a reasonable doubt*. Regardless of the outcome of the criminal case, when a criminal case is completed, it is also possible to be sued in a civil court.

A **civil action** protects individual rights and *results in payment of money* to the injured person (e.g., a back injury was sustained during a fall because spilled urine was not wiped up, causing the client additional treatment time, including physical therapy, pain, suffering, and loss of time from work). A civil action involves a relationship between individuals and the violation of those rights. A *tort* is a civil wrong. The two kinds of torts are intentional and unintentional, which are described as follows:

- **Intentional:** An **intentional tort** is intended to cause harm to the client (e.g., threat or actual physical harm).
- **Unintentional:** An unintentional tort did not mean to harm the client. "I did not mean to hurt the client" is no defense if you did not use the "Six Rights" and gave the client an incorrect medication, which caused injury.

Guilt on the part of the nurse can be established by a **preponderance** (majority) of the evidence. Table 7.1 provides a comparison of criminal and civil law.

Table 7.1 Comparison of Two Basic Classifications of Law

	CIVIL LAW	CRIMINAL LAW
Who the law generally applies to	Relationships between private individuals and infringements on individual rights	Relationships between individuals and the government (state)
Who is affected?	Individuals	Society as a whole
Sources of law	US Constitution, state and federal legislatures	US Constitution, state and federal legislatures
Punishment for breaking the law	Generally, payment of a monetary compensation. Other settlements could include a public apology or implementation of new safety standards	Death, imprisonment, fines, restrictions
How guilt is established	Proof by a preponderance of the evidence	Proof beyond a reasonable doubt
Examples of nursing liability	Contract Tort Unintentional Intentional Negligence	Murder, rape, larceny, homicide, manslaughter, assault and battery, embezzlement
Criminal infraction	None	Felony/misdemeanor/summary

Common law is judge-made law. A trial judge's ruling lays down a legal principle and sets a precedent. These principles are used to decide future cases. This type of law is continually adapted and expanded. *Statutory law is formal legislative enactment*. Law passed by Congress or enacted by state government. May be amended, repealed, or expanded by the legislature. The Nurse Practice Act is an example of statutory law.

Intentional Torts

Tort law is based on the premise that in the course of relationships with one another there is a general **duty** to avoid injuring one another. A tort is a wrong or injury done to someone that violates his or her rights.

Intentional torts require a specific state of mind; that is, that the nurse intended to do the wrongful act.

Assault and battery, false imprisonment and use of restraints, **defamation** that includes both libel and slander (discussed later), and physical and emotional abuse are examples of intentional torts. Not all insurance companies cover intentional torts in their malpractice insurance policies, so you should check your policy.

Assault and battery. **Assault** is an unjustified attempt or threat to touch someone. **Battery** means to cause physical harm to someone. (Students often confuse these two terms. To avoid this, remember that assault and attempt both begin with the letter "A"). When a client refuses a treatment or medication, forcing the client to take medication could result in an assault and battery charge against you. The client gives *implied consent* (permission) for certain routine treatments when entering the institution. Clients retain the right to refuse any treatment verbally and may leave the institution when they choose, unless they are there for court-ordered treatment. Nurses can also protect themselves from assault by a client but can use only as much force as is considered reasonable for self-protection.

Treating a client without consent is battery even if the treatment is medically beneficial. A health care provider might go to court to get a court order to allow a blood transfusion for someone who opposes it on religious grounds. If the client is fully competent, is not pregnant, and has no children, the court is likely to rule for the client even if a blood transfusion would save his or her life. When faced with a similar situation, the LPN/LVN respects the client's belief system and notifies the RN and/or supervisor for further guidance or interpretation.

False imprisonment and use of restraints. False imprisonment is keeping someone detained against his or her will. It can include the use of restraints or seclusion in a room without cause and without a health care provider's order. Restraint by verbal threats or physical harm is also included in this category. Chemical restraint (with medication) is defined as administering a PRN (from Latin, *pro re nata*, meaning "as needed") medication with a sedating side effect every 4 hours to keep the client tired and confined to a room. In this situation, the intent is to keep the client quiet and out of the way. The intended use of the medication has been circumvented to meet the nurse's need.

Defamation. Defamation means damage to someone's reputation through false communication or communication without their permission. Libel and slander are included in this category and are described as follows:

- **Libel** is defamation through *written* communication or pictures.
- **Slander** is defamation by *verbalizing* untrue or private information (gossip) to a third party.

The client has the right to expect you to speak the truth. Additional unnecessary conversation with coworkers and those outside the agency can result in a charge of defamation. The same is true for taking unwanted photographs or showing a client's injury, cancerous growth, or gunshot wound to others, students included, without the client's permission. Social media has escalated issues related to defamation. Posting any client information or "client story" on any type of social media site is prohibited unless written permission is obtained from the client and approved by your employer. Posting your clinical day experience even without using client names or specific information is prohibited. Review the pamphlet created by NCSBN, *A Nurse's Guide to the Use of Social Media* (https://www.ncsbn.org/brochures-and-posters/nurses-guide-to-the-use-of-socialmedia).

You often are privy to information about the personal lives of other nurses, health care providers, and other coworkers, and they are privy to information about you. Although the desire to repeat the information you hear may be tempting, it is best left unsaid. Later in the chapter, you will learn about the Health Insurance Portability and Accountability Act (HIPAA) and how that law defines privacy.

Physical and emotional abuse. Physical abuse is generally easier to identify, although the victim may find creative ways to hide the injuries for a period of time. Emotional abuse is more difficult to identify. The person doing the abusing may be very personable and attentive to the victim when out in public. A former student described how everyone thought her husband loved her and how fortunate she was. When they were alone, he would tell her she was ugly, worthless, and no one else would ever want her or love her. When she became pregnant, he would always take her to her health care provider appointment. He would answer the health care provider's and nurse's questions for her, and when she tried to speak, he would take over in gentle terms, doing the explaining. At no time was she alone with a health care provider or nurse.

In the course of your career in practical/vocational nursing, you will probably suspect or actually see the results of some types of abuse. As an LPN/LVN, you have a legal responsibility to report your suspicions or observations of abuse by following your facility's abuse policy. Note that a "suspicion" is a nagging doubt. Be empathetic (as opposed to sympathetic) so that your observations or report will be as objective as possible. Becoming a part of the client's emotions may lead you to jump to conclusions or accept a particularly convincing but untrue explanation. Whether the client is a child, woman, man, or elder, reputations are at stake. Once an accusation has been made, it is difficult to be truly free from it, even when it is proved groundless.

Refer to your state's abuse laws for specific rules that govern your responsibility for reporting abuse. Remember that you are a mandated reporter. You must report any suspected or observed physical or emotional abuse. Some state's laws may include a mandate that the individual who is suspicious of abuse contacts the government authority directly or, at a minimum, ensures the supervisor reported the event and follow-up has occurred. It is not sufficient to report to your supervisor and then move on, unsure if any investigation occurred. In addition, child abuse training may be mandated for licensure and licensure renewal in your state. Follow your facility's policy for reporting abuse. The social services department can help you report abuse. Offer concrete, specific observations. Quote the statements made and avoid offering a personal interpretation. Let the facts speak for themselves.

Unintentional Torts

An unintentional tort holds that the nurse did not intend to injure the client. However, the nurse did not maintain the nursing standard of care and did not do what a prudent nurse with comparable education and skills would do in a similar situation. Negligence and malpractice (professional negligence) are examples of unintentional torts.

Good Samaritan Act

The **Good Samaritan Act** stipulates that a person who renders emergency care in good faith at the scene of an accident is immune from civil liability for action taken while providing care. Details of each state's Good Samaritan laws vary. The state statutes are of particular interest to nurses and health care providers who provide emergency care when they are not in their employment setting. Check with your state's board of nursing or agency risk manager for information about your state's Good Samaritan laws. For example, in some states, a nurse has a choice of whether or not to give aid to someone during an emergency outside of a health care setting. A few states obligate health care professionals to assist at a scene of an accident requiring medical help. If, for instance, you provide pressure to stop severe bleeding and the client develops complications, you will not be held responsible as long as you acted without gross negligence. The law also permits the nurse to give aid to a minor at a sports event or accident scene before getting authorized consent from the parents. The LPN/LVN must have permission to treat the person, and verbal permission must be obtained from the victim. The person has the right to refuse. Once first aid is initiated, the nurse is obligated to continue until the victim can be turned over to someone with comparable or better training (Cherry and Jacob, 2019). The SAFEProject provides state information about Good Samaritan laws regarding assistance given to persons with drug addiction and overdosing (see https://www.safeproject.us/).

> **Try This**
>
> **Good Samaritan Act**
>
> Explain the protection that your state's Good Samaritan Act provides for the LPN/LVN.

NEGLIGENCE AND MALPRACTICE IN NURSING

NEGLIGENCE

Black's Law Dictionary (2014) defines **negligence** as "failure to use such care as a reasonably prudent and careful person would use under similar circumstances." A common type of negligence is personal injury. For example, your town has a law stating that sidewalks must be shoveled within 24 hours after a snowstorm. Your sidewalk has not been shoveled within 24 hours, and your neighbor falls in front of your house and breaks her arm. The neighbor sues you for negligence. Remember that in negligence the property owner did not intend to cause the injury to the neighbor, but knowing the risks and the law, he or she should have guarded against the injury. Good intentions do not enter in. It is your conduct, not your intent, that is the issue.

MALPRACTICE (PROFESSIONAL NEGLIGENCE)

Malpractice, the legal name for professional negligence, means negligence by a professional, in this case an LPN/LVN. The most common type of negligence in practical/vocational nursing relates to action or lack of action, not what you intended to do. These are often referred to as acts of commission or acts of omission. For example, you can give the wrong medication (commission) or forget to give a medication (omission).

Box 7.7 lists the most common sources of malpractice, according to Watson (2014). The top three closed claim sites per practice setting for the LPN/LVN are hospital-inpatient surgical service, client's home, and hospital-inpatient medical service (Watson, 2014). In addition, the LPNs/LVNs had an average paid indemnity of $83,213 (Watson, 2014). According to a PA-based Nurses Service Organization (NSO), which provides malpractice insurance to nurses, there has been an increase in the severity of closed malpractice claims impacted by closed claims that settled for $250,000 or more and involved infant and pediatric clients with tracheostomies (Relias Media, 2016). The charges of professional negligence (malpractice) listed could be avoided by good nursing practice (i.e., what a reasonable, prudent nurse would do in a similar situation). This includes knowing strategies to minimize

Box 7.7 Some Common Sources of Malpractice

- Medication errors
- Working while impaired
- Failure to follow standards of care
- Lack of observation and timely reporting about the client
- Failure to use a medical device accurately
- Failure to communicate
- Failure to properly supervise a client
- Negligent delegation and supervision
- Failure to act as a client advocate
- Failure to get informed consent

Five Most Common Allegations of Nursing Negligence

- Communication—failure to communicate in a timely manner
- Assessment—inadequate patient assessment or intervention to a patient problem
- Medication errors—administration of a medication not following the rights of medication administration
- Infection control issues—failure to follow the facility infection control policy and procedure in
- Equipment errors—unsafe or improper use of medical equipment

Modified from Watson E: Nursing malpractice: costs, trends, and issues, *J Legal Nurse Consult* 25(1):26–31, 2014 and Rokos C: Legal issues in nursing: the 5 most common allegations of nursing negligence 2025. https://www.clpna.com/lpn/lpn-knowledge-hub/part-4-legal-issues-in-nursing-five-most-common-allegations-of-nursing-negligence/.

errors required by entities such as TJC (The Joint Commission, 2019) (e.g., creating an institutional list of medications based on TJC's published list of commonly confused look-alike, sound-alike drug names). The student practical nurse/student vocational nurse (SPN/SVN) is held to the level of an LPN's/LVN's performance. Know your state's NPA and know essential standards of care.

There are occasions when the evidence is overwhelming and indicates the accused nurse is responsible for the client injury. Such an occasion is called *res ipsa loquitur*, meaning "the evidence speaks for itself." For example, a client develops a drop in blood pressure immediately after the nurse administered an injection improperly.

Malpractice Insurance for Nurses

More nurses are being named in lawsuits. Nurses assume **liability** for their own acts. Although the employing agency may assume responsibility for the nurse during a lawsuit, the agency can then turn around and sue the nurse. You can also be held responsible for the "neighborhood advice" you give, for example, telling a neighbor how to care for her sick child or emergency aid you provide in the community.

Each nurse must carefully consider whether or not it is necessary to purchase a malpractice insurance policy. Incidents of suing for malpractice continue, although your chances of being sued as an LPN/LVN compared with other health care providers are minimal. Given the inexpensive cost of malpractice insurance (approximately $100.00 per year for a recommended policy) for LPNs/LVNs, it is an important consideration. Malpractice insurance is provided for you as a student nurse, generally included in your total cost of attendance. Consider purchasing your malpractice insurance immediately upon graduation. Some reasons for having your own malpractice insurance are found in Box 7.8.

Try This

Malpractice Coverage

If you are currently assigned to a clinical area, find out what the agency policy is on malpractice coverage for practical/vocational nurses. If not required by the employer, consider reasons why an LPN/LVN working there should purchase malpractice insurance.

Four Elements Needed to Prove Negligence

Duty, **breach of duty**, **damages**, and **causation** are the four elements that must be present to cause an action for negligence against a nurse. Each of the four elements must be proved by the client to receive compensation. Box 7.9 explains the four elements needed to prove negligence.

Critical Thinking

Develop a scenario of an LPN/LVN who is being sued. Use the four elements needed to prove negligence as the basis for the suit.

Box 7.8 Reasons for Your Own Malpractice Insurance

- The jury's award could exceed the limits of your agency's coverage.
- Your *employing agency* could pay out an award to a plaintiff and then countersue you.
- You acted outside the scope of employment, and the agency argues it is not liable.
- Your employer's policy covers you only on the job.
- An agency might carry a policy that covers you only while you are employed by that institution. A suit may come up years after you have stopped working for the employer. It is suggested that nurses purchase occurrence coverage if malpractice coverage is desired, and not claims coverage. Occurrence coverage protects the nurse for each incident regardless of the present employer.
- The agency may decide to settle out of court. The plaintiff could then pursue a case against the nurse.
- Employer lapses in payment or renewal of policy.
- After a settlement, *insurers* could turn around and sue the nurse.
- If you have your own coverage, you will have your own lawyers, not the lawyers who are also defending the agency.

Box 7.9 Four Elements Needed to Prove Negligence

1. Duty refers to the nurse's responsibility to provide care in an acceptable way. The nurse has a duty based on education, as well as the policies and standards of the place of employment.
2. Breach of duty means that the nurse did not adhere to the nursing standard of care. What was expected of the nurse was not done (omission) or was not done correctly (commission). An expert nurse witness establishes the standard of care.
3. Damages mean that the client must be able to show that the nurse's negligent act injured him or her in some way. The client must prove actual damage.
4. Proximate cause means that a reasonable cause-and-effect relationship can be shown between the omission or commission of the nursing act and the harm to the client. Did the nurse's negligent act cause the injury in question? For example, an assistive personnel bumps the client's toe in the shower. The client has a history of diabetes mellitus. Despite prompt reporting, observation, and care of the toe, the toe becomes gangrenous and the foot requires amputation. The cause of the amputation was from the original "bump" of the toe.

STEPS FOR BRINGING LEGAL ACTION

Legal actions follow an orderly process. Remember that the nurse also has rights and is not considered guilty simply because someone filed a complaint. Steps for bringing a legal action by a client are found in Box 7.10.

DEPOSITIONS

Depositions are used to gather information under oath (fact finding). Once the deposition is scheduled, provide information on where and how you can be reached. The deposition usually takes place in an attorney's office. You may be able to request that it be in your attorney's office. (It will be helpful to have an attorney who understands nursing and is familiar with legal action against a nurse.) Opponents' attorneys may also be present. However, only one of the opponent's attorneys should be permitted to ask questions so as not to "tag team" (multiple attorneys firing questions at the nurse). A court reporter or stenographer will record your testimony.

Dress professionally, as you would for a job interview. Do your utmost to be calm and polite no matter how rude others, including the opposing attorney, seem to you.

ATTORNEY PROCEDURES

In preparation for a deposition, your attorney will do the following:

- Provide a checklist of basic instructions for the deposition.
- Practice likely questions that may be asked and critique your responses.
- Prepare you for types of questions that may slant your testimony.
- Suggest appropriate ways to respond, but not tell you what to answer.
- Use a practice deposition video (usually, not always).
- Meet with you in advance on the day of the deposition to answer any last-minute questions.

GIVING TESTIMONY

Here are some basics to keep in mind during a deposition:

- It is important to tell the truth, *always*. Avoid trying to be clever.
- A court reporter or stenographer can only record words, so questions must be answered verbally.
- Listen carefully to the question. If you do not understand the question, ask that the question be repeated or rephrased.
- Before answering, pause. This will give you an opportunity to consider the question. Think about what is being asked and how you will answer.
- Be specific in answering a question: If it is a "yes" or "no" question, then answer it that way. *Resist the urge to say more*. If you do not know the answer to a question, say so, and do not speculate. If you do not remember, say, "I do not remember."
- If your attorney instructs you to not answer a question, do not answer. Instruction to not answer a question is permitted under certain circumstances.

Box 7.10 Steps for Bringing a Legal Action by a Client

- The client believes that the nurse has violated his or her legal rights.
- The client seeks the advice of an attorney.
- The attorney has a nurse expert review the client's chart to see whether the nurse has violated the nursing standard of care. If it is determined that a standard of care has been violated, a lawsuit is filed.
- The client (the plaintiff) files a complaint that documents the grievance (violation of rules). This is served to the defendant (the nurse).
- The defendant responds in writing.
- The discovery period (pretrial activity) begins. Statements are taken from the defendant nurse, witnesses, nurse expert, client (plaintiff), and other caregivers. Policies and procedures of the health care facilities are reviewed.
- During the trial, important information is presented to the judge or jury. A verdict (decision) is reached. The plaintiff (the client) has the burden of proof (evidence of wrongdoing) during the trial. The award in a malpractice case is to make the aggrieved person whole. There is generally a monetary settlement. In addition, an apology or a safety initiative could be mandated by the court.
- An appeal (request for another trial) can be made if either the plaintiff or the defendant does not consider the verdict acceptable.

- Be careful not to reveal the content of any conversation with your attorney.
- Ask for a break, especially if you are tired or not thinking clearly. If there is a question pending, you will be expected to answer it before taking a break.
- You will not be permitted to take any notes during the deposition.
- A few weeks after the deposition, you and your attorney may be able to review the testimony and make corrections. You may be asked about the corrections during the trial.

LIABILITY

KINDS OF LIABILITY

Personal liability holds us responsible for our own behavior, including negligent behavior. This rule makes it impossible to completely shift responsibility onto someone else. **Vicarious liability** means responsibility for actions of another because of a special relationship with the other. The term *respondeat superior*, Latin for "let the master speak," is based on vicarious liability. It is applied in the following two ways:

1. *Borrowed servant doctrine* (e.g., the master/servant relationship between an employer [hospital] and an employee [nurse]). The employer (master) is assumed to be better able to pay for the injuries than the employee (servant). The employer may also be held responsible in a suit for the negligent acts of the employee performed during the time of employment. This provides incentive for health care agencies to hire carefully, as well as orient and supervise the work of the employee.
2. *Captain of the ship doctrine* (e.g., in an operating room). A nurse becomes the temporary employee of the health care provider doing the surgery. This doctrine assumes that in this situation the surgeon exerts control of the nurse in relation to specific conduct that caused client injury in the operating room.

Institutional liability is vicarious liability. It assumes that the health facility provides certain safeguards to keep the client from harm. This includes a safe facility to prevent physical harm (e.g., adequate supervision of staff, adequate staffing, and safe equipment).

COMMON CAUSES OF NURSING LIABILITY

Many of the errors leading to common nursing liabilities can be avoided by following the guidelines you learned in nursing school. The major areas of liability (responsibility/accountability) can be categorized as lack of safety, knowledge, skill, observation and reporting, documentation, and acceptance of responsibility for nursing actions, all of which are part of the usual clinical evaluation. The most common errors are drug errors, most of which can be avoided if you follow the guidelines you learn in basic nursing and practice in the clinical areas. One of the best defenses for prevention of legal liability is development of rapport with the client. If you treat clients with courtesy and respect, they are less likely to sue (unless you provide care below the nursing standard of care). Be honest, be nice, and be thorough. The very best defense is not to make a mistake in the first place. If you do err, the second-best defense is to immediately admit that you made an error and communicate freely all steps taken to prevent or minimize harm. Transparency is a must!

Professional Pointer

Ignorance of nursing law is not an excuse.

RESPONSIBILITY AND ACCOUNTABILITY IN NURSING

Nursing demands that you be responsible. This means being reliable and trustworthy. At no time can you expect a peer, supervisor, or client to say to you, "it's okay that you didn't come to work today because your car wouldn't start"; or "it's okay if we talk about just your problems today instead of the client's"; or "it's okay that you didn't do the work you were assigned because you're having a bad day." Nursing says, "I'm sorry that you have personal problems that are distracting you, but you have to resolve them because your priority in this profession is the client." Safe client care is essential.

The word *accountability* means that you are answerable. As a nursing student, you are answerable to yourself, to your assigned client, to the team leader, to the preceptor, to the health care provider, and to your instructor who constantly evaluates your work. As an LPN/LVN, accountability to the instructor is replaced by accountability to the employing agency. You are held accountable for all the nursing actions that you perform or are assigned to perform. The measures of accountability are the following nursing standards of practice:

- NPA of the state
- NAPNES Standards and Educational Competencies of Graduates of Practical/Vocational Nursing Programs (see www.napnes.org)
- NALPN Nursing Practice Standards for the Licensed Practical/Vocational Nurse (see www.nalpn.org)

They recommend minimal acceptable standards of nursing behavior for the SPN/SVN and the LPN/LVN.

LIABILITY OF STUDENT NURSES AND INSTRUCTORS

Student nurses are held accountable for the nursing care they give. They are held to the standards of an LPN/LVN. This emphasizes *the necessity to prepare for providing care for assigned clients in the clinical area*. The instructor has the responsibility to make client assignments based on the student's knowledge base and ability to give safe nursing care. The instructor is also expected to provide reasonable supervision for the

Box 7.11 Student Practical Nurse/Student Vocational Nurse Responsibilities for Client Care

- Prepare by reading the assigned client's chart/electronic health record, client profile, and established plan of care. Develop your own plan of care for the client to whom you are assigned, collaborating with the registered nurse (RN)/instructor. Research medical diagnoses, anticipated procedures, unfamiliar terminology.
- Research action, safety of ordered dose, side effects, nursing considerations, and contraindications for the assigned client's routine, PRN medications, and IV additives.
- Review how to perform ordered treatments.
- Compose a time sequence for care during your time with the client.
- When you arrive on the clinical unit, review your plan of care with the instructor before starting nursing care.
- Identify a need for and request additional help or supervision.
- Comply with agency and school of nursing policies.
- Document appropriately.
- Maintain client confidentiality.
- Communicate concerns, change in patient condition, questions to the instructor and the facility assigned nurse.

care given by a student. A list of your responsibilities is found in Box 7.11.

FUNCTIONING BEYOND THE SCOPE OF PRACTICE AND EXPERIENCE

As an LPN/LVN, you might be asked by an RN or health care provider to perform nursing duties that are beyond your scope of practice or experience. It is up to you to refuse. Box 7.12 contains examples of responses when asked to perform beyond your scope of practice. When seeking employment, check out the philosophy, mission statement, and policies of your potential place of employment. Ask what is included in your job, the period of orientation you will receive, what the orientation will cover, and who will do the orientation. If you discover during your inquiry that your work will cover more than you have learned or tasks that are beyond your scope of practice, say so. Listen also to your affective response: What is your intuition saying? Getting a job just to get a job may result in your being fired or losing your license. You may end up losing your job for something that was not your fault. The ideal is that everyone around you shares your ethics and demonstrates fairness, but the reality of ethics is sometimes quite different. Institutional policy and procedure is a critical resource for safe practice. Your employer can limit your scope of practice based on policy and procedure but may not expand it. For example, if you are employed in a state where LPN/LVNs are not permitted to administer IV medications via a central access device, then despite in-depth education and approval by your supervisor and institution, you may not perform that procedure.

Box 7.12 Possible Responses When Asked to Perform a Nursing Task Unfamiliar to You or Beyond Your Scope of Practice

- "I am not legally able to do something beyond the licensed practical nurse/licensed vocational nurse Nurse Practice Act."
- "I need to have a registered nurse (RN) immediately available for collaboration as the client's condition is unstable and changing."
- "I have never done this before. I will be glad to learn if you teach me, watch me demonstrate in return, and write a memo for my file that you have taught me to do this and watched a satisfactory return demonstration."
- "I was taught to do this while in school but did not have a chance to catheterize a real person. I observed the educational skills demonstration video on the Internet. Please observe me perform a catheterization and intervene if necessary. I welcome feedback so I can continually improve."
- "My orientation here did not include how to make daily assignments according to the skill level of staff. I need to be shown. Will you show me how to make assignments? I learn quickly, so it will be time well spent."
- "You have provided a detailed orientation, but I do not feel ready (or qualified) to assume a charge nurse position. I think I need more experience as a staff nurse, so I can function effectively and within my NPA."

SPECIFIC CLIENT SITUATIONS

A professional relationship between the nurse and the client is essential for the provision of nursing care. Legal precedent has established that the health care agency also has a responsibility to the client. Clients have become increasingly concerned and vocal about the quality of care they expect to receive. Many of the issues are directly related to privacy, confidentiality, and safety. These are also concerns of health agencies and health care workers, including nurses.

PRIVACY AND CONFIDENTIALITY

Privacy in health care means the right to be left alone and free from intrusion, including the right to choose care based on personal beliefs, feelings, or attitudes; the right to govern bodily integrity (accepting or rejecting treatment or exposure of the body); and the right to control when and how sensitive information is shared. **Confidentiality** in health care refers to the nondisclosure of information regarding clients.

INFORMATION THAT MUST BE REVEALED

Some laws require that certain client information must be reported without the client's consent. The purpose is to protect the public. Examples of client information that must be revealed are listed in Box 7.13.

CLIENTS' RIGHTS

Clients' rights in all types of institutions are mandated by the US Constitution and by state and federal

Box 7.13 Client Information That Must Be Revealed

In all situations, the supervisor (RN), director of nursing, and policy set by the facility are resources.

- **Communicable disease:** To the local health department or the Centers for Disease Control and Prevention. This includes AIDS, but the nature of the disclosure varies according to state law.
- **Vaccine-related adverse reactions:** To the Department of Health and Human Services. (Reporting of some reactions is mandatory; for others it is voluntary. Access Vaccine Adverse Event Reporting System at www.vaers.hhs.gov or call (800) 822-7967 for the VAERS Table of Reportable Events Following Vaccination.)
- **Criminal acts:** All states mandate reporting of rape cases. Some mandate reporting of injuries by gunshot or sharp instruments. Some states require reporting of blood alcohol levels (BAL) beyond the legal limit. Clarify your state's specific mandates. The local police department is a good place to clarify what is reportable *before* an incident occurs. Your institution policy can also be a source.
- **Equipment-related injuries:** When use of a medical device results in injury or death, it is reported immediately to your supervisor and health care provider. If emergency first aid is called for, follow the procedure you have been taught.
- **When there is a clear and present danger:** Health Insurance Portability and Accountability Act laws, for instance, mandate reporting of client mistreatment or professional misconduct. Report immediately to your supervisor or follow the policy manual for an emergency course of action.
- **Abuse and neglect of a client (child or elderly):** Report the incident immediately to your supervisor or director of nursing who will follow up by reporting to police and/or social services. It is your responsibility in many states to ensure a report has been made. Thus be sure that the required reporting has occurred.
- **Incompetence (including alcohol or drug impairment) or unprofessional acts:** As defined by state law. Facilities have policies for how to report and to whom. Report immediately to your supervisor, your director of nursing, or as directed in the facility's policy manual. Violation of nursing law will be reported to the state board of nursing.

laws. Legal rights vary depending on the health care agency and the client's competency. The American Hospital Association (AHA) developed *The Client's Bill of Rights* in 1972. It was revised in 2003 and renamed *The Client Care Partnership: Understanding Expectations, Rights, and Responsibilities*. It continues to be used in 2025. This is an ethical, rather than legal, document for hospitals recommending ways to guarantee client rights. It is intended as a model for states to develop rights statements. Some state legislatures have adopted client rights statements. Additional bills of rights have been developed for pregnant clients, nursing home residents, and mental health clients. The document is reviewed and revised yearly as needed. Box 7.14 provides *The Client Care Partnership* recommendations.

Box 7.14 *The Client Care Partnership* Excerpt: What to Expect During Your Hospital Stay

- High-quality hospital care
- A clean and safe environment
- Involvement in your care
- Protection of your privacy
- Help when leaving the hospital
- Help with your billing claims

From American Hospital Association: The patient care partnership, 2003. Available at: www.aha.org/advocacy-issues/communicatingpts/pt-care-partnership.shtml.

Try This

Clients' Rights

Obtain a copy of your state's or health facility's client rights statement. Briefly explain what is meant by each of the main topics. Identify the topics that are a part of what you have already learned in nursing.

HEALTH INSURANCE PORTABILITY AND ACCOUNTABILITY ACT

The US **HIPAA** rules took effect on April 14, 2003 for health insurance companies, hospitals, clinics, health care providers, pharmacies, and other health groups throughout the United States. The original intent of HIPAA was portability of insurance for employees from one job to the next. Portability is addressed in the law, but the main focus of the law is privacy. Changes to modify HIPAA privacy, security, and enforcement of rules are updated as technological advances dictate. The law gives clients rights over their health information. Basic HIPAA terminology is provided in Box 7.15.

Basics of the Health Insurance Portability and Accountability Act

The following are the three basic parts of HIPAA:

1. **Protection of privacy.** HIPAA provides a guide for health-related facilities and individuals to establish privacy standards based on the HIPAA model. This is intended as a national privacy standard throughout the United States. When discussing privacy, HIPAA uses the term *protected health information* (PHI) when referring to client information that should not be revealed. Proposed are rules to increase efficiency of the health care system by creating standards for use and dissemination of health care information.
2. **Administrative simplification.** The overall goal of administrative simplification is to reduce paperwork related to health care reimbursement (e.g., a goal is to develop a universal insurance claim form).
3. **Security standards.** The overall goal is to establish security standards for the protection of electronic (computer and fax) transmission of PHI (e.g., encrypted password protection when using a

Box 7.15 Basic Health Insurance Portability and Accountability Act (HIPAA) Terminology

- **HIPAA (not HIPPA):** Passed in 1996. Enforcement began April 14, 2003, Enforcement Rule started March 2006 to provide guidance on conducting investigations and issue civil monetary policies. The HITECH 2009 and Breach Notification rule started in 2009 to incentivize implementation of Electronic Health Records, and the Final Omnibus Rule was published March 2013, which filled gaps in existing HIPAA standards.
- **Portability:** Original intent of HIPAA was portability of health insurance for employees from one job to the next.
- **Protection of client privacy:** Main focus of HIPAA is protection of client health information.
- **Covered entity:** Health facilities that provide, bill, or receive payment for health care as a normal part of business.
- **Health care:** Any care, services, or supplies related to the care of a client.
- **Privacy officer:** HIPAA requirement that all covered entities designate a privacy officer.
- **Notice of privacy practices:** Each covered entity must develop a document written in plain language that explains the facility's privacy practices. It is distributed to all clients. The notice must also be posted in a prominent place to be read by all interested parties.
- **Department of Health and Human Services (DHHS):** The federal agency that oversees HIPAA.
- **Mandatory law:** Law that must be followed or penalties will be involved.
- **Breach rule:** All breaches of protected health information must be notified to affected individuals and to the DHHS Office for Civil Rights.

computer is a HIPAA requirement). Confidentiality and complete security requirements have increased since February 2010, including having a small health plan use a single national provider identifier.

The Department of Health and Human Services (DHHS) is the federal agency that oversees HIPAA. It has emphasized reasonableness as a guide to applying HIPAA regulations. Depending on the facility with which you are involved, interpretation of HIPAA ranges from reasonable to very strict. HIPAA rules and regulations have been reviewed and updated yearly since 2003. Details beyond the HIPAA discussion that follows can be found at update to https://www.hhs.gov.

? Critical Thinking

Client Privacy

List some examples of client information that could compromise client privacy if revealed.

The Notice of Privacy Practices

The main focus of HIPAA is protection of privacy. Each covered entity (health facility) must develop a written "Notice of Privacy Practices." The notice is made available to all clients, employees, and health-related companies with whom the facility does business (e.g., health insurance companies, medical equipment companies). The client receives a personal copy to read and sign. Signing the copy denotes understanding of, and agreement with, the use and disclosure of PHI for treatment, payment, and facility operation. This is not the same as consent for treatment. If the client is incompetent, state laws are followed. This usually means that the client's health proxy is treated as though he or she is the client.

What the Notice of Privacy Practices Addresses

The Notice of Privacy Practices must address the following in plain language:

1. **Access to medical records.** Clients have a right to a copy of their medical records and to review the records upon request. The facility determines under what conditions the records can be reviewed. Generally, this means reviewing the records with an RN or a health care provider present to translate medical terminology and answer questions. At no time does an SPN/SVN or LPN/LVN provide the records, or any part of them, to the client. The request must follow the protocol set up by the facility. The Notice of Privacy Practices must clearly state how to access the records. HIPAA allows up to 30 days for a facility to provide medical records for a client. A client may be charged for being provided PHI as hard copies or on electronic media, for example, the cost of a CD or flash drive/USB thumb drive.
2. **Amendments to medical records.** According to HIPAA, clients have the right to request changes in their medical records. All covered entities must appoint privacy officers. It is the job of the privacy officer to process a request for change in a client's medical records. The facility is obligated to consider the request and then notify the client of the final decision.
3. **Restrictions on the use of protected health information.** Clients can restrict use of their PHI as long as the requested information does not interfere with activities related to treatment, payment, or facility operation. The privacy officer usually makes the final decision. Rules include prohibition of the sale of PHI (without authorization) for use in marketing and fund raising.
4. **Access to an accounting.** Clients can request a list of the people, companies, or agencies that have received their PHI. The Notice of Privacy Practices lists steps for requesting an accounting on written request from a client. Rules exist restricting certain types of information to health plans.
5. **Confidential communications.** Clients may request that PHI be delivered in such a way that the sender cannot be identified. For example, the client may request that blood test results be mailed in a plain envelope without the agency's return address.

6. **Complaints about violations of privacy.** Clients can file a complaint if they think their privacy has been violated. The Notice of Privacy Practices tells them how to contact the privacy officer, as well as how to file the complaint. The Notice also provides information on how to contact the DHHS, the federal oversight agency for HIPAA. If a client is not satisfied with the outcome of filing a complaint with the facility's privacy officer, he or she may choose to contact DHHS. If DHHS determines there is a reason to investigate, it will do so and impose a fine on the covered entity if it has violated the HIPAA law.
7. **Minimum necessary rule.** This rule assists you in making an on-the-spot decision about how much client PHI you need to divulge. For example, if you are ordering a special bed for a client, you will need to include the client's height and weight. You will usually have no reason to include diagnosis, among other information.
8. **Telephone requests for PHI.** Nurses are often faced with telephone inquiries about a client. It is difficult to identify who is really making the inquiry and for what purpose. The HIPAA privacy rule permits a covered hospital to maintain a directory of client information including name, room number, and condition. More detailed information is available at www.cms.gov.
9. **E-mail and faxes.** To reduce the possibility of error during electronic transfer of information, the "minimum necessary" rule applies. Perhaps you have experienced sending an e-mail or fax to the wrong person. Think about the possible consequences of this happening with PHI. One safety feature is a disclaimer on an e-mail or fax that identifies the mail as confidential and explains how to notify the sender in case of error.

? Critical Thinking

Medical Records

Think of one or more reasons why, if a client removes or changes information in a medical record, it can affect a pending legal case.

Concerns That the Health Insurance Portability and Accountability Act Does Not Address

Additional concerns that the HIPAA does not address include discarding PHI that is not meant for the client's chart and hallway conversations (Box 7.16).

Try This

Maintain Client Confidentiality

Keep confidential the conversations you overhear in the clinical area that include personal information about a client and those that include more than the "minimum necessary" about a client. List one time that you were convinced to provide confidential information to an unauthorized person about a client. How can you avoid this in the future?

Box 7.16 Additional Concerns Not Addressed by Health Insurance Portability and Accountability Act (HIPAA)

- Protected health information not meant for the chart includes daily client assignments, nurse's personal notes about the client (used as the basis for charting), and anything else that could identify the client that is crumpled up and thrown in the wastebasket at the end of the shift. Many facilities have dealt with this by identifying a specific disposal area where the notes ultimately get shredded.
- Hallway conversation remains a problem. For example, a conversation about a client might not be overheard by the client involved but is often overheard by other clients or visitors. The same is true with conversation in lunchrooms, nursing desk areas, waiting rooms, and elevators.

Expect to find differences in interpretation of the HIPAA law. Find a copy of the facility privacy policy during each clinical rotation and do the same with each job you have after graduation. Note the differences and adjust to them. Question your employer if you do not understand why the differences exist. Seek to understand how the differences still meet HIPAA requirements.

CLIENT COMPETENCY

You can expect to hear increased use of the term *competency* in both a legal and a clinical sense. The following details provide a brief framework to help you use this term correctly.

Client competency has both a legal meaning and a clinical meaning. Some clients' rights issues are based on proof of competence or incompetence within the court system. *Legal* competency refers to a client who is:

- Eighteen years old or older.
- A pregnant or married woman.
- A self-supporting minor (referred to as a legally emancipated minor).
- Competent in the eyes of the law (incompetence is determined by the court).

Clinical competency refers to a client who is able to do the following:

- Identify the problem for which he or she is seeing the health care provider.
- Understand the options for care and the possible consequences.
- Make a decision.
- Provide sound reasons for the option he or she chooses.

CLIENT'S RIGHT TO CONSENT

The client's right to consent to or refuse treatment is a significant example of client autonomy (right to choose). It is advisable for a client to be accompanied by someone he or she trusts whenever he or she goes to a health agency for care. Clients are often stressed to the point that they do not "hear" what is being said to them. Words such as "cancer" and "heart attack" can cause sheer terror. Furthermore, some clients still are afraid to question the health care provider and therefore agree to procedures that they do not understand; "whatever you think is best" is a frequent response.

General (Implied) Consent

General (implied) consent for treatment is obtained on admission. It may be obtained by the LPN/LVN or by an admission clerk during a routine admission. The fact that a person has voluntarily sought admission to a health care agency and willingly signs a general admission form is an example of general consent. A client may revoke this permission verbally or in writing (e.g., you walk into a client's room with a syringe and explain that the health care provider has ordered Demerol for pain relief; the client might say, "I don't want a shot; I'm going home"). Institutional policy and procedure will confirm if the LPN/LVN can obtain general consent.

? Critical Thinking

Resolve Consent Issues

What steps will you take in the case of a client refusing to be turned every 2 hours?

Informed Consent

Informed consent must be obtained for invasive procedures ordered for therapeutic or diagnostic purposes (e.g., surgery). Informed consent means that the client is told the following in nonmedical language:

1. Diagnosis or suspected diagnosis
2. Purpose and description of treatment (some surgeons send the client home with a video or provide instructions to access a website that shows the surgery being performed before asking them to sign a consent form)
3. Expected outcome, expected benefits, and possible side effects or complications
4. Explanation of alternative treatments and their benefits, possible side effects, or complications
5. Names and qualifications of the people who will perform the procedure (treatment)
6. Prognosis if treatment is not done (when known)
7. Answers to questions client wants clarified
8. Explanation that the client has the right to revoke written permission at any time

The client must indicate comprehension (understanding) of the information. This means considerably more than just nodding the head. For example, have the client explain in his or her own words what he or she thinks is going to happen and the benefits and risks involved. Document the client's understanding of the information.

Informed consent is the responsibility of the health care provider because he or she must explain the implications and complications of the procedure to the client before written permission is obtained. *It is never the responsibility of the LPN/LVN or a student*. If you are in the room when the health care provider is obtaining informed consent, you might be asked to witness the signing. As a witness you are confirming that you observed the client give his signature willingly (no coercion) and the client appeared competent. As a student you are not allowed to be a witness.

If the LPN/LVN is present when the treatment is being explained and the informed consent signed, in most states the LPN/LVN may support the teaching that has taken place by the health care provider. Be sure to check your state's NPA and employer's policy.

Authorized Consent

Parents cannot give informed consent for the treatment of their children, but they can authorize treatment for their children up to a certain age; this is called **authorized consent**. Courts of law recognize that parents generally authorize what is appropriate for their children. In most states, "minor" is defined as younger than age 18. Some states allow minors to give their own consent for treatment of substance abuse, mental health problems, and sexually transmitted diseases (STDs). Emancipated minors (legal mechanism) are defined as those living on their own and managing their own finances or who are married and have children. They are competent to give their consent.

END-OF-LIFE ISSUES

PATIENT SELF-DETERMINATION ACT

The **Patient Self-Determination Act (PSDA)** (Teoli, 2021) is an amendment to the Omnibus Budget Reconciliation Act (a federal law). The PSDA requires many Medicare and Medicaid providers (e.g., hospitals, nursing homes, hospice programs, home health agencies, and health maintenance organizations [HMOs]) to give adult individuals, at the time of inpatient admission, certain information about their rights under state laws governing **advance directives**, including the following:

- The right to participate in and direct their own health care decisions
- The right to accept or refuse medical or surgical treatment
- The right to prepare an advance directive
- Information on the provider's policies that govern the utilization of these rights

ADVANCE DIRECTIVES

Two types of written advance directives are available to a client to give direction to health care providers about treatment choices in certain circumstances. The two types of advance directives are a living will and a durable power of attorney for health care. A good advance directive describes the kind of treatment that is desired by the person, depending on how sick he or she is. Usually the advance directive indicates what type of treatment is not desired. However, it can indicate that the person wants all possible measures used to prolong life. Information on advance directives can be found at MedlinePlus at https://medlineplus.gov/advancedirectives.html.

Living Will

A **living will** is a legal document that describes the kind of medical treatments or life-sustaining treatments the person would want if seriously or terminally ill. There are many issues that can be addressed, including the following:

- Transfusion of blood or blood products
- Cardiopulmonary resuscitation (CPR)
- Diagnostic tests
- Administration of medications
- Tissue or organ donations
- Dialysis
- Use of respirator
- Tube feeding
- Surgery
- Hydration, pain medication, food, and other comfort measures

A living will does not let the person select someone to make decisions for them. The living will is filled out by the individual and witnessed by a person who will not benefit by the death of that individual. Some individuals will use an attorney to develop a living will.

Living wills are recognized as legal documents in most states in the United States, the District of Columbia, and Guam. A few states do not recognize a living will as binding. The individual generally is advised to give a witnessed copy to the health care provider and a trusted friend or relation and to keep one copy in a location that is easily accessible. If a person is moving to or spending time in another state, he or she is advised to determine whether or not the living will is considered legal in that state. Otherwise, the person may discover too late that the written directive may not be honored. Blank forms are available from hospitals, other health care agencies, age-related organizations such as the American Association of Retired Persons (AARP), and attorneys' offices. Living wills can be revoked in writing or orally.

Durable Medical Power of Attorney (Advanced Health Care Directive)

A **durable medical power of attorney** (DPOA) is a legal document that is valid in all 50 states. It names a health care proxy (anyone at least 18 years old) to make medical decisions if that person is no longer able to make decisions. The DPOA is generally more useful than a living will. It becomes active anytime the person is unconscious or unable to make a medical decision. The DPOA may not be a good choice if the person has no one to trust to make these decisions.

> **Try This**
>
> **Legal Directives**
>
> Discuss the difference between a durable medical power of attorney and a living will.

DO-NOT-RESUSCITATE ORDER

A **do-not-resuscitate (DNR)** order is an advance directive based on the PSDA that gives a health care provider legal permission to write such an order. The health care provider may also write a DNR order for a client who no longer has decision-making ability but does not have personal advance directives written and signed. Commonly called a "no-code" order, it is a legal order to not resuscitate a client. The DNR order does not have to be updated unless the client changes her or his mind. If a written DNR order does not exist and the nurse does not try to resuscitate the client, the nurse is in effect making a medical decision. The nurse is essentially practicing medicine without a license and may be subject to a lawsuit. In addition, occasionally you may hear terms used such as "partial" or "slow" code. Generally, these terms may not be legal and can be viewed as unethical. All caregivers must know when a written DNR order exists. Check your state and agency policies regarding DNR orders because they vary considerably among states.

Sometimes providers ignore client advance directives. The client's instructions may be too vague, or the health care provider might assume that the client did not know about an available treatment, or simply defers to the wishes of family members. Sometimes clients have not discussed advance directives with their health care provider, or a facility has a policy that a written health care provider's order of DNR must be in the chart to comply with the client's wish. A survey by the California Health Care Foundation (2012) showed that only 7% of the respondents had spoken to their provider regarding end-of-life (EOL) wishes, despite the fact that 80% wanted to have a conversation. In the same survey, only 23% had put their EOL wishes in writing. Thus EOL dilemmas will occur in your practice. Additionally, it may be health care providers may find it difficult to initiate and facilitate these conversations. Chen et al. (2022) stated that it is critical for health care professionals to improve end-of-life communication practices to ensure that the patient dies "a good death."

For your legal protection, find out about your state's and facility's policies and if the client has a written advance directive of which the health care provider is aware. Do-not-hospitalize (DNH) orders may be more effective than DNR orders in limiting treatment and preventing unnecessary or unwanted client transfer *from* long-term care *to* an acute treatment facility. Most important for you, as an LPN/LVN, is to know your agency's policy. The Conversation Project provides a wealth of resources to assist people in having EOL conversations. More information can be found at https://theconversationproject.org/.

Physicians Orders for Life-Sustaining Treatment or POLST means that the order is valid outside the clinic or doctor's office. This form, often times printed on neon pink paper, tells all health care providers and first responders during a medical emergency what the client desires. It is for the seriously ill or frail client. It is more than a DNR order(https://polst.org/). For home care patients, the POLST form should be posted in an easy to see place, such as on a refrigerator or on the front door, so emergency responders will see it immediately before attempting resuscitation.

REMOVAL OF LIFE SUPPORT SYSTEMS

The health care provider must pronounce the client dead and document this status before the nurse turns off a ventilator. If the nurse removes a life support system before the health care provider pronounces the client dead, it can be considered an act of murder.

PRONOUNCEMENT OF DEATH

In many states the RN can also pronounce the client dead; however, this practice has been beyond the scope of practice for the LPN/LVN. However, the scope is changing, and in some types of care, such as home-based hospice care, a few states (PA, VA) have introduced legislation to allow the LPN/LVN to pronounce death. Check your SBON website for updates on this change.

PHYSICIAN-ASSISTED SUICIDE AND EUTHANASIA

Physician-assisted suicide (PAS) and **euthanasia** are not the same. "Physician-assisted suicide refers to a health care provider providing the means for death, most often with a prescription. The client, not the health care provider, will ultimately administer the lethal medication. Euthanasia generally means that the health care provider would act directly (for instance, by giving a lethal injection) to end a client's life" (Starks et al., 2013).

Both are different from the DNR order that a health care provider writes based on an agreement the health care provider makes with the client or the client's family. A DNR order is a passive action, with the goal of avoiding prolonging life unnecessarily, not actively ending it. Table 7.2 provides a comparison of active and passive euthanasia.

The following practices are also different from PAS:

- The practice of administering pain medication that may hasten death and relieve suffering for a terminally ill person has been held justifiable by courts (as long as the intent is to relieve suffering).
- The ANA (2013) position statement, *Euthanasia, Assisted Suicide, and Aid in Dying*, stated, "The ANA recognizes that assisted suicide and euthanasia continue to be debated. Despite philosophical and legal arguments in favor of assisted suicide it is the position of the ANA as specified in the Code that nurses' participation in assisted suicide and euthanasia is strictly prohibited."

ANA released a revised position statement in 2019, *The Nurses Role when a Client Requests Medical Aid in Dying*, which supersedes the 2013 statement. ANA states,

> *Knowledge of one's own stance helps clarify the boundary knowledge of between nonjudgment and respect for client's decisions, and imposition of personal values. Clarity about personal and professional values related to end-of-life options and care can also help nurses recognize the conditions to which they may conscientiously object. The nurse understands the distinction between medical aid in dying and euthanasia, and refrains from the sole intent to end life.*

ANA released a comprehensive statement in 2024: *Nurses' Roles and Responsibilities in Providing Care and Support at the End of Life*. The position emphasizes the importance of collaboration of the nurse with health care team members to ensure optimal symptom management for the patient and the family. Additionally it directs the nurse and health care providers to establish decision-making processes that reflect physiological realties, patient preferences, and the recognition of what clinically may or may not be accomplished. Check your state board of nursing or state nurses association websites often for updates on these controversial topics.

Death With Dignity Legislation

Oregon was the first state, in 1994, to have legislation to allow terminally ill residents to end their lives through

Table 7.2 Active and Passive Euthanasia

ACTIVE (ACTIONS THAT SPEED THE PROCESS OF DYING)	PASSIVE (DO NOTHING TO PRESERVE LIFE)
Actively end a person's life	Avoid prolonging a person's life
Initiate the dying process	Allow to continue a process that causes death
Morally wrong	Morally permissible
Legally not allowed	Legally allowed
Forbidden by professional organizations	Approved by professional organizations

the voluntary self-administration of a lethal dose of medications prescribed by a physician for that purpose (Oregon Health Authority, 2025). The **Death with Dignity Act** information is available at https://www.oregon.gov/oha/PH/ProviderPartnerResources/Evaluationresearch/deathwithdignityact/Pages/index.aspx.

According to the Death with Dignity National Center, as of 2025, 10 states have death with dignity statutes. Eighteen states are considering this legislation. To see the status of all states go to this link https://deathwithdignity.org/states/. In Oregon and Vermont, as of 2023, residency requirements were removed, with medical aid-in-dying (MAID) legislation.

Try This

Terminally Ill Clients

Divide into three groups. Choose a viewpoint about the terminally ill from the following descriptions. Be prepared to present reasons for the viewpoint. Choose a spokesperson to summarize the group's views.

- Group 1: Terminally ill clients have the right to choose death by PAS.
- Group 2: Terminally ill clients must wait to die of natural causes.Group 3: The nurse's personal ethics conflict with the decision of groups 1 and 2. Discuss the nurse's rights, roles, and responsibilities to the client.Refer to the critical thinking steps in Chapter 5 to assist you in making your decision.

ORGAN DONATION

Organ donations are voluntary. At this time, organs cannot legally be bought or sold. Although many clients and families give permission for organ donation after death, the demand for organs far exceeds the supply. You may have been asked to agree to personal organ donation when you received/renewed your driver's license. Many states participate in this effort. To increase the number of donors, it has been suggested that money be allocated to cover the donor's funeral expenses.

Body tissues that can be donated include skin, corneas, bone, heart valves, and blood. One example of an early successful body tissue transplant was the transplantation of umbilical cord blood for a rare genetic bone disease at the University of Minnesota in Duluth in 1995. Approximately one cup of blood, taken from a newborn's discarded umbilical cord and placenta, was donated. Donated body organs include the heart, liver, kidneys, lungs, and pancreas. Organ donation has raised both ethical and legal questions in some instances, for example, having a baby so that select organs or body tissues can be used to save a sibling.

END-OF-LIFE CARE

Many organizations and projects are devoted to establishing **EOL principles**. Numerous organizations, including the American Medical Association, TJC, National Hospice and Palliative Care Organization (NHPCO), and the National Association for Home Care and Hospice (NAHC), have adopted or support core principles for end-of-life care. The NHCPO describes hospice as focusing on caring, not curing when clients face a life-limiting illness (see https://www.nhpco.org/hospice-care-overview for more details). The Center to Advance Palliative Care defines palliative care as "specialized care for people with serious illness" (see https://www.capc.org/). Palliative care can be provided aside curative procedures. Palliative care and hospice care are common care modalities today. LPNs/LVNs are employed in home care and hospice units where this care is provided. The NAHC provides related resources at their website, https://www.nahc.org.

Get Ready for the Next-Generation NCLEX® Examination

Key Points

- The state's NPA is the most definitive legal statute or legislative act regulating nursing practice. It governs what you can and cannot do as a nurse in your scope of practice.
- Basic terminology in the NPA is standard in many states; however, scope of practice differs.
- Student nurses are held to the standard of an LPN/LVN, working under the supervision of the clinical instructor.
- Eight general categories of Board of Nursing disciplinary cases include fraud and deceit, criminal activity, negligence, incompetence, violation of the NPA or rules, disciplinary action by another board, unethical conduct, and alcohol and/or other substance use.
- Disciplinary action is based on rules of law. If guilty, the board may issue a public or private reprimand, such as probation, nonrenewal of license, suspension of license, revocation of license, or instruction to enter into a voluntary diversion rehabilitation program if the issue is alcohol and/or other substances.
- After successful completion of the NCLEX-PN® examination, the LPN/LVN may practice in the state of licensure. Some states accept licensure through interstate endorsement or the Nurse Licensure Compact.
- The nursing standard of care is what an ordinary, prudent nurse with similar education and experience would do in a similar situation.

- Ethics deals with rules of conduct; law provides regulations that control the practice of nursing.
- Common law is judge-made law that is useful in settling disputes such as tort law.
- The legislative branch of the state and federal government develops statutory law: The NPA is a statutory law.
- Civil action is related to individual rights; criminal action involves persons and society as a whole.
- Tort law has to do with a wrong or injury to someone that violates his or her rights.
- Intentional torts involve intended harm by the nurse, such as assault and battery, false imprisonment and use of restraints, defamation, and physical and emotional abuse.
- Unintentional torts mean no harm was intended by the nurse (e.g., professional negligence [malpractice]).
- Good Samaritan Acts hold that a person who gives emergency care in good faith at the scene of an accident is immune from being successfully sued. Some states have laws that make it mandatory to assist at the scene of an accident. A victim has the right to refuse aid.
- Elements necessary for negligence are duty, breach of duty, damages, and proximate cause.
- Personal liability holds us responsible for our behavior, including negligent behavior.
- Depositions are used to gather information under oath.
- When giving testimony, take your time; say "yes" or "no" when possible, *without adding details*; stick to the facts; and correct mistakes and misconceptions.
- Documentation is a legal expectation in nursing regardless of the method used. If it was not charted, it was not done, or it did not happen.
- Medication errors are among the most common errors related to nursing liability.
- Client competency has both a legal and a clinical definition.
- A client's right to consent is general, informed, or authorized, depending on the situation.
- Client rights include *The Client Care Partnership: Understanding Expectations, Rights, and Responsibilities;* the HIPAA Privacy Rule; and the PSDA.
- The PSDA includes advance directives (living will and durable power of medical attorney), written and signed by a client to state his or her wishes for EOL care.
- DNR orders written by a health care provider are legal orders to not resuscitate a client and are made possible because of the PSDA.
- Nurses may not remove a life support system until a client is declared dead by the health care provider, or RN where allowed.
- PAS involves a client voluntarily ending his or her life by self-administering lethal medication prescribed by a health care provider, especially for that purpose. In the United States this is legal in 10 states and more are enacting legislation.
- Active euthanasia entails health care providers directly administering a lethal medication to end a client's life. This is not legal in the United States.
- The ANA and AMA have evolving positions on nurse and health care provider participation in assisted suicide.
- Organ donation has cultural, religious, legal, and ethical constraints. In the United States, you can note on your driver's license if you wish to donate your organs.

Additional Learning Resources

Go to your Evolve website (http://evolve.elsevier.com/Carroll/success/) for the following FREE learning resources:

- Answers to Critical Thinking Scenarios
- Additional learning activities
- Additional Review Questions for the NCLEX-PN® examination
- Helpful phrases for communicating in Spanish and more!

Clinical Judgment and Next-Generation NCLEX® Examination-Style Questions

1. The SPNs/SVNs are discussing legal concepts. Which of the following indicates their understanding of the best reference that determines LPN/LVN legal guidelines for practice?

a. Institutional policy and procedure
b. State NPA
c. Employee handbook
d. School of nursing

2. The instructor is observing student nurses at a clinical site. Which situation most clearly illustrates negligence?

a. The student nurse became angry when the client would not stop screaming and slapped the client's face.
b. The student nurse inserted the urinary catheter, despite the client's refusal, because their bladder was visibly distended.
c. The student nurse decided to restrain an elderly client to prevent her from falling out of bed.
d. The student nurse forgot to lower the client's bed after completing colostomy care, and the client fell when trying to get out of bed.

3. A student nurse is assigned to a drug and alcohol rehabilitation unit. The preceptor recommends that the two students review several charts to compare various treatment strategies. While reviewing, the student nurse realizes that one of the charts is her ex-husband's chart. She decides to go visit him before she leaves for the day. Which statement best describes the outcome of this action?

a. Permissible as long as you do not look at his confidential records
b. A violation of the Affordable Care Act
c. A violation of HIPAA
d. Permissible because he is the student nurse's ex-husband

4. A nurse is asked to give testimony during a legal action. Which statement describes the nurse's best action in response to the lawyer's questions when giving her testimony?

a. Offer to tell what you believe really happened when the wrong medication was given.
b. Avoid referring to any documents to show how well you recall the incident.
c. Fill in silences with information about the health care provider who ordered the medication.
d. Be specific, answering "yes" or "no" whenever possible, without adding details.

5. **Which of the following are legal clients' rights? *(Select all that apply.)***
   - **a.** The right to revoke a signed informed consent verbally on the way to surgery
   - **b.** The right to take their medical records with them when they leave the hospital
   - **c.** The right to designate who will make decisions for them should they become incapable
   - **d.** The right to ask their health care provider to inject them with lethal medications that will end life
   - **e.** The right to file a suit for injury that they see as being the result of negligence

6. **Which of the following are needed to prove negligence? *(Select all that apply.)***
   - **a.** Deposition
   - **b.** NPA
   - **c.** Duty
   - **d.** Causation
   - **e.** Damages

7. **Highlight the information in the scenario that is essential for the nurse to take action differently before giving the morphine sulfate.** An LPN/LVN works nights on the med surgery/neurology unit in a small private hospital. During the night, a client who had cranial surgery began to have a great deal of pain. The nurse called the client's health care provider (HCP) and gave a brief review about the client to include type of surgery and recent medications. The nurse asked the HCP to come to the unit to evaluate the client's condition. The HCP gave an order for the client for morphine sulfate. The dose was large. The nurse repeated the order and questioned if the HCP meant the stated high dose. The HCP became angry and insisted the nurse immediately give the client the dosage as ordered and to repeat the dose in an hour. Then the HCP threatened to lodge a complaint against the nurse if orders were not followed. The nurse gave the client the morphine as ordered, and the client died. The nurse was charged with negligence. At the trial, the HCP testified that the nurse had never called. What could the nurse have done to protect both the client and the nurse?

Critical Thinking Scenario

Scenario 1

You walk in the day room on a psychiatric unit and there is a client on the floor, profusely bleeding from the facial area. A nursing assistant indicates that another client hit the injured client. Two other clients contradict this statement and state, "The nursing assistant pushed the client when the client would not start walking back to the client's room, and the client fell."

You are the LPN in the scenario described. Explain all actions you will immediately implement and all related follow-up. Explain your actions/provide rationales.

8 Effective Communication With Clients, Health Care Team, Faculty, and Peers

Objectives

On completing this chapter, you will be able to do the following:

1. Summarize key elements of the communication process, including influencing factors.
2. Discuss the difference between one-way and two-way communication.
3. Differentiate between verbal, nonverbal, and affective forms of communication.
4. Explain how communication strategies may be used every day during the practice of nursing.
5. Describe key blocks to communication and potential influencing factors.
6. Discuss common factors that impact the communication of the hospitalized client and communication strategies the nurse can implement to reduce client distress.
7. Analyze characteristics of effective communication with the health care team and faculty.
8. Describe the four steps of situation, background, assessment, and recommendation (SBAR) and an example of how SBAR can be used for health care team communication.
9. Discuss additional actions, beyond SBAR, included in the identify, situation, background, assessment, recommendation, and repeat back (ISBARR) method.
10. Discuss the various methods of digital communication and practice considerations.
11. Describe key conflict resolution strategies.
12. Differentiate various communication considerations across the lifespan.

Key Terms

acting disinterested
active listening
affective communication
belittling
closed-ended questions
commitment
communication blocks
empathy
false reassurance
feedback
focused questions
giving advice
honesty
humor
"I" messages
identify, situation, background, assessment, recommendation, and repeat back (ISBARR)
judging
knowledge
message
nonverbal communication
one-way communication
open-ended questions
patience
probing
purpose
receiver
respect
self-efficacy
self-esteem
sender
sensitivity
simple answers
situation, background, assessment, and recommendation (SBAR)
therapeutic communication
trust
two-way communication
verbal communication

Keep in Mind

Purposeful communication is an integral part of your personal and professional world. Taking the time to learn that language, verbal or written, is powerful may bring positive results. Social media presents new challenges to communication.

Two student practical nurses/student vocational nurses (SPNs/SVNs) are frustrated with their clinical instructor. One student says, "The instructor is never consistent. Their communication is confusing. We are never sure what is really expected until we are reprimanded for not meeting the clinical outcomes. I wish she could be more like our past clinical instructor, Mrs. Lopez." The other student agrees, stating, "She was tough and had high expectations; however, her communication was clear. Anytime I was confused, Mrs. Lopez would paraphrase and then ask a focus question. This helped me clarify my thinking. Then she listened to my plan of care and summarized it to ensure that I knew the plan of care before entering the

room. This really decreased my anxiety and improved my learning. I think Mrs. Lopez should teach the entire faculty how to communicate. Our lives would be much easier!"
As you read this chapter, think about why Mrs. Lopez's communication was so effective. How can you implement similar strategies in your professional and personal life to improve your communication?

COMMUNICATION PROCESS

ESSENTIAL COMPONENTS OF THE COMMUNICATION PROCESS

There are five essential components to effective communication (Cherry and Jacob, 2019):

1. Source/sender
2. Message
3. Method of transmission
4. Receiver
5. Feedback

All five components are required for effective communication. The **sender** must present a **message** clearly using an effective **method of transmission** to the one receiving the message; the **receiver** must give **feedback** concerning the message so the sender can be reassured the message was appropriately understood. In Fig. 8.1 you can see that communication is a circular process. Feedback is received by the sender, which may trigger the sender to send another message, prompting the receiver to give additional feedback. The circle of communication continues. There are multiple factors that can affect communication at any point in the process. A discussion of those factors follows.

FACTORS THAT AFFECT COMMUNICATION

Some common factors that can influence communication include:

1. Personal attributes of both the sender and receiver
2. Cultural characteristics
3. Situational influences
4. Context in which the message is sent or received

Personal attributes can include such elements as age, gender, income, and marital status. Life experiences, attitudes, personal opinions, and bias are other personal attributes. *Cultural characteristics* can involve personal space and distance, language and dialect, use and meaning of touch, values, meaning of gestures, and time of day. *Situational influences*, sometimes referred to as *noise*, can include the physical (i.e., pain) and emotional state (i.e., anxiety) of the client and nurse, the room temperature, interruptions, background noises, odors, environmental distractions, and client privacy concerns (i.e., family's/significant other's presence and Health Insurance Portability and Accountability Act, or HIPAA). *Context* can include the appropriateness or inappropriateness of the communication. "What can I do to make you more comfortable?" is an appropriate question directed to a dying client. Discussion with the family about who gets the belongings of a loved one while the person is dying and within hearing distance is inappropriate communication. As a student, it is easy to forget context as you are focused on your own learning. Be sure to stop and think before you speak in front of a client or their family/visitors.

ONE-WAY VERSUS TWO-WAY COMMUNICATION

An SPN/SVN walked into a client's room at the start of the shift without knocking on the door and said, "I'm going to measure your blood pressure. Give me your arm." The client gave the SPN/SVN a quizzical look but exposed his arm. When the SPN/SVN finally got the cuff on after having some difficulty, he had a flushed face. The SPN's heart was beating so hard that she could not hear the client's heartbeat.

Try This

Communicating With Your Client

1. What kind of communication did the SPN/SVN provide to the client?
2. What steps did the SPN/SVN skip that resulted in making the client being uncomfortable?
3. After reviewing this chapter, discuss or role play how the SPN/SVN may have handled this interaction with effective communication skills.

The SPN/SVN engaged in **one-way communication**, in which the sender (the SPN/SVN) controlled the situation by telling the receiver (the client) what the receiver was going to do (the message). The SPN/SVN offered no opportunity for feedback (response) from the client. Feedback would have provided the client

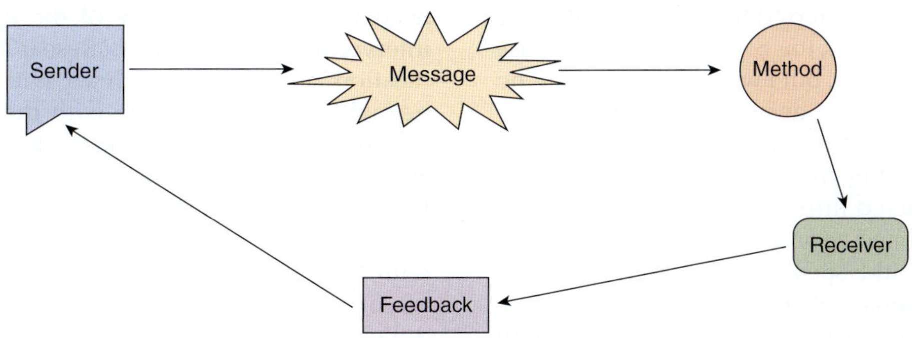

Fig. 8.1 Communication. (From Cherry B, Jacob S: *Contemporary nursing: issues, trends, and management*, ed 6, 2014, St. Louis: Mosby.)

with an opportunity to question, agree, or refuse the procedure. The SPN/SVN was so focused on herself and the tasks she was required to do that she omitted common courtesies, such as knocking on the door and introducing herself to the client, ensuring she was close enough to be heard and in a proper position, sharing the reason for being there. Best practice requires using two client identifiers to ensure client safety. The student created an unsafe environment by not using two client identifiers when engaging in the interaction. The client's unspoken response may have increased the student's discomfort.

One-way communication is used to give a command, as in military service, or give information when no feedback is expected. There are rare occasions when one-way communication is acceptable. An imminent or real disaster would be an example. Even during an urgent client situation, **two-way communication** generally creates a safer environment. A health care provider's oral order is repeated by the nurse, thus verifying the order for accuracy. Two-way communication is the usual form of conversation in health care. Each person contributes equally, and feedback is both expected and respected.

TYPES OF COMMUNICATION

The three types of communication are verbal (spoken or written word), nonverbal (body language), and affective (feeling tone). They may or may not all occur at the same time. When they do occur together, all three must mirror one another (be congruent) for the communication to be honest. This is the ideal but often does not occur. Individuals frequently send mixed messages. For example, a client has diarrhea and is incontinent for the third time that evening. He apologizes to the SPN/SVN. The SPN/SVN states, "No problem"; however, the client notes a sense of frustration in her face and voice. As a result, he feels more embarrassed and depressed.

VERBAL COMMUNICATION

Verbal communication is powerful. A client may accept what an SPN/SVN says as an absolute fact, appearing as clear evidence. The SPN/SVN should know in advance what can or cannot be discussed with a client and what should be referred to another health care team member. Sometimes the SPN's/SVN's response should be: "I do not know, but I will find someone who does." Evidence provides answers to many clients' questions. The SPN/SVN should be sure to use a valid source when answering clients' questions. Collaboration with the registered nurse (RN) to ensure communication is accurate and appropriate is vital.

SPNs/SVNs should speak as clearly as possible, using proper grammar. Slang is usually not appropriate and may have a different meaning to different people. Depending on age and culture, the client may not understand slang. Using out-of-date slang can also make the SPN/SVN come across as unprofessional or silly. Worse yet, the slang word may be considered no longer culturally acceptable.

Medical jargon is rarely helpful. If SPNs/SVNs truly understand medical terms, they can translate the words into everyday language. The use of colloquial (common) expressions will be appropriate with some clients (i.e., pediatric clients). For example, the word "urinate" may be understood by some children as pass water, tinkle, or pee-pee. SPNs/SVNs should use the word that the client understands. Clients need a professional he or she can look up to and one who will respect his or her individual differences; the client does not need the nurse to be a buddy.

SPNs/SVNs should maintain professional boundaries. A client will respect SPNs/SVNs and follow their directions if professionalism is displayed. The focus of conversation during care should be on the client and not personal concerns, such as a child's crisis at school or an argument with a classmate.

Some illnesses also affect a client's interpretation of verbalization. Clients with neurological disorders can experience diverse communication issues. Both expressive and receptive aphasia can occur. Expressive aphasia will contribute to each client's difficulty finding and saying the right word, phrase, or sentence. These clients will have great difficulty sending messages. Receptive aphasia can prohibit the client from understanding the spoken word. Thus their ability to receive a message is adversely impacted, reducing their ability to understand instructions. Clients with Alzheimer's disease also experience communication issues caused by memory impairment. Clients diagnosed with schizophrenia interpret words concretely (literally). They have trouble understanding abstract (inferred) meanings. For example, after using a stationary bicycle, a client was asked by the nurse, "How do you feel now?" He grabbed his buttocks and responded, "My butt is numb; that's how." The nurse had been trying to determine a change in his stress level. Instead, his response was based on literal interpretation of the question.

Individuals with intellectual, developmental, and cognitive disabilities can create a challenge for communication and high-quality health care. Nurses need to assess the nature of the disability and plan interventions accordingly. Researching the communication needs of individuals with various disabilities will provide students with the necessary critical information and interventions to manage these clients. For additional information, refer to the National League for Nursing's Advancing Care Excellence Series for Persons with Disabilities: Communicating with People with Disabilities (2024) at https://www.nln.org/education/teaching-resources/professional-development-programsteaching-resourcesace-all/ace-d.

Nurses must also be concerned with the health literacy of a client. Health literacy is the ability of an individual to obtain, understand, and use information and health care services to promote personal health (CDC, 2023). This may be impacted by their level of education, primary language spoken, ability to read and/or write, access to health information via the Internet and other technologies, or level of wellness (when individuals feel sick, they are less apt to listen well). Interpreters are effective for bridging any language gap between the nurse and client. Improving health literacy could improve health outcomes and access to health care services among clients. One goal of Healthy People 2030 is to improve the health literacy of individuals as an effort to improve health. Beyond verbal instruction, nurses can improve health literacy by providing written educational material that has simple instructions in a client's preferred language with culturally sensitive verbiage. By using two-way communication (discussed earlier in this chapter), a nurse is better able to assess the client's understanding of any teaching provided by the nurse. Verbal communication will be a challenge in many health care settings. Well-developed communication strategies and the ability to try multiple approaches will enhance communication with the client and their family.

Try This

Health Literacy

1. Review the Healthy People 2030 objective: Improve Health Communication at https://health.gov/healthypeople/objectives-and-data/browse-objectives/health-communication
2. Review the Center for Disease Control and Prevention's website regarding Health Literacy: https://www.cdc.gov/health-literacy/php/about/?CDC_AAref_Val=https://www.cdc.gov/healthliteracy/learn/index.html
3. Discuss strategies a nurse could implement when considering the health literacy of a client.

NONVERBAL COMMUNICATION

Commonly known as body language, **nonverbal communication** either supports or cancels verbal communication. Expressions, eye contact, posture, movements, touch, and gestures, whether the client's or the SPN's/SVN's, give important clues to the truth of the verbal communication. Careful observation of body language may clue the SPN/SVN into client discomfort, even though pain has been denied verbally. Gathering additional data will help clarify the real issue creating discomfort. The use of telehealth and social media communication modalities can further limit nonverbal communication, eliminating this potential piece of data. The SPN/SVN should implement all strategies to ensure a minimal impact on nonverbal behavior.

Nonverbal communication works both ways. Clients tend to observe the SPN/SVN closely, looking for clues regarding the seriousness of their illness. For example, a male client who is carefully watching an SPN/SVN review results of his diagnostic tests may conclude erroneously that he is acutely ill, because of a distressed look on the SPN's/SVN's face. How is he to know that the SPN/SVN just received a text from her child's school informing her of a verbal altercation involving her child?

Nonverbal communication also includes the volume and tone of voice that is used when communicating with one another. Some may perceive a loud voice as confident or enthusiastic and others may perceive it as anger. The tone of voice provides meaning to words as well. When SPNs/SVNs ask clients how they slept the previous night and they say "fine," is it a cold (not well, but don't want to talk about it), downcast (did not sleep well and maybe you should investigate further), or happy (they slept well) tone? Additionally, SPNs/SVNs may adjust their volume and tone based on the needs of the client. An elderly client with hearing loss may require a louder voice during interactions, and a newborn/babies may require a more soothing volume with a musical tone.

Physical appearance is a part of nonverbal communication. The client's appearance on admission provides signs of personal care plus important clues about the illness. Clients also quickly evaluate SPNs/SVNs and, based on what they observe, will draw conclusions about the SPN's/SVN's competence as a nurse. This is a major reason why most nursing schools continue to have a dress code. It is also the reason why instructors demonstrate appropriate dress and behavior to students.

Try This

Appropriate Dress Code and Behavior

Observe a client's response to different members of the health care team based on their dress and behavior. Describe what you observed. Explain the changes you will make based on your observations.

AFFECTIVE COMMUNICATION

"Affect" refers to mood or emotion. The feeling tone that people perceive when they approach a person or step into a room is real. For every thought a person has, there is a physiological response in the body. The same is true for the client and others in which a nurse encounters. The tendency may be to ignore this level of communication because it cannot be seen or heard. **Affective communication** is as significant as verbal and nonverbal communication. Truly honest communication integrates verbal, nonverbal, and affective communications so they all express the same message.

Critical Thinking

Affective Communication

1. Give an example of a time that you stepped into a room or approached a person and, before anyone spoke a word, experienced a feeling of excitement, happiness, sadness, anger, tension, or some other emotion. What was the outcome?
2. Think of a time when you were angry and tried to hide the feeling. Did anyone pick up on your feeling tone and ask you if you were angry? How did you deal with the question?
3. Give examples of how you try to be congruent (matching) verbally, nonverbally, and affectively in your communication. What do you need to improve to achieve more congruency?

STRATEGIES FOR THERAPEUTIC COMMUNICATION

There are many strategies for improving therapeutic communication in health care. Active listening is a strategy that shows respect for the sender and assists the receiver with hearing the correct message (Tennant et al., 2023). Therapeutic communication cannot exist without active listening behaviors. The nurse can demonstrate therapeutic communication when asking clients open-ended, closed-ended, and focused questions. A nurse's personal characteristics can advance therapeutic communication to clients.

ACTIVE LISTENING

Active listening is probably the most important part of communication, particularly **therapeutic** (health-related, purposeful) **communication**. Therapeutic communication is the interaction between the nurse and the client, focusing on the client's physical and emotional needs. These interactions require the use of effective communication strategies to provide support to the client.

Key factors in active listening include purpose, disciplined attention, and focus. The **purpose** refers to the health-related reason for gathering or giving information. *Disciplined attention* means that a person does not assume accuracy of information without checking it. SPNs/SVNs should clarify what they think they understand the client is saying and ask further questions, as needed. This applies both to gathering information and giving health-related information. *Focus* means that all your senses are alert to clues that the client may be communicating. A common mistake in listening is to listen to the words but not really hear the words, misunderstanding the meaning.

ACTIVE LISTENING BEHAVIORS

The most used active listening behaviors include restating, clarifying, reflecting, paraphrasing, encouraging minimally, remaining silent, summarizing, and validating.

- **Restating** refers to repeating in a slightly different way what the client has said, for example:
  Client: "My chest hurts. I can't sleep at night."
  Nurse: "You've been unable to sleep at night because of chest pain."
- **Clarifying** is asking a closed-ended question in response to a client's statement, to be sure the nurse understands, for example:
  Client: "My chest hurts."
  Nurse: "Exactly where does your chest hurt?"
- **Reflecting** is putting into words the information you are receiving from the client at an effective communication level, for example:
  Client: "I'm sick of seeing health care providers and not getting answers."
  Nurse: "You are upset with the lack of answers to your health problems."
- **Paraphrasing** refers to expressing, in one's own words, what the nurse thinks the client means, for example:
  Client: "I don't think I'm being told the truth about my condition."
  Nurse: "You believe you have not received all the important information about your health condition."
- **Encouraging minimally** involves using only sounds, words, or short phrases to encourage the client to continue, for example:
  Client: "It just happened so fast . . ."
  Nurse: "Yes . . . go on . . . and then what . . . hmmm . . . uh huh . . ."
- **Remaining silent** involves using pauses effectively. The normal tendency is to fill silence with chatter or speculation. Even 5 seconds of silence can seem like forever. However, avoiding silence may cause the client to "turn off" or change the story. Maintaining disciplined attention and focus during silence lets clients tell the story in his or her own way. Avoid making interruptions and doing busy work while the client is speaking. Practice using silence as a communication strategy.
- **Summarizing** means briefly stating the main data gathered, for example:
  Nurse: "This is what I heard you say... Is that correct?"
- **Validating** provides the client with an opportunity to correct information, if necessary, at the time of summary, for example:
  Client: "That is correct" or "No, you got this part wrong . . ." (This allows the client to correct the information.)

TYPES OF QUESTIONS

The three types of questions that are commonly used in therapeutic communication are open-ended, closed-ended, and focused questions. **Open-ended questions** permit the client to respond in a way that is most meaningful to him or her. The questions often begin with *what, where, when, how,* or *why*. For example, the nurse might ask, "What happened to your leg?" **Closed-ended**

questions require a specific answer. For example, the nurse might ask, "When did you first notice the pain?" **Focused questions** provide even more definitive information. For example, the nurse might ask, "On a scale of 1 to 10, with 10 being the worst possible pain, how would you rate your pain right now?"

PERSONAL ACTIONS

Communication is far more complex than just talking. Some of the many contributing actions are listed below with a brief description in the following learning exercise.

Try This

Self-Evaluation of Personal Actions

Evaluate the effectiveness of your actions when communicating with clients.

ACTIONS	DESIRABLE	SELF-EVALUATION
Eye contact	Usually 3–5 seconds. Cultural variations exist.	________
Respect for personal space	Approximately 1.5 feet, except for personal care. Cultural variations exist.	________
Appropriate touch	Gentle, but firm. Cultural variations exist.	________
Attitude	Nonjudgmental. Practices unconditional love.	________
Voice/tone	Moderate or according to growth and development needs. For example, individuals typically talk to infants with a cheerful tone.	________
Rate	Paced according to client's ability to comprehend.	________
Appearance	Models positive nursing image. Looks healthy and ready to deliver high-quality care.	________
Posture	Open, without folded arms or hands on hips.	________
	Stands or sits upright to increase confidence.	________
Gestures	Moderate to enhance conversation. Consistent with conversation.	________
Language	Speaks effectively and at client's level of understanding. Correct grammar.	________
Expression	Demonstrating understanding and rapport. Nonjudgmental.	________

Critical Thinking

A Plan for Change

List the personal actions that are impacting your communication. Develop a plan for change and for measuring improvement, using the phases of the nursing process (see Chapter 12).

COMMUNICATION CHALLENGES

COMMUNICATION BLOCKS

Communication blocks occur daily. Often, nurses are not even aware of the impact. Perhaps the client's visual image, voice, or behavior triggers a sad thought or biased experience. Workload, stress, and exhaustion can create blocks of effective communication for a nurse. Imagine it is a snowy night: three people call in sick to work and there are no replacements, resulting in a nurse struggling to meet the needs of the clients and performing priority tasks only. During medication administration, a client is silently sobbing and starts talking to the nurse, who is already beyond the state-allowed time period for safe practice. In addition, the client reminds the nurse of a friend with whom the nurse struggled to get along. It is easy to see that multiple blocks are present. It is unlikely, despite the issue, that real communication will occur without effort. The nurse wants to give every client the best care possible, regardless of personal response and the given circumstance. Although it is not easy, careful planning can minimize communication blocks even in difficult situations. Common communication blocks involve reassuring falsely, probing, judging, belittling, giving advice, providing simple answers, and acting disinterested.

Avoiding Communication Blocks

- **False reassurance** involves making unsupported statements to the client, such as saying "Everything will be okay," or "You'll be just fine," or "Don't worry about anything," or "We'll make sure you get well," or "This experience will make you stronger," or "You'll see the good in this someday." There is no way SPNs/SVNs can guarantee what they are telling clients.
- **Probing** means pushing for information beyond what is medically necessary to know. Curiosity takes over, and the client's privacy is no longer respected. Consider the value of the information and how the information can be used. Think twice before continuing with statements, such as "Let's get to the bottom of this once and for all."
- **Judging** client behavior, such as smoking, is of limited value to the client with severe emphysema or lung cancer. It could be possible that the client never smoked. An SPN/SVN can provide therapeutic care to the client without supporting the client's behavior.

- **Belittling** involves mimicking or making fun of a client in some way. It may include downplaying the importance of the symptoms, such as when a nurse says, "You could be having heart surgery! This is just a wart removal." As a health care provider once pointed out, "If you have a tonsillectomy, it's minor surgery; if I have a tonsillectomy, it's major surgery." It is all a matter of perspective.
- **Giving advice** when an individual knows what someone else should do is very tempting. Unsolicited advice is rarely beneficial in health care and closes the door to the client personally solving a problem. A more beneficial response, even when the client asks what the nurse would do is to say, "What ideas do *you* have? I'm sure you've thought of ways you might solve this problem." This also gives the nurse an opportunity to review any evidence that could help assist the client with decision making. The SPN/SVN should listen carefully, summarize what the client has said, and then support the client in identifying the next steps, while suggesting available resources, as needed. In doing so, the SPN/SVN will assist the client in maintaining autonomy and receiving quality health care.
- Providing **simple answers** such as "Everyone feels this way" may come so easily, but these answers make clients feel dismissed and misunderstood. Clients do not really care if everyone else feels this way. As far as they are concerned, these feelings are theirs alone. The client's concerns are different from everyone else's, and they need a comforting touch or reassuring words. Provide an appropriate response, such as "I'll be in the room when you return."
- **Acting disinterested** with comments such as, "I have several other clients who are very sick tonight, what do you need?" can negatively impact communication, even if it is true. Clients need to know that their issues are important.

Try This

Blocks to Communication

Discuss examples of communication blocks that have occurred in your personal or professional life. Give examples of how these interactions could have been handled differently.

Body Posture and Communication

Body posture is a powerful nonverbal form of communication that can create or dissolve blocks in communication. When people stand tall, with shoulders back and head held high, they are perceived to have confidence and control. Confidence is important in therapeutic communication. Research has demonstrated that people can be perceived as being confident when they display an upright posture, as well as give direct eye contact and present with a smile (Schieber et al., 2022). How the client perceives the SPN's/SVN's level of confidence could impact communication.

Try This

Power Pose

Visit https://www.ted.com/talks/amy_cuddy_your_body_language_shapes_who_you_are?language5en and discover how to improve your confidence resulting in more effective communication.

CULTURAL DIFFERENCES

Members of diverse cultures within our dominant culture embrace and value their beliefs and practices. The SPN/SVN needs to be respectful of these beliefs and practices to respond therapeutically. The SPN/SVN has an interest in learning about cultural differences in communication. These differences can be noted in spoken language, voice volume, pronunciation, eye contact, touch, use of silence, and the use of personal space. Individual client differences need to be identified. Chapter 10 provides more information about cultural diversity.

Try This

Cultural Differences

List and discuss two cultural differences of someone in the area in which you live that could impact communication.

1. ______
2. ______

Communication patterns change with time, vary with the situation, and differ in public or private settings. SPNs/SVNs are encouraged to learn as much as possible about the cultures frequently served in their area and be mindful that families may have been in this country for generations, yet differences may be nonexistent regardless of ethnic background.

COMMUNICATION WITH CLIENTS

When individuals become sick and require hospitalization, the new role of being a hospitalized client can influence their communication. What happens to clients who find themselves in a dependent position after having always been in control of their lives? The concerns they have go beyond the physical realities into areas we consider in the next section. The SPN/SVN needs to be aware of the client's perspective while implementing therapeutic communication.

Critical Thinking

Immediate Concerns Upon Hospitalization

Imagine yourself being hospitalized. List four immediate concerns you would probably have. Discuss how these concerns relate to your various roles in life.

1. ______
2. ______
3. ______
4. ______

Professional Pointer

Best practice requires using two client identifiers (e.g., name and birth date) to ensure safe practice. After the client states their name, ask the client what the client would prefer to be called and address the client consistently thereafter, as desired. However, always be sure to verify their formal name and utilize two client identifiers when required.

THE INTRODUCTION

The SPN's/SVN's communication, verbally, nonverbally, and affectively, sets the tone for rapport with the client. Showing respect to the client, the SPN/SVN will knock on the door and pause briefly to collect data *before* walking in. Nonverbal and affective communication clues can be assessed from the start of care. SPNs/SVNs are encouraged to address the client as *Mr.*, *Mrs.*, *Miss*, or *Ms.*, or by a professional title if it applies. SPNs/SVNs will provide their name, identify themselves as a student practical nurse/student vocational nurse (SPN/SVN), provide the name of their school, and state the purpose for being in the room.

It may sound something like this: "Good morning Mrs. Hill, my name is Koralynn. I am a student practical nurse/student vocational nurse from the Middle American Technical College. I am here to measure your blood pressure, temperature, pulse, and respirations. It is a part of the admission procedure. Would you please confirm your name and date of birth?" Two client identifiers are minimum safe practice standards for all client interactions. Clients may request that the SPN/SVN address them by his or her first name; the SPN/SVN should not assume this without permission. The hospital or other health agencies may have a policy regarding how employees introduce themselves. This will dictate the SPN's/SVN's actions.

NURSING JARGON

Using medical terms may sound impressive to the SPN/SVN and provide a feeling of having arrived, but using unfamiliar terminology with the client can increase the client fears and cause misunderstandings. Clients may respond, "What does it mean that I will have an IV started, have a WBC stat, and you'll be doing vitals q2h for now?" Health literacy, discussed earlier in this chapter, is affected when a client doesn't understand what is being said. When SPNs/SVNs really know something, they can explain words and symbols in terms the average layperson can understand. Now *that's* impressive!

FEAR OF THE UNKNOWN

Clients often have numerous unspoken fears about tests, procedures, and possible outcomes. These include, but are not limited to, pain, sleep, needle sticks, thirst, hunger, and being treated respectfully. Simple answers, such as "Everything will be fine," displays a lack of understanding of the depth of client fears. Clients may not ask questions because they think it might sound silly or that they are bothering the staff. An open-ended question from the SPN/SVN, such as "What questions do you have? If I don't know the answer, I'll try to find out for you," can open the way for expression of fears.

PERSONAL FACTORS

A client's illness rarely affects the client alone. Thoughts and concerns may extend to family, work, finances, and so on. For example, the parent of a newly hospitalized child was irritable and inattentive when the nurse was explaining the unit rules. Finally, the nurse stopped midsentence and said to the parent, "Is there something troubling you?" The parent looked at the nurse and then blurted out that there was another sick child at home, their spouse worked nights and slept days, and she had been up most of the last 3 nights. "Where should I be? Both kids need me, and my neighbor can only come in for 2 hours a day. I am so worried I don't know what to do." The parent could not begin to focus on the unit rules until there were solutions to the problems at home. The SPN/SVN may not have a solution, but the student can make needs known to the instructor or assigned nurse. Other health care team members may be aware of additional resources.

ENVIRONMENTAL FACTORS

Health care settings (whether clinics, hospitals, rehabilitation centers, or nursing homes) are very different to clients than their homes. There is no true opportunity for privacy. A variety of staff show up at different times throughout a 24-hour period; lights are on day and night; the nursing staff makes more noise than they realize; machinery is humming, buzzing, or beeping; nurses check out different parts of the body; bloodwork is drawn at early morning hours. A client may have put the call light on because of a need to go to the bathroom *now*. By the time someone arrives, it may be too late, much to the client's embarrassment.

Advance communication and planning can be beneficial for the client. Nurses need to make sure the client knows their plan of care and who their caregivers are, including their title and explanation of their role in the client's care. The client may reveal that he or she always has a snack of toast and tea at 9 pm, always gets up to go to the bathroom at 11 pm, or always has bran cereal and a banana at 6 am. Notes of this nature in the client's care plan can assist in the continuity of communication and care.

COMMUNICATING WITH INSTRUCTORS AND STAFF

Effective communication is essential for health care environments. Appropriate and courteous communication is important among instructors, staff, fellow students, and clients. Characteristics of effective communication involve respect, trust, honesty, empathy, sensitivity, humor, knowledge, patience, commitment, self-esteem, and the use of I messages.

CHARACTERISTICS OF EFFECTIVE COMMUNICATION

Respect

Respect involves both self-respect and respect for others. Nurses communicate self-respect by establishing a plan of self-care (healthy sleep, exercise, and nutrition) and by doing their best every day. When SPNs/SVNs treat themselves with self-respect, it becomes easy to extend respect to their instructors, staff, and clients. Clients quickly pick up on whether they are respected during conversation and physical care (e.g., verbal and nonverbal communication, such as eye signals between staff). In-depth personal conversation with peers while delivering care is a sign of disrespect to the client.

Trust

Trust begins with confidence in one's ability to make decisions. The SPN/SVN communicates this to instructors and staff by consistently doing the required preliminary preparation for assignments. This preparation and knowledge, along with the willingness to seek out information when needed, contribute to creating a trusting relationship with the client. Delivering on promises to the client also positively impacts trust.

Honesty

Honesty means that SPNs/SVNs will present themselves truthfully. For instance, scheduling additional time with an instructor to practice a procedure demonstrates this trait in communication, as it shows honesty in acknowledging personal needs.

Empathy

Empathy is the ability to understand and appreciate what someone else is feeling without experiencing the emotion itself. When individuals are sympathetic, as they would be with a family member or close friend, they share concern for that individual. Being *empathetic* permits an individual to understand how someone is feeling and why her or she feels that way, and involves maintaining control of emotions to think clearly. For example, an SPN/SVN might offer to help a staff member who is having a bad day perform client care (a practical intervention) instead of discussing the staff member with other members of the team.

Sensitivity

Focusing on nonverbal and affective communication helps the SPN/SVN verify verbalization or a lack thereof. Sometimes an individual can offend someone without being aware of it. The SPN/SVN should consider observing and listening for any cues that may have unknowingly offended a client or others. Sensitivity involves the ability to be aware of the present situation. Clarify, if needed, "Is there anything I said that upset or confused you?"

Humor

Healthy **humor** at the client's level of appreciation can help "lighten" a situation. Keep in mind that offensive humor and poking fun at a client or at other cultures or races is unacceptable. The staff sometimes privately laughs at something very serious or medically gross. Look for examples in movies and television programs with medical themes or at your clinical rotation. Reflect on how these behaviors impact client care and job satisfaction.

Knowledge

Knowledge is fundamental to gathering data and performing effective health-related communication. Instructors and staff quickly assess the SPN's/SVN's level of understanding. Instructors emphasize the importance of this trait by assigning tasks early, allowing SPNs/SVNs to research and prepare. SPNs/SVNs demonstrate their knowledge by being well-prepared for client care.

Patience

In today's fast-paced world, society often expects instant results and gratification. This can make it challenging to allocate the necessary time for developing communication skills. **Patience** is crucial in the SPN's/SVN's work with clients, as illness, growth, and development levels often require slowing down or repeating instructions. Both clients and SPNs/SVNs might be tempted to say "I know" when they do not. Initially, SPNs/SVNs may feel frustrated with personal communication attempts with clients. However, patience is a vital characteristic of communication and takes time to develop and perfect.

Commitment

Commitment means regularly incorporating all the previous characteristics into nursing communication practices. SPNs/SVNs need to conclude that they are learning the nursing profession because they really want to be here. Then, they need to do the work that needs to be done. Commitment shows, and it pays off.

> **Try This**
>
> **Code of Ethics**
>
> Review the National Student Nurses Association Code of Ethics for Students at https://www.dropbox.com/s/a229ong-58d5jx4p/Code%20of%20Ethics.pdf?dl50. Pay attention to communication and the key characteristics of communication in this document. Discuss how your class or clinical group can/do address these principles. What is your responsibility as an individual or as a group?

Self-efficacy (Self-confidence)

Self-efficacy (self-confidence) is an individual's belief that completion of a task is possible by taking action to fulfill a personal goal. Self-efficacy is valuable when communicating with others because unless the individual (the sender) has a goal of speaking confidently and takes action to do so, the receiver will doubt the ability of the sender. When individuals have self-efficacy, they recognize that they have something very special to offer in nursing communication, such as being able to communicate effectively with clients and the health care team. The SPN/SVN should consider the type of thoughts they create.

- Are thoughts positive or negative when they have personal thoughts?
- The two basic types of thought are random and active. Random thoughts just show up, but an individual initiates active thought. Random thoughts usually pass through, unless the person picks a thought and changes it into an active thought.
- To improve **self-esteem**, SPNs/SVNs should contemplate: What do my active thoughts say about me and the person I am? Do my thoughts support my sense of self, or do the thoughts tear me down?
- When individuals' thoughts are not serving them well, they should change them. If SPNs/SVNs make a mistake, they should learn from it and let it go. They should not continue to punish themselves.
- Daily, SPNs/SVNs should evaluate what they did well and give themselves a cheer for a job well done!
- Compliment peers for a job well done! It can be contagious.
- Thoughts also set the feeling tone for how SPNs/SVNs communicate with clients and other staff. How they feel about something creates actions that bring about results.
- Remember, as Socrates stated, "The unexamined life is not worth living."

Practice makes the SPN's/SVN's conversation meaningful, while increasing self-efficacy. SPNs/SVNs should make peace with silence; if they are talking just to fill in the silence, they should *stop!* They should learn to say what they mean, be direct in conversation, and remember that language is never innocent. SPNs/SVNs should listen before speaking. When they give clients information or directions, they should avoid medical jargon. Being long-winded just means that individuals do not know how to express themselves clearly. Asking clients what they think the SPN/SVN said can avoid misunderstandings. If SPNs/SVNs are on the receiving end of a lengthy conversation, they should remember that they can take control.

Willingness to Use "I" Messages

Remembering to use **"I" messages** whenever possible is important. Self-confidence will assist the SPN/SVN in using "I" messages effectively. When a message starts with "I," it allows the receiver time to respond without becoming defensive. Messages that begin with "you" often cause the receiver to become immediately defensive.

Try This

"I" Messages

Discuss how your immediate feelings differ if you receive each of the following messages:

"You make me want to scream when you do not answer the clients' call lights immediately."

"I am trying to understand why the call lights are not answered in a timely manner. Can you help me understand what the issue is?"

SITUATION, BACKGROUND, ASSESSMENT, RECOMMENDATION (SBAR)

Components of SBAR

Nurses are taught to be objective and detailed when providing information. Health care providers are more interested in the most important information. The communication process of **SBAR** was first developed in the military and has been adopted by many health care institutions to facilitate clear communication. For example, if you are calling a health care provider because of concern about a client, SBAR can be useful following these guidelines:

- **S**. Situation could include identifying the following about the situation:
  1. Who the nurse is
  2. The client's unit
  3. Client name and room number
  4. What the problem is (briefly), when it started, and how severe it is
- **B**. Background could include the following:
  1. Client's admitting diagnosis
  2. Date of admission
  3. Information related to current status, such as:
     a. Recent mental status
     b. Vital signs
     c. Oximetry
     d. Oxygen device and flow rate
     e. Current medication
     f. Allergies
     g. IV fluids, lab results
     h. Code status
- **A**. Assessment could include the following (collaborate with the RN as needed):
  1. What the licensed practical nurse/licensed vocational nurse (LPN/LVN) thinks is going on based on the evidence
  2. If appropriate, based on the signs and symptoms, if the LPN/LVN believes the problem is life threatening
- **R**. Recommendation involves what is needed from the health care provider. Terms like "could be" and "might be" are usually effective. Consider the following:
  1. Does the nurse want the health care provider to come and see the client?
  2. Does the nurse want the health care provider to place an order for medication?

3. Does the nurse want to transfer the client to a higher level of care?
4. Does the nurse need a consult with another member of the health care team?

Some facilities may utilize **ISBAR,** which starts with Identify (identify yourself, who the nurse is talking to, and who the nurse is talking about) to stress the importance of this information. A more advanced version of ISBAR is **ISBARR** in which another step is added after Recommendation called Repeat Back. If a nurse uses identify, situation, background, assessment, recommendation, and repeat back (ISBARR) to report a client's status change and the health care provider responds with a new order, then repeating back the order becomes valuable to confirm accuracy of the order.

SBAR for the Shift Report

SBAR is also a useful tool for providing the end-of-shift report, reporting off when a nurse leaves the clinical unit, or transferring a client to another unit. The process will have some differences, such as the following:

Situation: Additionally, the nurse could include the admission date, chief complaint, and diagnosis.

Background: Consider these relevant additions:

1. Client's medical and social history
2. Allergy status
3. Code status
4. If client is in isolation
5. Pain management strategies and response to interventions
6. Imaging studies
7. Lab results
8. Location of peripheral or central venous line access devices
9. Diet
10. Mobility

Assessment: Provide relevant information in a systematic manner using a systems approach (collaboration with RN as needed), including:

1. Vital signs and range of vital signs since admission
2. Pain assessment and client's pain goal
3. If a client has diabetes, how frequently monitored and results since admission
4. Diagnostic studies and results
5. If a client needs turning or other therapeutic/preventative measures, how often and whether client can turn self
6. Fall risk if it applies and any other precautions specific to this client
7. Medications prescribed and client response

Recommendations: Consider the following:

1. The client's goals of care
2. What needs to be done on the next shift
3. Any procedures that must be done
4. Client's education and discharge needs

Both the Joint Commission and the Institute for Healthcare Improvement support the use of SBAR in health care facilities.

> **Try This**
>
> **Using the SBAR Method**
>
> Write an example of how you will use the SBAR method when you give a report to your clinical instructor during a clinical rotation. Identify differences compared with the way you gave reports in the past. Practice giving a report to a peer utilizing the SBAR method and ask them to give you constructive feedback.
>
> If your clinical instructor gives you a task to complete, such as retake the client's vital signs, after you give the SBAR report, what action should you perform with your clinical instructor that would follow the ISBARR method to confirm accurate understanding of your clinical instructor's directions?

DIGITAL COMMUNICATION

Electronic Documentation

Electronic documentation (electronic health record [EHR]) ideally provides a location where all agency professionals involved in client care enter the most recent information. Electronic documentation may be part of basic nursing education for documenting medications and treatments, as well as obtaining client information. Each facility may have slightly different protocols; however, the underlying concepts are similar. Be sure to enter factual and timely information into the clients' EHR. Additionally, the client's HIPAA rights must be protected with electronic documentation with only authorized users having access.

E-mail

E-mail is a popular way of communicating with administration, within departments, and with other departments. Before getting involved in sending e-mail, SPNs/SVNs should review the basics of e-mail etiquette. Some people e-mail things they would never say directly to someone. Box 8.1 lists some e-mail essentials suggested by Pagana (2015). Lastly, SPNs/SVNs should be sure to adhere to the electronic communication policies of the health care institution. These policies will outline steps to enhance secure communication, thus protecting the client's and employee's private communication and information.

Cell Phones and Text Messaging

SPNs/SVNs are sitting in class or watching a clinical demonstration, when someone's cell phone rings. It certainly disturbs the chain of thought for both the students and the instructor. Although the phone can be set to vibrate, the shuffle to see who called is annoying. During this time, SPNs/SPNs may have missed something essential for the care of a future client.

Text messaging has been integrated into student life with astonishing momentum. Some students continue to text during class, providing a distraction to themselves and their peers. An additional concern is that some students are using cell phones to cheat on exams.

Many programs have adopted a rule of shutting off cell phones during class and clinical. As a matter of

Box 8.1 E-mail Etiquette

- Determine whether e-mail is the best way to send your message.
- Consider the content of the e-mail message and to whom you are sending it.
- Be sure to use the subject line. People read this first to decide whether the message is worth opening.
- Use effects, such as boldface and underlining, to emphasize points.
- Keep your sentences and paragraphs short.
- Skip a line to separate topics.
- Send your message to the right person. Determine if you wish to respond to all or just the sender.
- Be specific. Avoid useless information.
- Avoid using inappropriate language.
- Be cautious with humor. The person sees only the written word.
- Check your spelling and punctuation. Proofread all messages before sending them.
- Avoid typing an entire e-mail in uppercase or "red"; both "scream" at the recipient.
- Use capitalization. Lowercase letters make you look sloppy and lazy.
- Avoid sending confidential information unless the e-mail system is encrypted. Verify policy and procedure.

etiquette, it is considered disrespectful to classmates and the instructor to text during class. Cell phone access is restricted during any testing situation.

Personal cell phones are an unsecure network; client or employee personal information may be at risk. It is generally prohibited to use a personal cell phone at a clinical site or for any related activity.

Social Media

Every year there is an increase in the number of social media platforms available for organizations and individuals. Nurses should be aware of any social media policies instituted by their employer. Additionally, individual use of social media must not include any information that violates a client's HIPAA rights. For more information, refer to the National Council of State's Board of Nursing's (NCSBN) brochure on social media entitled *A Nurse's Guide to the Use of Social Media* at https://www.ncsbn.org/public-files/NCSBN_SocialMedia.pdf.

Try This

Digital Communication

1. Research digital communication policies that exist within your nursing program and/or clinical site(s).
2. Discuss individual components of the policies and develop a teaching plan to teach future students regarding appropriate practice and use of digital communications.
3. Assist with implementing and/or reviewing digital communication polices at your school of nursing.

CONFLICT RESOLUTION

In the health care setting, conflict can be related to many factors, such as stress, diversity, language, generation, and personality. The health care team is composed of multiple individuals that approach the care of the client based on the unique perspective of their discipline (Cherry and Jacob, 2019). Differences can be magnified in high-stress situations. Problems can translate into medication errors, client safety, and even client mortality. Individual or team communication issues can be a sign of a system-based issue. Many health facilities and educational institutions have developed educational programs to improve conflict negotiation skills, interdisciplinary communication, and collaboration. The SPN/SVN should consider the following basic steps to focus on a mutually beneficial solution based on shared interests.

1. Accept conflict as a natural part of life. Different points of view, needs, and beliefs are often involved.
2. Temper personal attitude and behaviors. Be aware of initial reactions and take a deep breath. (One's automatic defense system wants to automatically respond and fight.)
3. Take time to think critically before reacting. For example, did individuals think through what they were going to report before doing so, or did it appear that they were rambling?
4. Treat conflict as an opportunity to voice opinion and listen to the other side of the story. SPNs/LVNs may have to take the initiative to approach the health care team member regarding what is being seen as a conflict. They may not be aware of how you are being affected, and ultimately unresolved feelings may escalate. Job satisfaction may be negatively impacted, and client care may suffer.
5. Choose the approach wisely. A win-lose approach (one side wins, while the other side loses) will only escalate the intensity of the feelings involved. The best choice for a solution depends on the situation. There is no single correct way. A win-win approach (both sides wins) often involves active listening, creative thinking, and compromise.
6. Listen and learn. Conflicts are often based on assumptions and a lack of information. When nurses are wrong, they should apologize and find out how to correct personal mistakes in future incidences. They should not dwell on the mistake but move on.
7. Discover what is important or the core issue. It can range from hurt feelings to unmet needs. Getting to the root of the problem assists in resolving the conflict.
8. Respect one another. Conflict can be very emotional. Show respect despite the anger and hurt feelings. Stay away from name calling and blaming. Using "I" statements (for example, "I don't understand what you mean") lets a person own their own statements.
9. Find common ground to create the highest common denominator. In this case, it is generally for the client's highest good (see Chapter 17).

Try This

Resolving Conflicts

Think of a time recently when you experienced a conflict with someone. What was the outcome? Are you still upset with the other person, or was the issue resolved in a mutually beneficial way? What part of your behavior are you especially pleased with? What, if anything, would you do differently the next time?

Try This

Putting It All Together

TeamSTEPPS is another method for improving communication and teamwork in the healthcare setting.

1. Review The Agency for Healthcare Research and Quality's initiative to improve safety, communication, and teamwork skills among health care professionals entitled TeamSTEPPS at https://www.ahrq.gov/teamstepps/index.html
2. Review TeamSTEPPS curriculum materials at https://www.ahrq.gov/teamstepps/instructor/index.html

COMMUNICATION ACROSS THE LIFESPAN

Growth and development levels and medical conditions affect communication with clients. Each age group (whether infant, preschool, school-age, teenage, adult, or elderly) has different communication needs.

INFANTS

Infant communication includes crying, cooing, and body language. They act out their feelings with total body language. As their recognition of words grows, certain words act to soothe or trigger a reaction. Infants are influenced by the sound of voices. As one parent pointed out, "I used to put my baby to sleep each night by rocking them and reading the newspaper aloud in a soothing voice." Newborns respond favorably to a high-pitched voice, but this changes by the end of the first month; after that, calm, low tones are more soothing.

Parents (caretakers) are the best source for learning the meaning of different cries. They learn quickly to differentiate between wet, hungry, and uncomfortable. Rely on them to share specific information on an infant's communication style.

PRESCHOOLERS

For this information, toddlers are included in this category as early preschoolers. They are usually known for magnificent tantrums, and it is no wonder: they have learned some words, but when frustrated, they may not be able to put them together effectively. Thus the body acts out what the words cannot tell. Laughing at or trying to reason with the preschooler is counterproductive.

When these children have a tantrum, they should be removed from the immediate situation and audience. Once preschoolers are more composed, they can communicate by pointing, by showing on their bodies, or by pointing to a picture what made them upset. During procedures, the nurse should explain briefly and simply what is going to happen, while telling them what they can do during the procedure. For example, preschoolers will often assist and cooperate with receiving injections if they are patiently coached on exactly what to do (e.g., position, what to do with their feet and hands, how long they need to stay still, and what to expect during the injection).

SCHOOL-AGE CHILDREN

The vocabulary of school-age children has increased considerably. They are ready to be a part of most (but not all) discussions with their parents. Drawings or pictures can be used to explain an illness or procedure. Nurses should ask for feedback to avoid misconceptions: "Tell me in your own words what . . ." The child may not need to hear all the information. In that case, go with the parent to a separate area so the child will not overhear the conversation or parts of it, if possible. Whispering and misinterpretation can evoke new problems.

TEENAGERS

When ill, teenagers need to believe that someone knows more than they do and that someone is in charge. Nurses should deal with them with the same courtesy one would extend to adults, considering similar expectations of them. Teenagers may need encouragement to express their feelings, fears, and concerns. Their sense that nothing will happen to them has been shaken. The SPN/SVN should answer questions within their role, seeking answers when needed. The SPN/SVN should avoid hiding behind the nursing jargon. Using teen slang generally does not work well. Without real knowledge of the meaning, SPNs/SVNs may end up looking foolish instead of professional.

ADULTS

Many of the issues discussed in this chapter apply to adult communication. Collecting information at all three levels of communication (verbal, nonverbal, affective) is essential. The SPN/SVN should limit your questions to areas that are medically or safety (e.g., abuse) related. Pushing and probing based on curiosity may be harmful to the client (i.e., painful issues that have been suppressed). It does not work to probe and then leave clients to pick up the pieces of what they revealed under pressure. If SPNs/SVNs are concerned about conversation shared by clients, they should collaborate with the health care provider to discuss a potential consultation.

Clients with diminishing memory seem to have relatively preserved reading ability. Visual information seems to be more permanent. The health care worker or family member can try writing information of a size that is easy for the client to read. Written information seems to be more neutral and does not evoke the emotional reaction that words can.

Consider generational differences that may occur among adult clients. Most importantly, note what mode of communication they use. For example, Millennials or Generation Z individuals (see Chapter 1) may not return phone calls or possibly even e-mails. Their preferred mode of communication is texting. Thus if a nurse is attempting to contact a Millennial, a phone message may be ineffective. Conversely, a Baby Boomer would probably prefer a call or voicemail message. Keep in mind that these are general assumptions of the generations; individuals within a generation may have different preferences.

ELDERS

SPNs/SVNs should consider how they perceive elderly people. Unresolved parental issues, for example, can get in the way of quality care. If SPNs/SVNs see aging as just another part of the life cycle, they will be able to work effectively with elderly clients. At the start of care, SPNs/SVNs should assume that elderly clients can hear and communicate effectively. If the assessment produces different results, then accommodation is needed. Because the elderly may get tired by the evening hours, the nurse should consider detailed conversations to occur earlier in the day, if possible.

Hearing and vision can be impacted as individuals age. When hearing begins to diminish, it is easier for both men and women to hear lower-frequency sounds. The nurse should assess for hearing loss. If the hearing loss occurs only in one ear, then the care plan should include interactions accordingly. Age-related vision changes require the nurse to assess the elderly client for impairments and to interact based on the nature of the problem (i.e., blurry vision, lack of vision, lack of peripheral vision, etc.).

Communication is essential to ensure a smooth transition in care for the elderly. During a hospitalization, discharge begins with admission. The nurse takes advantage of teachable moments to interject information, demonstrate techniques, and have the client repeat the demonstrations. The nurse must respect the elderly person's autonomy while carefully evaluating who can assist them in understanding important directions regarding their health care.

Speaking directly to the client, unless the client requests otherwise, is important. Listening carefully when the client describes their home environment and available resources can assist with discharge planning. Will adaptive equipment be necessary? Will other health providers have to be involved in making the transition between this facility and home? The SPN/SVN should collaborate with your instructor and staff nurses to meet client's needs effectively. The National League for Nursing (NLN) Advancing Care Excellence for Seniors (ACES) provides information regarding care of the elderly at: http://www.nln.org/professional-development-programs/teaching-resources/ace-s.

Get Ready for the Next-Generation NCLEX® Examination

Key Points

- The communication process has five essential components: sender, message, method of transmission, receiver, and feedback.
- Communication involves verbal, nonverbal, and affective communication.
- The most important part of therapeutic communication is active listening. It involves purpose, focus, and disciplined attention.
- Common active listening behaviors involve restating, clarifying, reflecting, paraphrasing, minimal encouraging, remaining silent, summarizing, and validating.
- Questioning involves open-ended, closed-ended, and focused questions.
- Personal actions can influence therapeutic communication with others.
- Common blocks to communication involve reassuring falsely, probing, judging, belittling, giving advice, providing simple answers, and acting disinterested.
- Cultural differences in communication exist, especially with individuals who are new to the country and/or maintain their strong cultural beliefs and customs.
- Role changes for the client during an illness experience can be distressing. A focus on the proper introduction, nursing jargon, fear of the unknown, and personal and environmental factors can be helpful to the client.
- Communicating with the instructor and staff involves the same characteristics as communicating with a client. They include trust, honesty, empathy, respect, sensitivity, humor, knowledge, patience, commitment, and self-efficacy (self-confidence).
- Be alert to what your thoughts are saying, and if they help you or hinder you.
- Take your conversation seriously: Practice saying what you mean and know that your thinking affects your feelings and the way you communicate with clients and staff.
- SBAR is a way to give precise information when communicating to other members of the health care team or providing shift report.
- ISBARR is an advanced version emphasizing the introduction and the need to report back valuable information received after the report.
- E-mail etiquette is essential for effective and efficient electronic communication.
- Many programs have adopted a no private cell phone or text messaging policy during class or clinical.
- Be aware of and adhere to social media policies at your school and place of employment.
- Successful conflict management is based on a mutually beneficial solution through direct interaction among both parties.
- Lifespan communication differences are related to developmental and other issues, male/female differences, and medical problems.

Additional Learning Resources

Go to your Evolve website (http://evolve.elsevier.com/Carroll/success/) for the following FREE learning resources:

- Answers to Critical Thinking Scenarios
- Additional learning activities
- Additional Review Questions for the NCLEX-PN® examination
- Helpful phrases for communicating in Spanish and more!

Clinical Judgment and Next-Generation NCLEX® Examination-Style Questions

1. **What is an appropriate response by the nurse to a client when the nurse identifies that the client is angry?**
   a. Leave the room and report observations to the team leader immediately.
   b. Lighten up the situation by sharing some funny e-mail jokes with the client.
   c. Provide observations of nonverbal behavior and encourage the client to talk about their feelings.
   d. Continue with the present plan, but do it silently and leave as soon as possible.
2. **What statement most accurately reflects a nursing communication difference that is age related?**
   a. Speaking in a loud, high voice to make it easier for an elderly client to hear
   b. Discussing with school-age clients their illness in age-appropriate terms
   c. Giving a toddler, who is having a tantrum, a special treat
   d. Using medical jargon and current slang to help a teenager see the nurse as human
3. **A nursing student's first clinical experience is at a long-term care facility. The student wants to do everything correctly and feels comfortable because the student spent time in the past with their elderly grandmother. For each action, specify if the interaction promotes a positive or not positive interaction with their assigned resident.**

Action	Positive Interaction	Not Positive Interaction
Face the resident when discussing the options for breakfast.		
Walk in the room with exaggerated enthusiasm and say, "Hi, how are you doing?"		
Talk loudly in the client's left ear, assuming the client will have hearing difficulties.		
Say, "Good morning, my name is___________, I am a nursing student from___________ and I will be caring for you today."		
Knock on the door before entering.		

4. **A health care provider has reprimanded the SPN/SVN at the client's bedside. The SPN/SVN feels an instant flash of anger but says nothing. When the healthcare provider leaves the room, the SPN/SVN follows the provider to talk to the provider. What is an appropriate response by the SPN/SVN? *(Select all that apply.)***
   a. "Dr. Jones, I wish to speak with you privately."
   b. "How dare you shame me in front of a client?"
   c. "Please explain what you wanted me to know."
   d. "In the future, please ask to talk to me privately, not at the bedside."
   e. "I am going to report you to my nursing supervisor."
5. **A nurse had a challenging day at work due to a difficult client assignment and coworkers that were not supportive and did not help. The nurse decided to verbalize their frustration on social media about their coworkers by calling the coworkers unfair and rude. What agencies would consider the nurse noncompliant? (*Select all that apply*)**
   a. The Health Insurance Portability and Accountability Act (HIPAA)
   b. NCSBN's *A Nurse's Guide to the use of Social Media Guidelines*
   c. Health care facility where the nurse is employed
   d. State law where the nurse holds a primary license.
   e. National Student Nurses Association Code of Ethics for Student Nurses.
6. **A nurse is caring for a 62-year-old client in a long-term facility who has osteoarthritis to both knees and hypertension:**

Nurses' Notes	
1000	Client is complaining of dull constant bilateral knee pain this morning. Vital signs: T: 98.0°F (36.7°C), P: 92, RR: 20, BP: 146/94. Pulse Ox reading: 98% on room air.

   What focused question should the nurse ask the client?
   a. "On a scale of 1 to 10, with 10 as being the worst possible pain, how do would you rate your pain right now?"
   b. "Why do you think you have knee pain?"
   c. "When did the pain begin?"
   d. "How are you coping with your knee issue?"
7. **Continuing with the scenario in question 6, for each statement made by the nurse listed below, check the box to indicate whether the statement promotes therapeutic communication or blocks therapeutic communication.**

Nurse's Statement	Therapeutic Communication	
	Promotes	Blocks
a. "I will be caring for you today. How are you feeling?"		
b. "Your doctor is the best knee surgeon."		
c. "If I were you, I would have knee surgery."		
d. "Is there anything else I can do for you?"		
e. "I am leaving in 10 minutes. Are you OK?"		

8. A nurse calls a physician regarding a new issue with a client. What order should the following statements occur if the nurse follows the ISBARR format during the phone call?

a. "Administer meloxicam 10 mg by mouth now and then daily starting tomorrow."
b. "Hello, Dr. Lopez. My name is Mindy Johnson, the LPN/LVN caring for Deborah Manes, at Memorial Nursing Center, in room 239."
c. "Her right knee is swollen and warm to touch, which is a new finding since she came to our facility."
d. "Could it be that she needs a stronger NSAID order?"
e. "She has osteoarthritis to both knees as well as hypertension."
f. "I'm calling because she is complaining of increased right knee pain, 7/10, even after receiving the ordered amount of ibuprofen."

Critical Thinking Scenarios

Scenario 1

The instructor has discussed using SBAR when reporting off at the end of clinical. You have had a chance to practice this in class using a case study provided by the instructor. The case study indicates that the client is 78 years old and has a diagnosis of exacerbation of congestive heart failure. The client is short of breath when speaking. Their spouse died 4 weeks ago. The client is crying as you enter the room. Discuss your approach to caring for this client.

Scenario 2

A resident in the long-term care facility is used to having things done their own way and is critical of everything the staff nurses are doing. A student nurse has been assigned to administer the resident's medications this morning. When the SPN/SVN enters the room, the resident demands to know what the student is doing there. What should the SPN/SVN say?

9 Assertive, Nonassertive, and Aggressive Behaviors: A Personal Choice

Objectives

On completing this chapter, you will be able to do the following:

1. Describe nonassertive behavior, including the outcomes that may result.
2. Describe assertive behavior, including the outcomes that may result.
3. Discuss strategies for using the problem-solving process to promote assertiveness.
4. Describe aggressive behavior, including the outcomes that may result.
5. Analyze contributing factors that may lead to aggressive behavior, including nursing actions that could reduce the risk of aggressive behavior.
6. Discuss how negative coping mechanisms lead to aggressive behavior, including nursing strategies to avoid them.
7. Describe various work issues related to aggressiveness in nursing and nursing actions to address them.
8. Explain different forms of aggression for which a nurse may file charges.
9. Discuss strategies for reducing incivility in the academic setting.

Key Terms

aggressive
assault
assertiveness
bullying
choice
compensation
denial
incivility
lateral violence
manipulation
nonassertive (passive)
problem solving
projection
rationalization
sexual harassment
vertical violence

Duke and Kamy, two student practical nurses, are discussing their care plan assignment. Duke remarks loudly to Kamy, "Do you even know what you're doing?" Embarrassed, Kamy takes a deep breath to calm herself before responding. Then she replies, "I feel embarrassed by your comment. I want to provide safe care to clients just like you do. Can we discuss our strategies for creating care plans so we can both learn from each other?" In this situation, Kamy started her response with an "I" statement to avoid an uncivil comment to Duke. In this chapter, you will learn about different types of behavior, how they affect client care, and practical approaches to change the actions of others.

? Critical Thinking

Personal Expectations

Imagine that the nurse–client roles are reversed, and you are the client. What are your expectations of the nurse assigned to you? List the rationale for each expectation you identify.

EXPECTATIONS	RATIONALE
____________	____________
____________	____________
____________	____________

This exercise should give you some insight into why a nurse must be assertive. After reading this chapter, consider reviewing this exercise and evaluating any changes in your expectations.

Verbal, nonverbal, and affective communication (discussed in Chapter 8) translate into three major behavior patterns. You will *hear, see*, and *feel* the message acted out. The most effective communication or behavior is open, honest, and courteous due to promoting positive relationships, providing a healthy sense of self, and establishing trust. Ineffective communication or behavior is hurtful as it leads to blame, attacks, or denial, as well as being harmful to self.

The three major behavior styles are nonassertive (passive), assertive, and aggressive. The desired behavior style for effective nurses is assertive behavior. An *assertive* style of behavior separates the person from the issue. Most importantly, the nurse speaks out of **choice**. *Nonassertive* (passive) and *aggressive* styles of behavior may involve emotion and uncontrolled reactions. Let's begin by identifying nonassertive behavior.

NONASSERTIVE (PASSIVE) BEHAVIOR

Nonassertive (passive) or fear-based behavior is an emotionally dishonest, self-defeating type of behavior. Nonassertive nurses attempt to look the other way, avoid conflict, and take what seems to be the easiest way out; they are never full participants in the health care team. Nonassertive individuals do not express feelings, needs, and ideas when others deliberately or accidentally infringe upon their rights. There may be a lack of eye contact, swaying and shifting from one foot to the other, complaining, and hesitancy when speaking. The overall message is "I do not count. *You* count." This personal pattern of behavior can be reflected in nursing care as well. Consequently, nurses who demonstrate nonassertive behavior are unable to recognize and meet client needs. Some examples of nonassertive behavior are shown in Box 9.1.

Try This

Nonassertive Behavior

Identify nonassertive behaviors in which you have been involved. Describe how each behavior worked or did not work for you or the client. How did these behaviors make you feel?

Box 9.1 Nonassertive Behavior

Telling another nurse how "foolish" the health care provider is for ordering a certain type of treatment

Complaining about a nurse manager to another staff nurse, instead of approaching the nurse manager directly

Routinely telling clients who ask many questions about their illness, etc. to "Ask the health care provider" or "Ask the RN" to take the easy way out

Assuming, without checking, that the client wants to skip daily personal care when a visitor drops in, to avoid conflict

Experiencing a feeling of being "devastated" when a health care professional criticizes nursing skills, interpreting criticism of work as criticism of self

Responding to a client's in-depth questions about the nurse's personal life and that of other staff for fear of not being liked by the client, leaving the professional role and assuming a social role instead.

When asked by another nurse to assist with the care of assigned clients, responding by saying, "Well, uh, I guess I could," although already too busy, hesitating and repressing own wishes

Needing help with an assignment but saying nothing, refraining from expressing own needs

After making an error, overexplaining, continually apologizing, or placing blame on staffing issues, etc., ignoring the reality of making a potential mistake, of the need for taking responsibility for it, and of the value of learning from the error

After making an error, planning on finding a new job for fear of the outcome and administrative response, avoiding conflict

Getting angry when being yelled at by the health care provider in front of a client, but not saying anything, refraining from expressing own opinion, and internalizing anger

By not taking risks and not being honest, nonassertive nurses typically feel hurt, misunderstood, anxious, and disappointed. They often feel angry and resentful later. Because they do not allow their needs to be known, they are the ones who lose out. Their clients can also be impacted adversely.

? Critical Thinking

Nonassertive Behavior

Develop a plan of change for correction using each one of the nonassertive behaviors that you identified to better produce satisfactory outcomes.

ASSERTIVE BEHAVIOR

Assertiveness (assertive behavior) involves acting confidently toward others, while supporting and respecting the other individual. According to Merriam-Webster's Dictionary (2024), assertive is defined as "disposed to or characterized by bold or confident statements and behavior." Nurses work in a setting that requires them to speak frankly and openly to others in such a way that personal rights are not violated. Assertiveness is a tool, not a weapon.

As with any new behavior (or skill), becoming truly assertive will take time and practice. Nursing students should avoid being harsh with themselves or giving up just because old behaviors emerge when they are under pressure. They should resolve to try again until assertive behavior is integrated as a part of their being. Although it is not the nurse's intent to hurt others deliberately, it is unrealistic to be inhibited to the point of never hurting anyone. Some people are hurt because they are unreasonably sensitive, and some people use their sensitivity to manipulate others.

Assertiveness is not only what individuals say but how they say it. Examples of assertive body language include standing straight, steady, and directly facing others when speaking, while maintaining eye contact; speaking in a clear voice, loud enough so others can hear; and speaking fluently without hesitation and with confidence. Practicing an assertive response in the mirror can be very beneficial. Asking a colleague for feedback will also improve the effectiveness of an assertive approach.

Nurses have a right to express their own thoughts and feelings. To do otherwise would be insincere. Assertive nurses claim responsibility for their own feelings, thoughts, and actions. Using "I" at the start of statements shows acceptance of responsibility for personal thinking, feeling, and doing. For example, "I feel frustrated when…" instead of "You are making me feel frustrated when… ." Assertiveness, then, is a way of expressing oneself without insulting others. It communicates respect for the other person, although not necessarily for that person's behavior. The overall message is, "I count, and you count, too." Being assertive does not guarantee that an individual will get their way. What it does guarantee is that the individual will experience a sense of being in control of their emotions and responses. Win or lose, the person gave it their best shot. The real bonus is freedom from residual feelings of fear and anger. Exceptions to these concepts are included later in this chapter concerning potentially violent situations.

Box 9.2 shows examples of assertive behavior.

Keep in Mind

Assertiveness is an expectation in nursing. This is your responsibility as a client advocate.

Try This

Identify Assertiveness

List examples of assertiveness you can identify in your own behavior or in people around you. Role play with another person with some of the examples listed above. How do you see yourself responding in an assertive manner in similar situations in the future? Reflect on strategies to remain assertive.

USING THE PROBLEM-SOLVING PROCESS TO DEVELOP ASSERTIVE BEHAVIOR

The poem entitled *"Myself,"* found in Box 9.3, captures the reason for working toward assertiveness and improving self-confidence as an individual continues personal growth. Changing behavior is difficult. After all, personal behaviors have been practiced and perfected for years. It is so much easier to tell others what *they* should do to change. The decision to change must come from inside a person so it becomes their decision alone. Using the problem-solving process can help guide the change more effectively.

The Problem-Solving Process

The **problem-solving** process is a series of steps used to solve problems and can be valuable for improving assertive behavior. There are similarities between the problem-solving and the nursing process. The nursing process is a more focused method of using the problem-solving steps. Knowing how to solve problems allows an individual to appropriately speak and act confidently, growing in assertive behavior.

Box 9.2 Assertive Behavior

Requesting to talk to a health care provider privately about a questionable order and then presenting evidence for questioning the order, thereby offering a direct statement of information

Sitting down near and facing a client, while saying, "Mr. Smith, I would be interested in knowing how you are feeling. I have noticed that whatever I do, you are critical of my work." This involves listening attentively and responding nondefensively with direct statements of feelings, without interpreting the client's criticism as a personal attack

Responding, "I do not know, but I will find out for you" when a client requests information with which a nurse is unfamiliar, regarding their illness. Following through by checking with the appropriate staff and determining who is responsible for informing the client, thereby respecting the client's right to know

Saying, "I know it is uncomfortable, but I will walk along beside you. We can stop briefly any time you like. I will also teach you how to do a relaxation technique that you can use while you are walking" (after a health care provider orders the client to walk for 10 minutes out of each hour and the client complains that it hurts, not wanting to walk). Also, making sure that pain medication is given before the walk in an appropriate time to maximize pain relief, thereby respecting the client's feelings while supporting the need to carry out the health care provider's order

Asking a client directly if care should be provided or postponed when unexpected visitors arrive at the time care was to begin. If the care is delayed, stating the time that the nurse will be available to assist with care, thereby respecting the client's autonomy (right to choose), without compromising the care

Saying, "Please clarify. I want to be sure I understand" when a nurse has been criticized for their work. If it is the nurse's error, asking for suggestions to correct it or offering alternatives, thereby separating criticism of performance from criticism of self

Responding, "I feel both embarrassed and angry because you criticized me in front of a client. Next time, please ask to talk to me privately" when a health care provider criticizes a nurse's work in front of a client, thereby standing up for the nurse's rights without violating the rights of others

Saying, "That information is personal, and I do not choose to discuss it" when a client asks for personal information about a nurse (or another staff member), thereby standing up for personal rights without violating the rights of others

Saying, "Our institution's policy will not allow me to assist you in this manner. Can I call the case manager for you to see if she can assist?" This uses a direct statement without excuses when a client asks a nurse to pick up some personal items from the store

Saying, "I have to leave now, but I'll be glad to listen to you during our lunch break tomorrow" when a peer approaches you about a personal problem, as an attempt to compromise

Saying, "I would like to speak with you privately today before 3 pm. What time is convenient for you?" when you approach a team leader who has been "on your case" constantly, thereby using a direct statement of wishes

Saying, "I am not sure you realize that the line begins at the entrance of the coffee area" when another staff person moves ahead in the cafeteria line, thereby standing up for personal rights

Responding, "I am also busy today. Let's discuss all the client's priorities and come up with a plan to deliver the best possible care together for all the clients," thereby compromising when being pressed by other staff members to help with assignments

Saying, "I know you would like all of this done today. There is no way I can get it all done. What are your priorities?" to the team leader when the workday is overwhelming, thereby providing a direct statement of information and requesting clarification

Box 9.3 Myself

I must live with myself and so,
I want to be fit for myself to know.
I don't want to stand with the setting sun
And hate myself for the things I've done.
I want to go out with head erect.
I want to deserve all men's respect.
But here in this struggle for fame and self,
I want to be able to like myself.
I don't want to look at myself and know
That I'm bluster and bluff and empty show.
I never can fool myself, and so
Whatever happens, I want to grow
More able to be more proud of me,
Self-respecting and conscience free.

Edgar Albert Guest

The problem-solving process is a conscious growth-producing method of dealing with challenges in a person's life.

Step 1: Define the problem. Identifying ill-mannered behavior can help define personal behavioral problems. It may be helpful to look objectively at the gains and losses associated with personal behaviors. For example, blaming someone else for an individual's personal behavior may provide the individual with sympathy and concern from others. However, that individual produces no gain because he or she did not take responsibility for personal behavior or dealing with others in a growing way. A person's way of responding to others is developed as a response to past anxiety-producing situations in life. The behavior may have its roots in childhood.

Try This

Keep a Daily Journal

Maintain a confidential daily journal to help pinpoint specific situations that create worry, fear, anger, and rage in you by answering the following questions about those situations:

1. What happened?
2. When did it happen?
3. How did you feel physically?
4. How did you feel emotionally?
5. What would you have liked to have done instead?
6. What kept you from doing it?

Critical Thinking

Gains and Losses

Answer the following questions in your confidential journal: What are you gaining from maintaining your nonassertive behavior? What are you losing from maintaining your nonassertive behavior?

When people change the way they act toward others, others will often change their actions back. What has been a predictable reaction will no longer be predictable. If a person persists with their new, effective way of responding to situations, the behavior of others will gradually change. Identifying personal behavioral challenges is the first step to promoting change in others.

Collecting data of personal behavior will help define personal problems. Writing a problem statement based on this information is valuable. Collecting data needs to be done in an objective manner, as though observing someone else. Asking colleagues or family to assist in identifying behaviors can be very helpful. Listening with an open mind is worthwhile when defining personal behavioral problems. An example of a problem statement would be *I remain quiet when a doctor enters a client's room with me because I am uncomfortable talking to the doctor.*

Critical Thinking

Defining the Problem

Review the data you have collected for 3 to 4 days in your daily journal. It will give you an insight into the pros and cons of your current behavior. Develop a problem statement that is personal and specific for you. Before writing the problem statement, read the following:

Sample

I am afraid to say what I mean for fear that others will get angry with me.

This behavior is demonstrated in the following situations:

- Saying "yes" to requests to babysit or go out with friends when I need the time for homework.
- Not asking for help with household chores, even though I am a full-time student plus a parent with two children.
- Saying "yes" to added requests not related to the responsibilities for school that I must complete on my own time.
- Feeling tired and resentful most of the time and eventually becoming angry over something insignificant.

Step 2: Decide on a goal. To create a goal, individuals should review their problem statements and consider what should be done differently. Often it is more useful to decide on a long-term goal (the ultimate desired change or outcome) and several short-term goals (smaller changes or outcomes needed to eventually achieve the long-term goal). All goals should be SMART goals: **s**pecific (well-defined), **m**easurable (results can be measured), **a**ttainable (realistic), **r**elevant (appropriate for the desired outcome), and **t**ime-referenced (a deadline is provided when the results should occur and/or be evaluated)

Critical Thinking

Deciding on a Goal

Write a SMART goal about assertiveness for yourself. Before you write the goal, read the sample that follows:

Sample

LONG-TERM GOAL	SHORT-TERM GOAL
I will say what I mean without fearing that others will be angry with me by _______ (within 6 months).	I will say "no" to babysitting requests or going to a family event when I need the time to do homework by _______ (within 2 weeks).

After you have written your goals, consider these questions:

Are they **s**pecific?

Are they **m**easurable?

Are they **a**ttainable?

Are they **r**elevant to the change needed?

Is there a **t**ime frame provided to see desired results?

Note that each goal should begin with the phrase "I will." This phrase signals a personal commitment to working on the goal.

Changes or outcomes may not occur by the projected date. Individuals may need to revise the goals or goal dates from time to time. Most importantly, the targeted date provides a time frame for evaluation of whether the goal was met. As individuals accomplish each short-term goal, they can cross them out and then go on to the next one. Continuing to record personal progress in a confidential journal is helpful for obtaining valuable information. Its value now lies in keeping a record of the process as changes take place. This allows individuals to fully appreciate their work and progress. Many changes may be subtle but will not be accomplished without effort.

Step 3: Choose alternatives. Alternatives are the approaches that a person will use to attain each of the established goals. When making a list of alternatives in a personal journal, one should consider letting their imagination run wild. One should consider all the possible interventions to support the goals, from serious to humorous. This may even provide some comic relief from the serious challenge of creating positive change. Including "do nothing" in the list of alternatives makes the list realistic. Doing nothing is a *choice* and therefore an alternative.

Critical Thinking

Personal Alternatives

Write alternatives to support the short-term goal(s) you chose in the Deciding on a Goal exercise. Before you write in your journal, read the sample that follows:

Sample

Alternative action: Practice in front of a mirror. In an even tone of voice, say, "No, I will not be able to babysit tonight, but try again another time." If the person persists, say, "No, I do not have the time tonight." Repeat as needed until heard. Compliment yourself for not giving in.

After you have written your alternatives, consider this question:

Does the alternative action correspond to the short-term goal, assisting you to meet the goal?

Step 4: Try out the alternatives. The initial plan has been made. It is now time to put the plan into action. For many, taking the first step of implementing the plan is harder than creating the plan. It may be far easier to offer ideas to peers than to take the first step with a personal plan.

It is a good idea to create personal incentives to help promote new assertive approaches. Individuals often slip back into old familiar ways of behaving. One should not be dismayed. This is normal. Simply reinstituting a newly planned approach provides an appropriate response for continued growth. The more one practices new approaches, the more comfortable one becomes with implementing change. Ultimately, new assertive behaviors will replace old nonassertive or aggressive behaviors. Identifying a mentor or peer, who can provide feedback and assist with debriefing situations, can be valuable.

Try This

Celebrate Meeting Your Goals

Identify a worthy incentive to celebrate meeting your goal. To make it work, the incentive must be within your budget. Otherwise, the incentive may cause new problems for you to solve.

Step 5: Evaluate the effectiveness of your approach. Evaluating goals is a key part of problem-solving. Each goal, along with its alternative actions, should be assessed at the specified time to determine if it was achieved. If the goal hasn't been met, the nurse can consider extending the deadline. Setting a 3-week evaluation period allows enough time for change, as it typically takes at least 3 weeks to establish new behaviors. However, it may take up to a year for a new behavior to become fully integrated into a person's routine.

Try This

Review Your Journal

As a part of the evaluation process, review your entire confidential journal. This is an excellent source of information for what happened, how you dealt with it, and whether the present course was, and continues to be, effective.

Step 6: Repeat the process if the solution is not effective. The last step, step 5, provided information about whether one should continue the established course of action. If changes are needed, one should go back to step 3, identify additional alternatives, or perhaps choose alternatives that were originally identified but not used, and continue through the problem-solving process.

As individuals pursue an assertive way of behaving, they should monitor nonverbal messages. Nonverbal communication is even more powerful than words. It is possible to utilize correct words but to sabotage the words by hesitating, using a sarcastic tone of voice, or emphasizing certain words. One should practice in front of a mirror, listening to the verbal communication. Recording oneself could help an individual review and criticize his or her actions. A good strategy is to ensure that the last word of a sentence is no higher in pitch than the word before it, so the sentence does not sound like a question.

Posture plays an important role: individuals should sit up straight, walk with their shoulders back, and display a confident stride. Making eye contact when speaking is important. Periodically looking away can ensure a person is not perceived to be staring. Confidence is not perceived when someone displays annoying habits (staring, nail biting, finger or foot tapping, or fidgeting), plays with their hair, chews on a pencil or glasses, offers nervous laughter, and puts hands in and out of pockets. Another appropriate approach to display confidence would be to determine a certain spot on the body to place hands (e.g., folded on the lap, or lightly sitting on the hip). Amy Cuddy in a 2012 TED talk emphasizes how "power posing" can impact a person's confidence. Consider visiting the website and viewing the talk. It only takes 2 minutes to benefit from the "power pose" (https://www.ted.com/talks/amy_cuddy_your_body_language_may_shape_who_you_are).

When someone asks about opinions or appropriate actions, one should consider offering an answer. Instead of saying, "I really do not know," "Whatever you like," or "It does not matter," one should take the risk and express an opinion. Life is an adventure. All ideas count. The more a person expresses opinions, the easier it becomes to develop assertive behaviors.

Nurses enjoy working in long-term care when they have self-motivation, feelings of empowerment, and ownership of their working position (Aloisio et al., 2021). Learning assertive behaviors can help licensed practical nurses/licensed vocational nurses (LPNs/LVNs) promote personal value, feelings of empowerment, and professional growth. LPNs/LVNs should be assertive and promote their value. An example would be LPNs/LVNs requesting to attend institutional meetings because of their in-depth knowledge of the clients and their care.

The following three rules are helpful, overall, in the development of assertiveness:

1. Acknowledge personal feelings. Do not blame others for personal feelings.
2. Make personal feelings known by being direct and confident. Begin statements with "I."
3. Ensure nonverbal communication matches the verbal message.

Box 9.4 Aggressive Behavior

After a nurse asks to go to a conference, a supervisor responding, "Why should you go? Everyone else has worked here longer than you have," thereby attempting to make the nurse feel guilty for making a request

Pointing out another nurse's error in front of staff and adding, "Where did you say you graduated from?" thereby attempting to humiliate the nurse

After a peer approaches a nurse with a problem, the nurse saying, "If it isn't one thing, it's another with you. Why don't you get your act together?" thereby disregarding their feelings

After a staff nurse approaches a nurse manager about not liking a new rule, the nurse manager saying, "That's tough; this is the way it's going to be from now on," thereby disregarding the feelings and rights of others

Responding to a client who has had their call light on frequently throughout the morning by saying, "I have had it. You have had your light on continuously for nothing all morning. Do not put your light on again unless you are dying, or I will take it away," thereby displaying hostile overreaction out of proportion to the circumstance as well as verbal abuse

Parking in a handicapped parking spot because it is raining and the individual does not want to get wet, thereby displaying rudeness and disrespect to those who need the spot

AGGRESSIVE BEHAVIOR

When an individual speaks out without consideration of others, **aggressive** behavior is displayed. Aggressive (anger-based) behavior violates the rights of others. It is an attack on the person rather than on the person's behavior. The purpose of aggressive behavior is to dominate or put other people down. This behavior, although expressive, is self-defeating because it quickly distances the aggressor from other staff and clients. Examples of aggressive body language include leaning forward with glaring eyes, pointing a finger at a person to whom one is speaking, shouting, clenching fists, putting hands on hips, and shaking one's head. The overall message is, "You do not count. I count." The examples in Box 9.4 show how aggressive behavior can be recognized.

Try This

Aggressive Behavior

Identify aggressive behaviors that you have observed. How could you address the aggressor in these scenarios?

Critical Thinking

Aggressive Behavior

Develop a plan for dealing with the aggressive behaviors you identified in the previous learning exercise (Try This: Aggressive Behavior).

Aggressive behavior certainly is a way of saying what an individual means, while producing a temporary relief from anxiety. The feeling, however, does not last. Very often the aggressive person is left with residual anger that simmers until the next stressful situation or person comes along. Aggressive nurses are unable to function as true advocates for clients because they are too busy taking care of their perceived personal needs.

CONTRIBUTING FACTORS

Several factors may lead to aggressive behaviors among nurses, such as personal factors, workplace practices, environmental factors, and risk diagnoses. All areas of nursing are vulnerable to these factors.

Personal Factors

Personal factors that may influence aggressive behavior include nurses' attitudes, behaviors, as well as verbal, nonverbal, and affective communication. A negative display of these areas could be perceived as aggressive behavior. One's attitude and body language may be considered more powerful than verbal communication. Clients may respond negatively to aggressive behavior by nurses. A nurse can reduce the risk of aggressive behavior from clients with confident, effective communication skills. Hence the avoidance of aggressive behaviors is vital for effective client care.

Workplace Practices

Workplace practices that are aimed at improving safety for health care workers are critical. The quality, performance, and availability of security personnel is a key strategy. Officers convey authority when wearing a uniform more than when they wear casual attire, a nonverbal form of communication. Aggression management skills are vital for reducing aggressive incidents. Nurses may seek support from their union representatives to enhance the safety of the workplace and address any current issues if they do not feel supported by the administration. If an incident should occur, nurses should document the objective information immediately following the incident as this may be helpful if the perpetrator denies what occurred.

Environmental Factors

The location of a care facility (e.g., high-crime risk area) may determine the type of clients admitted to the facility. An important risk factor at hospitals and psychiatric facilities is the carrying of guns by clients, family, or friends of the client. Other issues include early release of acute or chronic mentally ill clients, the right to refuse psychotropic medication, the inability to voluntarily hospitalize mentally ill persons (unless there is an immediate danger to oneself or others), and hospitalizations of criminals instead of using incarceration. According to the Bureau of Labor and Statistics, psychiatric aides reported personal injury that were caused by clients' actions (US Bureau of Labor Statistics, 2024). Nurses should educate themselves on facility policies against workplace violence; administration should support active reporting of incidences (Kafle et al., 2022). Workplace violence will be discussed further in this chapter.

Risk Diagnoses

Harm to health care workers is often perpetrated by a small number of clients. A client's history of previous violence is a strong indicator of potential risk, but sometimes this information is not available to the staff. Clients may feel that they are placed in a vulnerable position by virtue of entering the health care system. This may elicit unwarranted behaviors by the client that he or she normally would be able to control through normal coping mechanisms.

Nurses need to learn how to read cues of potential risk for violence in clients (and others) with whom they are dealing. Some diagnoses may promote a possible risk, such as affective disorders, paranoid delusions, chemical abuse/dependence, dementia, impulse control disorders, and personality disorders, as well as situations in which clients/family are undergoing extreme stress.

If you find yourself in potential danger, take the following immediate steps:

- Have an escape route in mind.
- Stand at the side of the door; do not block a door. Always keep your back to the door.
- Maintain an open position: hands out of pockets, uncrossed arms and legs, hands visible.
- Call the person by name.
- If the person's voice is raised, speak softly and maintain a quiet, controlled voice.
- Remain calm; sit or stand still; do not fidget.
- Keep 5 to 7 feet of distance between you and the person.
- Do not touch, point, order, argue, plead, belittle, threaten, or intimidate the person.
- Never turn your back on the person.
- Make eye contact.

Many other practical suggestions are available from experienced nurses like your instructor. Consider valuable tools such as those developed by the Occupational Safety and Health Administration (OSHA; www.osha.gov). These tools and resources can be found at https://www.osha.gov/dsg/hospitals/workplace_violence.html. This is a time to keep a cool, calculating head (function now, shake later). Consider enrolling in a workshop aimed at teaching staff how to deescalate a client and use self-defense techniques in the health care setting.

Try This

Evaluate Protection Against Potential Dangers

Do the health care agencies where you receive your clinical experience educate their employees in management of harmful behavior and/or gentle self-defense? Is harmful behavior at this facility reported to the police? Under what circumstances are charges pressed against the perpetrator?

Investigate where in your nursing program you learn about identifying signs of possible danger as well as techniques of gentle self-defense to protect yourself.

Critical Thinking

Preventing Possible Harm

Depending on what you discovered in the previous learning exercise, create a plan for learning what you need to know to better protect yourself from potential harm.

Professional Pointer

If you feel unsafe, follow your intuition and remove yourself from the situation. Immediately notify your instructor or supervisor and **then** provide for the client's safety, if able.

NEGATIVE COPING MECHANISMS THAT LEAD TO AGGRESSIVE BEHAVIOR

When individuals experience ambivalent situations, they often develop coping mechanisms that lead to aggressive behavior. A discussion follows regarding negative coping mechanisms used by nurses.

Projection is a coping mechanism during which individuals attribute their own weaknesses to others. The interaction can be characterized as "My education is better than yours," "I'm more competent than you are," or "You're only a practical nurse." Unfortunately, this negative, aggressive interaction wastes energy that could be used on client care. Nurses who are confident and assertive enhance one another's knowledge base and legal responsibility. The client benefits from assertiveness.

Rationalization, another negative interaction, can occur between a client and a nurse when a logical but untrue reason is offered as an excuse for behavior. For example, a nurse quickly informs others that a client is a "troublemaker," a "manipulator," or "uncooperative." If other nurses incorporate this information into their transactions with the client, the client will never be seen as his or her true self. Anything the client does can be interpreted within the context of the label given by the nurses. A vicious circle can ensue. If the client's needs are not met because of this labeling, this increases his or her frustration. This in turn is a threat to self, resulting in anxiety. An honest, assertive response by the nurse could eliminate misunderstandings about the client (Box 9.5).

Box 9.5 A Potential Outcome of Rationalization

A young adult, who was paralyzed from the waist down because of a car accident, was due to be transferred from one care facility to another. A transfer form arrived at the new facility before the client did. The information on the form created immediate anxiety for the nurses before they met the client. The form labeled the client as *manipulative*. It stated that *the client will be pleasant and polite at first but watch out because it is a trick. When she has won you over, you will see her true colors.* The nurses discussed the prospective admission. They expressed gratitude that their colleagues in the other nursing home had warned them. After all, that is what colleagues are for. They felt "forewarned is forearmed."

When the client arrived and tried to talk to the nurses, the nurses abruptly interrupted her and made her wait for care. The nurses intended to show the client that they would not be manipulated. As the client's frustration and discomfort increased, she began to demand that their treatment be done on time. The client shouted angry comments at the nurses when they finally arrived to provide care. The nurses called the client "demanding" and "hostile." The original label of "manipulative" was supported when the client asked the roommate to engage the call light to get help to take her to the bathroom. Each day seemed worse than the day before.

The situation escalated when a long-time nurse announced they were leaving and would not return until the client was transferred to another facility, even offering to write the client's transfer note. Other nursing staff threatened to do the same. Finally, the administrator decided to transfer the client. The nurses congratulated one another for having worked together. Perhaps this could have been avoided if the nurses would not have rationalized (given false reasons for) the client's behavior.

Critical Thinking

Negative Interactions

Answer the following questions about the above story, A Potential Outcome of Rationalization:

1. What factors contributed to the client's behavior?
2. What factors contributed to the nurses' response to the client?
3. How could this situation have been handled differently?
4. Was the behavior of the nursing staff passive, aggressive, or assertive? Explain your answer.
5. Is it an ethical or a legal risk to "label" clients?

Denial is another negative transaction that involves keeping (denying) information from a client who has a right to know (e.g., a client being told that he or she will be transferred from a skilled nursing home facility to an intermediate nursing home facility). Application of this principle would be statements such as "I've got a secret," "It is not my responsibility," "They will be upset," or "They are too weak to figure out what is going on." The responsibility of informing the client about their condition or transfer plans is not carried out so the present staff does not have to deal with the full impact of the client's reaction to the information. The nurse refuses to recognize the existence and significance of the client's personal concerns. The nurse also uses denial as a way of excusing personal responsibility: "The health care provider should tell them," or "It's the team leader's responsibility." Although the decision may not be entirely the LPN's/LVN's, it is clearly their responsibility to check out what portion of the information they should give. **Compensation** occurs when a nurse guides the focus away from themselves as a means of covering up personal (real or imagined) inadequacies. *Gossip* is a common action of compensation that nurses may use to distract from their own weaknesses. If the focus is on another person's negative attributes, then the focus will not be on themselves. Gossip conversations can begin with, "Did you hear…" or "I just found out…" These conversations guide the focus, but they can also be destructive and ruin the reputation of both clients and personnel. Furthermore, time spent socializing at work is time away from providing high-quality client care. A listener can end this damaging interaction by saying assertively, "I will work on a good relationship between us, but I would prefer you do not talk to me about others." Today, gossip can also spread through social media.

? Critical Thinking

More Damaging Interactions

1. What other damaging interactions, among staff or between clients and staff, exist?
2. Provide examples of how continuation of this type of interaction is supported by others.
3. What can you do or say to avoid being drawn into these interactions?
4. Think about a recent scenario in your class when a peer tried to engage you in gossip. Self-reflect on how you responded in the situation. How should you act to avoid negative behavior in the future?
5. How does social media contribute to gossip? Remember that all client information is confidential.

Manipulation is a negative interaction in which an individual disregards the other person's feelings or needs. The examples in Box 9.6 show how manipulation can be recognized.

In dealing with manipulators, nurses must learn to take care of themselves. In turn, the nurse will be more effective in meeting the clients' needs. In taking care of oneself assertively, a nurse can serve as a positive role model for coworkers, those you lead and manage, and clients.

Box 9.6 Manipulation

The *seducer* initiates a relationship with someone (e.g., a nurse with a supervisor). The seducer shares what seems to be common goals and insights. Ultimately, the seducer asks for special favors or privileges. If denied, the seducer promotes guilt, saying, "I thought you liked me" or "I thought we understood each other." The other person is left feeling guilty, angry, or both.

The *passive-aggressive* manipulator, a health care provider, might point out a nurse's errors or personal problems in front of a client or other staff. The nurse is left feeling guilty, angry, embarrassed, or all these emotions. The health care provider focuses on the nurse's weaknesses and uses this knowledge to exploit or create anxiety for the nurse.

The *divide-and-conquer* manipulator, a community member, confides half-truths, rumors, or innuendo to a department head that a new employee cannot be trusted. By the time this information proves to be untrue, valuable time has been lost in client planning and care. A skilled manipulator can sever work relationships by sowing seeds of distrust. As the staff squabbles, there is less energy to unite and focus on common client issues.

? Critical Thinking

Negative Manipulative Interactions

Describe a situation when you feel that you were manipulated.

1. Describe the verbal and nonverbal communication that occurred in the interaction.
2. How did the encounter make you feel?
3. What behaviors can you change to prevent this from occurring again?

AGGRESSIVE BEHAVIOR AND WORK-RELATED ISSUES

Nurses are entitled to work in a healthy and safe environment. The American Nurses Association (ANA) promotes the importance of nurses working in an environment that is "safe, empowering, and satisfying" (ANA, n.d.). Standards for Establishing and Sustaining Healthy Work Environments were established by the American Association of Critical Care Nurses. The Nurses Bill of Rights, created by the American Nurses Association, can be found at www.nursingworld.org/practice-policy/work-environment/.

Workplace Violence

Workplace violence is defined by four categories (NIOSH, 2024):

1. Label 1: Criminal (perpetrator has no relationship with the workplace)
2. Label 2: Client-customer (involves abuse by a client, family member, or visitor)
3. Label 3: Coworker (current or former employee)

Box 9.7 Signs of Workplace Violence

INITIAL SIGNS OF WORKPLACE VIOLENCE
- Unusual behavioral change
- Lack of cooperation with nurses, other clients, or family members
- Hostile forms of communication, including cursing
- Episodes of anger occurring easily with frequent arguments
- Gossip or rumors being spread to harm others deliberately
- Uninvited sexual remarks
- Hostile responses to other nurses, clients, or family members
- Sleep disturbances mentioned at work
- Increased irritability and anxiety

SECONDARY SIGNS OF WORKPLACE VIOLENCE
- Conversation focused on "poor me, the victim"
- Notes with threats, violence, or sexual content
- Verbalization that includes plans or a desire to harm someone
- Occurrence of stealing workplace property
- Less interest in work and workplace assignments
- Increased arguments
- Increased physical accidents or injuries

4. Label 4: Domestic violence (personal relationship)

The most common category is Label 2: client-customer. Most abuse reported by nurses involved a client, family member, or visitor (NIOSH, 2024).

Signs of workplace violence. Nurses should be alert to signs of violence in clients, family members, visitors, and coworkers. Early signs of workplace violence are shown in Box 9.7. As the anger intensifies, and if conflicts remain unresolved, the result could be violence against oneself or other. Behaviors directed toward oneself may include depression or suicidal threats. Behaviors directed toward others may include physical fighting, property destruction, or use of a weapon to harm others. By recognizing the warning signs of workplace violence, nurses could intervene by reporting these to a nurse supervisor.

Prevention of workplace violence. Prevention is key and entails management commitment and employee involvement. Prevention begins when each nurse:
- Makes a personal commitment to follow prevention guidelines
- Participates in the training and refresher courses offered by the health care agency
- Takes advantage of programs offered by the police department or other agencies
- Remembers that his or her focus is on *gentle self-defense*, not offense
- Is prepared before workplace violence becomes an issue
- Is familiar with his or her workplace policies that cover forms of violence, as well as harassment

Box 9.8 Some General Safeguards for Preventing Workplace Violence

- Do your part to promote a supportive, congenial, yet professional work environment.
- Whenever possible, resolve conflicts as they arise. Know that there are times when you must back off. However, most of the time people want to have their point of view heard. A technique called *creative communication* encourages you to do the following:
- Listen carefully to the other person's point of view.
- Ask questions to clarify what you do not understand. (Remember that this step is not a sneaky way to argue or interject your own opinion!)
- Tell the person what you think he or she said and what you think he or she is feeling. If your version is inaccurate, have the person repeat the explanation. When you can repeat back accurately what the person thinks and feels, then it is your turn to present your view.
- Use these steps as well when you present your point of view.
- Deal directly with unwanted or unwelcome behavior, including uninvited sexual advances.
- Review your own behavior to determine whether:
- A clarification of the person's signals is in order.
- Limits must be stated clearly and firmly on what you consider unacceptable behavior.
- Supervisor or management intervention may be needed.
  - Get to know your fellow workers and look out for one another.
  - Promote workplace integrity. Treat one another, your clients, and their families with respect, courtesy, and professionalism. Negative comments by clients and relatives usually are a response to their fear of the unknown. Rarely are the comments meant to be personal. Check out the fear. What are the questions? What can you do to help find answers?
  - Be alert to changes in behavior that may signal violence.
- Avoid putting yourself in obvious danger. Make use of security guards for escorts to parking lots and out-of-the-way areas. Listen to your intuition. This is making conscious use of affective communication.

- Is alert to warning signs and has thought through what he or she can do to prevent an escalation
- **Takes all threats seriously**, reports them to management, and encourages others to do the same
- Advocates assertively for implementing prevention guidelines in the facility (Box 9.8)

? Critical Thinking

Personal Violence Prevention Plan

What additional ideas do you have to put into action to defuse or prevent violence of any kind in the workplace? Create an assertive approach.

Incivility, Bullying, Lateral Violence, and Vertical Violence

Some of the worst attacks on nurses are from within their own professional community. The attacks range from offensive words and vicious threats to physical harm. Many nurses accept the violence as the norm and do not report an attack to their supervisor.

Incivility is common terminology used to describe hostility among health care workers. Cynthia Clark writes extensively about civility in nursing. Review her journal articles and visit her blog at http://musingofthegreatblue.blogspot.com for details. Incivility in health care can be a detriment to safe client care (Clark, 2025). All nurses should self-reflect on their personal actions and continually try strategies to avoid incivility in the workplace, to promote positive client outcomes.

> **Try This**
>
> **Personal Reflection on Civility**
>
> Complete the Clark Workplace Civility Index, found in Fig. 9.1, from a student's perspective as if your educational institution is your workplace. Identify three areas that you could improve and then determine strategies for doing so.

Bullying is described as negative acts perpetrated by others, typically from a higher level of authority. It includes behaviors such as intimidation, malice, insults, or abuse of power by an individual or group against others. These behaviors are humiliating and threatening, and they can undermine self-confidence. Visit http://stopbullyingtoolkit.org for resources to implement strategies aimed at decreasing bullying in education.

Lateral violence is negative acts that occur between nursing colleagues. It includes both overt and covert physical, verbal, and emotional abuse by one nurse against another. The most common forms of lateral violence are shown in Box 9.9.

Vertical violence is negative acts that occur between people of unequal power. For example, it might occur between a staff nurse and a student; a nurse manager and a student; an instructor and a student; an instructor and a staff nurse; or a new nurse and a seasoned staff nurse. The behavior humiliates and undermines confidence. The person who is bullied ends up feeling fearful and unsafe.

Assault

Workplace violence has a long history of existing in health care facilities. The increase in violence is drawing attention among nurse leaders. **Assault** is the intentional act of causing harm or threatening to cause harm to another individual. Nurses are frequent targets of assault in the form of violence, hostility, sexual harassment, and discrimination. The American Nurses Association (2017) conducted a health risk appraisal over 3 years with over 10,000 nurse and student nurse respondents; 25% of the respondents had been assaulted by a client or a client's family member, and 9% were concerned about their physical safety at work. A nurse's response to a client can decrease the potential for violence. Being assertive but not aggressive can de-escalate a client or peer.

The US Bureau of Labor Statistics (2020) reported that health care workers suffer more than five times the incidents of assault compared to other occupations. According to OSHA (n.d.), health care and social assistance workers reported a 40% increase in injury and illness, which is more than other private workplaces. In March 1996, OSHA released its first *Act of Violence Prevention Guidelines* (1996) geared toward protecting health care and social service workers on the job. Unfortunately, incidences of work-related assaults continue to exceed the overall industry norm. As a result, in 2016, OSHA published *Guidelines for Preventing Workforce Violence for Health Care and Social Service Workers* to improve the safety of the workplace (Box 9.10).

Not all agencies have complied with the OSHA guidelines, but some state nurses' associations are working toward increasing penalties against those guilty of assaulting a health care worker or establishing task forces to study workplace violence. The New York Senate bill (Violence Against Nurses) made into law that an assault against a registered nurse (RN) or LPN on duty is a class C or class D felony (New York State Senate, 2010). California passed a law in 2018 requiring health care employers to have a violence prevention plan in the workplace (Castillio, 2018). Many states have passed laws concerning workplace violence in health care (Pollack, n.d.). In 2021, the *Workplace Violence Prevention for Health Care and Social Service Workers Act*, which would require employers to implement workplace violence prevention plans to protect employees from incidence of violence, was passed by the House of Representatives in Congress. When the bill was received by the Senate, it was passed on to the Committee on Health, Education, Labor, and Pensions. No further national action has been taken to date (Congress.gov, 2021). Further action is needed to finalize national legislation on this issue.

> **Try This**
>
> **Aggressive Behavior and Work-Related Issues**
>
> 1. The ANA *Nurses Bill of Rights* states, "Nurses have the right to safe work environments that prioritize and protect nurses' well-being…." Research what your state nurses' association is doing to minimize risks of violence in the workplace.
> 2. Review and discuss OSHA's *Guidelines for Preventing Workforce Violence for Health Care and Social Service Workers* at https://www.osha.gov/Publications/osha3148.pdf.
> 3. Review and discuss the *AACN Standards for Establishing and Sustaining Healthy Work Environments* (2016) at https://www.aacn.org/WD/HWE/Docs/HWEStandards.pdf.
> 4. Does your nursing program or clinical site have a workplace prevention program? Research and discuss.
> 5. Describe your experiences of healthy and/or unhealthy work environments. What strategies were most effective? What recommendations can you make for improvement?

Clark Workplace Civility Index©

SOURCES:

Clark, C.M., Sattler, V., & Barbosa-Leiker, C. (2018). Development and psychometric testing of the Workplace Civility Index: A reliable tool to assess workplace civility, *Journal of Continuing Education in Nursing, 49*(9), 400-406.

Clark, C.M. (2025). *Creating and sustaining civility in nursing education, 3rd ed*, Sigma Theta Tau International Publishing.

To complete the index, consider the 20 statements listed below. Read each statement carefully. Using a scale of 1- 5; (5) almost always, (4) usually, (3) occasionally, (2) rarely, (1) almost never, select the response that most accurately represents how true each statement to be. Enter the score for each item; then add the numbers to determine the overall health of your workplace. Scores range from 20-100.

Ask yourself, how often do I: (5) almost always (4) usually (3) occasionally (2) rarely (1) almost never

1.	Extend goodwill and think the best of others	1	2	3	4	5
2.	Include and welcome new and current colleagues	1	2	3	4	5
3.	Communicate respectfully (by e-mail, telephone, online, face-to-face) and really listen	1	2	3	4	5
4.	Avoid spreading negative gossip and rumors	1	2	3	4	5
5.	Keep confidences and respect others' privacy	1	2	3	4	5
6.	Encourage, support, and mentor others	1	2	3	4	5
7.	Avoid abusing my position or authority	1	2	3	4	5
8.	Use respectful language (no racial, ethnic, sexual, gender, weight, age, ability, or religiously biased terms)	1	2	3	4	5
9.	Attend meetings, arrive on time, participate, volunteer, and do my share	1	2	3	4	5
10.	Avoid distracting others (misusing media, side conversations) during meetings	1	2	3	4	5
11.	Avoid taking credit for another individual's or team's contributions	1	2	3	4	5
12.	Acknowledge others and praise their work/contributions	1	2	3	4	5
13.	Take personal responsibility and accountability for my actions	1	2	3	4	5
14.	Speak directly to the person with whom I have an issue	1	2	3	4	5
15.	Share pertinent or important information with others	1	2	3	4	5
16.	Uphold the vision, mission, and shared values of my organization	1	2	3	4	5
17.	Seek and encourage constructive feedback from others	1	2	3	4	5
18.	Demonstrate approachability, flexibility, and openness to other points of view	1	2	3	4	5
19.	Bring my 'A' Game and a strong work ethic to my workplace	1	2	3	4	5
20.	Apologize and mean it when the situation calls for it	1	2	3	4	5

Scoring the Workplace Civility Index: Add up the number of 1-5 responses to determine your 'civility' score
90-100—Very civil
80-89—Civil
70-79—Moderately civil
60-69—Minimally civil
50-59—Uncivil
Less than 50—Very uncivil

Fig. 9.1 Clark Workplace Civility Index. (From Clark CM: *Creating and sustaining civility in nursing education*, ed 3, 2025, Sigma Theta Tau International Publishing, Indianapolis. A license to use the Clark Workplace Civility Index can be obtained at www.boisestate.edu/research-ott/civility-matters/works/ or by contacting techtransfer@boisestate.edu.)

Sexual Harassment

Sexual harassment is about abuse of power. It is not about sex or passion. Sexual harassment against nurses is a significant dilemma around the world (Draucker, 2019). Most nurses do not report the incidents, mostly for fear of losing their job, embarrassment, or fear that he or she will not be believed. According to the Equal Employment Opportunity Commission (EEOC),

Box 9.9 Lateral Violence in the Workplace

- Nonverbal innuendo such as eye rolling or eyebrow raising intended to belittle another nurse
- Verbal affronts
- Undermining activities
- Withholding information including critical information regarding clients
- Sabotage
- Infighting
- Scapegoating
- Backstabbing
- Failure to respect privacy
- Broken confidences

Box 9.10 Occupational Safety and Health Administration Guidelines for Preventing Workforce Violence for Health Care and Social Service Workers

VIOLENCE PREVENTION PROGRAMS

- Management commitment and worker participation
- Worksite analysis and hazard identification
- Record analysis and tracking (identify patterns of assaults or near misses and how controls can decrease)
- Job hazard analysis
- Employee surveys[a]
- Client surveys[a]
- Hazard prevention and control
- Substitution (substitute hazard with a safer work practice)
- Engineering controls and workplace adaptations to minimize risk (e.g., physical barriers, door locks, panic buttons, metal detectors, better/additional lighting, more accessible exits)
- Postincident procedures and services (identify "root cause")
- Investigation of Incidents
- Safety and health training
- Understand the concept of "universal precautions for violence"
- Training topics
- Training for supervisors and managers
- Training for security personnel
- Evaluation of training
- Recordkeeping and program evaluation

[a]Help identify new or previously unnoticed risk factors and deficiencies or failures in work practices. From OSHA: Occupational Safety and Health Administration Guidelines for Preventing Workforce Violence for Health Care and Social Service Workers, 2016. https://www.osha.gov/Publications/osha3148.pdf.

sexual harassment includes unwanted sexual advances or other verbal or physical conduct of a sexual nature, such as a condition of employment or advancement, or a hostile environment where the advances intimidate, offend, or interfere with the nurses' ability to do their work. The keyword is "unwanted." A distinct difference is made between consent and unwanted.

If a nurse is the target, the nurse can confront the person who is harassing. An assertive response is to tell the person clearly what he or she is doing, that this behavior is offensive and unwanted. The nurse should be sure that their response is firmly assertive. The message must be congruent with verbalization, body language (nonverbal), and affective communication. Mere words do not justify a physical response. A nurse should document what happened, as well as what the individual said and did.

Employers have the responsibility to correct unwanted behavior that they know about or should know about in the workplace. If unwanted behavior does not cease, the nurse should report it to the supervisor, union representative, or department head, as needed, until the message is heard. Evidence of personal documentation may be helpful. If the employer is convinced that someone is harassing the nurse, the employer can reprimand, require counseling, demote, transfer, deny a promotion or raise, or dismiss the harasser. The seriousness of sexual harassment can no longer be ignored. The nurse's work is usually affected, and some will even leave their jobs to get away from it. For others, their emotional and/or physical health is affected, sometimes with long-term consequences.

Try This

Sexual Harassment Policy

Locate your school and clinical site policy regarding sexual harassment. Discuss with a peer some common types of sexual harassment in a workplace setting.

Critical Thinking

Personal Plans for Safety

Create a plan for yourself on how you will deal with any harassment attempts during future employment.

Insidious Aggression

Insidious aggression is aggressive behavior in the workplace, such as incivility, interpersonal issues, and hostile acts, that are not obvious to others. For example, nurses do not generally report that they are being ignored by several staff members or that a staff member is not speaking to them. This can result in more job stress, less job satisfaction, less job commitment, less satisfying relationships, higher levels of anger and anxiety, and lower levels of overall well-being (Luo et al., 2024). Individuals who are subjected to insidious aggression are more likely to leave the workplace.

A lack of action on the part of the nurse gives approval and permission for the perpetrator to continue the behavior. Nurses have the responsibility to act assertively, with the cooperation of other nurses, to advocate for a safe workplace.

Critical Thinking

1. Think of a time that you might have experienced insidious aggression. What were your feelings during that time? Did your quality of work suffer? Did the experience affect your health? How did you ultimately resolve the situation?
2. Review the document from *The Joint Commission's Sentinel Event Alert Issue 59* and the resources provided within the alert at https://www.jointcommission.org/resources/sentinel-event/sentinel-event-alert-newsletters/sentinel-event-alert-59-physical-and-verbal-violence-against-health-care-workers/. Identify how workplace violence is described, the prevalence, contributing factors, and the suggested actions. How does this information compare to the policies you have reviewed on this topic and have experienced in the workplace? What areas need to be improved? How can nurses assist with this problem in their workplace or within the profession?

COUNSELING AND FILING CHARGES

Often, only physical injuries are treated. All employees who have been verbally or physically assaulted should receive postincident debriefing sessions. Hospital managers should implement violence prevention programs as recommended by OSHA (2016). If a nurse is harmed or threatened by a client or a client's family member, the nurse has the option to file charges. Some agencies will do this for the nurse after a review board hearing or provide support if the nurse files legal charges themselves.

ACADEMIC INCIVILITY

Incivility can also occur in nursing education programs, which will affect both students and faculty. Uncivil behaviors can occur between faculty/instructor and students, between clinical instructor and staff nurse, between two or more students, and between two or more faculty. These uncivil behaviors (incivility) and the disruptions they cause create a negative learning environment (classroom, simulation lab, or clinical), which impacts student learning and faculty performance (Carroll, 2018). Nursing students can effectively learn how to handle uncivil situations when faculty provide learning experiences that include cognitive rehearsal, simulation, evidence-based scripting, deliberate practice, and debriefing (Clark, 2019). The NLN Vision Series: *Creating Community to Build a Civil and Healthy Academic Work Environment* (2018), available at https://www.nln.org/docs/default-source/uploadedfiles/professional-development-programs/vision-statement-a-vision-for-creating-community-to-build-a-civil-and-healthy.pdf?sfvrsn=2ca7ab0d_0&pdf=VisionSeries-CreatingCommunity, offers valuable insights on how faculty and students can collaboratively create civil learning environments.

Critical Thinking

Academic Incivility

Think about a time when you witnessed incivility at your learning institution or during a clinical experience. How did that experience make you feel? What strategies could be implemented to prevent incivility at your school or during clinical experiences?

Get Ready for the Next-Generation NCLEX® Examination

Key Points

- Communication translates into behavior.
- Assertiveness is honest and open behavior. It considers others' feelings and needs. It is based on choice. Communication statements begin with "I."
- Nonassertive (passive) and aggressive behaviors are based on emotional hooks. These styles are ultimately damaging to both parties involved. Be alert to unresolved feelings leading to a cycle of worry → fear → anger → rage.
- Using the steps of the problem-solving process can change undesirable behaviors and interactions. Verbal, nonverbal, and affective interactions must be dealt with during this change.
- Violence in the workplace has always been present. Health care institutions are not an exception.
- OSHA has established national guidelines to deter violence toward health care workers.
- Violent incidents are more common when nurses and security lack assertive management skills.
- Some client diagnoses provide clues to potential violence.
- Legal compensation is available to nurses who are injured during physical violence on the job.
- Insidious aggression on the job includes incivility, interpersonal conflict, and hostile acts.
- Learning to be assertive in nursing benefits both the nurse and the client.

Additional Learning Resources

Go to your Evolve website (http://evolve.elsevier.com/Carroll/success/) for the following FREE learning resources:

- Answers to Critical Thinking Scenarios
- Additional learning activities
- Additional Review Questions for the NCLEX-PN® examination
- Helpful phrases for communicating in Spanish and more!

Clinical Judgment Questions

1. What is the best description of assertiveness that a nurse manager can share in a unit meeting?

a. A level of communication that few nurses attain
b. Outspoken, anger-based, honest communication
c. An indirect method of getting others to do what you wish
d. Taking a positive stand without violating others' rights

2. Which scenario does the nurse recognize as the best description of potential sexual harassment?

a. Coworkers have been sharing jokes since they started working.
b. The immediate supervisor has asked a nurse (alone) to meet for dinner at his house to discuss a potential promotion.
c. A client asks a nurse if the nurse is willing to go out on a date after the client is discharged.
d. A coworker is upset because a peer has refused to meet him socially for a drink.

3. A supervisor is talking to a nurse about problems with another nurse on the unit. What statement indicates an assertive response by the nurse?

a. "I am honored that you trust me to try to resolve this issue with you."
b. "Maybe you and I can meet over coffee after the shift so it will be more private."
c. "I am happy to assist in problem solving the broad issue, but I am uncomfortable discussing my peer's behavior with you without them present."
d. "If you don't tell anyone of our conversation, I'll tell you what I know."

4. What recommendation should the nurse offer to the unit's safety committee to promote a safe workplace?

a. "Our department needs to examine how staff attitude, body language, and the environment can impact unit/institution safety."
b. "Safety is an issue that must be placed solely in the hands of nonuniformed, outside security staff."
c. "It is necessary to go back to the strict visiting rules and limit hours and visitors to family."
d. "Violence is a part of our current culture, and there is very little you can do to effect change."

5. Which of the following is an example of an "I"-centered, assertive statement? *(Select all that apply.)*

a. "I feel you are not quite working up to your potential."
b. "I think that you could improve the accuracy of your work."
c. "I feel that you are concerned for your safety."
d. "I will watch you demonstrate inserting a catheter today."
e. "I hope that you will be able to work tomorrow."

6. A health care organization is taking active steps to promote a safe, civil, and healthy environment for all employees. What scenarios should the nurse know as examples of insidious on-the-job-aggression and those that promote a healthy work environment?

ACTION	INSIDIOUS ON-THE-JOB AGGRESSION	NOT INSIDIOUS ON-THE-JOB AGGRESSION
As one nurse was talking to the health care provider, another nurse interrupted me to report on my client.		
A nurse states, "I am routinely assigned the heaviest client on the unit each morning."		
When a nurse is asked to go to lunch with someone, the nurse explains that studying for classes is a priority over the lunch break.		
A nurse is busy caring for their clients and cannot assist another nurse when requested.		
One group of nurses is bullying the new nurse on the unit.		

7. An LPN, who works in a long-term care facility, shares this information with the unit manager.

"I have been working with Dorine, another LPN on our unit, for the last several weeks. She seems to be struggling lately. She comes to work 15 minutes late, often without an excuse. Her uniform is wrinkled but appears clean. She seems tired when she arrives and doesn't want to hear the change-of-shift report from the previous shift. I overheard her talking to a resident about the "sloppy" work that one of the assistive personnels performed the day before. She was talking about her son to one of the residents this morning, indicating that he was struggling in school. I feel bad that she is going through a hard time. Is there anything I should do for her?"

What are the three priority actions the unit manager should perform (select three)?

a. Council the LPN for reporting this information about Dorine.
b. Discuss the late policy with Dorine.
c. Reprimand Dorine on coming to work without looking professional.
d. Instruct Dorine on practices that promote sleep.
e. Discuss the importance of collaboration with Dorine.
f. Confront Dorine about the report of her gossiping.
g. Provide supportive strategies for parental involvement with child-learning.

8. Continuing with the scenario is question 6, complete the following sentence:

Dorine has the potential for demonstrating __(A)__ as evidenced by __(B)__.

A options:
vertical violence
denial
workplace violence
rationalization

B options:
professional appearance
tardiness
gossiping
weak parenting skills

Critical Thinking Scenarios

Scenario 1

An RN was recently appointed as the unit manager in a long-term care facility. The staff thought this new manager was an excellent choice for the unit because the manager is smart and outwardly charming to visitors and healthcare providers. One day, an LPN opened a door to a resident's room and heard the unit manager yelling at the resident, "You are so stupid, and either you do as you're told or I will see to it that you are taken out of the home." Neither the RN nor the client heard her open the door, so the LPN backed out quietly, unsure of what she should do. What are the LPN's options and the rationale for each option?

Scenario 2

A new LPN is eager to do well in his or her new job at a medical clinic. The new LPN is also trying hard to fit in with the rest of the staff (an advanced practice registered nurse [APRN] and a medical technologist). The LPN is responsible for greeting the clients, getting a brief statement of why the client came in, measuring vital signs including the height and weight, and charting findings in the electronic health record. What suggestions could be offered to the LPN?

10 Cultural Uniqueness, Sensitivity, and Competence

Objectives

On completing this chapter, you will be able to do the following:

1. Describe the key characteristics of culture.
2. Discuss the danger of ethnocentrism, prejudice, and discrimination and how to mitigate them.
3. Discuss nursing strategies for developing personal cultural competency in the health care setting.
4. Summarize key patterns of cultural diversity and how a nurse could assess these patterns.
5. Identify how cultural differences may affect communication, including nursing strategies to reduce misunderstandings.
6. Discuss how nurses can increase personal knowledge of culturally diverse groups of people.
7. Perform a cultural assessment using the Giger and Davidhizar's Transcultural Model.
8. Describe how nurses can effectively plan care for culturally diverse clients.

Key Terms

assimilation
complementary and alternative medicine (CAM)
cultural bias
cultural competence
cultural diversity
cultural sensitivity
culture
customs
discrimination
enculturation
ethnic groups
ethnocentrism
melting pot
nonjudgmental
prejudice
stereotype
wellness and illness
worldview

Hilary and Jamal, two student practical nurses, sat in the lounge area studying for the next class. Hilary struggled to focus as Jamal chatted with other classmates and played music. Hilary grew up in a household in which she was the only child, so she was used to a quite environment when she studied at home. When she approaches Jamal, she says, "Hey, Jamal, I've noticed I get distracted when we study together. I'm used to studying in silence. It's hard for me to focus with the background noise."

Jamal paused, realizing the issue. "I get it. At home, my four siblings and I always study with music or conversation. It helps me feel connected, but I see how it might be distracting for you." Hilary and Jamal determined that they both wanted to be good students in the practical nursing program, but their differences cause them to approach studying in a different manner. In this chapter, you will learn how to identify and deal with the differences of others and find commonalities, which are valuable skills in nursing.

Keep in Mind

With knowledge comes responsibility. With knowledge of cultures, that responsibility entails a respect for differences.

Licensed practical nurses/licensed vocational nurses (LPNs/LVNs) have chosen a career that will give them an opportunity to meet people who are different from themselves.

- Some of these people will be clients.
- Some will be peers at school.
- Some will be coworkers.
- Some will be at different ages.
- Some will belong to a different social class.
- Some will have disabilities.
- Some will have different health care beliefs about what causes them to get sick.
- Some will have different values.
- Some will have different cultural backgrounds because of ethnic group status.

Regardless of cultural background, some differences will be the result of a growing diversity in their individual and family lifestyles.

Student practical nurses/student vocational nurses (SPNs/SVNs) will discover that people think, feel, believe, act, and see the world differently than themselves and their family and friends. Log on to www.minoritynurse.com/about/index.html to check out featured articles about issues facing nurses.

SPNs/SVNs are encouraged to review the standards of the National Association for Practical Nurse Education and Service, Inc. (NAPNES) at www.napnes.org, and the National Association of Licensed Practical Nurses (NALPN) at www.nalpn.org. Both organizations have embraced statements that describe the need of the LPN/LVN to provide health care to all clients regardless of race, creed, cultural background, disease, or lifestyle. This is an ethical expectation.

The states' Nurse Practice Act (NPA) informs that failing or refusing to render nursing services to a client because of the client's race, color, sex, age, beliefs, national origin, disability, or sexual orientation is listed as unprofessional conduct. The ethical expectation now becomes a legal mandate. Nurses could risk legal suits because of an ignorance of **culture** that could result in poor nursing judgment.

Not only do LPNs/LVNs need to provide care for all individuals and communities; they also need to provide culturally competent care. **Cultural competence** is the *continuous* attempt of LPNs/LVNs to gain the knowledge and skills that will allow them to effectively provide care for clients of different cultures. Cultural competence is not gained by reading a chapter in a textbook or by looking up a culture in a reference book. It is obtained by developing an awareness of different cultures (**cultural sensitivity**) and continually learning about people who are different. Giger and Powell-Young (2025, p. 7) describes cultural competence as "a dynamic, fluid, continuous process whereby an individual, system, or health care agency finds meaningful and useful care-delivery strategies based on knowledge of the cultural heritage, beliefs, attitudes, and behaviors of those to whom they render care."

When differences are identified in a health care situation, the LPN/LVN needs to suggest adaptations to the plan of care, so the plan recognizes these differences. In doing so, the client will be encouraged to follow suggestions, avoid treatment failures, and return to health as quickly as possible. LPNs/LVNs will then be able to say that they have truly met the client's needs.

CULTURE

Culture is a way of life. It is the total of the *ever-changing* knowledge, ideas, thoughts, beliefs, values, communication, actions, attitudes, traditions, customs, and objects that a group of people possess and the ways they do things. Culture also involves standards of behavior and sets of rules by which to live. **Customs** are the generally accepted ways of doing things that are common to people who share the same culture.

CHARACTERISTICS OF CULTURE

An important point about culture is that it is learned behavior. The culture of a group is passed on from generation to generation. From the moment a person is born, he or she begins to learn about the culture of the group into which he or she was born. The process of learning the ways of a culture (the way a group does things) is called **enculturation**. The result of enculturation is a **worldview** that is generally shared by individuals with the same cultural background. The worldview, or similar ways of seeing and understanding the world, becomes the reality of the group. This reality fills every aspect of life. It is a **cultural bias** (a mental leaning) that is never proved or questioned by the individual. The value of everything, either within or outside the group, depends on whether it fits the worldview of the cultural group. One's worldview can lead to ethnocentrism, prejudice, and discrimination, unless it is modified by knowledge and experience.

Socialization is the process by which a person of one culture learns how to function in a larger culture. SPNs/SVNs are being socialized into the career of practical/vocational nursing because they are learning how to think and act like an LPN/LVN.

DANGERS: ETHNOCENTRISM, PREJUDICE, AND DISCRIMINATION

People who belong to the same cultural group may develop an attitude, through their worldview, that their way of doing things is superior, right, or better than that of groups with different cultures (**ethnocentrism**). The group uses its culture as the norm against which to measure and evaluate the customs and ways of others. The group can be uncomfortable with people who display customs and behaviors that differ from their cultural group. Ethnocentrism is common to all cultural groups. When intolerance of another cultural group occurs, **prejudice** results. When rights and privileges are withheld from those of another cultural group, this is called **discrimination**.

This chapter will provide strategies for developing cultural competency in the health care setting. It is important for SPNs/SVNs to avoid false assumptions or stereotypes, when caring for culturally diverse clients to avoid ethnocentrism, prejudice, and discrimination. A **stereotype** is an assumption used to describe all members of a specific group without exception. It is an expectation that all individuals in a group will act the same in a situation just because they are members of that group. Stereotypes ignore the individual differences that occur within every cultural group. Members of any culture may have modified the degree to which they observe the values and practices of their culture. Box 10.1 provides a guide on how to avoid stereotyping culturally diverse clients.

SPNs/SVNs are encouraged to think like an anthropologist. Anthropologists are scientists who study physical, social, and cultural characteristics of human groups. It is helpful to understand how these scientists conduct their studies:

- Anthropologists start the study of cultural groups by identifying common trends in a cultural group.

Box 10.1 How to Avoid Stereotyping Culturally Diverse Clients

STEREOTYPE REPLACEMENT
Become aware of the stereotypes you hold and create non-stereotypical alternatives to them

COUNTER-STEREOTYPIC IMAGING
Remember or imagine someone from a stereotyped group who does not fit the stereotype

INDIVIDUATING
See each person as an individual, not a group member; pay attention to things about them besides the stereotypes of their group

PERSPECTIVE-TAKING
Imagine the perspective of someone from a group different than your own ("Put yourself in the other person's shoes.")

CONTACT
Seek ways to get to know people from different social groups. Build your confidence in interacting with people who are different from you. Seek opportunities to engage in discussions in safe environments, spend time with people outside your usual social groups, or volunteer in a community different than your own.

EMOTIONAL REGULATION
Reflect on your "gut feelings" and negative reactions to people from different social groups. Be aware that positive emotions during a clinical encounter make stereotyping less likely.

MINDFULNESS
Keep your attention on the present moment so you can recognize a stereotypic thought before you act on it

Adapted from U.S. Department of Health and Human Services Office of Minority Health. (n.d.). Combating implicit bias and stereotypes. https://thinkculturalhealth.hhs.gov/assets/pdfs/resource-library/combating-implicit-bias-stereotypes.pdf.

These common trends found in the group are called *generalizations*.

- Then anthropologists gather data to determine if the common trends (generalizations) apply to all individuals within that cultural group.

Automatically generalizing cultural information about a group's health practices to one person in that group might be creating a false assumption. Does the individual follow the traditional practice of the group? Has the individual rejected the practice? Does the individual use the practice only in certain situations? If so, what situations? Is the person an immigrant? How recently?

When people immigrate to a new country, culturally different groups do adopt some of the culture of the new country. The process of giving up parts of their own culture and adopting parts of the culture of the dominant group is called **assimilation**. Complete assimilation, however, rarely occurs. Members of the generations that follow the original immigrants may retain some elements of their original culture in addition to partially assimilating the new culture. For these reasons, *generalizations help explain observed behavior, but they do not predict behavior.*

Try This

Avoiding Stereotyping

Nurses should avoid stereotyping clients because it can lead to ethnocentrism, prejudice, and discrimination. Using Box 10.1, create a plan of action with rationales on how you can avoid stereotyping clients who appear different than you to implement now and when you are an LPN/LVN.

DEVELOPMENT OF CULTURAL COMPETENCY IN THE HEALTH CARE SETTING

The American Nurses Association developed their eighth Standard of Professional Performance, called Culturally Congruent Practice, to focus on the importance of nurses providing culturally competent care (Marion et al., 2016). All levels of nurses should strive to provide culturally competent client care. To develop cultural competency in the health care setting, nurses should perform a self-assessment, identify cultural commonalities, identify cultural differences, expand personal knowledge regarding culturally diverse groups of people, modify the workplace environment, perform a cultural assessment of the client, and effectively plan care for culturally diverse clients.

SELF-ASSESSMENT

To become aware of different cultures, SPNs/SVNs need to be aware of their own cultural standing first before delivering culturally competent client care. Several activities in this chapter are designed to help SPNs/SVNs develop cultural self-awareness. A self-assessment is the first step toward developing cultural competency, a necessary skill for nurses. SPNs/SVNs should consider evaluating personal cultural beliefs, values, and worldview and how they influence thoughts and actions. Some elements of culture are obvious, such as language, celebrated holidays, and food preferences and preparations. However, other aspects of culture may be hidden. Elements such as aspects of communication, beliefs, attitudes, values, sex roles, use of space, concept of time, structure of the family, and family dynamics may be more difficult to recognize and discuss. A deep understanding of personal culture is a valuable foundation for giving culturally competent care to others.

LPNs/LVNs need to guard against making judgments about people who are culturally different. This does not mean the nurse must adopt differences as part of their behavior. It means being open-minded and **nonjudgmental**. It means taking the difference at face value, accepting people as they are, and giving high-quality care. *LPNs/LVNs should be aware of their own attitudes, beliefs, values and hidden biases as they can* *affect their ability to give high-quality care.* LPNs/LVNs should become sensitive to cultural differences and acknowledge that they exist. All nurses should gather knowledge about personal biases and try to modify them to provide more culturally competent care.

Try This

What Makes You Unique?

Let your uniqueness show! Divide the class into small but equal-sized groups. Find one item that makes you unique from other members of the group using Giger and Davidhizar's Transcultural Model (2002) as a reference. Share with your class the item that makes you unique.

IDENTIFICATION OF CULTURAL COMMONALITIES

Because of our genes, each individual is different from every other person in the world. (The only exception is identical twins.) Before considering cultural difference among people, it is a good idea to think about what people have in common.

Try This

What We Share In Common

When you are among a group of your peers (e.g., eating lunch in the cafeteria or walking to the parking lot), take a few minutes to play the "What We Have in Common" culture game. Excluding sex, age, marital status, and culture group, try to find five items you have in common with each member of the group. This activity is especially helpful when the group includes classmates you perceive as "different" from you.

1. ______________________________
2. ______________________________
3. ______________________________
4. ______________________________
5. ______________________________

In a class situation, discuss the items you have in common. Did any item you had in common with other members of the group surprise you?

Did you discover any stereotyping in *your* thinking regarding your peers?

IDENTIFICATION OF CULTURAL DIFFERENCES

In the nineteenth century, waves of immigrants from all over the world came to the United States. The United States was eventually called a **melting pot**, meaning that these immigrants had given up their native cultures and adopted the culture of the American people.

At the beginning of the twentieth century, most immigrants to the United States were of European ancestry. This trend has changed and is impacting the overall trend of the U.S. population. According to the United States Census Bureau in 2021, 57.8% of the U.S. population was White (down from 63.7% in 2010), 18.7% Hispanic or Latino, 12.1% Black, and 11. 4% for the remaining groups: Asian, American Indian/Alaska Native, and Native Hawaiian/other Pacific Islander (Jensen et al., 2021). If current trends continue, the U.S. Census Bureau predicts that minorities will make up 56% of the U.S. population by 2060 (United States Census Bureau, 2020). The concept of the melting pot has been replaced by the concept of **cultural diversity**, which refers to the many differences of culture in the people groups in American society.

Components of cultural diversity include racial and **ethnic groups**. The concept of race as a means of categorizing people by biologic traits has come under attack by social scientists. These scientists suggest using ethnicity as a more accurate means of capturing the great diversity found in the world. Members of ethnic groups are a special type of cultural group, composed of people who are members of the same race, religion, or nation, or who speak the same language. Examples of ethnic groups in the United States include Italian Americans, African Americans, American Indians, Asian Americans, German Americans, Mexican Americans, Jewish Americans, Arab Americans, Greek Americans, Finnish Americans, and many more.

Nurses need to be aware of patterns of cultural diversity among clients, which could include family structure, food preferences, religious beliefs, concept of time, communication, educational background, economic level, wellness and illness beliefs and practices, modesty, mental illness, pregnancy and birth beliefs and practices, and terminal illness and death beliefs and practices. The following is a discussion of these patterns of cultural diversity.

Family Structure

No matter what culture is being discussed, the family is the basic unit of society. One of the roles of the family is to have children, if desired or possible, and to raise them to be contributing members of the group. Actual child-rearing practices vary from culture to culture. Families generally socialize the young to the culture of the group. They meet the physical and psychological needs of the young in culturally specific ways. Some cultures expect only the nuclear family (mother, father, and children) to live in the same house. Others may expect the extended family (the nuclear family plus the grandparents and other relatives) to do so.

The single-parent family continues to challenge the traditional nuclear family as the typical family structure. A parent may become a single parent on the death of a spouse, by electing not to marry at the time of pregnancy, by divorce, or through in vitro fertilization (IVF). The blended family and same sex parent families represent a growing trend in our society. Health care workers who have not been in the same situation may be unaware of, and be insensitive to, the different ways of life of others.

Try This

Cultural Pattern: Family Structure

Respond to the following statements. Your responses will help you discover your own cultural patterns regarding the family.

1. Describe your family structure (nuclear, extended, or alternative lifestyle).
2. Describe the role of children, if any, in your family.
3. Discuss who makes major decisions for your family (e.g., hospitalization)
4. List factors that influence the decision of your family members to visit or not visit the hospital when a member is ill. If visiting is acceptable, how long does your family think it is appropriate to visit?
5. Describe the effect that your hospitalization today at 4 pm for emergency surgery would have on you and your family.

Food Preferences

All cultures use food to provide needed nutrients. However, what people eat, when people eat, and how people eat differ vastly by cultural group. Knowledge of nutrition as a science differs by culture. It is interesting that the soil of some cultures (e.g., Mexico) encourage the growth nutrient-rich foods (two complementary foods that together make up a basic protein source: corn and beans) and became a staple of that culture's diet. Specific foods in different cultures have different meanings. All cultures use food during celebrations. Through generations of experience, different cultures have learned to use different foods to promote health and cure disease.

Try This

Cultural Pattern: Food

To assist you in identifying your own cultural patterns about food preferences, respond to the following statements or questions.

1. What is your favorite food?
2. Identify one special occasion on which your cultural group participates. What foods, if any, are part of this celebration?
3. Describe your favorite recipe or meal from your mother and from your grandmother. What special ingredients or techniques are used to make the recipe? Is there a written recipe?
4. Discuss with a classmate your food preferences that are unknown to you in your culture. Learn from each other.
5. Plan a lunch/dinner at school in which everyone brings a cultural food item to share and discuss the origin of the recipe/food.

Religious Beliefs

Religious beliefs are personal to the individual. Religion is an important aspect of culture but can have different meanings in people's lives. For some, religion is a brief, momentary, and sporadic part of daily life. For others, it may influence every aspect of life, while having a profound effect on personal perspective and on how one lives his or her life. For yet others, religion may not play a part in their lives at all. (Chapter 11 deals with spirituality and religious differences.) There is a close relationship between religious beliefs and the concept of wellness and illness in some groups. LPNs/LVNs need to be aware of their own religious beliefs, obligations, and attitudes. They need to know whether these beliefs and attitudes influence the care they give to clients.

Concept of Time

Some people follow *clock* time. An hour has a beginning and an end (after 60 minutes). People who follow clock time eat, sleep, work, and engage in recreational activities at definite times each day. Other people live on *linear* time. For them, time is a straight line with no beginning and no end. People who follow linear time eat when they are hungry and sleep when they are tired.

Try This

Cultural Pattern: Time

The questions that follow give you an opportunity to discover your own cultural patterns regarding time.

1. What determines when it is time for you to eat or sleep?
2. When you are not in the clinical area, do you keep track of time?
3. Are you on time for appointments?

Communication

Chapter 8 introduced you to the types of communication and potential barriers to the communication process. As mentioned earlier in this chapter, a major barrier to communication in health care is when the client speaks a different language. A person's language gives a view of reality that may differ from others. The following is a list of areas of communication that may vary for people who are culturally different.

Forms of hellos and good byes

- A nurse may greet a client and want to get right down to business.
- The client might expect some light conversation before getting to the matter at hand.
- In some cultural groups, people take an hour to say good-bye, whereas people from other cultures may get up and leave without saying anything.

Appropriateness of the situation

- Some groups prefer people to sit, not stand, while they converse.
- In some groups, the sharing of food is a good way to relate to others and get them to verbalize.

Confidentiality

- All the information the client gives the nurse is considered confidential.
- Some clients do not want their spouse questioned or informed about their problems with the reproductive organs. They fear the spouse may think they are less desirable sexually.
- See Chapter 7 for HIPAA-related content.

Emotions and feelings and their expression

- Emotions are universal, but the cues to those emotions vary considerably. A lack of awareness of this fact can cause unnecessary stress between the client and the nurse.
- In some cultural groups, people cannot display affection in public, show disapproval or frustration, or vent anger.
- A nurse may show dissatisfaction with other members of the health care team by approaching them directly, whereas some team members may show dissatisfaction by being polite to one's face but then complaining about them to the rest of the staff.

Pain expression

- Pain has two parts: sensation and response. All individuals experience the same sensation of pain.
- One's culture influences the definition of pain and the response to the sensation.
- Pain is whatever the person says it is. It exists whenever the person says it does.
- One's culture provides guidelines for approved ways of expressing one's response to the pain sensation and ways to relieve the pain.
- Some cultures teach individuals that it is acceptable to cry, moan, and exhibit other behavior that calls attention to the pain. These behaviors may be considered a cure for pain in their culture.
- Other cultures encourage uncomplaining acceptance of pain and passive behavior when pain is experienced (stoic behavior).

Tempo of conversation

- A nurse may tend to speak quickly and expect a quick response.
- The client may be accustomed to pausing and reflecting before giving a response.

Meaning of silence

- Silence can mean anything from disapproval to warmth, but generally it does not indicate tension or lack of rapport.
- Silence can be difficult for some nurses to tolerate. Nurses should resist the temptation of jumping in during a pause in the conversation and instead force themselves to concentrate on listening and reflecting on the discussion.

? Critical Thinking

Stoic Behavior in Clients

Discuss some nursing situations in which a stoic (seemingly unaffected by pain) reaction to pain could have negative consequences if an LPN/LVN lacked knowledge of cultural differences in pain expression (e.g., a woman in labor or a client having a heart attack).

Try This

Cultural Pattern: Communication

Develop an awareness of your own cultural patterns in communication by answering the following questions:

1. What is your first (native) language?
2. Do you speak additional languages?
3. What facial or body habits are you aware of in yourself while you are talking?
4. How do you greet people, and how do you say good-bye?
5. How do you express the following emotions?
   a. Love
   b. Hate
   c. Fear
   d. Excitement
   e. Disappointment
   f. Dissatisfaction
   g. Humor
   h. Anger
   i. Sadness
   j. Happiness
6. Do you make eye contact when talking to people?
7. Do you touch people while talking?
   a. If so, how do they react?
   b. How do you react when people touch you while they are talking to you?
8. How do you express pain? How do you react to pain?

Educational Background

Nurses need to consider differences in educational background and literacy when teaching clients. According to the U.S. Department of Education (2019), one in five U.S. adults has difficulty when completing tasks that require comparing/contrasting and making low-level inferences. This equates to 43 million Americans. Of this 43 million, 8.4 million are considered English illiterate. When in the clinical area, SPNs/SVNs need to assess the client's level of understanding and adapt explanations accordingly. Keep in mind that other factors, such as pain or illness, may cause even the most educated person to have trouble concentrating or understanding what the nurse is teaching.

Try This

Cultural Pattern: Educational Background

Your responses to the following statements will help you identify your own beliefs and practices regarding education.

1. Calculate the number of years of education you have.
2. State your ultimate educational goal.
3. Discuss the role education plays in your life.
4. Describe your feelings toward a person who has less education than you.
5. Describe your feelings toward a person who has more education than you.
6. Describe your feelings if you were referred to your school's tutor/skills development center/remediation center.
7. Discuss the effect of your cultural background on your values and practices with regard to education.
8. Who in your family has graduated from high school, technical school, junior college, or a college or university?
9. Did you identify any related bias?

Economic Level

Economic level is often related to educational background. Sociologists use these two factors to determine the social class of individuals. SPNs/SVNs will meet clients who are very wealthy and clients who are at or near the poverty level. Others have mid-level incomes. Clients' annual incomes can have an impact on the type of house they live in, the neighborhood where they live, the availability of food, and the ability to participate in certain types of preventive health care. LPNs/LVNs need to consider the client's economic level when reinforcing client teaching and should adapt their approach accordingly when needed.

Try This

Cultural Pattern: Economic Level

Identify your personal patterns regarding economic level by responding to the following statements or questions.

1. Describe how your economic background affects your daily life in the following areas:
   a. Availability of food
   b. Availability of shelter
   c. Availability of clothing
   d. Amount and type of recreation
2. Discuss your feelings toward a person who has less money than you.
3. Discuss your feelings toward a person who has more money than you.
4. Describe how these feelings fit with those of your cultural group.
5. Discuss your ability to afford to go to a health care provider when you get sick.
6. If you work, do you have health insurance benefits?
7. Discuss the implications as they relate to Maslow's hierarchy of needs theory.

Wellness and Illness Beliefs and Practices

Wellness and illness can have different meanings for people who are culturally different. *Wellness* and *illness* are relative terms. What is good health to one person can be sickness to another. Wellness may not be a high-priority matter to some clients.

Preventing illness. Some clients believe that illness can be prevented; they practice elaborate rituals and engage special individuals to carry out those rituals to prevent disease. Other clients look at prevention, negatively, as an attempt to control the future; they may consider this an impossible feat in the way they view their lives. They may wonder about the necessity of seeing a health care provider for preventive care, such as immunizations or cancer screening. Others may think prevention is tempting fate and following through with prevention is risky.

Curing illness. When disease does occur, some people blame pathogens (germs), some blame spirits, and others blame an imbalance in the body. Some cultural groups have folk medicine practices, such as rituals, special procedures (e.g., rubbing the skin with the edge of a coin to release the toxins causing illness), and special people in the group to help cure disease (e.g., health care provider, herbalist, shaman). Some groups believe that special foods or food combinations (e.g., "cold" foods for "hot" illness) and herbs (e.g., Echinacea and Feverfew) can prevent or cure illnesses. Others see no relationship between diet and health.

Complementary and alternative medicine. The dominant health care system in the United States is biomedicine (Western medicine). Biomedicine focuses on symptoms, with the goal of finding the cause of a disease and then eliminating or relieving the problem. Over 50% of Americans seek methods that avoid side effects from medications and treatments and/or that focus on the whole body and not just symptoms when treating disease. They are spending billions of dollars a year, mostly out of pocket, on complementary (used in conjunction with biomedical treatments) and alternative (a substitute for conventional medicine) medicines.

Complementary and alternative medicine (CAM) focuses on assisting the body's own healing powers and restoring body balance. The diversity of non-Western health care practices among the many cultural groups in the United States has helped increase the interest and use of CAM. Common examples include massage therapy, acupuncture, or the use of herbs. The National Center for Complementary and Integrative Health (NCCIH), part of the National Institutes of Health, conducts research and evaluates the effectiveness and safety of CAM. Visit the NCCIH's website at https://nccih.nih.gov/ for more information about CAM.

Modesty

Individuals in some cultures are embarrassed when they must discuss bodily functions or allow certain body parts to be examined during a wellness or illness examination. Hygiene practices vary according to beliefs, living conditions, personal resources, and physical characteristics.

Mental Illness

Some cultural groups attach a stigma to mental illness and psychiatrists but are accepting of impairments to physical health. Other groups believe that mental health responses are a healthy reaction to an emotional crisis. Yet others believe that the mind and body are united and are not separate entities. These cultures may have traditional healers who are experts at healing both the mind and the body. Some people may seek out traditional healers to heal the mind, while at the same time consult Western medicine to heal the body.

Try This

Cultural Pattern: Wellness Beliefs and Practices

To assist you in identifying your own cultural patterns regarding wellness beliefs and practices, respond to the following statements and questions.

1. Describe what it means to you to be in good health.
2. What are some of your own practices or beliefs about staying well?
3. Describe what it means to you to be sick.
4. List some foods in your diet that you believe help prevent illness.
   a. How does eating these foods prevent illness?
   b. What are some foods you must avoid preventing illness?
5. List some foods in your diet that help you recover when you are sick.
   a. What illnesses do these foods cure?
   b. How do these foods cure illness?
6. Discuss CAM used by your family.
7. If you use CAM and biomedicine, do you inform the health care provider of CAM use, including herbs, during a clinic visit?
8. Describe your attitude toward mental illness.
   a. Describe what you think causes mental illness.
   b. Who do you think should treat mental illness?
   c. How do you believe mental illness is best treated?

Pregnancy and Birth Beliefs and Practices

Different cultures welcome a new member into the world in different ways. The *Try This: Cultural Patterns: Pregnancy and Birth Beliefs and Practices* box helps identify personal beliefs about pregnancy and birth.

Try This

Cultural Pattern: Pregnancy and Birth Beliefs and Practices

To assist you in identifying your own cultural patterns regarding birth beliefs and practices, respond to the following statements and questions about your family's customs regarding pregnancy and birth.

1. Do the women in your family receive prenatal care?
2. How is "discomfort" expressed during labor?
3. Who attends the birth?
4. Where does birth take place?
5. Who delivers the baby?
6. Is bonding encouraged?
7. What special practices take place after birth and during the postpartum period?
8. Are there special practices regarding the placenta and umbilical cord?
9. Is breastfeeding encouraged?
10. Are there precautions regarding breastfeeding?
11. Is birth control encouraged? Is it permitted?

Terminal Illness and Death Beliefs and Practices

Generally, death and terminal illness bring out strong emotions in most people. Be aware that some cultures have special taboos and prohibitions when a death occurs. Roles that family and friends carry out at the time of death may vary. There are many differences in the way different cultures handle terminal illness for a member. When death does occur, the rituals practiced are numerous and varied. It is important for nurses to listen to their clients and client's family to learn of their needs during terminal illness and death.

Try This

Cultural Pattern: Terminal Illness and Death Beliefs and Practices

To assist you in identifying your own cultural patterns regarding terminal illness and death beliefs and practices, respond to the following statements and questions pertaining to a death in your family.

1. Is it acceptable to tell a terminally ill family member the diagnosis? If yes, who tells the family member?
2. Would your family engage in palliative or hospice care for themselves or their loved one?
3. Where does an anticipated death usually occur (at home, in a hospital)?
4. Who should be present when the death occurs?
5. Does your family require specific treatment of the body after death?
6. Does your family permit/encourage autopsy or organ donation?
7. Who makes the burial arrangements?
8. Describe what you believe happens to you after death.
9. Does your family permit cremation?
10. Does your family have a funeral or memorial service?
11. Do you have a get-together after the burial? If so, for whom? What occurs during the get-together?
12. How does your family remember the dead?

Try This

Areas of Cultural Diversity

With your peers, discuss your answers to statements and questions about various areas of cultural diversity, especially wellness and illness, birth, and death practices.

Regardless of which cultural group you belong to, these exercises about cultural diversity have given you the opportunity to think about the many ways you and your peers differ. You will observe some of these differences in clients in the clinical area and learn from them. Along with that awareness of and sensitivity to differences, a tolerance may develop of the different beliefs and actions of others without thoughts of prejudice or discrimination.

EXPANSION OF PERSONAL KNOWLEDGE REGARDING CULTURALLY DIVERSE GROUPS

Nurses who provide health care today and in the future need to be able to accommodate clients of many different cultural backgrounds. An expansion of personal knowledge regarding culturally diverse groups of people is essential. A failure to develop sensitivity to and competence in handling this diversity could lead to misunderstandings between the nurse and the client, resulting in stress for both. The plan of treatment for the client could fail. Nurses could make false assumptions based on generalizations. Nurses might label clients as difficult or uncooperative when their lack of cooperation with the plan of care could be related to a conflict with their personal health belief system. Clients may experience less-than-adequate care when cultural diversity and the differences it represents are overlooked or misinterpreted. Examples of areas of cultural diversity that may be taken for granted in client situations would include food preferences, religion, educational background, economic level, wellness and illness beliefs and practices, the birth experience, and terminal illness and death beliefs and practices. Clients have the potential for the best outcomes when nurses consider the client's cultural preferences and provide culturally competent care.

Professional Pointer

Respect Cultural Differences

Many factors are responsible for differences in clients. They may think and behave differently because of personal income, religion, ethnic background, or personal choice. Regardless of these differences, all clients have the right to receive high-quality nursing care. As an LPN/LVN you cannot decrease the quality of the care you give because of differences you observe or perceive.

No one can be an expert on every culture in the world. Even those who are experts on a particular culture do not like being labeled as such. These people are aware of the ever-changing nature of cultures and of the important individual variations that occur within any cultural group. Experts are always cautious about stereotyping people in any cultural group.

Try This

Your Area's Cultural Groups

Implement five or more of the following learning activities to increase your knowledge about cultural diversity groups:

1. Hear stories from peers about various cultural groups (Think beyond the more traditional cultural groups, based on ethnicity and consider the disabled, elderly, single parents, alternative lifestyles, and so on.)
2. Read about the different cultures that are served in your area. Use the References and Suggested Readings for this chapter, Internet sources in the text, and the resources of your learning resource center (LRC) as suggested in Chapter 2 to find texts and articles about specific cultural groups. Google a specific group to obtain information (www.google.com) and remember to verify your sources.
3. View documentaries on television or on the Internet about cultural groups.
4. Attend community events sponsored by cultural groups.
5. Attend graduations, weddings, birth celebrations, and funerals of different cultures when the opportunities present themselves.
6. Attend a religious service of a cultural group.
7. Read novels involving different cultures.
8. Attend seminars about cultural groups.
9. Invite a member of a cultural group to class to talk about the health/illness beliefs of the group of whom he or she is a member.
10. Participate in diversity training or an international type of club, if offered by your institution or clinical affiliate.

MODIFICATION OF THE WORKPLACE ENVIRONMENT

The health care environment can be made more welcoming to culturally diverse clients. Many of these changes require little cost or time to implement, but the results can promote better health and compliance among culturally diverse clients. Box 10.2 presents suggestions for modifying the workplace environment for the LPN/LVN working in health care agencies with culturally diverse clients.

Box 10.2 Modifying the Environment to Accommodate Culturally Diverse Clients

- Identify the various cultural groups that use the health care facility.
- Post welcome signs in the languages of the groups you serve.
- Arrange for messages on answering machines to include the languages of the clients you serve. Place magazines in waiting rooms that reflect the diversity of the clients you serve.
- Include background music that reflects the diversity of the clients you serve.
- Provide handouts, appointment cards, and client education materials in the languages of the clients you serve.
- Decorate the environment (pictures, posters, objects, etc.) to reflect the diversity of the clients you serve.
- Stock adhesive bandages that do not match any specific skin tone; for example, Walt Disney characters for children and fluorescent or varied colors for adults.
- In waiting areas, provide books, toys, and multicultural videos for children that promote acceptance of diversity. Sesame Street and SpongeBob SquarePants themes are especially effective and accepted.

Adapted from Reinhardt E: *Through the eyes of others—intercultural resource directory for health care professionals*, Minneapolis, 1995, University of Minnesota School of Public Health, pp 19–20.

Try This

Modification of the Workplace Environment

Using the suggestions for modifying the workplace environment found in Box 10.2, develop an action plan that you hope to implement when you become an LPN/LVN in a long-term care facility.

CULTURAL ASSESSMENT OF THE CLIENT

Everyone is unique and a product of their experiences, cultural norms, and beliefs (Giger and Powell-Young, 2025). Giger and Davidhizar's Transcultural Model (Box 10.3) provides a framework for caring for clients in a variety of settings focused on their unique personal identity. Nurses need strong assessment skills

Box 10.3 Giger and Davidhizar's Transcultural Assessment Model

CULTURALLY UNIQUE INDIVIDUAL

1. Place of birth
2. Cultural definition
   What is…
3. Race
   What is…
4. Length of time in country (if appropriate)

COMMUNICATION

1. Voice quality
   A. Strong, resonant
   B. Soft
   C. Average
   D. Shrill
2. Pronunciation and enunciation
   A. Clear
   B. Slurred
   C. Dialect (geographical)
3. Use of silence
   A. Infrequent
   B. Often
   C. Length
      1. Brief
      2. Moderate
      3. Long
      4. Not observed
4. Use of nonverbal
   A. Hand movement
   B. Eye movement
   C. Entire body movement
   D. Kinesics (gestures, expressions, or stances)
5. Touch
   A. Startles or withdraws when touched
   B. Accepts touch without difficulty
   C. Touches others without difficulty
6. Ask these and similar questions:
   A. How do you get your point across to others?
   B. Do you like communicating with friends, family, and acquaintances?
   C. When asked a question, do you usually respond (in words or body movement, or both)?
   D. If you have something important to discuss with your family, how would you approach them?

SPACE

1. Degree of comfort
   A. Moves when personal space invaded
   B. Does not move when space invaded
2. Distance in conversations
   A. 0 to 18 inches
   B. 18 inches to 3 feet
   C. 3 feet or more
3. Definition of space
   A. Describe degree of comfort with closeness when talking with or standing near others
   B. How do objects (e.g., furniture) in the environment affect your sense of space?
4. Ask these and similar questions:
   A. When you talk with family members, how close do you stand?
   B. When you communicate with coworkers and other acquaintances, how close do you stand?
   C. If a stranger touches you, how do you react or feel?
   D. If a loved one touches you, how do you react or feel?
   E. Are you comfortable with the distance between us now?

SOCIAL ORIENTATION

1. Normal state of health
   A. Poor
   B. Fair
   C. Good
   D. Excellent
2. Marital status
3. Number of children
4. Parents living or deceased?
5. Ask these and similar questions:
   A. How do you define social activities?
   B. What are some activities that you enjoy?
   C. What are your hobbies, or what do you do when you have free time?
   D. Do you believe in a Supreme Being?
   E. How do you worship that Supreme Being?
   F. What is your function (what do you do) in your family unit/system?
   G. What is your role in your family unit/system (father, mother, child, advisor)?
   H. When you were a child, what or who influenced you most?
   I. What is/was your relationship with your siblings and parents?
   J. What does work mean to you?
   K. Describe your past, present, and future jobs.
   L. What are your political views?
   M. How have your political views influenced your attitude toward health and illness?

TIME

1. Orientation to time
   A. Past-oriented
   B. Present-oriented
   C. Future-oriented

Continued

Box 10.3 Giger and Davidhizar's Transcultural Assessment Model—cont'd

2. View of time
   A. Social time
   B. Clock-oriented
3. Physiochemical reaction to time
   A. Sleeps at least 8 hours a night
   B. Goes to sleep and wakes on a consistent schedule
   C. Understands the importance of taking medication and other treatments on schedule
4. Ask these and similar questions:
   A. What kind of timepiece do you wear daily?
   B. If you have an appointment at 2 pm, what time is acceptable to arrive?
   C. If a nurse tells you that you will receive a medication in "about a half hour," realistically, how much time will you allow before calling the nurses' station?

ENVIRONMENTAL CONTROL

1. Locus-of-control
   A. Internal locus-of-control (believes that the power to effect change lies within)
   B. External locus-of-control (believes that fate, luck, and chance have a great deal to do with how things turn out)
2. Value orientation
   A. Believes in supernatural forces
   B. Relies on magic, witchcraft, and prayer to effect change
   C. Does not believe in supernatural forces
   D. Does not rely on magic, witchcraft, or prayer to effect change
3. Ask these and similar questions:
   A. How often do you have visitors at your home?
   B. Is it acceptable to you for visitors to drop in unexpectedly?
   C. Name some ways your parents or other persons treated your illnesses when you were a child.
   D. Have you or someone else in your immediate surroundings ever used a home remedy that made you feel sick?
   E. What home remedies have you used that worked? Will you use them in the future?
   F. What is your definition of "good health"?
   G. What is your definition of "poor health"?

BIOLOGICAL VARIATIONS

1. Conduct a complete physical assessment noting:
   A. Body structure (small, medium, or large frame)
   B. Skin color
   C. Unusual skin discolorations
   D. Hair color and distribution
   E. Other visible physical characteristics (e.g., keloids, chloasma)
   F. Weight
   G. Height
   H. Check lab work for variances in hemoglobin, hematocrit, and sickle cell phenomena if Black or Mediterranean
2. Ask these and similar questions:
   A. What diseases or illnesses are common in your family?
   B. Has anyone in your family been told that there is a possible genetic susceptibility for a particular disease?
   C. Describe your family's typical behavior when a family member is ill.
   D. How do you respond when you are angry?
   E. Who (or what) usually helps you cope during a difficult time?
   F. What foods do you and your family like to eat?
   G. Have you ever had any unusual cravings for:
      1. White or red clay dirt?
      2. Laundry starch?
   H. When you were a child what types of foods did you eat?
   I. What foods are family favorites or are considered traditional?

NURSING ASSESSMENT

1. Note whether the client has become culturally assimilated or observes own cultural practices.
2. Incorporate data into plan of nursing care:
   A. Encourage the client to discuss cultural differences; people from diverse cultures who hold different world views can enlighten nurses.
   B. Make efforts to accept and understand methods of communication.
   C. Respect the individual's personal need for space.
   D. Respect the rights of clients to honor and worship the Supreme Being of their choice.
   E. Identify a clerical or spiritual person to contact.
   F. Determine whether spiritual practices have implications for health, life, and well-being (e.g., Jehovah's Witnesses may refuse blood and blood derivatives; an Orthodox Jew may eat only kosher food high in sodium and may not drink milk when meat is served).
   G. Identify hobbies, especially when devising interventions for a short or extended convalescence or for rehabilitation.
   H. Honor time and value orientations and differences in these areas. Allay anxiety and apprehension if adherence to time is necessary.
   I. Provide privacy according to personal need and health status of the client (Note: the perception of and reaction to pain may be culturally related).
   J. Note cultural health practices:
      1) Identify and encourage efficacious practices.
      2) Identify and discourage dysfunctional practices.
      3) Identify and determine whether neutral practices will have a long-term ill effect.
   K. Note food preferences.
      1) Make as many adjustments in diet as health status and long-term benefits will allow and that the dietary department can provide.
      2) Note dietary practices that may have serious implications for the client.

From Giger JN, Powell-Young YM: *Transcultural nursing: assessment and intervention,* ed 9, California, 2025, Elsevier.

to identify the cultural values of clients. An effective cultural assessment of the client is the first step in the nursing process when providing competently competent client care. Giger and Powell-Young (2025) describe six cultural phenomena that are critical to the client assessment to promote effective decision making with culturally competent care. See Fig. 10.1 for details. These six phenomena include communication, space, social organization, time, environmental control, and biological variations.

Communication

Communication differences include spoken language, verbal behaviors (i.e., voice quality and pronunciation), nonverbal behaviors (e.g., direct eye contact, touching), and the use of silence. Communication is a cornerstone to effective client care. Thus, research supports the critical need for an interpreter, when a nurse and client speak a different language. Communication and language assistance is listed as one of the National Standards for Culturally and Linguistically Appropriate Services in Health and Health Care (U.S. Department of Health and Human Services, n.d.). The purpose of CLAS is to "provide effective, equitable, understandable, and respectful quality care and services that are responsive to diverse cultural health beliefs and practices, preferred languages, health literacy, and other communication needs" (U.S. Department of Health and Human Services, n.d.). The standards highlight the need to ensure the competence of an interpreter among other initiatives.

Potential Health Insurance Portability and Accountability Act (HIPAA) violations should be considered if family assists. In most cases, children should not be used as interpreters because of the subject matter; women may also not be acceptable because of the cultural view of women in some cultures (Rimmer, 2020). The local community may offer interpreter services. In addition, entities such as LanguageLine Solutions exist to meet this need (www.languageline.com). The LPN/VPN should review institutional policies and procedures and implement them accordingly.

Space

Space refers to the degree of comfort when speaking or interacting with people around us in a two person or a group setting. For example, most nurses generally feel comfortable with a small space zone of 0 to 18 inches (Cherry and Jacob, 2019). This can be necessary for the delivery of care to a client. This can vary significantly in some cultures. Nurses need to assess this aspect of culturally sensitive care when establishing a relationship with a client.

Social Orientation

Social orientation refers to the family unit, the client's affiliated religious or ethnic groups, and their political views. Family can be interpreted differently across

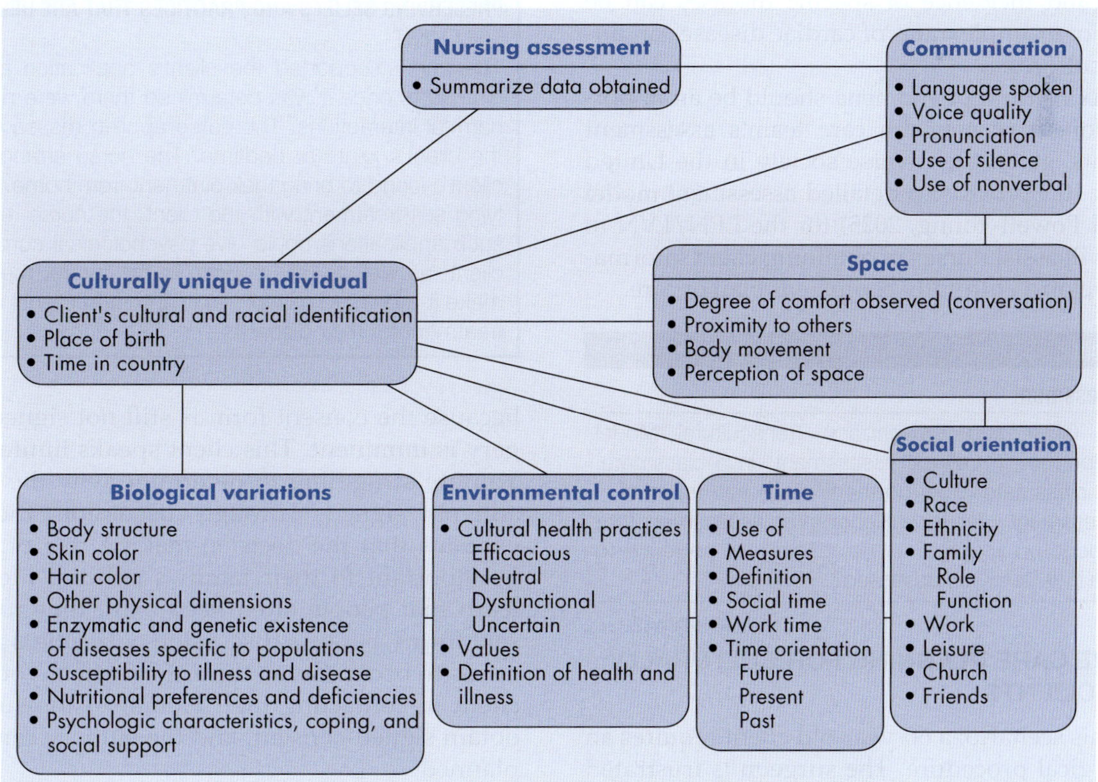

Fig. 10.1 Application of cultural phenomena to nursing care and nursing practice. (From Giger JN, Powell-Young YM: *Transcultural nursing: assessment and intervention*, ed 9, California, 2025, St Louis: Elsevier.)

cultures. For example, a person of another culture may call someone a sister, even though there may not be a relation by blood but instead by friendship or experience.

Time

Time orientation differs across cultures. People and cultures can be described as present-, past-, or future-oriented. People who live in the present live in the "moment." They move on to the next task when the time is right (Cherry and Jacob, 2019). This can contrast greatly with someone who lives in the past or future. People living in the past often look to their ancestors for wisdom and guidance and value previous experiences. Punctuality is often not a priority for those who have a past-oriented time reference. Lastly, those who live in the future are generally punctual and strong planners. Long-term health care goals are important.

Environmental Control

Environmental control refers to whether the person has an internal (power is within them) or external locus of control (fate plays a large role in outcomes). The person's belief or lack of belief in supernatural forces can also vary across cultures.

Biological Variations

Biological variations across cultures can be visible or invisible. Genetic tendencies related to body build and body structure, hair type, eye shape, and skin characteristics can be easily visible. In contrast, nutritional variations and incidence of specific diseases can be invisible. For example, rates of cardiac disease can differ across cultures.

These six cultural phenomena should be an important component of a health care team's assessment of all clients, given the diverse society in the United States. Box 10.3 provides a detailed assessment model (Giger and Powell-Young, 2025) for the LPN/LVN to use. This will assist nurses in obtaining client information to develop a culturally competent plan of care.

Try This

Cultural Assessment

Using the Giger and Davidhizar's Transcultural Model Box 10.3, perform a cultural assessment on a classmate, a friend, or classmate. How do the findings you found during the assessment interview differ from an assessment that would be done on yourself? What actions can you take to support the individual you assessed?

Box 10.4 Preserving the Beliefs and Practices That Are Helpful to the Client

SITUATION

A 72-year-old was admitted to Brent Hospital with pneumonia and advanced osteoarthritis. An LPN is the nurse and cannot understand how anyone can get to such a state of ill health without seeing a health care provider. The nurse is especially upset because the client could have prevented much of their disability from arthritis if the client had followed a preventive program when first diagnosed with this disease.

CULTURAL HEALTH BELIEFS IN THIS SITUATION

The client has lived in poverty for their entire life. As with any person in this situation, their main concern in life has been the present and getting through their problems on a day-to-day basis. The client's time orientation is the moment (present), not the future; therefore, preventive regimens have not been central to their way of thinking. People with similar backgrounds and situations delay care until the disease interferes with their ability to work or results in a disability.

It cannot be said that clients ignored their condition. Clients participated in self-treatment by using cultural health practices in the form of topical application of oils and ointments to their aching joints. These self-treatments helped the client deal physically and psychologically with his condition. The client looks at their disability as a punishment from God, who let something get into their joints. The client's belief stems from the wellness and illness beliefs brought to this country from their homeland. These beliefs center on wellness as a state experienced when one is in harmony with nature. Illness is experienced as a state of disharmony with nature.

PRESERVING BELIEFS AND PRACTICES THAT ARE HELPFUL TO THE CLIENT

The nurse supported the client's application of oils and ointments once it was determined there were no potential harmful interactions. The nurse applied massage lotion to the client's joints at bedtime. The nurse arranged for the client's friend to bring their ointment from home. After clarifying self-treatment with the client, the nurse realized that such applications could give psychological comfort to the client, as well as relieve pain. In the future, the nurse will make it a point to ask all newly admitted clients about self-treatment for their diseases.

EFFECTIVE CARE PLANNING FOR CULTURALLY DIVERSE CLIENTS

Imagine this scenario: a 60-year-old client requires an urgent surgical procedure. The surgeon is frustrated because the consent form is still not signed and surgery is imminent. This client speaks limited English. You are struggling to determine why the consent is still not signed. Through discussion, the husband explains that the decision-making role of the elders is important to their family's cultural lifestyle. You learn that people often need extra time to sign consent forms, because discussion with elders and family needs to occur. Given this information, you assist the client in contacting their elders, so the surgeon can obtain signed consent, and the surgery can occurs as planned.

Understanding cultural preferences can improve client care. For more resources on caring for different cultural groups, nurses could:

- access the resource library provided by the U.S. Department of Health and Human Services at https://thinkculturalhealth.hhs.gov/resources/library. The website provides practical how-to-guides and checklists to effectively provide culturally competent client care.
- access the free online training by The U.S. Department of Health and Human Services, Office of Minority Health (n.d.), *Culturally and Linguistically Appropriate Services (CLAS) in Nursing*, designed to assist nurses in providing culturally competent client care. Visit https://ccnm.thinkculturalhealth.hhs.gov/ to access this training.

Remember that general group behavior *sometimes explains* observed behavior, but it is *not predictive* of individual behavior. Assumptions based on generalizations should not be made. When using this information, SPNs/SVNs should avoid stereotyping clients.

Nurses may consider suspecting cultural differences when a client is not following the plan of care, refuses treatment, is labeled by some erroneously as a "problem" client, and so on. Asking a client questions about their ADLs and wellness and illness beliefs could reveal cultural attitudes and beliefs, which could be valuable for care planning.

Jackson (1993) suggests ways of co-creating a treatment plan with culturally diverse clients. Nurses could consider the following strategy for incorporating cultural beliefs into a client's plan of care:

1. *Discover the health beliefs of the individual.* Be respectful and open-minded when questioning the client about the cause of the health problem, the moment it began, its severity, its course, the problems it has caused in the client's life, and the treatment the client thinks will cure the disease. *Avoid assuming anything.* When unsure of anything, ask! In situations of cultural diversity, our clients are the teachers and nurses are the students.
2. *Co-create treatment plans with the client.* Avoid trying to change clients' beliefs. Cultural health practices can be deeply respected by the client. Involve the client in making decisions about his or her own care. Do so in a way that does not threaten the client's beliefs and practices or conflict with them. Explain from the biomedical point of view the cause of the disease, how the disease alters the body, the role of treatment, and the expected outcome. Then compare the client's belief system with that of biomedicine to help ensure the client's cooperation with the plan of care.
3. *Preserve the beliefs and practices that are helpful to the client.* Starting in 1993, the Office of Alternative Medicine of the National Institutes of Health began to identify, study, and bring together the best healing practices of other cultures with those of Western medicine. In 1998, the National Center for Complimentary and Integrative Health was established to focus on determining the usefulness and safety of complementary and integrative health interventions and their roles in improving health and health care. Many of the beliefs and practices of non-Western health beliefs have proved beneficial. Acupuncture and acupressure are now a common practice in the United States and many more alternative treatment modalities continue to emerge. LPNs/LVNs can collaborate with the RN about clients' practices that have not yet been researched or found effective. If the practices seem to help the client and do no harm, then they can be included in the plan of care, regardless of the nurse's ability to see the benefit of the practice. Box 10.4 provides an example of preserving the beliefs and practices that are helpful to the client.
4. *Repattern harmful practices.* Harmful practices that are prevalent in Western society include smoking, diets high in fat, refined grains, and refined sugar, and lack of exercise, which can cause high blood pressure and heart disease. Extreme dietary restrictions during pregnancy can lead to maternal toxemia and poor fetal development. Nurses should explain reasons for opposing harmful practice and offer alternatives.

When nurses listen and learn with sensitivity and humility about the cultures of all people, they can deliver exceptional client-centered, culturally competent care. All nurses should perform a self-assessment, identify cultural commonalities, identify cultural differences, expand personal knowledge regarding culturally diverse groups of people, modify the workplace environment, perform a cultural assessment of the client, and effectively plan care for culturally diverse clients to develop cultural competence in the health care setting.

Try This

Cultural Care Planning

Access the resource library of the U.S. Department of Health and Human Services at https://thinkculturalhealth.hhs.gov/resources/library.

What resource do you find helpful for providing culturally competent client care?

How will you implement what you learned during your clinical experiences?

Get Ready for the Next-Generation NCLEX® Examination

Key Points

- A good place to start learning about how people are different is to remind yourself that all people are unique but have similarities as well.
- Giger and Davidhizar (1991) describe six cultural phenomena: communication, space, social organization, time, environmental control, and biological variations that are critical to the assessment of clients and provision of culturally competent care.
- One guideline in health care is the philosophy of individual worth; that is, the confidence that all people are unique and have value regardless of the way they view their world and that they deserve the best nursing care you can give.
- Awareness of cultural diversity is important for LPNs/LVNs, so they can avoid false assumptions and misunderstandings about the clients in their care.
- The first step in understanding other people's culture is to understand your own culture. Be aware of your personal beliefs and practices in the areas of family, religion, communication, educational background, economic level, pregnancy, wellness and illness beliefs and practices, and death and dying.
- Some ways to learn about cultural diversity include reading about different cultures, especially those found in your geographic area, and actively listening to reports from your peers and clients who are culturally different.
- Cultural characteristics of groups are not predictive of behavior of individuals in a group. They are generalizations. *Always allow for individual variations within specific groups*.
- Performing a self-assessment, identifying cultural commonalities, identifying cultural differences, expanding personal knowledge regarding culturally diverse groups of people, modifying the workplace environment, performing a cultural assessment of the client, and effectively planning care for culturally diverse clients can help SPNs/SVNs develop cultural competence in the health care setting.

Additional Learning Resources

Go to your Evolve website (http://evolve.elsevier.com/Carroll/success/) for the following FREE learning resources:

- Answers to Critical Thinking Scenarios
- Additional learning activities
- Additional Review Questions for the NCLEX-PN® examination
- Helpful phrases for communicating in Spanish and more!

Clinical Judgment Questions

1. A group of LPNs/LVNs are discussing culture-related terms. What should be avoided when studying different cultures?

a. Stereotyping
b. Socialization
c. Enculturation
d. Assimilation

2. What statement best illustrates the philosophy of individual worth?

a. All individuals are unique and have value regardless of their differences in how they meet daily needs.
b. People who belong to ethnic groups have different daily needs in most needs' categories.
c. People of different cultures need to be approached as if their culture is the best of all culture groups in the area.
d. Empowerment is culturally dependent.

3. An Asian American client in a nursing home does not want to follow the nursing care plan regarding diet. What describes the nurse's best course of action?

a. Insist the resident accept the diet as ordered.
b. Document the stubbornness of this resident.
c. Avoid making an issue of his noncompliance.
d. Consider the possibility of cultural differences.

4. A client, a member of a culture that values being stoic, was admitted to the medical floor with a diagnosis of angina. The client has an order for nitroglycerin PRN (as needed) for chest pain. What statement describes the priority concern of the LPN/LVN who is administering pain medication to this client?

a. The drug should be kept in a dark container to protect it from light.
b. The drug is always kept with the client when he is walking.
c. Nonverbal signs of pain should not be overlooked in this situation.
d. The client's pain level should be assessed at the beginning of the shift.

5. LPNs/LVNs use culture and nursing care guides to gather information about different cultures. What suggestion applies to the use of culture reference guides and other electronic resources? *(Select all that apply.)*

a. Avoid applying information automatically to all members of a culture.
b. Variation between any member of the same cultural group does not occur.
c. Assume that all members of a cultural group are the same in all aspects.
d. Information obtained explains behavior but does not predict behavior.
e. Once you gather data for one client, this information can be applied to others.

6. An SPN/SVN wants to provide culturally sensitive care to clients. What order could the following steps be taken to develop cultural competency?

a. Identify cultural differences
b. Effectively plan care for culturally diverse clients
c. Perform a self-assessment
d. Modify the workplace environment
e. Identify cultural commonalities
f. Perform a cultural assessment of the client
g. Expand personal knowledge regarding culturally diverse groups of people

7. Indicate whether the following nursing actions represent culturally competent care or not.

NURSING ACTIONS	CULTURALLY COMPETENT	NOT CULTURALLY COMPETENT
a. Obtain various skin-colored adhesive bandages		
b. Perform a self-assessment		
c. Select All-American food for a client's meal		
d. Teach clients to avoid alternative medicine practices		
e. Predict customs of Native American clients		

Critical Thinking Scenario

A female client who is from a culture that values "being stoic" and values the male role in decision making was admitted to the hospital after experiencing 3 days of intermittent chest pain. She does not like being on bedrest and has attempted to walk down the hall several times. Using gestures only, the client has been indicating that she is in pain, but she consistently refuses medications. During visiting hours, the client's husband, children, sisters, brothers, and parents visit. The health care provider plans to order a diagnostic study to evaluate the client's coronary arteries. The health care provider asks the husband for permission, and he refuses. The client has another stroke, and after two days, the health care provider tells the husband that the client must go to a long-term care facility. He is horrified to hear this news.

Why did the client wait 3 days before coming to the hospital?

Why did she attempt to walk down the hall when she knew she should be on bedrest?

Why did she refuse medications for pain?

Why were there so many visitors?

Why did the spouse refuse coronary artery studies for the client?

Why did the spouse become upset when nursing home placement was suggested for the client?

11 Spiritual Needs, Spiritual Caring, and Religious Differences

Objectives

On completing this chapter, you will be able to do the following:

1. Describe holistic nursing care.
2. Define spirituality.
3. Discuss the role of the licensed practical nurse/licensed vocational nurse (LPN/LVN) in providing spiritual care to the client and the family as a member of the health care team.
4. List members of the health care team who can help provide spiritual care for clients.
5. Discuss key nursing interventions to meet the spiritual needs of clients.
6. Discuss personal religious and/or spiritual beliefs, or the absence of them, and how these beliefs will influence nursing practice.

Key Terms

agnostic
atheist
compassion
emotional needs
faith
holistic nursing care
hospice nurse
intentional presence
layperson
moral distress
palliative care nurse
parish nurse
pastoral care team
religious beliefs
religious denomination
rituals
spirit
spiritual care
spiritual dimension
spiritual needs
spirituality
transcendence

> **Keep in Mind**
> If you were hospitalized, is it important to you that the staff be informed of your spiritual practices?

The evening nurse found a client, age 32, sitting up in bed, crying and moaning with what they interpreted as pain after a testicular biopsy that was positive for cancer. After assessment, the nurse volunteered to get the client some pain medication, but they refused. The client shouts, "Why did I have to get cancer? Why me?" Then says, "Never mind. No one understands. Just leave me alone." The nurse quickly and quietly leaves the room so the client can be alone.

SPIRITUALITY IN HOLISTIC CARE

Providing client-centered care is an essential part of building a therapeutic nurse–client relationship. A holistic approach of caring for body, mind, and **spirit** is a well-recognized, vital component to quality, client-centered care. In its *Nursing Diagnoses:* 2024–2026 edition, the North American Nursing Diagnosis Association (NANDA) includes nursing diagnoses related to spirituality (i.e., readiness for enhanced spiritual well-being; risk for one's moral distress) and a separate diagnosis related to religiosity (Herdman et al., 2024). In the foregoing situation, the client was in distress. A minister, priest, other spiritual/religious individual, or **layperson** might have been able to address the client's problem, but the client needed immediate spiritual care. It would have been helpful to the client if the nurse had offered to spend time with them and encouraged them to talk about what they were thinking and feeling at that time. It is a privilege for nurses to be invited into the spiritual realm of the client, and it is an integral part of **holistic nursing care**. Despite the NANDA-I diagnoses, some nurses are uncomfortable with matters of the spirit while understanding the important client benefits of such nurturing. Many nurses feel unprepared and lack training and understanding of diverse beliefs. Nurses also face barriers such as time constraints or lack of institutional support in providing **spiritual care**. Inadequate spiritual care could affect patients' decision-making, mental well-being, and physical capability for health (Murgia et al., 2022).

SPIRITUALITY

Spirituality is an essential part of being human. The word comes from the Latin word *spiritus*, which means "breath" or "air." The spirit is the very essence of a person. It includes the beliefs and value systems that give people strength and hope. Miller et al. (2023) describe a connection with self, others, and/or a higher power as central to human spiritual experiences. This includes a sense of purpose, a reason for living. Lukovsky et al. (2021) identify connectedness, **transcendence**, and meaning in life as core components of spirituality that shapes one's purpose. The spirit gives meaning to life. For some, **faith** and **religious** beliefs are the foundation to spirituality, whereas others relate spirituality to traditions, relationships, and purpose. One's personal experiences and faith/cultural background significantly shape an individual's view on what brings hope and peace. Thus spirituality is highly variable from person to person. Many people simply describe spirituality as believing in something larger than themselves (Carson and Koenig, 2008). The spiritual self grows and changes throughout one's lifespan. Regardless of how one expresses their spirituality, spiritual well-being has overall positive health benefits that include lower anxiety and pain levels and lower risk of suicide, stress, and depression (Diego-Cordero et al., 2022). However, if spiritual needs are not met, individuals experience higher risks of depression, diminished quality of life, and lack of spiritual peace (Cosentino et al., 2020).

SPIRITUAL VERSUS EMOTIONAL DIMENSION

Meeting the spiritual needs of clients through spiritual caring differs from providing emotional support. The **spiritual dimension** of a person gives insight into the meaning of life, suffering, and death. This dimension refers to the relationship of an individual with a higher power or sense of purpose in life. **Emotional needs** include how people respond and deal with feelings of joy, anger, sorrow, guilt, remorse, and love. The spiritual dimension of a client's life requires the same emphasis that other daily needs receive. When **spiritual needs** of clients are met, licensed practical nurses/licensed vocational nurses (LPNs/LVNs) can say they have cared for the total person.

IMPORTANCE OF SPIRITUAL CARE

Spiritual care involves helping clients develop an awareness of and improve the following:

- Inner strength
- Self-awareness
- Life's meaning and purpose
- Relationship to others
- Relationship to a higher power

Florence Nightingale, Mary Seacole, and Clara Barton, among others, have encouraged nurses to be instruments of **spiritual caring** in all situations. Nurses should avoid waiting for crisis situations to occur before they become concerned about spiritual care. The Joint Commission (TJC) requires that spirituality is assessed for all clients; however, TJC does not define exactly what should be included. TJC suggests questions such as the following when accessing spirituality (2022): "Who or what provides you strength and hope?" "How do you express your spirituality?" "What are your spiritual goals?" "What does suffering mean to you?" "Do you use prayer in your life?" "How does faith help you cope with illness?" "What type of spiritual/religious support do you desire?" Spiritual care is supported by organizations worldwide. As an LPN/LVN, you have the responsibility to ask these questions in providing spiritual care to clients and families.

> **Try This**
>
> Free Download of the FICA Spiritual Assessment Tool through The George Washington University Institute for Spirituality & Health (GWish). Dr. Christina Puchalski is the founder of the institute and author of this well-known tool that helps clinicians assess client spiritual histories and preferences (© Copyright Christina Puchalski, MD, 1996, updated 2025. All rights reserved. No excerpts, translations, or adaptations may be created without written permission).

PROVIDING SPIRITUAL CARE

WHO NEEDS SPIRITUAL CARE?

An individual's spiritual dimension can be a very personal area. Although all people have a spiritual dimension, needs that arise in this area depend on a variety of situations and the individual's ability to cope with them. An example of nurses who routinely recognize spiritual needs are nurses who work with clients in various church settings in a health ministry. The goal of these **parish nurses** is to integrate health and healing by treating the whole person: body, mind, and spirit within a faith community. Parish nurses recognize the relationship between spirituality and health and encourage spiritual growth in their clients. **Palliative care** and **hospice nurses** are often referred to as spiritual care generalists who focus care on being present, actively listening, assessing for spiritual concerns, and collaborating with clergy and spiritual leaders. This requires the nurse to be spiritually self-aware due to the significant exposure to client sadness, health crises, and trauma (Miller et al., 2023).

Crisis situations occur in all health care situations, but they especially arise in acute health care. Clients' beliefs and values can profoundly affect their response to these crises, their attitude toward treatment, and their rate of recovery or peace with their prognosis. Be alert to the following client situations that may intensify the need for spiritual care for clients and families:

- Hospitalization
- Clients who are in pain
- Clients who have a chronic or incurable disease
- Clients who are dying

- Families who have experienced the death of a loved one
- Clients who are facing an undesirable outcome of illness, such as an amputation
- Clients who have significant emotional needs during a crisis

Cosentino and Colleagues (2020) describe how nurses are perfectly positioned to provide spiritual care due to extensive direct client interaction. Clients may benefit from the efforts of nurses to meet spiritual needs, yet nurses are often inconsistent in initiating spiritual assessments and interventions. A detriment to spiritual care is lack of spiritual care training. Even if a nurse feels uncomfortable, spiritual care is part of holistic nursing care, and neglect of this area prevents a client's full manifestation of their spiritual being. Training, beginning in nursing school and continued in practice, is important in building confidence for providing unbiased, client-centered care.

GATHERING DATA FOR SPIRITUAL ISSUES

The first step to providing spiritual care for clients is to strive to become more comfortable with spiritual matters and more aware of your own spirituality and purpose in life. Gather data about your spiritual self. The exercise in "Try This: Your Personal Spirituality" box can help expand your awareness of your own spirituality.

Try This

Your Personal Spirituality

1. How do you cope?
2. Who is your source of support?
3. Who are the significant people in your life?
4. With whom do you laugh?
5. Do you feel loved?
6. Do you have someone with whom to cry?
7. What gives your life meaning?
8. What brings joy to your life?
9. Do you believe in the power of prayer?
10. What are your beliefs about a higher power?
11. Do you have a relationship to a higher power?
12. Do you have a religious affiliation? If so, how do your religious beliefs affect your spirit?
13. What is your philosophy about life and death?

Critical Thinking

My Spiritual Sensitivity

1. Have you ever said or heard others say, "My spirit is broken"? What does this remark mean to you? Talk to a peer and discuss similarities and dissimilarities.
2. How would you respond if a client states that their health issues or pain are punishment from God or a higher power? Where would you begin? With whom would you suggest a consult?
3. What would you say to a client who states they have lost all hope? What concerns would you have for this client?

MEETING THE SPIRITUAL NEEDS OF CLIENTS AND THEIR FAMILIES

Once you know your spiritual self, you will be better able to help others meet their spiritual needs. Nurses have spiritual care needs that stem from both personal and professional experiences. Reflecting on the suffering and pain in the world and in the work setting often affects one's own spirituality and the spiritual care or lack thereof to clients. Taking time for self-care, self-compassion, and strengthening your own spiritual life is an essential part of preventing burnout and providing holistic client care. This care includes mindful, **intentional presence** for clients and practicing **compassion**. Practicing compassion goes beyond empathy and includes deliberate action to minimize suffering (Harris and Tao, 2022; Miller et al., 2023). These actions may include therapeutic listening, silent presence, respectful care, kindness, prayer, assessing spiritual needs, recognizing concerns, and being available (Lukovsky et al., 2021). There are other ways to provide spiritual care and practice compassion. Take some time and be intentional to clients, families, and yourself. The questions in the "Your Personal Spirituality" box can also be used to gather data for clients' spiritual condition. Respect for the belief system of clients and families can give strength, hope, and meaning to their lives. When working with clients and families, try to do the following:

- Ask questions to help clients and families verbalize beliefs, fears, and concerns, such as "What do you think is going to happen to you (your father/mother)?" and "Who is your source of support?"
- Show interest and kindness through supportive statements (see Chapter 8).
- Listen with an understanding attitude. Be sure your body language and affective response reflect what you are saying.
- Respond as naturally to spiritual concerns as you do to physical needs.
- Help clients cope with the reality of a terminal illness without abandoning hope.
- Encourage the client's active involvement in self-care, which can help uphold hope.
- Allow families to participate in caregiving (e.g., offering fluids/ice chips, when allowed; wiping the client's brow).
- Avoid false assurances such as "Everything will be okay."
- When a client faces death, you can help make the remaining days meaningful by attending to needs, respecting their beliefs and death practices, and approaching the client in a supportive and empathetic manner. Feeling cared for helps bring peace to the dying.

Box 11.1 lists spiritual care interventions that can be used by LP/LV nurses.

Box 11.1 Spiritual Care Interventions

- Ask open-ended questions.
- Actively listen to the client. Sit beside the client. Make eye contact as appropriate.
- Expect to learn from clients.
- Be nonjudgmental of clients and their responses.
- Don't give advice or a lecture to the client.
- Avoid being a proselytizer (i.e., a person who tries to convert another person to one's religion).
- Be aware of nonverbal messages from the client.
- Understand the feelings of the client, but avoid adopting those feelings for yourself. (See Chapter 8 for a discussion of sympathy vs. empathy.) Stay with the client after the person has received an unfavorable diagnosis.
- When clients request help with prayer, offer to pray with them or find someone who will pray with them if uncomfortable.
- When a client requests help with specific readings, offer to read to him or her.
- Help the client participate in desired religious/spiritual rituals.
- Protect the client's religious/spiritual articles.

PASTORAL CARE TEAM

The **pastoral care team** is made up of ministers, priests, rabbis, consecrated religious women (i.e., nuns/sisters), representatives of other religious and spiritual organizations, and laypersons. All are educated to meet spiritual needs, in addition to religious needs, in a health care setting. The members of this team are allies with nurses in providing spiritual care. You can notify this team if a client requests a visit. When members of the pastoral care team come to the unit to fill the request, inform them of the client's background and condition. Describe the interventions you have incorporated into the client's care to provide spiritual care. Remember that the pastoral care team does not relieve you of your responsibility to provide spiritual care.

By visiting, talking, and listening, the pastoral care team explores the clients' fears, hopes, and sources of strength. Because of federal privacy standards (see the Health Insurance Portability and Accountability Act [HIPAA] in Chapter 7), the health care facility may not make a client's name available to church representatives without the client's permission. Before being hospitalized/admitted, clients can personally notify their spiritual leader regarding a planned hospitalization and desire for a visit. If an admitted client requests a visit of personal spiritual leader, follow the facility directive for arranging this request. Agency policies vary.

HOW CLIENTS MEET SPIRITUAL NEEDS

CLIENTS' SPIRITUAL PRACTICES

Regardless of religious beliefs, or lack of them, *all* clients have a spiritual self. They also have spiritual needs and personal spiritual practices to meet those needs. Spiritual practices help individuals develop an awareness of self, an understanding of the meaning and purpose of life, and an appreciation of their relationship to a higher power. Examples of personal spiritual practices may include gardening, reading inspirational books, listening to music, meditating, watching select TV shows and movies, communing with nature, walking, practicing breathing techniques, enjoying art, enjoying fresh flowers, volunteering, expressing gratitude, counting blessings, talking with friends, relatives, and loved ones, and participating in crafts and hobbies.

Try This

My Spiritual Practices

Identify the spiritual practices that you use to meet your spiritual needs.

RELIGION AND THE CLIENT

The religious self refers to the specific beliefs an individual holds regarding a higher power. Some clients help meet their spiritual needs through a religious faith or denomination. A **religious denomination** is an organized group of people who share a philosophy that supports their concept of God or a higher power, as well as worship practices and experiences.

People who are agnostics hold the belief that the existence of God can be neither proved nor disproved. **People who are atheists** do not believe that a higher power exists. People who are Christian, for example, may find comfort and solace in their refuge in God, including passing into another life after death. The person who is an atheist may not have this belief. It may be difficult for the nurse who believes in a higher power to relate to a person who does not or for the nurse who does not believe in a higher power relate to the fervent faith of a client. The spiritual aspect, however, is present in all individuals. Spiritual assessment and interventions are appropriate for all clients. Encourage all clients to express personal feelings about life, death, separation, and loss.

Professional Pointer

Avoid imposing your personal beliefs and values on the client. Reexamine your own beliefs regularly. Knowing your own personal beliefs is critical to providing unbiased spiritually focused care.

VALUE OF RITUALS AND PRACTICES

The different rituals and practices of a religious faith are stabilizing forces for the client. **Rituals** in certain faith settings are a series of actions that have religious meaning. They can bring the security of the past into a present crisis. Concrete symbols such as pictures, icons, herb packets, rosaries, statues, jewelry, religious texts, and other objects can affirm the client's connection with a higher power or purpose.

The value of clients' rituals and religious practices is determined by their faith. Value is not determined by scientific proof of their benefit. As an LPN/LVN, you need to develop an awareness of the general religious philosophy of the client's belief system. If membership is claimed in a specific denomination, question the client about the rituals and exercises that the client believes in and practices. **Moral distress** can be observed in clients who are unable to practice their religious rituals or who experience a conflict between their religious and spiritual beliefs and the prescribed health regimen (e.g., a client who is Jehovah's Witness and had a hemorrhage and is encouraged to accept a blood transfusion; this client may or may not struggle with moral distress depending on how the faith is practiced).

THE CLIENT AND PRAYER

Prayer is a spiritual practice of some individuals. They may be members of a faith-based religious organization or may be unaffiliated. Prayer can put a client in touch with a higher power. Sometimes prayer can decrease anxiety as effectively as medication. Prayer helps some clients cope with their illness or situation. Honor the request of the client who wants to pray privately. If the client requests prayer, the nurse needs to support the client by being present or seeking assistance in this matter. When clients express an interest in praying, ask what prayer they would like to say. Try to accommodate the request.

In her book Spiritual Dimensions of Nursing Practice (1989), Carson comments on conversational prayer, one of the many forms that prayer can take. In this type of prayer, the specific concerns and needs of the client are included in the prayer. Carson provides the following interaction between a client awaiting a cesarean section and a nurse who noticed the client had been crying. It is an excellent example of the simplicity and effectiveness of conversational prayer that you can use as a guide if comfortable. If you are not comfortable, find someone who is or consult the pastoral care team.

Nurse: You have been crying. What's wrong?

Client: I wanted to see my minister this morning, but they will not be able to get here before my surgery. I wanted them to pray for me and my baby.

Nurse: Well, I'd be happy to pray for you and the baby. Would that be okay?

Client: Oh, yes, would you please? This surgery really scares me.

Nurse: Dear God, please comfort this parent as they enter surgery. Lift her fear, and in its place give her peace and strength. Let her know that you are with her and the baby.

Client: Thanks so much. That really means a lot to me.

THE RELIGIOUS AMERICAN

Try This

Investigate three religious faiths from the following list with which you are not familiar. Identify ways to incorporate this information into your spiritual care toolbox. Examples of religious faiths in America include Hindu, Judaism, Buddhism, Islam, Lutheran (Evangelical Lutheran Church in America, Wisconsin Synod, Missouri Synod, and English Synod), Catholic (Roman Rite, Eastern Rite as Ukrainian Catholic, and Greek Catholic), Eastern Orthodox (Russian Orthodox and Greek Orthodox), Religious Society of Friends (Quaker), Presbyterian, Methodist, Church of Christ, Amish, Mennonite, Seventh-Day Adventist, Assembly of God, Brethren in Christ, United Brethren, Church of the Brethren, Christian & Missionary Alliance, Church of Latter Day Saints, Baptist (Independent, National, Progressive National, Southern Baptist Convention, and German Baptist), Pentecostal, Unitarian, Wiccan, Jehovah's Witness, Episcopalian, African Methodist Episcopalian, Christian Methodist Episcopalian, Christian Science, United Church of Christ, Moravian, Evangelical, Salvation Army, and nondenominational. This is not an exhaustive list. Take time to research and familiarize yourself with other faiths as well.

The First Amendment of the US Constitution allows the free exercise of religious choice. America has a long history of religious freedom and tolerance. The United States is religiously diverse.

RELIGION IN THE UNITED STATES AND WORLD

There are 372 faith groups and over 350,000 congregations in the United States (U.S. Religion Census, 2020). Thus as an LPN/LVN it will be impossible to know the key beliefs of each of these entities. Christians represent 29.72% of the world population, followed by Muslims at 24.41%, unaffiliated at 16.88%, Hindus 14.17%, and Buddhists at 6.21% (World Statistics, 2025). Globally, a fifth or more adults are switching from the religious faith of their upbringing to another faith or to nothing, also known as unaffiliated (PEW Research Center, 2025). Although rare in countries like Israel and India, in North and South American, Western Europe, and East Asia switching faiths is more common (PEW Research Center, 2025). Around 62% of the US population identify as Christian; however, the percentage of religiously unaffiliated, also referred to as the "nones," has nearly doubled since 2007. The "nones" include persons who identify as atheists, agnostics, or those who identify as "nothing in particular" (PEW Research Center, 2025).

In the United States, 23% of Christians identify as Evangelical Protestant with the majority being Baptist (8%). Catholics make up 19% of Christians, whereas 11% of Christians are considered mainline Protestant. Methodists are the largest group of mainline Protestants at 3% (Pew Research Center, 2025).

AVOIDING FALSE ASSUMPTIONS AND STEREOTYPES

The suggestions presented in Chapter 10 regarding the avoidance of false assumptions and stereotyping when caring for culturally diverse clients also apply when caring for clients of different religions. Some nursing students may find a guidebook that supplies nursing interventions when caring for clients who belong to different religions. However, as with different cultures, this type of approach can lead to false assumptions and stereotyping. Not only is there diversity among religious groups, but there is also diversity among members of a specific religion or group.

It is a false assumption to expect that all individuals of a specific religion or belief system will believe exactly the same just because they are members of that religion or belief system. Avoid assuming that all Protestants, Catholics, Jews, Muslims, Buddhists, and Hindus, for example, believe in and follow all the aspects of their formal religion/belief system. *Individual differences occur in every religious or belief systems group*. Members may have modified the degree to which they observe the practices of their religion or belief system based on age, experience, education, socioeconomic, and social group. Avoid judging clients if their religious beliefs do not conform to the traditional ones for that religion. Data must be gathered about each client's specific beliefs and religious practices.

Each religion has specific beliefs and practices. Sometimes an individual will adapt them to fit their own circumstances. Clarify with the client the specific beliefs and practices that offer comfort to them and that they prefer. Develop an awareness of health issues and decisions that may involve religious or philosophical beliefs.

Get Ready for the Next-Generation NCLEX® Examination

Key Points

- The practical/vocational nurse has a responsibility to care for the total person, including their physical, emotional, and spiritual needs.
- Spiritual needs of clients arise from their desire to find meaning in life, suffering, and death.
- Gathering data about spiritual needs and providing spiritual care are routine parts of all clients' care, not only in times of crisis.
- To meet the spiritual needs of clients, you need to be aware of the client's personal spiritual beliefs.
- Members of the health care team who assist the LPN/LVN in providing spiritual care to clients are the minister, priest, rabbi, chaplain, the pastoral care team, and other representatives of religions, groups, and philosophies.
- Many clients meet their spiritual needs by participating in an organized religion.
- Spirituality is highly variable among individuals and may or may not include a religious faith.
- Moral distress can occur when clients cannot fulfill the rituals and practices of their religion/beliefs or when they experience conflict between their spiritual beliefs and their health regimen.
- LPNs/LVNs need to develop an awareness of religious differences and an understanding of the basic beliefs, rituals, and practices of the many religious denominations, groups, and philosophies that exist today. But, be aware to avoid stereotyping.
- Avoid assuming that clients who belong to a specific religion or belief system adopt all the beliefs and practices of that religion or belief system.
- Clarify personal spiritual and religious beliefs and practices for all clients.

Additional Learning Resources

Go to your Evolve website (http://evolve.elsevier.com/Carroll/success/) for the following FREE learning resources:

- Answers to Critical Thinking Review Scenarios
- Additional learning activities
- Additional Review Questions for the NCLEX-PN® examination
- Helpful phrases for communicating in Spanish and more!

Clinical Judgment and Next-Generation NCLEX® Examination-Style Questions

1. The nurse has identified the need to engage a pastoral care team in the care of a client. Which statement describes the role of the pastoral care team?

a. The pastoral care team is the social services department in acute care facilities and extended care.
b. The pastoral care team works with the nursing staff to help meet the spiritual and religious needs of clients.
c. Religious care and spiritual support are offered by pastoral care only to seriously ill and dying clients by the pastoral care department.
d. The pastoral care team is only needed for the discharge planning of the client.

2. The nurse is caring for a client prior to surgery, and the client requests to receive a special blessing/prayer prior to surgery from a spiritual leader. What is the LPN's/LVN's appropriate response?

a. Reassure the client they are not going to die.
b. Notify the client's family that their condition has changed.

c. Call the client's health care provider to report a change in mental status.
d. Notify the pastoral care team and/or the client's spiritual advisor of their request.

3. An LPN/LVN and nursing assistant are bathing a client in a long-term care facility that has a terminal illness. The client looks at the nurse and says, "I am afraid to die because I don't know what will happen to me afterward." Identify which LPN/LVN responses are appropriate versus inappropriate or the LPN/LVN.

RESPONSE	APPROPRIATE	INAPPROPRIATE
Tells the client that everything is going to be OK		
Asks the client if they would like to meet with the pastoral team or their spiritual advisor		
Hugs the client and tells them they are safe.		
Asks the client if they would like to discuss their feelings		
Stays with the client after the bath and recites a prayer that he or she knows		

Critical Thinking Scenarios

Scenario 1

What faith groups are frequently seen in your community? Discuss how you would avoid stereotyping and making false assumptions about a client who is dying.

Scenario 2

An older adult client in a long-term care facility appears sad every Sunday morning. There are no religious or spiritual services offered at this facility on Sunday, and the client verbalizes that they miss attending. The client sits in their room quietly and refuses to join their friends for breakfast. Discuss what steps you could initiate.

The Role of the Nurse: Implementation of the Nursing Process and the NCSBN Clinical Judgment Measurement Model

12

Objectives

On completing this chapter, you will be able to do the following:

1. Describe the steps of the nursing process, including the role of the licensed practical nurse/licensed vocational nurse (LPN/LVN) in each step.
2. Differentiate between The NCSBN Clinical Judgment Measurement Model and the Nurse Process.
3. Discuss how an LPN/LVN could apply The NCSBN Clinical Judgment Measurement Model to develop clinical judgment.

Key Terms

analysis
assisting
data collection
dependent role
desired client outcome
evaluation
goals
implementation
independent role
interdependent
intervention
NCSBN Clinical Judgment Measurement Model
nursing diagnosis
nursing interventions
nursing process
objective information
outcome
planning
subjective information
taxonomy
validate information

Several students are debating about the licensed practical nurse/licensed vocational nurse (LPN/LVN) role in the nursing process, particularly regarding assessment. One student says, "Of course LPNs/LVNs can assess the client. They could never plan care and evaluate the client without assessing the client." However, another student reminds them, "The LPN/LVN could collaborate with the registered nurse during the assessment and then continue to develop the plan." A third student, overhearing the conversation, states, "Let's be real. I work in a long-term care facility on the weekends. If the LPN/LVN is not able to assess the resident, no one would assess the resident. It is not realistic because of the low number of registered nurses working in long-term care facilities." One student concludes, "Maybe that is happening; however, LPNs/LVNs need to be sure they are working within their scope of practice (a term used that usually refers to the Nurse Practice Act). Each state's Nurse Practice Act has different regulations. Generally, there are some restrictions on assessment, particularly the initial assessment. Therefore the LPN/LVN needs to collaborate with the registered nurse as indicated. This results in safe, high-quality client care."

As you learn about the nursing process and The NCSBN Clinical Judgment Measurement Model, think of this dialogue. How will you prepare for this issue as a new graduate?

> **Keep in Mind**
>
> The **nursing process** and the National Council of State Boards of Nursing **(NCSBN) Clinical Judgment Measurement Model** provide a common strand that unites all nurses in their delivery of relationship-centered care, at the individual, family, and population levels. They provide a process for nurses to communicate with each other for identification of what the nurse will do to safely help the client reach their desired outcomes. They promote the continuity of safe, relationship-centered care.

Understanding the nurse's role in providing system-based health care is essential. Nurses must provide client-centered care that is safe and not harmful. To do this, nurses must develop skills beyond a strong knowledge base. Knowing basic principles in how to care for an individual with a particular medical condition is valuable, but applying that information to a unique client requires the nurse to think, plan, act, and evaluate with strong clinical judgment. Various tools provide all nurses with strategies for developing critical thinking and clinical judgment. Two tools that will be discussed in this chapter are the nursing process and The NCSBN Clinical Judgment Measurement Model.

Some of the tasks and skills performed by nurses (LPNs/LVNs and registered nurses [RNs]) can be completed by assistive personnel (AP). It is the LPN's/LVN's ability to critically think by utilizing the nursing process and The NCSBN Clinical Judgment Measurement Model that separates the LPNs/LVNs from the AP. These distinctions make LPNs/LVNs a strong member of the health care team. The LPN/LVN today uses critical thinking to develop clinical judgment, by using the nursing process and The NCSBN Clinical Judgment Measurement Model, to carefully identify client needs, health issues, expectations, and risks involved through focused thinking.

LPNs/LVNs also use these same skills to identify wellness strategies in the community aimed at improving the community's health. Judgments are based on evidence rather than assumptions and minimal training. The LPN/LVN thinks before acting and collaborates with the RN, who uses the nursing process and The NCSBN Clinical Judgment Measurement Model at a higher skill level based on education and makes final decisions on nursing diagnoses and the creation and application of client care plans. The LPN/LVN is both a "doer" and, more importantly, a "thinker."

THE NURSING PROCESS

Try This

The Nurse Practice Act

Using the internet, review the Nurse Practice Act (NPA) in your state, territory, or country. Your role in the nursing process and The NCSBN Clinical Judgment Measurement Model is dictated by this law. As you read the law/regulations, discuss with a peer any areas of your state regulation that are not clear. Seek assistance from your instructor as needed. There are variations within the states, territories, and countries. The NPA defines your scope of nursing practice. It is your legal responsibility to know and practice within that scope.

In 2002, the National Council of the State Boards of Nursing (NCSBN) integrated the nursing process into all areas of the National Council Licensure Examination for Licensed Practical Nurses (NCLEX-PN®). By doing so, the council validated the significance of the nursing process and critical thinking for LPNs/LVNs to do their work in nursing. The nursing process remains integrated throughout the clients' needs categories and subcategories in the 2023 NCLEX-PN® detailed test plan, which now includes The NCSBN Clinical Judgment Measurement Model. This discussion will continue by focusing on the nursing process and will follow, later in the chapter, on The NCSBN Clinical Judgment Measurement Model. The NCSBN recognizes that LPNs/LVNs must utilize the nursing process, also called a clinical problem-solving process, "to collect and organize relevant health care data, assist in the identification of the health needs/problems throughout the client's life span and contribute to the interdisciplinary team in a variety of settings (NCSBN, 2023, p. 3).

The nursing process for the LPN/LVN, under the supervision of an RN, consists of the following (NCSBN, 2025):

- **Data collection** (assessment) is a systematic gathering and review of information about the client; abnormal findings are communicated to appropriate members of the health team.
- **Analysis** is a process of **assisting** the RN in determining if the abnormal findings connect with the medical condition of the client.
- **Planning** involves assisting the RN in the development of nursing diagnosis, **goals**, and interventions for a client's plan of care while maintaining client safety.
- **Implementation** is the provision of required nursing **intervention** to accomplish established client goals.
- **Evaluation** compares each actual client **outcome** with the expected outcomes, which are then communicated to members of the health care team.

There are differences between the role of the LPN/LVN and the RN regarding the nursing process. Governed by the state's Nurse Practice Act (NPA), the LPN's/LVN's role in the nursing process can be limited. The LPN/LVN acts in a more **dependent role** when participating in the planning, analysis, and evaluation phase of the nursing process but acts in a more **independent role** when participating in the ongoing data collection (assessment) and implementation phases of the nursing process. However, LPNs/LVNs always work collaboratively with the RN or health care provider. Because RNs are taught in-depth assessment skills as part of their basic education, their skills include client interview and physical assessment of all body systems. LPNs/LVNs continually gather data about the client, family, environment, and the community (when indicated) by taking vital signs, checking therapeutic responses to medications and treatments, and collecting data on symptoms of health problems, among other functions. The RN and LPN/LVN function in an **interdependent** manner as they work together to provide care for clients.

STEP 1: DATA COLLECTION

Data collection begins with admission and continues with each client encounter. The client is the primary source of information in data collection. After all, clients know themselves and their body better than anyone else. All interview questions should be directed to the client unless he or she is unable to respond. The RN interviews the client to obtain the health history and assesses body systems. The LPN/LVN assists in the assessment process by collaborating with the RN.

- **Subjective information** is based on the client's opinion and what the client says. Some refer to subjective information as *symptoms*. This usually includes information obtained based on the client's responses, such as feelings of physical discomfort, anxiety, and mental stress that are more difficult to measure. The nurse cannot experience or objectively measure subjective symptoms. Subjective information will be charted as "Client states . . . ."

- **Objective information** includes data that the nurse can verify; it is also known as *signs*. A physical assessment provides objective data. The terms *check*, *observe*, *monitor*, *weigh*, *measure*, *smell*, *touch*, and *hear* provide cues for objective data collection. Obtaining some initial data, such as vital signs, height, and weight, may be assigned to the LPN/LVN. Objective information helps support or cast doubt on subjective information. For example, a client's subjective statement about feeling feverish (subjective) can be verified by measuring their temperature (objective). Objective information, such as temperature, pulse, respiration, blood pressure, weight, and skin color, will be charted as what is observed and measured without judging or drawing conclusions. Florence Nightingale said that if you do not observe your client, you should not be a nurse (Nightingale, 2009). The LPN/LVN is always collecting data on therapeutic responses to treatments, interventions, and medications (Box 12.1). With each contact, the LPN/LVN must see, hear, smell, and touch the client when necessary, using all the senses to gather data about the client and the environment. Continual data collection is vital because the client's condition may change throughout the day. This is why accuracy in measuring vital signs; describing vomitus, bleeding, or skin lesions; and determining level of consciousness are so important. For example, has the client's skin lesion changed since the last time the nurse checked the lesion? How has it changed? How much has it changed? Did the nurse use objective assessment skills (i.e., measuring the lesion)? Every piece of data is important to assist the client in achieving the best possible health outcome.

Box 12.1 Examples of Practical/Vocational Nurse Data Collection

These examples can apply to acute care, long-term care, or community-based care:

- Observing for results of medication or treatment administration (i.e., laxative, enema)
- Observing for signs of congestive heart failure for a client taking furosemide (Lasix) and digoxin (Lanoxin)
- Observing an ulcer on the lower leg of a diabetic (i.e., size by measuring, location, appearance, drainage)
- Observing behavior for signs of disorientation or confusion
- Observing the client self-administering insulin following a teaching demonstration
- Observing the client's position in bed (acute care)
- Observing gait and posture (community care)
- Observing whether a 76-year-old client is showing signs of ego integrity or despair (Although the client should be at ego integrity, the client is not capable of being there. Because of a cerebrovascular accident [CVA], the client must be washed, fed, and lifted everywhere. The client is also incontinent. The client's needs remind the nurse of those of an infant. The nurse will work at establishing trust in the client instead of ego integrity.)
- Observing family interactions
- Observing the environment for need for safety factors: spills, bed rails, glasses on table, hearing aids, dentures, and so on
- Observing the client's urine for color, odor, amount, and other characteristics

Chapter 8 elaborates on communication techniques that will assist student practical nurses/student vocational nurses (SPNs/SVNs) in making the best use of the limited time available for obtaining needed data from a client.

SPNs/SVNs should keep in mind that barriers exist that may hinder data collection, such as insufficient time, cultural differences, poor skills in data collection, personal bias by the nurse, and communication failure (i.e., situations that involve a comatose client, a client who presents with a language barrier, the presence of distractions, or a client who is too sick to speak well.)

STEP 2: ANALYSIS

Analyzing information is an important step in the nursing process for nurses to **validate information**. LPNs/LVNs should determine if the data collected make sense. Could the findings be inaccurate? Should the vital signs be retaken? Do the collected findings match the client's clinical situation? Should the abnormal findings be reported to an RN or a provider, or are the abnormal findings expected, according to the client's condition and progress? Consider differentiating between subjective and objective data. Remember that decisions must be based on evidence, not assumptions. The client's subjective comments are important. Confirm with evidence, whenever possible. Clients can express a subjective feeling (i.e., "a feeling of doom") before a change in vital signs. Nurses should continue to monitor the client when subjective comments do not match objective data. LPNs/LVNs should compare the findings with the RN and other staff involved with the client, as well as the medical record. SPNs/SVNs should ask their instructor or an RN for guidance on how to analyze the clinical findings to advance personal analytical skills.

STEP 3: PLANNING

Planning includes assisting the RN to develop *nursing diagnoses*, *client outcomes*, and *nursing interventions*. A nursing care plan is typically the tool used to show the plan of care. The focus is on client functions that will benefit from nursing interventions. After the problems are identified and organized, the RN selects appropriate nursing diagnoses. The LPN/LVN and the RN collaborate to create the plan of care.

There are different types of care plans available in the clinical setting:

- *Individualized written care plans* are created uniquely for each client (see Table 12.1).
- *Standardized care plans* are based on research of the best possible options for a nursing diagnosis (nursing problem) and applied to a variety of clients. To individualize a standard plan, the nurse will cross out interventions that do not apply to the client and add appropriate interventions that do apply.

Table 12.1 Nursing Diagnosis, Nursing Problem, Outcome, and Interventions

NURSING DIAGNOSIS	NURSING PROBLEM	OUTCOME
Altered nutrition: eating less than the body needs.	Eats only 5% of each meal related to loss of appetite and weakness.	The client will eat 1500 calories of ground foods and drink 2000 mL of liquids during each 24-hour period. (The problem is reversed and stated positively.)
Interventions		
1. Six small, ground meals at 8 am, 10 am, noon, 2 pm, 4 pm, and 6 pm. Client seated in an easy chair with minimal assistance. Encourage self-feeding. Assist only if needed.		
2. Offer 240 mL of liquids at 6 am, 9 am, 11 am, 1 pm, 3 pm, 5 pm, 7 pm, and 9 pm. Vary choices: likes Jell-O, ice cream, 7-Up, chocolate milk, and pineapple juice. Drinks herbal tea with meals.		

- *Computerized care plans* are generally part of the electronic medical record. Individualized plans can be entered into the computer.
- *Multidisciplinary (collaborative) care plans* work well in settings in which staff from varied professions and disciplines are involved with the care of the client. This is true in many settings today as interdisciplinary care is an expectation, such as in a long-term care, psychiatric setting, or medical-surgical unit. Plans are developed by a multidisciplinary team and reflect specific interventions used by each discipline (e.g., physical therapist, social worker, nutritionist, nurse, and health care provider). Progress is usually documented on a common document to provide easy access for all involved with the plan.
- A *clinical pathway* is another type of multidisciplinary plan that schedules clinical interventions over an anticipated time for a specific type of client health problem. The clinical pathway is frequently used for high-risk, high-volume, high-cost care. Often, care is documented right onto the clinical pathway.

A *concept map*, as another type of care plan, is a diagram of a client's condition and treatments. Concept maps can be used to plan care for clients and are increasingly employed in all types of nursing education programs. Concept maps may be valuable for planning interventions and monitoring client progress. From a student perspective, concept maps encourage critical thinking and can enhance learning. See Fig. 12.1 for an example of a concept map of caring for a client with chronic cancer pain.

Try This

Assisting With Planning

In the planning phase, the SPN/SVN takes the nursing diagnosis and states it as a nursing problem with which the client presented. SPNs/SVNs state the problem, set outcomes, list interventions, and then list data collection for care plans. This process seems to be the opposite of the RN's process, but remember that LPNs/LVNs do not have the initial responsibility for data collection (step 1). The SPN/SVN does not study North American Nursing Diagnosis Association International (NANDA-I) lists in most nursing programs and relies on the RN for the final nursing diagnosis. To demonstrate understanding of the nursing diagnosis, the LPN/LVN states the nursing diagnosis in objective and specific terms as a nursing problem in the client's care plan (Table 12.2).

Nursing Diagnosis

RNs will identify the client's **nursing diagnosis** or list of problems, which provides a basis for the creation of the client's plan of care. The RN uses an established list of current nursing diagnoses developed by NANDA-I (Visit www.nanda.org for details). NANDA-I was developed as a standardized, orderly, systematic language (**taxonomy**) that would provide a common language for nurses to communicate with one another. In LPN/LVN programs, students may create client care plans using a problem list in lieu of the approved nursing diagnosis list. In clinical, an instructor may ask students for their "top five." This is a method to assist students in identifying existing and emerging client problems in the clinical setting and assist them in learning to prioritize. Nurses often use Maslow's hierarchy of needs (see Chapter 13) to assist in prioritizing client needs. Keep in mind that some health care settings are starting to move away from NANDA-I-approved nursing diagnoses and use problem lists instead.

Critical Thinking

The Seven Survival Needs

Write an example of a problem for each survival need.

1. Food
2. Air
3. Water
4. Temperature
5. Elimination
6. Rest
7. Pain

Possible Answers

1. Not enough or too much food intake
2. Shortness of breath
3. Dehydration caused by vomiting
4. Temperature above or below normal
5. Diarrhea
6. Sleeping too much or too little
7. Pain that interferes with functioning

Client Outcomes

Client outcomes state a general intent on what could be accomplished. The focus of a client outcome should be on the client, not the nurse, and should begin with "the client will . . . ." It may be easier for an SPN/SVN to

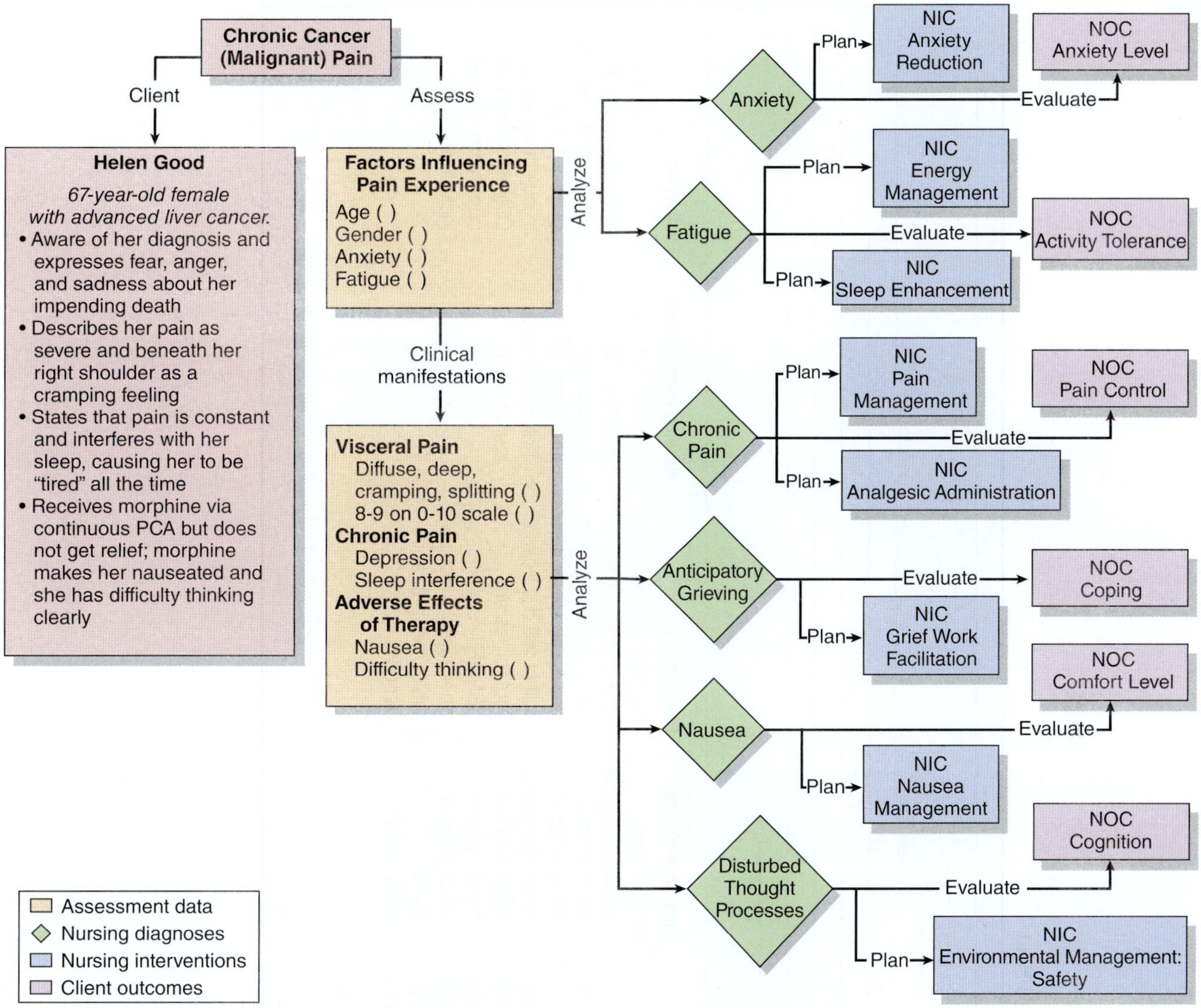

Fig. 12.1 Concept map of a client with chronic cancer pain.

use the phrase desired (or observable) client outcome. This focuses directly on what the client will accomplish rather than on what the nurse will do. A good strategy for developing appropriate client outcomes or goals would be to develop SMART goals, which have the following characteristics:

- Specific (clearly, precisely stated)
- Measurable (objective, able to be monitored)
- Achievable (realistic for the client)
- Relevant (focused on the client's problem)
- Timely (includes an estimated deadline for evaluation of the outcome)

To state an observable client outcome as a student, reverse the problem and state it in positive terms.

The statement tells what the client **will** do to overcome the problem rather than what the client will **not** do. Here are some examples:

- Observable outcome: The client will eat 1500 calories of ground foods and liquids during each 24-hour period.
- Unclear statement: The client will not miss any feeding during a 24-hour period.

The client and the client's family are important partners in attaining outcomes. Building on client and family strengths provides a sense of contribution and some control for the client and family.

Nursing Interventions

Nursing interventions identify specifically what the nurse will do to assist the client in reaching the **desired client outcomes**.

- Sometimes this means encouraging the client to do certain activities, such as self-feeding.
- Interventions are also called *nursing approach*, *nursing action*, or *nursing care*.
- When nursing interventions are clearly written, all nursing staff members, according to their skill level and if within their legal role, will be able to carry out the nursing action. *It needs to be identified on the care plan if the RN, LPN/LVN, or AP will carry out the intervention.*
- Nursing interventions should be evaluated: Are they objective and specific as written? Interventions that SPNs/SVNs will develop in their care plans are

Table 12.2 Example of a Student Assignment Sheet and Client Care Plan

Student__________
Client Initials__________ Room__________
Health Care Provider__________ Allergies__________
Age__________ Marital Status__________ Religion__________ Occupation__________
Admission Date__________
Date of Surgery__________ Diet__________
MedicalDiagnosis__________
Meaning in Own Words__________
Surgical Procedure__________
Meaning in Own Words__________
Primary Nursing Problem__________

Categories of Human Function	Data collection	Nursing problems	Outcomes	Nursing intervention	Evaluation
Protective (e.g., personal care and hygiene, environment, surgery) Sensory-perceptual Comfort, rest, activity, and mobility (e.g., sleep and rest, body alignment) Nutrition Growth and development (e.g., identify Erikson developmental stage) Fluid-gas transport Psychosocial cultural (e.g., emotional support, spiritual support, diversion, and recreation) Elimination (e.g., urinary and gastrointestinal elimination) Need for community resources	You will: Check, observe, monitor, weigh, and measure. Collect data (1) at beginning of shift for baseline, aligned with NPA and institutional policy. (2) periodically during shift, and (3) right before reporting off duty.	What is the problem, in your own words? Be specific and objective. May use nursing diagnosis as confirmed by RN assessment.	The client will: (Reverse the problem and state positively what health care provider client will do. Ensure outcomes are (SMART) specific, measurable, achievable, relevant, and timely).	The nurse will: (Be objective and specific. What will the nurse do to help client meet outcomes?)	What progress is client making toward outcomes? Results of data collection in objective terms. Clients' subjective comments can be included.

NPA, Nurse Practice Act; *RN*, registered nurse.

based on courses taken, additional reading, collaboration with the health care team, and information from alternate sources.

- Developing interventions require critical thinking and collaboration. (See Chapter 2 for information on academic resources.)

Keep in mind that the intervention needs to support the client's ability to meet the desired client outcomes.

STEP 4: IMPLEMENTATION

When *implementing* nursing interventions, LPNs/LVNs need to refer to the nursing care plan to provide safe care. By continually evaluating the data collected as care continues, LPNs/LVNs critically think and remain appropriate with nursing interventions. LPNs/LVNs need to follow the institution's policies and procedures when performing nursing skills in the clinical setting, reviewing them before providing care, if needed. Client teaching before giving care could ease a client's anxiety and promote cooperation during an intervention.

LPNs/LVNs should reinforce teaching of principles, procedures, and techniques for maintenance and promotion of health. For example, if the client has been newly diagnosed with diabetes mellitus type 2, the LPN/LVN can reinforce foot care that the RN taught earlier in the morning and continue to observe for any client knowledge deficit. The LPN/LVN should be alert to questions that the client has and seek answers to the questions, as needed. SPNs/SVNs should consult their instructor when they are unsure of client teaching or procedures.

LPNs/LVNs should consider the following strategies to ensure client safety:

- Use safe and appropriate techniques during client care. For example, check the client's position before lifting the safety rails to ensure arms are not between the bed and the rail. Always survey the room for safety violations before leaving the client (i.e., bed in high position, call bell out of reach).
- Use precautionary and preventive interventions when providing care to clients. Make sure that wheelchair wheels and bed wheels are locked before moving the client from the chair to the bed and back again.
- Institute nursing interventions to compensate for adverse responses. If the client gets weak while standing, assist him or her to lie or sit down and, if sitting, place the client's head between his or her knees (if not contraindicated by physical condition). Ease the client to the floor if necessary to avoid injury from a fall.
- Initiate life-saving interventions for emergency situations. For example, if the client begins to choke on food, perform the Heimlich maneuver.
- Monitor care given by unlicensed personnel. The charge LPN/LVN is responsible for the care provided by the assistive personnel.
- Collect data during every client contact. Be alert to even minor changes in skin color, breathing, respirations, and so on, even if assisting with minor tasks.
- Collect further data when necessary. If nurses observe abnormal symptoms, then they should collect additional data. For example, if the client is beginning to perspire profusely for no apparent reason, measure their vital signs and obtain their blood sugar.
- Report observations to relevant members of the health team. Report urgent findings immediately to the RN. Report all daily observations before leaving the unit.
- Document the client's response to nursing intervention, therapy, or teaching. Document all interventions, responses, and changes. Use the care plan as a guide for documentation and reporting.

Try This

Implementing the Plan of Care

As an SPN/SVN, the next phase is implementing the plan of care that you have developed with your instructor's supervision. Did you remember to include the client strengths you identified during your data collection? *Which interventions are within the LPN/LVN role?*

STEP 5: EVALUATION

In the *evaluation* phase, LPNs/LVNs assist the RN in determining client progress based on client findings, using the following strategies.

- Collect data during every client contact. If the client outcome is written correctly and the data collection list is complete, evaluation will be the result of the daily data collection. The continual collection of data makes daily evaluation a part of the natural flow of good nursing care (Table 12.3).
- Compare actual outcomes with desired client outcomes. If progress is being made toward meeting the outcomes, continue the plan as is.
- Assist in determining the client's response to nursing care. If the client is not meeting the outcome, check the way the outcome is written. Is it specific, measurable, achievable, relevant, and timely (SMART)? If an outcome is difficult to evaluate, the

Table 12.3 Data Collection, Outcome, and Evaluation

DATA COLLECTION LIST	OUTCOME	EVALUATION
Check intake: Amount and type of liquid in milliliters Amount of food taken at each meal	The client will eat 1500 calories of chopped foods and drink 2000 mL of liquids during each 24-hour period	By day 2, the client was able to consume 1500 calories in ground meals and 1600 mL of liquids during a 24-hour period (Outcome was partially met)

outcome probably is not appropriate. If necessary, change the portion that needs revision, or restate the entire desired outcome.

- Assist in identifying factors that may interfere with the client's ability to implement the plan of care. Talk with the client to see if he or she can share, from his or her perspective, why progress is not being made. Review daily data collection notes for patterns that could emerge. Consider whether the client's strengths have been considered in the care plan. Are they stated as observable outcomes less than or beyond what the client can accomplish? Are they realistic/achievable? Is the focus on evaluating nursing care, as opposed to evaluating client progress toward meeting desired outcomes? If necessary, revise nursing interventions that are not working.
- Document the client's responses to care, therapy, or teaching.
- Report findings to relevant members of the health care team.

Consider how heavily dependent each step of the nursing process is on the others and how the steps are often occurring simultaneously. Although some desired outcomes are met, other problems may emerge. According to Maslow's hierarchy, regression may occur with illness. As observable outcomes are achieved at the lower level (when the client begins to improve), higher levels of needs begin to emerge. Be aware that the client may be functioning on more than one level. Continual communication with the client and their family will identify needs as they emerge and improve overall client outcomes.

Keep in Mind

Evaluating Client Progress

The time-referenced portion of the desired outcome states the approximate date by which the client will attain an observable outcome. It is an educated guess on the part of the RN, based on education, experience, and client input. The SPN/SVN makes an educated guess on the care plan assignment regarding the time it will take the client to meet his or her outcome. As an SPN/SVN, your daily data collection assists the interdisciplinary team in evaluating how far the client has progressed and identifies any difficulties. A complete daily data collection list is essential and, as pointed out, is the basis of the data collection during every client contact. Further assessment and analysis of that data in collaboration with the RN and other members of the interdisciplinary team result in revisions in the plan of care as indicated.

THE NCSBN CLINICAL JUDGMENT MEASUREMENT MODEL

The NCSBN continues to research the skills needed for novice nurses, RNs, and LPN/LVNs. Critical thinking is essential but not the only skill needed for new nurses of all levels. Clinical judgment is the ability to critically think and analyze situations but then take steps to provide safe, effective care, as needed. Clinical judgment and effective decision-making are essential for the nursing profession. National exams need to test knowledge as well as clinical judgment to promote public safety (Betts et al., 2019). In agreement, NCSBN determined that the NCLEX® needed new testing questions, Next-Generation NCLEX® (NGN) questions, to show a better measurement of clinical judgment among graduates to reduce errors made by novice nurses, RNs, and LPNs/LVNs. This brought a change of approach to nursing education. The NCSBN Clinical Judgment Measurement Model serves three purposes: it helps nursing students learn, educators teach, and NCSBN test clinical judgment processes. Empowering novice nurses with better decision-making skills on the first day of employment may reduce the rate of errors with client care.

THE NCSBN CLINICAL JUDGMENT MEASUREMENT MODEL EXPLAINED

See Fig. 19.1 for a diagram of The NCSBN Clinical Judgment Measurement Model. This may look overwhelming at first, but you will see that at the base of the model is the nursing process. This model supplements the established processes of nursing. As you look at the figure of the model, you will want to *start at the bottom and continue upward* to work through the process of how nurses effectively make appropriate clinical decisions for meeting client needs.

Nursing Process

Along the base of the figure, the nursing process is displayed. The nursing process, as described earlier in this chapter, is still the foundation for developing clinical judgment.

Layer 4

As you move up to Layer 4, you will see that nurses provide client-centered care, when nurses consider the environmental and individual factors that come into play with each client in providing effective care. There are examples provided, but this is not an exhaustive list within the figure. As LPNs/LVNs care for more clients, they will learn from the environmental and individual factors that influence client care.

Layer 3

This layer may be the most important layer in the figure to understand The NCSBN Clinical Judgment Measurement Model well. These steps, discussed later in this chapter under "More Details of Layer 3 in The NCSBN Clinical Judgment Measurement Model," advance as one moves from left to right across the figure and mirror the steps of the nursing process.

Layer 2

As the nurse works through the steps within Layer 3, the nurse will form hypotheses (educated guesses), redefine hypotheses, and evaluate outcomes. If the outcomes are unsatisfactory (goals are not met), the nurse continues to work through this process at this level.

Layer 1

If the outcomes are satisfactory (goals are met), then the process of clinical judgment is complete. The nurse has finished the cycle of critical thinking and decision-making to provide appropriate care.

Layer 0

Clinical decision-making has been successful, and the client's needs have been met by the nurse using clinical judgment.

MORE DETAILS OF LAYER 3 IN THE NCSBN CLINICAL JUDGMENT MEASUREMENT MODEL

Layer 3 provides a cognitive, practical approach for developing strong clinical judgment. The NCSBN focuses on this level with the new NCLEX® NGN questions (see Chapter 19 for more details). Nursing students need to understand the process of this layer to be successful in decision-making and to be competent in NCLEX® NGN questioning. To obtain clinical judgment skills cards to help learn this process, visit: https://www.nclex.com/clinical-judgment-measurement-model.page.

See Fig. 19.1 for a figure of The NCSBN Clinical Judgment Measurement Model. Progression of Layer 3 in this model advances as one navigates from left to right across the figure.

Recognize Cues

Considerations: Nurses obtain information from a client when they gather subjective and objective information. Nurses will need to know what information is important and, thereby, what information is a concern by identifying abnormal findings by recognizing cues.

Example: A nurse obtains vital signs on a client who had an appendectomy on the previous day. The vital signs are temperature: 101.5°F (38.6°C), Pulse: 96, Respirations: 24, Blood pressure: 124/72, Pain level: 6/10 (scale 1–10, with 10 being the highest pain). What vital signs should the nurse anticipate as important and a concern? During this step, nurses simply identify information that is not normal for this client: elevated temperature, pulse, respirations, and pain level.

Analyze Cues

Considerations: When nurses establish abnormal findings, they will need to organize and compare the information with the client's clinical situation. Do the cues support or contradict the condition? Consider multiple aspects of the situation during this step.

Example: Continuing with the above situation, the nurse will consider linking the cues to the client's situation. Post-op pain would explain the elevated pain, as well as the elevated pulse and respirations. The elevated temperature could be a concern because this is a post-op client.

Prioritize Hypotheses

Considerations: Next, nurses will want to evaluate and rank hypotheses (educated guesses) of what is happening, to prioritize them. What explanation is most concerning? Is the nurse able to prioritize concerns?

Example: The elevated temperature is the highest concern because the client had surgery the previous day and has a risk of a post-op infection. The elevated pain level, pulse rate, and respiratory rate could be from the post-op pain.

Generate Solutions

Considerations: Now, nurses identify potential nursing interventions for desired client outcomes. Nurses should try not to limit their thinking, coming up with as many as possible. Additional assessment of findings could be an intervention, if needed.

Example: Requesting an order for a blood culture and sensitivity could help determine if there is a concerning post-op infection. Assessing whether an antibiotic has already been ordered would be helpful to know when contacting the provider. Assessing the surgical dressing and site, if able, could provide more information about the potential for an infection at the incision. Assessing lung sounds could determine if there is fluid development in the lungs, a potential site for infection. Assessing the last time when the client had pain medication would indicate if additional medication could be administered. Providing pain medication, if able, could reduce the pain and then reduce the heart rate and respiratory rate. Assessing the pulse oximetry could help determine the peripheral oxygenation status to further explain the elevated respiratory rate. Keep in mind that an elevated respiratory rate could be a compensatory measure due to hypoxemia, which may be occurring due to potential blood loss from the surgery.

Take Actions

Considerations: During this step, nurses consider the list of interventions, determining which interventions are most appropriate to address the highest-priority actions needed as well as implement them. What priority action should nurses take?

Example: In the case above, priority interventions are those that address the elevated temperature. After those actions are underway, then nurses can administer pain medication. Keep in mind that pain is uncomfortable for clients, but if physiological concerns exist, then they become the priority (Maslow's Hierarchy of Needs, from Chapter 13). The nurse may want to assess additional relevant clinical findings before contacting the surgeon for further orders.

Evaluate Outcomes

Considerations: After performing interventions, nurses evaluate the expected outcomes. Were the nursing actions effective to meet the goals? Did the client show improvement, a declining status, or no changes?

Example: Following the interventions ordered by the provider, the nurse will evaluate if the temperature reduced and whether the assessment findings improved, declined, or were unchanged.

Following the steps of Layer 3 in The NCSBN Clinical Judgment Measurement Model allows nurses to form hypotheses, refine hypotheses, and evaluate outcomes to effectively make clinical decisions and provide safe care to clients. Chapter 19 will discuss how the structure of the NCLEX® NGN questions will follow Layer 3 in The NCSBN Clinical Judgment Measurement Model.

LPNs/LVNs use critical thinking to develop clinical judgment by using the nursing process and The NCSBN Clinical Judgment Measurement Model to provide safe client care.

Try This

Compare and Contrast the Nursing Process and Layer 3 of The NCSBN Clinical Judgment Measurement Model

There are five steps to the nursing process and six steps to Layer 3 of The NCSBN Clinical Judgment Measurement Model. Create a chart or concept map showing how these compare (and contrast) with each other. Include a clinical scenario and how you will follow through each process showing the similarities of client care for both.

Get Ready for the Next-Generation NCLEX® Examination

Key Points

- The NPA of your state/territory or country identifies your legal role in the nursing process as an LPN/LVN. Take time to read it and question what you do not understand.
- In 2002, the nursing process and critical thinking were integrated throughout the NCLEX-PN®. The steps of the nursing process for LPNs/LVNs were redefined. The additional step, nursing diagnosis within the planning step, is considered the exclusive responsibility of the RN.

Step 1: *Data collection.* Client data are gathered and reported to appropriate personnel.
Step 2: *Analysis.* The nurse determines if the data collected should be reassessed, is related to the client's clinical condition, and is a concern.
Step 3: *Planning.* The LPN/LVN assists the RN to develop the nursing diagnosis, outcomes, and interventions for the client's plan of care.
Step 4: *Implementation.* Nursing interventions in the care plan are put into action. This includes maintaining client safety.
Step 5: *Evaluation.* Actual outcomes of the interventions are compared with desired client outcomes (emphasis is on client progress toward meeting outcomes). Results are reported and documented.

- Critical thinking, the nursing process, and the NCSBN Clinical Judgment Measurement Model are essential for SPN/SVN education and NCLEX-PN® success.
- A variety of nursing care plans are implemented in clinical settings.
- In 2023, NCSBN implemented the NCSBN Clinical Judgment Measurement Model to create NGN (Next-Generation NCLEX®) questions. Clinical judgment is essential for nursing students to provide safe client care. Critical thinking involves thinking beyond what is obvious; clinical judgment involves taking appropriate action based on what the critical thinking revealed.

Step 1: Recognize Cues: Identify abnormal assessment findings.
Step 2: Analyze Cues: Evaluate if the abnormal findings match the client's clinical condition and are a concern.
Step 3: Prioritize Hypotheses: Rank hypotheses (educated guesses) of what is happening with the client and what is most concerning.
Step 4: Generate Solutions: Brainstorm potential nursing interventions for expected client outcomes, including additional assessments.
Step 5: Take Actions: Determine high-priority nursing actions and implement.
Step 6: Evaluate Outcomes: Determine if the expected client outcomes were reached and whether assessment findings are improved, declined, or unchanged.

Additional Learning Resources

Go to your Evolve website (http://evolve.elsevier.com/Carroll/success/) for the following FREE learning resources:

- Answers to Critical Thinking Scenarios
- Additional learning activities
- Additional Review Questions for the NCLEX-PN® examination
- Helpful phrases for communicating in Spanish and more!

Clinical Judgment and Next-Generation NCLEX® Examination-Style Questions

1. Some RNs and instructors have questioned the value of teaching SPNs/SVNs the nursing process and clinical judgment. Which statement provides a valid reason for including both in the SPN/SVN curriculum?

a. Knowledge of the nursing process and critical thinking encourages postgraduate education so that one day the LPN/LVN can be an RN.

b. LPNs/LVNs and RNs collaborate, assisting the client to meet their outcomes. A common language and thought process provides an organized way of understanding what is to be done.
c. Learning the nursing process and critical thinking provides the opportunity to be working on both LPN and RN levels of nursing at the same time.
d. Learning the nursing process and critical thinking provides a cookbook method of learning and provides time to deal with job stresses.

2. An LPN/LVN is working with an RN in a long-term care facility. Which request by the RN will the LPN/LVN refuse to do because it is beyond the LPN/LVN scope of practice?

a. Updating a plan of care for a resident and discussing with the RN
b. Catheterizing a resident and reporting the total output to the RN immediately
c. Checking a resident's pressure sore on the right hip for changes since admission
d. Assisting the RN by performing the assessment of a client newly admitted to the unit

3. The LPN/LVN observes a client demonstrating signs of aspiration and choking while eating a piece of meat. What is the best action within the LPN/LVN scope of nursing practice?

a. Ask someone to get help as you move quickly toward the client to perform the Heimlich maneuver.
b. Ask another client to straighten up the client while you go to get an RN or other qualified staff member.
c. Immediately call the client's health care provider for permission to perform the Heimlich and mention you are an SPN/SVN.
d. Because you do not know if this client has a do-not-resuscitate order on the chart, send someone to check.

4. An LPN/LVN is collecting data from a 75-year-old female client who arrives at the health care provider's office following a recent fall. What data requires verification?

Nurses Note: Client states she fell yesterday at home when she tripped while in the kitchen. Spouse states the client fell off a step stool in the kitchen. Was able to get up with assistance from their spouse. No injuries noted at the time of the fall. Today, she noticed swelling in the right wrist. Client denies pain with movement but supports wrist gingerly; facial grimaces are noted when attempting to move the wrist. Right wrist with edema is noted. Capillary refill and sensation to fingers are positive.

5. An LPN/LVN understands the steps needed to develop clinical judgment when the LPN/LVN prioritizes the following steps (indicate the order of Layer 3 in the NCSBN Clinical Judgment Measurement Model).

a. Recognize cues received when assessing a client.
b. Generate solutions of possible interventions to meet client outcomes.
c. Analyze cues to determine which abnormal findings are a concern.
d. Prioritize hypotheses (educated guesses) to determine what finding is of most concern.
e. Take action by implementing high-priority interventions.
f. Evaluate outcomes to determine client progression and whether outcomes have been met.

Critical Thinking Scenarios

Scenario 1

You overhear a conversation among peers stating that the NCSBN Clinical Judgment Measurement Model is a waste of time. Someone states, "Nurses know intuitively what a client needs because of their love for clients. After all, this is the reason a person becomes a nurse." You have decided to engage in the conversation. What evidence will you share to support why you believe the NCSBN Clinical Judgment Measurement Model is valuable for delivering high-quality client care?

Scenario 2

A nursing student wants to improve their grades. The student learned about using the nursing process during class a couple of days ago. "If it works for planning client care, why can't it work for me? I am going to give it a try."

Answer the following questions about what the student can do for each step of the nursing process to improve their grades:

1. How might the student **gather data** on their study habits?
2. In the **analyzing** stage, the student evaluates whether their study habits could directly impact their grades. What is a possible correlation between reduced studying and poor results?
3. In the **planning** stage, the student discovered that they periodically fell asleep while studying (maybe because they was studying in bed). The student was surprised to see that they had a total of 30 cell phone calls or text messages during that time. They spent time talking on the cell or texting in response. They did not even finish the chapter they was trying to study. What changes could they **implement** to ensure future success?
4. How would the student **evaluate** their success?

Now, apply this same situation to the steps of the NCSBN Clinical Judgment Measurement Model. Do you have similar responses?

13 Nursing Theory, Research, and Evidence-Based Practice

Objectives

On completing this chapter, you will be able to do the following:

1. Differentiate key nursing theories as they relate to the nursing process.
2. Explain the importance of nursing research, including the two types of research.
3. Discuss the importance of evidence-based practice (EBP) while demonstrating how best evidence for practice is determined.
4. Discuss the role of the licensed practice nurse/licensed vocational nurse (LPN/LVN) in EBP.

Key Terms

evidence-based practice (EBP)
Leininger's culture care theory
Maslow's hierarchy of needs theory
nursing research
nursing theories
Orem's self-care deficit theory
Peplau's interpersonal relations theory
qualitative research study
quantitative research study
Rosenstock's health belief theory
spirit of inquiry
Watson's theory of human care

In a clinical rotation at a skilled nursing facility, Trinh, a student practical nurse, was assigned to a client who had an order for wet-to-dry dressing changes. Trinh was questioning this type of dressing. When he approached the nurse caring for the client, the nurse said, "This is a typical dressing change order in our facility."

Later, Trinh discussed the situation with the clinical instructor, who suggested that he review research studies to determine current evidence-based practice (EBP). Trinh realized that advocating for change in nursing practice requires not only understanding how to obtain current research findings but also finding the courage to speak up when nursing practices need to change to improve client care.

Keep in Mind

Becoming acquainted with terminology allows a nurse to perform at the highest level for critical thinking possible in the nursing career.

NURSING THEORIES

Numerous **nursing theories** have been developed to provide a basis for research on the effectiveness of nursing care.

It is important to discuss nursing theories because they provide a framework for nursing education and clinical practice. Furthermore, understanding nursing theories allows the licensed practice nurse/licensed vocational nurse (LPN/LVN) to develop critical thinking.

FLORENCE NIGHTINGALE: THE FIRST NURSING THEORIST

Florence Nightingale, in 1860, was the first to emphasize the client's environment: ventilation, warmth, noise, light, and cleanliness. Nightingale is considered the first nursing theorist. She strongly believed that environmental issues influenced the outcome of illness. She also saw the nursing role as a provider of health care, not as a "handmaiden." She was the first to collect data and use evidence to make clinical decisions. Nightingale determined that an environment that was warm, clean, well lit, and quiet resulted in a decreased death rate for soldiers. Consequently, when she instructed her nurses to adhere to these standards, the soldier death rate plummeted.

ABRAHAM MASLOW'S HIERARCHY OF NEEDS THEORY

Although Abraham Maslow was a psychologist, **Maslow's hierarchy of needs theory** has been adapted by many professional programs, including nursing programs, as a framework for education. Here is a general description of the theory:

1. Certain internal, external, physical, and psychological needs are common to all people.
2. Common needs are arranged in a hierarchy.
3. Unmet needs create tension, which motivates the person to react to meet the need.
4. When needs are met, the person is no longer aware of the need, and the need (now met) no longer motivates them.

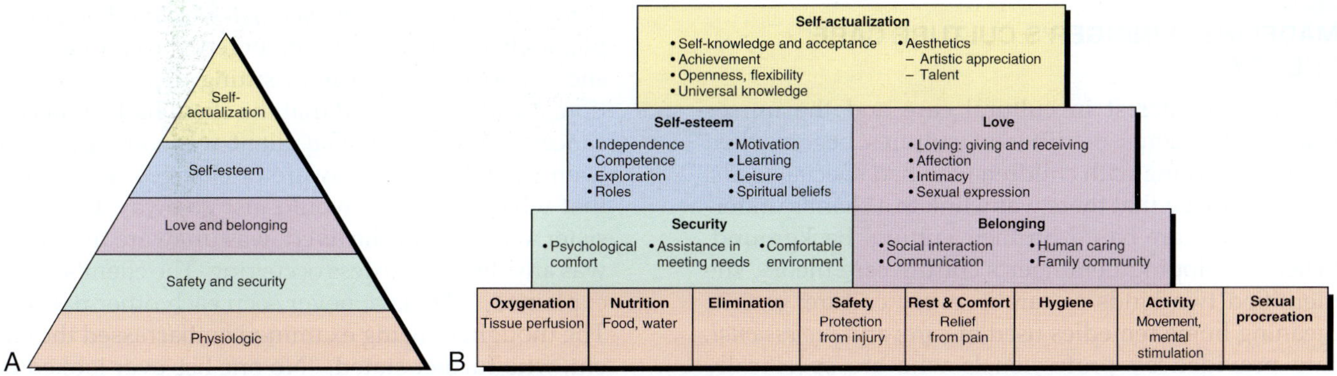

Fig. 13.1 **(A)** Maslow's hierarchy of human needs. **(B)** Evolving hierarchy of needs adapted by nursing.

5. Dominant needs that matter to a person can vary in life.

Fig. 13.1 identifies the client hierarchy for needs and adaptation to the nursing profession. In general, lower-level needs must be met before higher-level needs can be considered. Remember that a person may be functioning within more than one level of need at the same time. Individuals may go back to the physiologic level periodically to satisfy basic needs, for example, nutrition.

Applying Maslow's Hierarchy of Needs Theory to the Nursing Process

The LPN/LVN understands the value of assessing the following needs to prioritize care:

- *Physiologic:* Oxygen, food, water, elimination, safety, sleep, activity, mental stimulation, and sexual procreation. (For example, the nurse collects data on whether a client is eating enough to maintain their strength and health.) Then, the nurse can focus on safety and security needs.
- *Safety*: Security, freedom from harm, and protection. (For example, data are collected on real or imagined safety needs, such as whether the client needs more than one nurse to safely transfer from the bed to the toilet.) The primary areas that involve hospital nursing care are the first two levels: physiologic and safety needs.
- *Love and belonging:* Love, affection, and companionship (for example, data are collected on whether the client has a support system to assist with care after the client is discharged from the hospital). This is a part of discharge planning to ensure that the client has the support needed to meet his or her needs at home. Engaging the client's family in their care and assisting them in understanding the possible behavior changes that the client may experience (such as a flat affect following a stroke) may help the family share love to the client. The nurse may be involved in doing follow-up care in the home after hospitalization (home health, visiting nurse service, etc.).
- *Esteem:* Respect and recognition (for example, data are collected on what the client is doing or can do that will assist in earning a positive sense of self). Is the client able to do volunteer work to help others, such as participating with a retired senior volunteer program? Can the client join a senior center that has activities, as well as meals at a reasonable price? A parish nurse, case worker, or another member of the health care team may be providing care at this level. Once esteem needs are met, the individual may be ready to focus on self-actualization.
- *Self-actualization:* This is the highest level of need. This involves realization, creativity, and fulfillment of the individual's potential. (For example, data are collected on whether the client expresses self creatively or demonstrates personal fulfillment in life.)

OREM'S SELF-CARE DEFICIT THEORY

Dorothea **Orem's self-care deficit theory** is a general theory that consists of three subtheories:

1. *Self-care:* This involves a goal that is directed toward a safer environment for life, health, and well-being. (Ideally, individuals learn to respond to health cues in themselves or the environment as a means of maintaining personal health as independently as possible.)
2. *Self-care deficit:* Individuals do not meet their self-care demands. (The individual does not recognize or know what to do about personal health situations.)
3. *Nursing system:* Nurses help meet the client's self-care demands until the client can do so independently. (Nurses respond to the client's care needs totally, partially, or in a supportive role according to the need.)

Orem's theory is concerned with growth and development needs, as well as physiologic and psychosocial needs. Nurses can use the data collection step of the nursing process to identify specific self-care deficits. By working with the client, nurses can then choose interventions that will have the desired outcomes for the client. During the last several decades, many hospitals, particularly rehabilitation hospitals, have used Orem's self-care deficit theory to guide their practice.

MADELINE LEININGER'S CULTURE CARE THEORY

Leininger's interest in cultural care and the nurses respond to clients of different cultures began when she was working with children who had special needs. She recognized that there was a link to a client's understanding of care based on their cultural background. When developing Leininger's culture care theory, she identified two kinds of care in every culture: *generic*, meaning home remedies used in care; and *professional*, care provided by professionals who are specifically trained in providing care.

Leininger proposed three modes to guide nursing decisions when providing care:

1. *Cultural care preservation or maintenance*. This means assisting individuals in maintaining personal, cultural values in an effort to maintain health or restore health. As an example, some cultures use periodic cupping, which is a localized suction technique on the skin, to relieve symptoms of hemochromatosis (excess iron deposits throughout the body). Another cultural practice is to periodically give blood at a blood blank to reduce the hematocrit (the percentage of your blood that is made up of red blood cells). The nurse *accepts* the client's cultural practice.
2. *Cultural care accommodation or negotiation*. This means adjusting the cultural practices to a more accepted practice. In some cultures, Vicks VapoRub is placed in the nostrils, which has the potential of leading to aspiration and then aspiration pneumonia. A cultural care accommodation would involve a home health nurse placing Vicks VapoRub on the chest and neck, rubbing it in a soothing manner. The vapor's fumes relieved the congestion. The nurse suggests a change in the cultural practice that is an *accepted compromise*.
3. *Culture care repatterning or restructuring*. Leininger's theory is concerned with respecting cultural differences and yet providing a safe and protective environment. For example, in some cultures, mud is placed on an infant's umbilicus after delivery. Because of the risk for local and systemic infection, a visiting nurse could provide clean pads. The nurse demonstrates their use, how to clean the area, and how to leave the area uncovered, for a designated time, so the umbilicus could be exposed to the air. The nurse respectfully promotes a *new* practice to promote client safety.

Applying Leininger's three modes when providing nursing care develops a foundation for providing culturally competent or congruent care.

ROSENSTOCK'S HEALTH BELIEF THEORY

Irwin Rosenstock developed **Rosenstock's health belief theory**, which tries to explain why a person will not take action to prevent or detect illness. According to this theory:

1. *Perceptions vary and may not match reality*. For example, a client came to the emergency room because she experienced pain with sitting. Upon examination, it was determined that the client had advanced cancer of the vulva. The client was very shy, and even though she was aware of changes, she hoped that whatever it was would just go away. Even her sister, with whom she lived, was unaware that there was any disease process occurring. The client's sister explained, "We have never seen each other naked." The thought of being examined embarrassed the client, who further stated, "No one has ever looked at me down there." **Misguided perceptions may not reveal the necessity of health care.**
2. *Beliefs are connected to existing barriers*. For example, a client views a preventive or treatment activity as expensive, painful, or inconvenient. If there are fewer perceived negative aspects, the possibility of doing something is higher. Conversely, if more negative aspects exist, a person is more likely not to act. For a further example, an 82-year-old client began to have gastrointestinal symptoms and asked her son to make a health care provider's appointment for her. The son made the appointment and drove 8 hours to take his mother to the appointment. Upon arrival to the medical office, the client refused to go in, explaining, "I've changed my mind. It's nothing." This went on several more times over a period of years before the client was so uncomfortable that she finally kept the appointment.

   The client was diagnosed with advanced cancer of the colon. She explained that she already had seven surgeries and did not want to put up with another uncomfortable healing process. Because of the pain she was having now, the client agreed to surgery. The surgery was palliative, which gave relief from pain, but she was told that she probably had 6 months to live. **Personal beliefs can cause barriers to health care.**
3. *A cue to action is seen as necessary*. For example, significant pain, a news story, or a reminder call from the health care provider's office can prompt a client to make an appointment. The cue for the client in the above scenario was the pain she began to experience. **Identifying the reason why clients seek health care is important.**

This theory can be useful when using the nursing process to promote health. *Assessing perceptions and beliefs* can reveal misunderstandings and barriers. Discussing *health consequences or reasons for seeking care* can motivate clients toward illness-prevention initiatives. The nurse can consider assessment findings to determine educational interventions and outcomes. This theory can be beneficial for promoting yearly examinations, vaccinations, and wellness classes.

JEAN WATSON'S THEORY OF HUMAN CARE

According to **Watson's theory of human care**, health is harmony between the body, mind, and spirit. It also involves self-perception and how the self is experienced. Illness is a lack of harmony within the self and the soul. The nursing role is a caring process to help the client regain harmony and health. Through nursing care, the client develops self-knowledge and self-healing. The enabling actions allow the client to solve problems and grow. Both the client and the nurse grow through this process.

We have only presented a few classic nursing theories. Countless other theories, such as Hildegard **Peplau's interpersonal relations theory**, Sister Callista Roy's Adaptation Model, and Pat Benner's theory from novice to expert, are used in nursing practice and nursing education. If you want to learn more about theories, visit www.nursing-theory.org. In addition, most nursing fundamental and foundations textbooks have a chapter devoted to theories and models.

> **Try This**
>
> Look at the clinical paperwork that you complete in your nursing program to see if any of these theories are implemented. Do you need to assess or create interventions for any of the following?
> - Environment (Nightingale)
> - Needs: Physiologic, safety, love and belonging, esteem, and self-actualization (Maslow's Hierarchy of Needs)
> - Self-care deficit (Orem's self-care deficit theory)
> - Culture (Madline Leininger's culture care theory)
> - Perceptions about health, beliefs/barriers, and cue to action/reason for seeking care (Rosenstock's health belief theory)
> - Mind, body, and spirit (Watson's theory of human care)

NURSING RESEARCH AND EVIDENCE-BASED PRACTICE (EBP)

NURSING RESEARCH

Research in any profession supports existing knowledge and develops new knowledge based on observation and experimentation. Nursing research strengthens the nursing profession. Starting with Nightingale's study of soldier morbidity and mortality data during the Crimean War and continuing today's emphasis on EBP, **nursing research** has improved existing nursing knowledge and generated new knowledge that has influenced nursing practice. Research studies in nursing are important because they:

- Identify specific nursing interventions that are proven effective and not merely based on tradition. "That is the way we have always done it" should no longer be the sole reason for nursing actions.
- Provide evidence that supports the quality and cost effectiveness of what nurses do.
- Generate knowledge for clinical practice and nursing education.

Nurses of all educational levels are encouraged to participate and promote nursing research in varying degrees (Cherry and Jacob, 2019). These are the two main types of research studies done in nursing: quantitative research and qualitative research.

Quantitative Research

A **quantitative research study** is an objective study in which *numerical* data are valuable for analysis. In this type of research, a response to an action is typically evaluated. One *variable* is the event or action the researcher is trying to measure. One group of participants receive the intervention and the other group of participants that does not receive the intervention. Numeric data are collected and measured using statistics to describe variables, examine relationships among variables, or determine cause-and-effect interactions between variables. A randomized control trial is an example of quantitative research. A more specific example follows: A study is conducted to determine the effect of a new medication to treat Alzheimer's disease on the progression of dementia-like symptoms. One group of clients (experimental) receives the new medication, and another group (control) receives the current standard of treatment. The observed effect (identified symptoms) is measured and compared within each group. A number is assigned to each observed effect to calculate the data *numerically* (*quantitative* research).

Qualitative Research

A **qualitative research study** is a subjective study in which *communicatio*n data are valuable for analysis. Data are gathered through interviews and/or direct observations. Themes found in the words collected or words used to describe observations are identified. The study can be a narrative description of the "lived experience" of individuals or possibly groups. An example would be a study focusing on understanding how nursing students' confidence is increased in the clinical setting. The data are analyzed by looking at the (*quality of the*) *communicated* themes presented during student interviews (*qualitative* research).

All research methodologies contribute to the development of the science of nursing and can assist in establishing nursing as an independent science.

EBP

Background of the EBP Movement

At the start of the 20th century, proven effective health care was noted to be essential. Here is a chronological journey of this development:

- Dr. Archie Cochrane (1901–1988), a British epidemiologist, challenged the public to only pay for medical care that was proven to be effective. He advocated the use of randomized, controlled trials (RCTs) as a means of reliably influencing health care practices. In 1993, the Cochrane Collaboration, an independent, not-for-profit organization, was established to prepare and promote the accessibility of *Cochrane Reviews*, a collection of evidence-based health care interventions obtained by systematic reviews of research.

- In 1999, the Institute of Medicine (IOM), now known as the National Academy of Medicine (NAM), issued the report *To Err Is Human: Building a Safer Health System*, which discussed the incidence of medical errors in health care and the need for health care reform.
- In 2001, the IOM issued *Crossing the Quality Chasm: A New Health System for the 21st Century*, calling for consistent, high-quality health care for all people. IOM promoted health care that is supported by available scientific knowledge.
- During the last two decades, insurance companies began to pay for health care practices only if their effectiveness is supported by scientific evidence.
- During the last decade, Medicare has been denying payments to hospitals when complications develop if evidence-based guidelines were not followed.
- Clients and families are seeking the latest evidence on websites about the most effective treatment for illnesses and diseases.
- Large national research projects, funded by the federal government and other partners, seek to identify client outcomes. An example of a research project that studied nursing student outcomes is the National Council of State Boards of Nursing (NCSBN) study aimed at examining the relationship between clinical simulation in nursing schools and nursing program outcomes.
- Today, countless sites exist allowing quick easy access to current EBP guidelines, such as evidence available from NCSBN, National League for Nursing (NLN), NAM, the Joint Commission on Accreditation of Healthcare Organizations (JACHO), and JBI, formally known as the Joanna Briggs Institute.

Guidelines for Determining the Best Evidence for Practice

Best evidence is determined through a complex, rigorous process:

- Individuals seeking EBPs develop a clinical question in an objective, concise manner. For example, a nurse may want to research, "Is there a higher incidence of aspiration pneumonia among clients with G-tubes vs. J-tubes during hospitalizations?"
- Using professional resources, nurses can obtain the latest, most relevant research evidence that pertains to the clinical question. The information in Box 13.1 will provide a list of acceptable, professional resources.
- An expert or panel of experts conducts a systematic review, which is a summary of results from the selected studies.
- Specific practice recommendations are derived from the summary of research articles.

Box 13.1 Systematic Reviews Used to Develop Evidence-Based Practice Guidelines

PUBMED (http://pubmed.gov)

The U.S. National Library of Medicine (NLM) database of biomedical citations and abstracts. An abstract is a summary of the research completed.

- Medline is the largest component of PubMed and is freely accessible. (https://www.nlm.nih.gov/bsd/medline.html).

CUMULATIVE INDEX OF NURSING AND ALLIED HEALTH LITERATURE (CINAHL)

- A source for practical/vocational nurses for evidence-based practice (EBP) interventions.

COCHRANE REVIEWS (https://www.cochrane.org)

- Each review addresses a clearly formulated question. All the existing research on a topic that meets certain criteria is searched for and collated and then assessed using stringent guidelines to establish whether or not there is conclusive evidence about a specific treatment. The reviews are updated regularly, ensuring that treatment decisions can be based on the most up-to-date and reliable evidence.

AGENCY FOR HEALTHCARE RESEARCH AND QUALITY (AHRQ) (https://www.ahrq.gov)

- An agency of the U.S. Department of Health and Human Services

JBI (FORMERLY THE JOANNA BRIGGS INSTITUTE) (https://jbi.global/)

- An international not-for-profit membership-based organization. The institute develops methods to appraise and synthesize evidence, conducting systematic reviews and analyses of the research literature to provide the best available evidence to inform clinical decision making.

Try This

Read the abstract (the summary of a research study) from the following article: https://pubmed.ncbi.nlm.nih.gov/37227191/. Does this article support the use of G-tubes for enteral feedings in the hospital? This research provides evidence (findings from research) for nursing practice in the clinical site.

EBP in Nursing

Nursing care based on comments such as "This is how we do this procedure here" or "This is how I was taught to do this nursing intervention 20 years ago" is not sufficient in today's health care environment. Nursing interventions such as cleansing wounds with Betadine or hydrogen peroxide and massaging over bony prominences are examples of common nursing interventions in past years that have been proven through research to be potentially harmful (Ackley et al., 2008). EBP is the clinical practice of nurses based on scientific knowledge that demonstrates proof that the knowledge is effective.

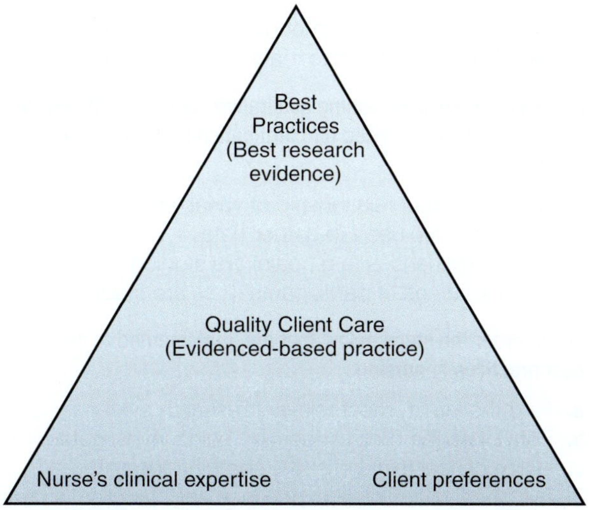

Fig. 13.2 The triangle of evidence-based practice.

Research provides the foundation for evidence-based nursing practice. **Using critical thinking, nurses use research findings, combined with clinical experience and the client's preferences or values, to promote EBP (Fig. 13.2).** All nurses need to stay up to date with current EBPs to provide safe, effective client care.

Further implementation of EBPs can be found in utilization review and quality improvement measures. **It is not enough to determine research results; nurses must promote EBPs by evaluating the care provided and improving the quality of care based on research findings.**

Try This

Start a Journal Club with your classmates. Select a topic and find two to three research articles on the topic. Meet as a group to discuss the research results, share what you know from your clinical experience, and talk about how different client preferences or values may change nursing care regarding the research findings. Refer to Fig. 13.2.

The Role of the LPN/LVN in EBP. In 2010, the NLN established competencies for nursing graduates at all levels. The competency that addresses nursing research and EBP is **spirit of inquiry**. A nurse with a spirit of inquiry is one who asks questions, challenges current practices, and promotes resolution of problems. The role of the LPN/LVN regarding research is to question the basis for nursing actions by considering research, evidence, tradition, clinical experience, and client preference. Student practical nurses/student vocational nurses (SPNs/SVNs) participate in the nursing research process by reviewing current articles from professional resources as part of their student learning experience, while supporting EBP in care plans and nursing interventions. The National League of Nursing developed Core Competencies for nurse educators to strengthen the learning of nursing students.

Health care institutions promote EBPs by creating and updating protocols, policies, and procedures. *Protocols* are processes that are approved for health care workers to follow, for example, urinary catheter care for clients with urinary catheters (like standing orders but for certain nursing interventions). *Policies* are general guidelines used to manage a clinical situation, for example, infection control with wound care. *Procedures* include the detailed steps of nursing interventions for implementing the policy, such as step-by-step instructions regarding dressing changes using aseptic technique. SPN/SVNs and LPN/LVNs must follow an institution's protocols, policies, and procedures, while critically thinking about EBPs. If evidence supports a contrary procedure than the established guidelines, then the SPN/SVN or LPN/LVN can provide research findings to promote change.

Try This

An LPN/LVN is working in a nursing home and is concerned about the risk involved for clients to leave the facility and go to physician appointments, such as increased infection potential, risk of an accident in travel, and overexertion of the client. The LPN/LVN feels that telehealth appointments could be of value and wants to research the evidence on this topic. Roleplay the LPN/LVN and use the websites found in Box 13.1 to research the benefits of telehealth in health.

Get Ready for the Next-Generation NCLEX® Examination

Key Points

- Nursing involves many different theories. Choosing the appropriate theory can improve client care and nursing curriculum.
- Nursing research is a scientific process that validates and refines existing knowledge and generates new knowledge that influences nursing practice.
- The clinical practice of nurses needs to be based on scientific knowledge with proof that the knowledge is effective.
- Research provides the foundation for EBP in nursing.
- The elements of EBP are best research evidence, resources including nurse's clinical expertise, and client preferences.
- All research methodologies contribute to the development of the science of nursing and can assist in establishing nursing as an independent science.
- A quantitative research study involves the collection and analysis of numerical data to evaluate the effects of an intervention, often using control and experimental groups to determine cause-and-effect relationships. A qualitative

research study involves analyzing communication data gathered through interviews or observations to identify themes and describe the "lived experiences" of individuals or groups, such as understanding how nursing students' confidence increases in clinical settings
- A qualitative research study involves analyzing communication data gathered through interviews or observations to identify themes and describe the "lived experiences" of individuals or groups.
- Spirit of inquiry for an LPN/LVN means a nurse who asks questions, challenges current practices, and promotes resolution of problems.
- LPNs/LVNs participate in the nursing research process by reviewing current articles in professional sources, supporting clinical interventions on care plans with evidence-based nursing practices, collecting data for research studies as requested by the registered nurse, following protocols and procedures of the agency in which they are employed, and providing objective data gathering to evaluate the effectiveness of selected EBPs.
- LPNs/LVNs need to stay up to date on current evidence-based practices EBPs to provide safe, effective client care.

Additional Learning Resources

Go to your Evolve website (http://evolve.elsevier.com/Carroll/success/) for the following FREE learning resources:

- Answers to Critical Thinking Scenario
- Additional learning activities
- Additional Review Questions for the NCLEX-PN® examination
- Helpful phrases for communicating in Spanish and more!

Clinical Judgment Questions

1. Each member of a group of SPNs/SVNs are providing examples of elements needed to provide EBP. What example best indicates that the SPN/SVN requires additional instruction regarding the elements needed for evidenced-based practices?

a. Best research evidence
b. Nurse's clinical expertise
c. Client preferences
d. Tradition in agency

2. What statement describes quantitative research?

a. The researcher focuses on the words of the participants to determine themes.
b. Numeric data are collected and measured using statistics.
c. Interviews are conducted to gain insight into a problem.
d. The research study is subjective.

3. What statement is accurate regarding theories useful to nursing?

a. Orem's interpersonal theory defines roles and steps in developing a therapeutic relationship.
b. Maslow's culture care theory is concerned with how to meet cultural needs through nursing care.
c. Rosenstock's needs theory focuses on meeting client needs that may have no basis in fact.
d. In Maslow's theory, unmet needs create tension, which motivates the person to react to meet the need.

4. A student nurse is explaining qualitative research to a peer. What response indicates a need for clarification regarding qualitative research?

a. A cause–effect relationship of variables is confirmed.
b. Interviews are used to gather data.
c. Lived experiences (e.g., pain) are studied.
d. Problem areas of participants' lives are studied.

5. List in order the steps below that are implemented to identify best practices in nursing.

a. Find the latest, most relevant research evidence.
b. Formulate the clinical question being investigated.
c. Using critical thinking skills, combine the gathered evidence with clinical experience and the client's preferences and values when providing client care.
d. Evaluate the validity and relevance of the evidence found and determine how you can apply the evidence to the clinical situation selected.

6. Select the items that describe the LPN's/LVN's role in nursing research and EBP. *(Select all that apply.)*

a. Collect data for research studies as requested by the registered nurse.
b. Collaborate to formulate clinical questions that need to be investigated for validity.
c. Follow protocols and procedures of the place of employment.
d. Gather data for evaluation of the effectiveness of EBPs.
e. Support clinical interventions in practice with evidence-based nursing practices.

7. Indicate whether the following nursing actions are evidence-based practice EBP or not:

NURSING ACTION	EVIDENCE-BASED PRACTICE	NOT EVIDENCE-BASED PRACTICE
a. Cleanse a wound with hydrogen peroxide		
b. Wash hands upon entering a client's room		
c. Massage bony prominences		
d. Encourage a post-op client to cough and deep breathe		
e. Elevate head of bed at least 30 degrees for clients with G-tube feedings		

8. All nurses should stay up to date with_______, to effectively provide_______.

personal rest	weather information
evidence-based practices	nutritious food
vacation time	worthy trust
personnel gossip	safe client care

Critical Thinking Scenario

An SPN/SVN has a medical/surgical clinical experience in a hospital that uses EBPs. The clinical instructor reviewed the student's care plan and noted one intervention as: 5 mL of air will be instilled into the client's gastric feeding tube while auscultating over the epigastric area for a "swooshing" sound to ascertain proper tube placement. (The client is receiving intermittent tube feeding.) The instructor questions the student's source of information, and the student states that she found the information on the internet. If you were the instructor, what would you discuss with the student?

14 The Interdisciplinary Health Care Team: The Role of the Practical/Vocational Nurse

Objectives

On completing this chapter, you will be able to do the following:

1. Differentiate the roles and settings associated with the members of the interprofessional health care team, including why the licensed practical nurse/licensed vocational nurse (LPN/LVN) needs to know this information.
2. Differentiate the educational requirements and the roles of the various nursing positions.
3. Distinguish between the different methods for the delivery of nursing care in acute care settings, including why the LPN/LVN needs to know this information.

Key Terms

associate degree nursing (ADN) program
Bachelor of Science in Nursing (BSN) program
case management method
certification
certified nursing assistant
client-centered care
clinical pathways
diploma program
electronic health record (EHR)
functional method
general supervision
independent
interdependent
licensed practical nurse/licensed vocational nurse (LPN/LVN)
nurse manager
nursing case management
patient (client) outcomes
primary care method
registered nurse
skill mix
standards of care
student nurse
team method
total patient (client) care
unit clerk
unit manager
unlicensed assistive personnel (UAP)

> **Keep in Mind**
>
> You cannot identify the members of a health care organization without having structure to the health care delivery. This chapter identifies the members of the health care team. Consider creating a chart or concept map of each health care team member, the education required for their role, and the importance of their role in caring for clients.

PROGRESSION OF CARE THROUGH THE HEALTH CARE SYSTEM: AN INTERDISCIPLINARY APPROACH

A 75-year-old client is taken to surgery for a right hip repair following a fall on their 200-acre farm. Under general anesthesia during surgery, the client's blood pressure reached dangerously high levels but quickly stabilized under the anesthesiologist's interventions. Despite this setback, the client was discharged after 3 days in the hospital. The client and the family agreed that physical therapy was necessary to learn how to function at home. Therefore the client was admitted to a rehabilitation facility. Two weeks later, the client was discharged from the rehabilitation facility to the client's home.

This sounds like just another success story for nursing, doesn't it? We will follow this client as she progresses through the health care system and then decide who should get credit for the client's discharge back to the farm.

EMERGENCY CARE

Following the client's fall, their daughter calls the emergency squad to transport the client to the nearest hospital. The hospital is located 20 miles away in a city with a population of 98,000 people. The three people manning the emergency squad are *emergency medical technicians* (EMTs). Each EMT has taken an approximately 150-hour course in basic life support skills and has been certified as an EMT after passing a national examination. The EMTs are currently taking an 18- to 24-month paramedic course, which is preparing them to provide more advanced life support skills. On the way to the hospital, the EMTs monitor the client's blood pressure, pulse, respirations, and level of consciousness, while keeping the right leg immobilized. The EMTs maintain contact with the hospital emergency department (ED) by means of a two-way radio or cell phones.

On arriving at the ED, the EMTs provide the *registered nurse* (RN) with verbal and/or written reports of the client's status. The ED health care provider examines the client and orders an x-ray of their right hip. The *x-ray technician* brings the x-ray equipment to the ED and takes the right hip x-ray. This x-ray technician has taken a 2-year program conducted by a hospital or technical college to prepare them to perform diagnostic measures involving radiant energy. The *radiologist* on duty reads the x-ray of the right hip. Based on the physical examination and the results of the x-ray, the ED health care provider diagnoses a fracture of the right proximal femur. The ED health care provider notifies the client's *family health care provider* and an *orthopedic surgeon* whom the client and family requested.

The RN receives the client in the ED, performs an assessment, and provides care until she is admitted to the hospital. The RN is a graduate of a **Bachelor of Science in Nursing (BSN)**, associate degree, or diploma program. This nurse has passed a national examination, the National Council Licensure Examination for Registered Nurses (NCLEX-RN®), to become an RN. RNs who work in the ED participate regularly in continuing education courses at the hospital and at seminars, given regionally and nationally, for ED nurses, and often achieve certification as an emergency nurse practitioner (ENP-BC). This RN prepares the client for surgery.

To be qualified to oversee the medical care of this client, the family physician is a health care provider who has attended 4 years of college, 4 years of medical school, and a 3-year residency program. Medical school consists of a program that provides the basic knowledge and skills needed to be a medical physician. The residency program prepares physicians for practice in a specialty. The specialty in this situation is family medicine. Most hospitals have a position called *hospitalist*, for managing the medical care of clients during the hospitalization, like the family physician performed in the past for their hospitalized patients. Family physicians, as well as other medical specialties, fill the hospitalist position. Instead of working in an outpatient practice, hospitalists only work in the hospital, caring for the patients during hospitalizations.

The ED physician, the radiologist, and the orthopedic surgeon had the same education as the family physician, before starting the residency experience. The ED physician completed a residency program in emergency or trauma medicine. The radiologist completed a residency program in radiology, the reading and interpretation of x-rays. The orthopedic surgeon completed a 3- to 5-year residency in performing surgery for problems of bones and joints. These physicians have passed the board examinations, which license them as health care physicians and allow them to practice under the state medical practice act. Each health care physician in this scenario is board certified in their specialty area.

This client also has visits from health care provider extenders who are working in collaboration with the physicians. These extenders are generally nurse practitioners (NPs) or physician assistants (PAs). An NP is an advanced practice RN. These nurses have a minimum of a Master of Science in Nursing (MSN) degree, which often is a 2-year program of study at the graduate level, beyond the bachelor's degree. Organizations such as the American Association of Colleges of Nursing (AACN) recommends NPs be educated at the doctoral level. They are licensed specifically as an NP and have a unique role as defined by the Nurse Practice Act (NPA) in their state.

A PA has a minimum of a bachelor's degree and health care experience prior to attending a PA program. A PA is nationally certified and state licensed as a health care provider. Although still acting as a member of the interdisciplinary team, NPs in some states can function in an autonomous manner. PAs and NPs in other states must work in collaboration with a physician for some activities, such as prescribing medication.

Laboratory studies are ordered preoperatively. *Lab personnel* draw blood for these studies. Lab personnel have varied educational backgrounds. Some have on-the-job training to obtain blood samples. A medical lab technician has 2 years of education. A medical technologist (MT) has more than 4 years of education and can be certified by a national examination. Lab personnel are responsible for collecting the specimens needed for lab tests, performing the tests, and reporting the results to health care providers and staff.

The family members request that their parish *priest* be contacted to give the client the sacrament of the sick (see Chapter 11). Because surgery is imminent, the pastoral care department is notified. A Roman Catholic priest, a member of the pastoral care team, anoints the client with holy oils, prays with them, and gives them Holy Communion. To be able to meet the client's spiritual needs, the priest has had 4 years of college and 4 years of theological school before being ordained.

Assistive personnel (AP) cares for the client in the ED. These can be certified nursing assistants (CNAs), transport aides, client-care technicians, or various other support care staff (i.e., admissions representatives). These individuals have completed short-term training (2–16 weeks), specific to their job role. Training is often provided by the employer but can be achieved through a community-based educational program. These health care workers may need to be listed on a statewide registry.

THE SURGICAL EXPERIENCE

In the ED, the nurse *anesthetist* prepares the client and family for the anesthesia part of the surgical experience. This nurse is an RN with a Doctor in Nursing Practice degree, who has studied an additional 7 to 8 years including an approved school of anesthesiology, has passed a national exam to be a certified registered nurse anesthetist (CRNA), and works collaboratively with an anesthesiologist. The nurse anesthetist provides anesthesia to clients undergoing surgery. The client is transferred to the surgical suite, where she undergoes a right hip pinning procedure under general anesthesia. This type of anesthesia will put the client in a state of unconsciousness.

During surgery, the nurse anesthetist monitors the client's vital signs continuously while the client is unconscious. The *surgical technicians* set up the sterile environment in the operating room and assist the orthopedic surgeon. This health care worker makes sure the surgeon's instruments and supplies are available when the surgeon requests them for the pinning of the right hip. The surgical technician is a graduate of a 1- to 3-year diploma program or associate degree program at a local technical or community college. An RN who has a minimum qualification of a BSN coordinates the overall functions of the surgical team.

During surgery, the CRNA notes that the client's blood pressure is rising to a dangerous level. The CRNA contacts the anesthesiologist STAT (i.e., immediately!). The *anesthesiologist*, a physician who completed a residency in anesthesiology, orders antihypertensive medications (i.e., medications that lower the blood pressure). The situation is quickly brought under control. Surgery is completed, and the client is sent to the postanesthesia care unit (PACU).

POSTANESTHESIA CARE UNIT

The purpose of the PACU is to monitor the client's vital signs, level of consciousness, movement, pain, and any special equipment required by clients after surgery. When the client's conditions are stable, she is transferred to her hospital room. After 1.5 hours, the PACU RN, who went to nursing school for 2 years (associate degree), 1 to 3 years (diploma), or 4 years (BSN degree), determines that the client is ready to leave the PACU. Because of the episode involving high blood pressure during surgery, the surgeon orders the client to go to the intensive care unit (ICU) overnight for closer observation instead of going to the postoperative surgical unit. A *transport aide*, who is trained on the job, and a *staff nurse (RN)* from the PACU transfer the client to the ICU.

ICU: TIME FOR CLOSE OBSERVATION

The ICU is staffed with RNs who went to school for 2 years (associate degree), 1 to 3 years (diploma), or 4 years (BSN degree). Each nurse has taken the same national examination (NCLEX-RN®) to become an RN. Most institutions prepare an RN for the responsibilities of this unit through in-services, a nurse externship, postgraduate, or continuing education courses after a minimum amount of nursing experience. The client's nurse (a 2-year graduate or an RN with a BSN degree), is responsible for the care and observation of two clients.

The family is unable to answer some additional questions about the client's medical history. The family physician asks the *unit clerk* to obtain the client's medical records from the medical records department or through the **electronic health record (EHR)**. The unit clerk assumes responsibility for many of the clerical duties that are a necessary part of any client care area. The unit clerk learns these skills by taking a course that varies in length, depending on the area of the country. The course can average one semester of theory and clinical experience.

The *medical records department* is staffed by personnel who have attended a Health Information Technology or Health Information Management Program of study at the associate degree level or bachelor's degree level and learned the skills required for indexing, recording, and storing client electronic health records, which are legal documents. The client's old records are received or scanned into the EHR so the family physician receives answers to his medical questions. Minimal paper charts are currently utilized in the United States, due to the availability and portability of the EHR.

The surgeon creates postoperative orders for the client in the EHR, including an order for client-controlled analgesia (PCA) to control postoperative pain. The hospital *pharmacist* has studied for approximately 8 years (doctoral level) to become licensed to prepare, compound, and dispense medications prescribed by a health care provider or dentist. The pharmacist fills the order for the medications and IV solutions.

A referral is sent to the respiratory therapy department. The *registered respiratory therapist* (RRT) evaluates the client's respiratory status and suggests treatment to prevent respiratory problems. Health care workers in the respiratory therapy department can be certified respiratory therapists (CRTs) or registered respiratory therapists (RRTs) based on their level of educational preparation and performance on the national exams: Therapist Multiple Choice Examination (TMC) and the Clinical Simulation Examination (CSE). Today, respiratory therapists are educated at a minimum of a bachelor's level, inclusive of course work specific to the specialty area. Within 24 hours of admission to the ICU, the client is evaluated to be in stable condition. A *transport aide* and an *ICU staff member* transfer the client to the surgical unit.

SURGICAL UNIT: PREPARATION FOR DISCHARGE

The **nurse manager** in the surgical unit at this hospital is an RN who has graduated from a BSN program (4 years) or higher degree. As the nurse manager of the unit, this nurse is responsible for all the care given to clients and the overall functions of the nursing unit, including budgetary responsibilities. The client's *team leader* is an RN who studied for 2 years (associate degree), 1 to 3 years (diploma), or 4 years (BSN degree). This RN is responsible for formulating a plan of care for each of the assigned clients, collaborating with other members of the team to execute the plan, and modifying these plans as needed.

The team leader receives a verbal report and the current plan of care for the client from the ICU personnel. The team leader begins assessing the client for admission to the unit. The ***licensed practical nurse/licensed vocational nurse* (LPN/LVN)** assists the client to bed and immediately assesses their vital signs. The

LPN/LVN is a graduate of a 1-year practical/vocational nursing program. The LPN/LVN has passed a national examination (NCLEX-PN®) to become licensed. The LPN/LVN is assigned to the client to provide bedside care and administer medications. In some states, the NPA limits the LPN/LVN role in IV therapy administration and initial assessment of the client.

A referral is sent to the physical therapy department. The *physical therapist* (PT) assesses the strength of the client's unaffected extremities. The PT sets up a program of exercises and ambulation with no weight bearing on the right extremity. The goal of treatment is to restore function and prevent the development of complications. Physical therapy establishes an exercise regimen to strengthen the unaffected leg until the client can bear weight fully on the right side. The PT is educated at the doctoral level (5–6 years of college). The *physical therapy assistant* (PTA) has been educated in a 2-year community college or technical school setting. The PTA carries out the plan of care developed by the PT.

The client may also have an *occupational therapist* (OT), educated at the master's or doctoral level, working with the client to rebuild skills needed for everyday activities, such as activities of daily living (ADLs). In addition, other health care members may assist in providing care, such as an *occupational therapist assistant* (OTA) who has been educated in a 2-year community college or technical school setting.

Soon after the client is transferred to the surgical unit, the *social worker* or *case manager,* who could be an RN, visits the client and family to discuss discharge plans. Although discharge planning begins from the moment the client is admitted, there will be a focused effort on the transition of care at this point in the client's recovery. The social worker or case manager suggests that the client stays in an extended-care or rehabilitation facility for 2 weeks to participate in extensive physical therapy before returning to the farm. In addition, the social worker or case manager begins to assess what care and services the client might need following their stay at the extended-care or rehabilitation facility and provides for the transition of care from the hospital to home, ultimately. A focus on relationship-centered care is instrumental to successful client outcomes, a reduction of complications, and a readmission to the hospital. The financial impact of the care is also discussed. Social workers obtain a bachelor's degree in social work in 4 years and a master's degree in 1 to 2 additional year(s). The social worker talks to the client, PT, and the family. The family will be able to care for the client at home after the client receives an exercise program and skills training.

An ***unlicensed assistive personnel* (UAP)** member, often called a *client care technologist* (PCT) in a hospital setting, is assigned to take the client's vital signs. APs or PCTs perform treatments and skills assigned to them by the RN or the LPN/LVN. APs and PCTs are trained by the hospital for the specific duties they can perform. Training involves classes (sometimes virtual or self-study classes) and a clinical component. The training that APs and PCTs receive is short, varying among facilities. Alternative job titles, such as *assistive personnel* (AP), *nurse's aide* (NA), *nursing assistant*, and *client care assistant,* are used in some facilities. Minimum educational hours and core content are mandated by the federal government if the NA is employed in a facility receiving Medicare payments for services.

Because the client is 50 pounds overweight, the health care provider orders a weight-reduction diet. The *dietitian* teaches the client and the family the elements of weight reduction that will be continued when the client returns to the farm. A hospital dietitian is responsible for planning the meals and supplementary feedings for clients as well as the cafeteria meals for staff. The dietitian also supervises the preparation of food and instructs the clients and their families about nutritional issues and therapeutic diets. This health professional is educated in a 4- to 6-year college program, followed by a year of internship in a health care agency.

The *housekeeper* cleans the client room and bathroom every day during the hospitalization. Maintaining cleanliness is an effort to maintain medical asepsis (absence of germs) and provide a pleasant environment. The housekeeper receives training in the skills needed by the employed institution or through a short course in a technical school.

Finally, the client is discharged from the hospital, leaving by *Medi-Van* and is transported to the extended care or rehabilitation facility.

EXTENDED-CARE UNIT: ON THE ROAD TO REHABILITATION

The client's roommate in the subacute extended-care or rehabilitation facility is an 80-year-old individual who has had a stroke. The roommate is also preparing to go home after additional physical therapy. The PT conducts an initial assessment of the client and incorporates the hospital physical therapy plan of care with their findings. The *physical therapy assistant* (PTA) assists the client daily with exercises and ambulation, while using a walker, and minimum weight bearing on the right leg. A CNA is assigned to assist the client with personal care. CNAs are educated to give bedside care through courses of a minimum of 75 hours. Successful completion of this course of study makes the NA eligible to take a certification examination. When the exam is passed, the NA is placed on the state registry as a CNA.

A referral is sent to the occupational therapy department. The OT completes an assessment of the client. The OTA carries out the plan of care. The goal for the client is to be as *independent* as possible when returning to the farm, despite their physical limitations. Occupational therapy helps clients restore body function through specific tasks and skills, involving activities of daily living. Educational requirements of the OTA include a 2-year program to prepare OTAs for their roles.

The client receives their newly prescribed blood pressure medication from the *LPN/LVN*, who is also functioning in the expanded role as charge nurse in this facility. The *day supervisor*, an RN with a BSN, checks the client daily to monitor their progress. In addition, a physician or an NP collaborates with the staff to carefully assess any complications and monitors the client's progress. Ten days later, the client is ready to be discharged back to the farm. The client is pleased with her progress and is confident about going back home. The client knows that at this time she is unable to gather the eggs each day, but she is looking forward to cooking in the kitchen.

HOME CARE: SMOOTH TRANSITION TO PREVIOUS ROLES

Home care is coordinated care between physical therapy, occupational therapy, and nursing. The OT will assess the home for safety hazards and provide recommendations to improve the client's outcomes. These recommendations could include installation of safety devices (i.e., grab bars) and removal of safety hazards (i.e., floor rugs, loose boards on a deck, insecure entrance ways) throughout the home. The PT will continue evaluating strength and function after the client has returned home, if continued therapy is needed. An LPN/LVN or RN may also be a member of the home care team to assist with medication administration/management, treatments, and other supportive services. A *home health aide* can assist the client with activities of daily living (ADLs).

THE BENEFITS OF AN INTERDISCIPLINARY APPROACH

A primary goal of health care is to restore optimal physical, emotional, and spiritual health to clients. This goal is accomplished by promoting health, preventing further illness, and restoring health when illness or accident has occurred. Health care includes many specialized services. It is necessary for these health care workers to work together to integrate care to provide safe, high-quality, comprehensive health care (Fig. 14.1). These groups of health care workers are called the interprofessional *health care team*.

For the above-mentioned client to be rehabilitated after her fall, it took a minimum of 130 years of education for all the health care workers in this scenario to learn how to perform their respective jobs. The x-ray technician's x-ray confirmed the presence of a right hip fracture. The pharmacist supplied a narcotic pain reliever that relieved pain after the surgical procedure, allowing the client to move more freely and avoid complications. The treatment by the rapid response team (RRT) helped prevent pneumonia. The PTs, OTs, and nursing staff helped restore the client's health and prevent further illness by avoiding complications. The dietitian's expertise allowed the client to receive the basic nutrients she needed to maintain health, heal the fracture, and lose weight. Weight reduction education promoted health by pointing out the importance of keeping the client's weight within acceptable limits.

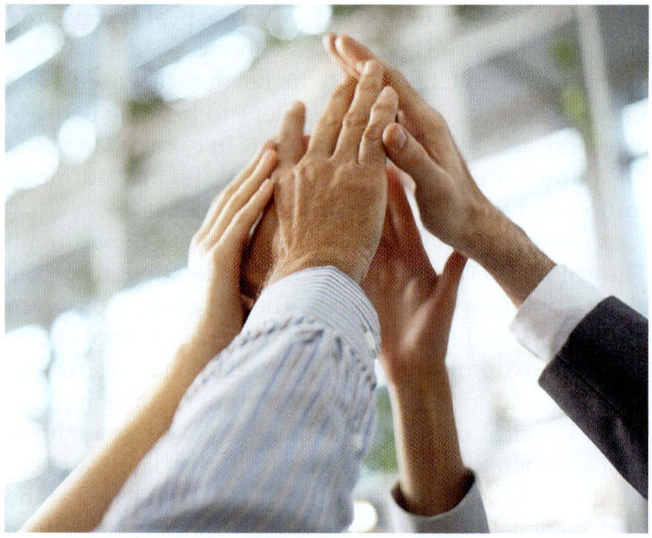

Fig. 14.1 All members of the health care team working together achieve great client outcomes. (From GlobalStock/iStock.)

As you can see from this case, each member of the interprofessional health care team, because of their specific preparation in a field of study, can increase the quality of health care for a client. It is impossible for one person to provide the knowledge, expertise, and skills that the health care team can provide. Everyone needs to work together. It is a team effort. The nurse is an important member of this team, often coordinating client care.

The members of the interdisciplinary health care team are generally on duty in acute or residential health care organizations 24 hours a day, 7 days a week. Some members of the team may not be scheduled at night or on weekends or holidays. Some team members are available on an on-call basis. In the community, health care workers' hours vary depending on the site of employment. Some sites are open Monday through Friday, during daytime hours only, whereas others also offer services in the evening. Other sites are open 7 days a week and sometimes 24 hours a day.

Each member of the interdisciplinary health care team needs to have good communication skills to ensure care is coordinated for the client's benefit (see Chapter 8). Fragmentation of care can be avoided. Each team member must be able to anticipate problems and avoid them, when possible, by using critical thinking skills. Nurses are encouraged to deepen their thinking by following the National Council of State Boards of Nursing (NCSBN) Clinical Judgment Measurement Model (see Chapter 12). When problems do occur, the team needs to use problem-solving skills to find solutions in the process of delivering care. In this way, the quality of client care is continuously improving. The team must strive continually to keep its client care relationship centered. The team needs to realize that cooperative effort is needed to reach client goals.

? Critical Thinking

Who Is Responsible for the Client's Recovery?

Who is responsible for the client's return to the farm? What value did each health care team member have in this client's recovery after her fall?

THE NURSING TEAM WITHIN THE HEALTH CARE TEAM: AN INTRAPROFESSIONAL ANALYSIS

Virginia Henderson, a nursing theorist, stated, "The unique function of the nurse is to assist the individual, sick or well, in the performance of those activities contributing to health or its recovery (or to peaceful death) that he would perform if he had the necessary strength, will, or knowledge" (Vera, 2024). Henderson refers to nursing's interest in illness and wellness. The direction of LP/LV nursing has been channeled by this definition. For an overview of "what is nursing" provided by the American Nurses Association, visit https://www.nursingworld.org/practice-policy/workforce/what-is-nursing/. It is necessary for LPNs/LVNs to understand their own role in the client's care, as well as understand the education, licensure, roles, and responsibilities of the varied members of the interdisciplinary health care team.

Nursing staff on the interdisciplinary health care team, who are focused on providing **client-centered care**, include *advanced practice nurses, RNs, LPNs/LVNs, student nurses, CNAs, assistive personnels,* and *unit managers*. Unit clerks, although not nurses, are an important part of the unit staff. Most people are unaware of the different types of nurses on the health care team. Some RNs do not know the educational requirements for LPNs/LVNs, and some LPNs/LVNs do not know the educational requirements for RNs. A common question from the public is: "What is the difference between a registered nurse and a licensed practical/vocational nurse?" Members of the health care team generally, and nursing specifically, need to know about one another. For this reason, general information about the education and roles of nurses is provided in this section.

REGISTERED NURSES

Education

The RN is a member of the largest group of health care workers in the United States. More than 3 million RN jobs existed in the workforce in 2023 (BLS, 2024). The graduates of the three types of educational programs for professional nurses currently take the same licensing examination. On successful completion of the NCLEX-RN® examination, these graduates hold the title of RN.

Associate degree in nursing program

- An **associate degree nursing (ADN) program** is a 2-year educational program that can be found in community colleges, junior colleges, and technical schools.
- The ADN program includes general education courses (e.g., courses in biological, behavioral, and social sciences), nursing courses, and clinical practice.
- Upon graduation, the nursing graduate receives an ADN and is eligible to take the NCLEX-RN® examination to become an RN.

Diploma program

- A **diploma program** is a 1- to 3-year educational program conducted by a hospital-based school of nursing.
- The diploma program comprises the same general education courses as 2-year programs, with nursing courses and clinical practice. Diploma programs traditionally emphasized clinical experience.
- Today, many diploma nursing schools have a university educational partner. The nursing student is likely to be dual enrolled (e.g., enrolled in a diploma nursing program and the university).
- Upon graduation, the nursing graduate receives a diploma in nursing and is eligible to take the NCLEX-RN® examination to become an RN.

Bachelor of science in nursing program

- A BSN program is typically a 4-year nursing program that can be found in public and private colleges and universities.
- The bachelor's program emphasizes course work in the liberal arts, sciences, and nursing theory. Clinical practice is included.
- Upon graduation, the nursing graduate receives a BSN and is eligible to take the NCLEX-RN® examination to become an RN.

Role of Registered Nurses

Graduates of all three nursing programs are prepared for entry-level staff nursing in a hospital, long-term care, or community setting upon passing the NCLEX-RN® examination. Although you may find 2- and 3-year RNs in supervisory and administrative positions, RNs with a BSN have been specifically prepared in their nursing education programs for advancement to these positions, as well as beginning positions in public health agencies.

According to the 2022 National Nursing Workforce Study, 47% of new RNs reported having a BSN degree when entering the nursing career (NCSBN, 2024). This education trend is expected to continue as the complexity of client care increases. Some demographic locations require a BSN to obtain employment in a hospital setting. This is particularly true for Magnet-designated institutions. Research supports the hiring of BSN-prepared RNs (AACN, 2019; Porat-Dahlebruch et al., 2022).

All RNs function under the NPA of the state of employment. RNs use the nursing process to identify client problems, formulate nursing diagnoses/identify concerns, and plan and evaluate care. The NCSBN Clinical Judgment Measurement Model offers a framework for advanced clinical decision making. **Standards of care** are used instead of care plans in some acute care agencies. These standards include the priority nursing diagnosis or concerns for each client, with appropriate assessments, nursing interventions, and expected outcomes (goals). Standards provide minimum guidelines for a consistent approach to delivering client care. The RN uses standards as a reference when individualizing client care.

RNs delegate the routine care of stable clients to assistive personnel. This allows RNs to do the following:

1. Plan care
2. Coordinate all the activities of care, including care from interdisciplinary health care team members
3. Provide care that requires more specialized knowledge and judgment
4. Teach clients, families, and other members of the health care team
5. Act as a client advocate

Box 14.1 Nursing Management and Executive Roles

Supervisor: Bachelor of Science in Nursing (BSN) preferred; deals with specific problems with nursing personnel; makes rounds to all nursing units on assigned shift to ensure clients' needs are met according to organization's procedures; acts as a clinical resource for collaborative decision making.

Nurse manager: Middle management position; Master of Science in Nursing (MSN) preferred; leads a specific clinical department (e.g., medical services); responsible for personnel, quality of care, safety, and unit budget.

Director: Entry level of executive role; MSN or master's degree in business or health-related field typically required; coordinates the development and implementation of strategies to initiate new programs and improve current services of several departments.

Chief nursing officer (CNO): Highest-ranking administrative nurse in a health care organization; MSN, master's in business or health-related field typically required; doctorate may be required in larger organizations; organizes and coordinates the nursing department; carries the responsibility for excellence in nursing that is consistent with the mission, vision, and values of the organization.

Independent role of the registered nurse. RNs function in an **independent** role in nursing by initiating and carrying out nursing activities. For example, RNs assess clients with an order to be on bed rest to identify potential complications in the respiratory and circulatory systems. The RN identifies the need for a turning routine, deep breathing and coughing, leg exercises, and range-of-motion exercises. If not contraindicated by the client's diagnosis and/or treatment, RNs add these nursing interventions to ordered care. Because of their level of education, RNs can identify which clients can and cannot receive these nursing interventions. In the community, RNs will initiate dietitian and social worker referrals. *It is the independent role in decision making that distinguishes RNs from LPNs/LVNs.* RNs have the ultimate responsibility for the nursing care given to clients.

Interdependent role of the registered nurse. When RNs carry out the legal orders of another health professional (e.g., the health care provider), they are functioning in an **interdependent** role. RNs function interdependently (collaboratively) when carrying out decisions about client care that are made jointly by members of the interprofessional health care team. The complexity of care delivery warrants collaboration to maximize high-quality client outcomes.

Advanced Education and Roles for Registered Nurses

The 21st-century health care system requires RNs to possess leadership skills to promote positive change. Effective nurse leaders, whether in a management position or not, possess the ability to develop a shared vision with nursing staff on quality, safety, and cost control that will help improve client outcomes. The typical four levels of nursing management are *supervisor*, *nurse manager*, *director*, and *chief nursing officer* (CNO) (Box 14.1). The practical/vocational nurse's role as charge nurse is discussed in Chapter 17.

The postgraduate educational opportunities available to RNs, to prepare them to be competent nurse leaders, are presented here, to explain the various RNs found in the health care team.

Bachelor of science in nursing program. After passing the NCLEX-RN® examination, associate degree and diploma graduates can enroll in an RN to BSN program. Programs vary in length, content, and mode of delivery, including online and competency-based programs.

Accelerated bachelor of science in nursing program. Individuals with a bachelor's degree in another discipline can earn a BSN in approximately 15 months. The 15-month program is very intensive, and when completed, the graduate is eligible to take the NCLEX-RN® examination.

Certification. Passing the NCLEX-RN® examination provides initial licensure in nursing and ensures basic competence for entry into nursing practice. After gaining work experience, RNs can receive **certification** from numerous professional nursing groups. The certification, which is awarded after passing a comprehensive examination, indicates the nurse has demonstrated competence in a select area of practice. The American Nurses Credentialing Center (ANCC), a subsidiary of the American Nurses Association (ANA), makes certification available to all RNs.

A certification as an advanced practice registered nurse (APRN) requires the completion of a designated MSN degree. Because certification needs to be renewed periodically, a certification allows the RN to demonstrate ongoing competence in a selected area of nursing. In addition, the National League for Nursing (NLN) offers a certification for nurse educators called the CNE (www.nln.org).

Master of science in nursing program. MSN programs prepare RNs for a specialty area in nursing, such as medical-surgical, pediatrics, leadership, nursing education, psychiatric/mental health, family care, and geriatrics. The MSN degree is a minimum requirement for teaching in many nursing programs. Generally, nurses with BSN degrees are the only nursing graduates who may elect to do graduate work in nursing at the master's and doctoral levels. However, MSN programs exist that offer an MSN degree to nurses with an undergraduate degree in an area other than nursing. The MSN degree then becomes the entry degree into nursing. Various nursing educational pathways exist, encouraging nurses to be lifelong learners.

Advanced practice registered nurse. With an additional degree, RNs can pursue expanded roles, called *advanced practice*. These nurses, who acquire specialized nursing knowledge and skills, demonstrate a greater depth and breadth of nursing knowledge and an increased complexity of skills and interventions. The term *advanced practice registered nurse* identifies the advanced practice roles of a clinical nurse specialist (CNS), an NP, a nurse anesthetist, and a certified nurse-midwife (CNM). Each of these nurses has a minimum of an MSN, obtained in a 1- to 2-year program of study.

- **Clinical Nurse Specialist** This RN has a minimum of an MSN in a specialty area (e.g., medical-surgical nursing). CNSs are a clinical expert in nursing practice based on the latest research and have certification as a CNS. When employed by health care organizations, CNSs serve as mentors, role models, and resources for staff by setting standards for nursing care. They provide direct care in challenging client situations and share knowledge, experience, and resources with staff. They are employed by hospitals, clinics, nursing homes, nursing schools as instructors, and in other community settings. In all sites of employment, CNSs can serve as educators, consultants, researchers, and administrators.
- **Certified Registered Nurse Practitioner (CRNP)** This RN has a minimum of an MSN and certification by a national body. Additional studies can include the Doctor of Nursing Practice (DNP), preparing the APRN for the highest level of clinical practice. Some states may mandate a doctoral degree. There are many areas of specialization for NPs, such as acute, adult, gerontological, pediatric, and psychiatric/mental health. Some NPs provide primary care in the community, in health care providers' clinics or in their own offices. Others provide acute care services in hospitals and long-term care settings. NPs order and interpret lab and diagnostic tests, develop medical diagnoses, and prescribe treatments, including medications, for acute and chronic diseases. State regulations differ for NPs regarding prescriptive privileges and other responsibilities. Review the state NPA for details.
- **Certified Nurse-Midwife** This RN has a minimum of an MSN and certification as a nurse-midwife. The CNM provides holistic maternal/family-centered health care in the areas of prenatal low-risk pregnancy, childbirth, the postpartum period, care of the newborn, and family planning at home, in hospitals, and birthing centers and in the gynecologic care of women. CNMs diagnose and treat illness, as well as prescribe medications.
- **Certified Registered Nurse Anesthetist** This RN has a minimum of an MSN, is a graduate of an accredited nurse anesthesia educational program, and has certification as a nurse anesthetist. CRNAs work in every setting where anesthesia is given, such as operating rooms, clinics, and outpatient surgical centers. CRNAs prepare clients for anesthesia; induce and maintain local, regional, and general anesthesia; provide post anesthesia care, including pain management; and provide emergency resuscitation.

Doctoral nursing program. The AACN advocates for advancing the nation's health by promoting doctoral programs in nursing to advance the profession of nursing in the clinical and educational settings (AACN, 2023).

There are two types of doctoral programs in nursing:

- Research-focused: These programs lead to an academic doctorate (PhD) or professional doctorate (DNS or DNSc). Most DNS or DNSc programs have transitioned to PhD programs to better meet the needs of the nursing industry. Graduates are prepared as scientists and do rigorous investigations into, for example, clinical or educational issues, to help build the science of nursing (NLN, 2024).
- Practice-focused (DNP): These programs graduate nurses who are considered nursing expert clinicians (nurses working in health care agencies) and most effective practice leaders who will facilitate changes in practice that enhance quality care (AACN, 2023).

Try This

Get to Know the Nursing Team

During an unhurried moment in the clinical area, ask RNs with whom you are working about the educational requirements to be employed in their positions. If there are initials of credentials behind their names, ask for them to be explained. Ask them why and how they achieved the certifications identified by the initials.

LICENSED PRACTICAL NURSES/LICENSED VOCATIONAL NURSES

According to the U.S. Bureau of Labor Statistics (2024), 630,250 LPN/LVN jobs existed in 2023, which is a drop from 724,500 in 2016. The LPN population contributes to the diversity of the nursing profession with over one-third of LPNs/LVNs identifying as racial minorities (NCSBN, 2024). LPNs/LVNs work in a variety of diverse care settings in collaboration with the interprofessional health care team.

Education

The educational program for LPNs/LVNs varies from 12 to 18 months. Part-time study can extend the program a few months longer. The LPN/LVN program can be public or private, located in trade, technical, vocational schools, and community colleges.

LPN/LVN education concentrates on clinical care at the bedside, based on fundamentals of biological sciences. Courses in basic nursing care, behavioral sciences, and biological sciences are included. Basic nursing care includes the administration of medications, inclusive of IV therapy in some states. LPN/LVN programs emphasize critical thinking, the development of clinical judgment, and the LPN's/LVN's assisting role in the nursing process as determined by each state's NPA. Clinical experiences in acute care facilities, long-term care facilities, and the community are included. At the completion of the program, the graduate receives a diploma in practical nursing and is eligible to take the NCLEX-PN® examination. Upon passing this examination, the graduate becomes an LPN/LVN.

Role of LPNs/LVNs

LPNs/LVNs must be aware of the content of the NPA of the state in which they are employed. The LPN's/LVN's role and scope of practice is found in this law, which differs from state to state. Administrative rules and regulations as well as interpretations of the state's Board of Nursing provide more specific details and clarification. Some NPAs list specifically what LPNs/LVNs can do, but others are written more broadly to allow for changes in the evolving role of the LPN/LVN. This eliminates the need for state legislatures to reopen the act and revise it each time a change is required. However, it also can cause the blurring of professional boundaries. It is the LPN's/LVN's responsibility to be aware of the law of the state in which employed. Generally, the role of the LPN/LVN includes the following:

- Caring for clients within the scope of the state's NPA while upholding clinical standards
- Providing care in basic and complex client situations under the **general supervision** of an RN, health care provider, podiatrist, or dentist, as determined by the state NPA, regardless of the site of employment
- Providing primary responsibility in the care of vulnerable populations with chronic, stable conditions
- Providing safe client care, serving as a client advocate, teaching clients, and communicating effectively, all while functioning as a collaborative member of the health care team

Employers expect LPNs/LVNs to think critically and solve problems in client care situations. LPNs/LVNs function interdependently when they offer input to the RN about the effectiveness of client care or offer suggestions to improve care. When LPNs/LVNs provide actual care at the bedside in acute care situations, their collection of data is valuable in determining whether progress is being made to meet client outcomes.

A major criterion in differentiating between the roles of the RN and LPN/LVN is that the LPN/LVN does not function independently. LPNs/LVNs must function safely and be accountable for their actions. They function interdependently (collaboratively) with other members of the health care team, while assisting the RN in client care. They should assume responsibility only for nursing actions that are within their legal role and that they feel competent in carrying out. Table 14.1 identifies the differences between the LPN/LVN and the RN roles.

? Critical Thinking

The Licensed Practical Nurse/Licensed Vocational Nurse Role in Assisting with the Nursing Process

Identify the major difference between the RN's and LPN's/LVN's roles in the nursing process. How is the LPN's/LVN's role in the nursing process determined? How does the LPN/LVN contribute to the plan of care?

Expanded Role of LPNs/LVNs

In some settings, LPNs/LVNs are being used in their expanded role. An example of the expanded role of the LPN/LVN is the charge nurse position in long-term care facilities. During implementation of care by the LPN/LVN, the RN is available for collaboration, assisting with decision-making when questions arise, either onsite (direct supervision), virtually, or by phone (general supervision). See Chapter 17 for further discussion of the expanded role of the LPN/LVN.

? Critical Thinking

Expanded Role of the Licensed Practical Nurse/Licensed Vocational Nurse

Refer to your state's NPA. Describe care situations in which the LPN/LVN should immediately collaborate with the RN or health care provider.

STUDENT NURSES

Student professional and practical/vocational nurses come to the clinical area under the supervision of clinical instructors. The clinical area is an extension of the classroom and skills laboratory. It provides an opportunity

Table 14.1 Differences Between the Roles of Registered Nurses and Licensed Practical Nurses/Licensed Vocational Nurses

FIVE NURSING ROLES	ROLES OF RN AND LPN/LVN
Professional	
Registered nurse (RN)	Can join and be involved in American Nurses Association (ANA) at state/local levels.
Licensed practical nurse/licensed vocational nurse (LPN/LVN)	Can join and be involved in the National Association of Licensed Professional Nurses (NALPN) and/or National Association for Practical Nurse Education and Service (NAPNES) at state/local levels (see Chapter 18).
Provider of Care	
RN	This is an independent and interdependent role. Initiates all phases of nursing process; formulates nursing diagnoses/concerns.
LPN/LVN	This is a dependent and interdependent role. Assists with all phases of the nursing process. Works with established nursing diagnoses. Identifies possible new nursing problems and reports them to the RN.
Manager of Care	
RN	Controls decisions regarding staff and the care of clients.
LPN/LVN	First-line manager in long-term care and other community settings. Responsible to RN nurse manager or health care provider.
Teacher	
RN	Initiates all health teaching.
LPN/LVN	Initiates health teaching for basic health habits (e.g., nutrition and cleanliness). Reinforces and assists with health teaching as directed by the RN in other areas.
Researcher	
RN	Theory is included in the 4-year program. All levels interpret and implement evidence-based practice guidelines. Participates in the research process.
LPN/LVN	Assists in implementing evidence-based practice guidelines. Collects data, as instructed, for research studies.

to apply theory into practice. When assigned to clients, **student nurses** have a responsibility to give safe care and function responsibly under the supervision of the instructor. Students are in the clinical area to learn, not to give service. It is possible that a clinical instructor can remove students from the assigned clinical site at any time for additional learning experiences.

Student nurses are members of the interdisciplinary health care team. They are expected to assist other team members in addition to performing their client assignments, supporting a safe clinical environment. Examples of such assistance include delivering trays, answering call lights in acute care and long-term care situations, and assisting clients and staff in the community. These activities assist students in developing communication and team-building skills.

Student practical nurses/student vocational nurses (SPNs/SVNs) are responsible for giving the same safe nursing care that LPNs/LVNs provide. This is a legal matter. Therefore the student role demands preparation and supervision.

CERTIFIED NURSING ASSISTANTS

CNAs are trained for their positions by combining federally mandated classroom instruction with close supervision by RNs while in the clinical area. Vocational and private schools offer programs that last a minimum of 125 hours and are up to 12 weeks in length, depending on state regulations. These programs combine classroom or virtual instruction with clinical practice. At the completion of the course, testing for competence occurs to meet federal Omnibus Budget Reconciliation Act (OBRA) requirements. When test results are satisfactory, the individual is placed in a registry and obtains the title of **CNA**.

CNAs function under the direction of RNs or LPNs/LVNs. CNAs, who work in hospitals, specialty hospitals, subacute units, and long-term care settings, assist in providing personal and comfort needs of stable clients. They are assigned routine tasks, sometimes involving housekeeping duties. Many CNAs are employed in long-term care settings. The supply of CNAs does not meet the demands of employers. According to the US Bureau of Labor and Statistics (2024), the projected percent increase in employment for NAs/orderlies is 4% from 2023 to 2033, equaling the average growth rate for all occupations. People in some areas of the country refer to male NAs as orderlies.

Some states offer an advanced NA course that teaches more complex skills. These skills can include tasks that are performed by an LPN/LVN. The demand for home health care workers continues to increase. CNAs are allowed to perform a wider variety of skills in the home as home health care workers. Some states offer a postgraduate course for CNAs to prepare them for the transition to home care. The comprehensive home care program may also be available to individuals without NA experience.

Keep in Mind

Diversity of Age for Coworkers on the Nursing Team

In addition to a diversity of educational preparation, the nursing team needs to contend with several different generations of its members. The different generations of personnel on the nursing team can have different goals, priorities, and work preferences (Tussing et al., 2024). Awareness and understanding of these differences are necessary for successful communication and working as a team. (See Chapter 1 for details.)

ASSISTIVE PERSONNEL

To use health care workers more efficiently and effectively, health care organizations have added another level of workers to the health care team. APs are trained by health care organizations to function in an assistive role to RNs and LPNs/LVNs. Some health care organizations require applicants for AP positions to be registered as CNAs. These workers learn selected skills by classroom or virtual methods, combined with some clinical teaching. Actual skills learned depend on which skills are needed in specific client-care units. APs are also known by the terms *patient (client) care technician*, *patient (client) care associate*, *nurse extender*, and *multiskilled worker*.

UNIT CLERKS

The job of the **unit clerk** is like an administrative assistant role, but the duties vary from site to site. Given the increase in the use of the EHR, the role of this clerk is changing. However, their skills continue to assist nurses and other members of the interdisciplinary health team. Unit clerks are trained on the job or in programs of several months' duration in technical schools or community colleges. Clerks prepare, compile, and maintain client electronic records on a nursing unit. Duties include scheduling lab tests, x-ray procedures, and surgeries; scheduling other appointments for services; routing electronic health records on client transfers or discharges; compiling the client census; answering the telephone; maintaining established inventories of supplies; distributing mail to clients; and generally ensuring that the unit functions smoothly.

UNIT MANAGERS

Some large health care organizations have a **unit manager** to supervise and coordinate management functions for client units. A college degree and supervisory experience are desirable for this position. This job is combined with on-the-job training for specific duties. Responsibilities include budgeting, supervision, assignment, and evaluation of all staff on the unit; coordination with all members of the interdisciplinary health care team; responsibility for client and unit outcomes, including satisfaction and quality ratings; and clarification of hospital compliance with insurance requirements, including Medicare. If a health care organization does not have unit managers, the unit clerk and the nurse manager assume these duties.

Critical Thinking

Know Your Health Care Team

During clinical, list the various members of the interdisciplinary health care team with whom you have contact. Draw a concept map describing their role on the team and education required for their job.

NURSING CARE DELIVERY METHODS: ORGANIZATIONAL PERSPECTIVES

With the goal of providing optimal care, the nursing team uses different methods to assign clients to staff. The methods evolved as a response to changing needs of the health care system, including staffing. Each of the methods is discussed in its general form as it was intended to function. Health care organizations modify these methods to fit their individual needs.

TOTAL PATIENT (CLIENT) CARE (CASE METHOD)

At the turn of the 20th century, families hired nurses to meet a client's special needs in the home. By the 1920s, private-duty nursing was popular. This **total patient (client) care** or case method of client care continued in various degrees into the 1960s. Reduced forms of case method, or a one-to-one relationship with a client, are found today in acute care situations and described as total client care (comprehensive care). In the case method, one nurse is assigned to one or two clients and is responsible for planning, organizing, and carrying out the care for these clients. Today, total care nursing occurs in intensive care or special care units. Nursing instructors frequently use the total client care method when assigning nursing students to the acute care clinical area.

FUNCTIONAL NURSING

During World War II, the **functional method** was a popular method for client assignments. RNs were in scarce supply because of the war. Hospitals increased the number of LPNs/LVNs and NAs to provide care to clients. The functional method of client care is task oriented. The tasks that must be done for clients are divided among the staff. For example, one person might measure all vital signs, another might do all treatments, and still another might make all the beds. This method's emphasis on efficiency and division of labor is based on the assembly-line-production concept found in industry.

Long-term care facilities create resident assignments by the functional method. A CNA helps the client with their physical care. An LPN/LVN administers medications and performs treatments. In addition to assuming responsibility for all care given to residents, the charge nurse, an LPN/LVN, has managerial (e.g., staff evaluations) and nonnursing duties (e.g., inventory of supplies).

Functional nursing can easily overlook holistic care, especially around psychosocial needs. This results in fragmentation of care. Although this method is efficient and appears to be less costly to implement, it can discourage client and staff satisfaction. The functional method, however, may work well in times of critical shortages or the need for large numbers of personnel, such as disaster situations and emergencies.

TEAM NURSING

After World War II, the shortage of RNs continued. The **team method** of client care was introduced and aided by the increasing number of LPNs/LVNs and NAs. The team consists of members with different levels of educational preparation, comprised of a **skill mix**. The team method is based on the belief that goals can be achieved through group action. The clients on a unit are divided into small groups. Small teams are assigned to care for the clients in each group. Assignments are based on the needs of each client and the skills of the team members. The team leader, an RN, leads the team. The RN continues to have the final responsibility of planning, coordinating, and evaluating the implementation of care for each client as well as supervising the personnel giving the care. In long-term care settings, the LPN/LVN can lead a team, with the collaboration of an RN supervisor.

In team nursing, the capabilities of each team member are used effectively. This increases the quality of care for the client and the satisfaction of the team members. An integral part of the team method is the team conference. During this conference, which should be held daily, team members share information about specific clients. Client problems are identified and solved, whereas plans of care are developed and revised. At times, alterations may be needed. When the unit is busy, changes may be needed, such as the team leader administering medications and performing treatments, team conferences being postponed, and the team method switching to a functional method for assigning care.

Because of the recent nursing shortage created by nurses leaving the workforce (from burnout due to the COVID-19 pandemic, Baby Boomer nurses continuing to retire, an increasing number of elderly in society, and the increasing need for health care for elderly), health care institutions, as permitted by the NPA, offer more responsibilities to the LPN/LVN in acute care settings. This change provides stability in the workplace and helps improve work environments.

PRIMARY NURSING

Hospitals adopted the **primary care method** several years ago to replace the team method for assigning care. The intention was to increase the quality of care for clients. This method was instituted in the 1970s because of the dissatisfaction of professional nurses with their lack of direct client contact and the fragmentation of care that resulted from functional and team nursing. In primary nursing, RNs individualize client care and accept responsibility and accountability for total client care, generally eliminating the need to delegate to other licensed staff. Ideally, staffing for this method requires a nursing staff composed entirely of RNs. Each nurse is assigned a maximum of four to six clients in a hospital setting. It is unlikely to see the primary nursing model used in a long-term care setting. There are no team leaders in this method. Each primary nurse is a bedside nurse, who has received the assignment from, and in turn reports to, the nurse manager.

The major characteristic of this method is the responsibility and accountability of the primary nurse. The primary nurse is assigned to a client on admission, develops the nursing diagnoses after the admission interview and assessment, develops a plan of care, and is responsible for the care of that client 24 hours a day until he or she is discharged. When the primary nurse is off duty, an associate RN continues the care as planned by the primary nurse. If any changes are contemplated in client care, the primary nurse must be contacted. LPNs/LVNs are used as assistive nurses in primary care situations.

Although primary nursing facilitates continuity of care, there are disadvantages. Positive aspects of the primary method can include shorter hospital stays for clients, improved communication among staff, and a more holistic focus of care. The challenge of recruiting enough RNs is one negative aspect, but the greatest drawback is the cost of a staff composed entirely of RNs. However, research by nursing experts reports that the use of BSN-prepared nursing staff improves client outcomes, such as client mortality rates (Porat-Dahlerbruch et al., 2022)

NURSING CASE MANAGEMENT

In acute care, **nursing case management** focuses on achieving **patient (client) outcomes** within a specified time frame. **Clinical pathways** or critical paths are used as tools by all health care workers involved with the client's care to identify incidents that must occur at specific times to achieve patient outcomes within an appropriate length of stay. These pathways provide a blueprint for care that includes a time frame of significant events that are expected to occur each day during the hospitalization.

Nursing case management became popular in the 1980s in response to the increasing complexity of client care, the need to use scarce nursing resources, and the meeting of client needs in a cost-effective manner in acute care. Depending on patient needs, this method uses all types of RNs, LPNs/LVNs, CNAs, and assistive personnels in varying ratios to deliver nursing service.

Some institutions use care maps, which are a combination of care plans and critical paths. The case manager keeps an eye on timely discharge and continuity of care in the community by planning, directing, and evaluating care throughout the client's hospitalization. The strength of the **case management method** for delivering nursing services is its focus of delivering cost-effective, quality care to clients with complex needs. Quality, service, and cost are timely considerations for health care in the 21st century.

Understanding these methods for providing nursing care is important for LPNs/LVNs. *Whether leading a team in a long-term care facility or working with an RN in a hospital, LPNs/LVNs can use their knowledge of care delivery methods to contribute new ideas, demonstrate their value to the health care team, and promote safe client care.*

? Critical Thinking

Care Delivery Method at the Clinical Setting

Make a list of the different clinical settings that your nursing program uses for clinical. Then identify the care delivery method used at each location. As an LPN/LVN, what changes could you suggest to the nurse manager if you had the opportunity?

Get Ready for the Next-Generation NCLEX® Examination

Key Points

- Each member of the interprofessional health care team provides a valuable service to clients. All members are equal in importance to each other.
- Members of the nursing team are RNs, LPNs/LVNs, student nurses, CNAs, APs, unit clerks (support staff), and unit managers.
- To understand where the LPN/LVN fits into the interprofessional health care team, be aware of the educational background, role, responsibilities, and possible licensing requirements of all levels of personnel on the team.
- To understand your position on the interprofessional health care team, keep current regarding new levels of health care workers and the method of delivering nursing care in your health care agency.
- Functional, team, and primary nursing are examples of methods used to deliver nursing care in acute care and long-term care facilities.
- Nursing case management focuses on achieving client outcomes within a specified time frame using clinical pathways.
- LPNs/LVNs can use their knowledge of care delivery methods to contribute new ideas, demonstrate their value to the health care team, and promote safe patient care.

Additional Learning Resources

Go to your Evolve website (http://evolve.elsevier.com/Carroll/success/) for the following FREE learning resources:

- Answers to Critical Thinking Scenarios
- Additional learning activities
- Additional Review Questions for the NCLEX-PN® examination
- Helpful phrases for communicating in Spanish and more!

Clinical Judgment Questions

1. An LPN/LVN hears the following discussion just prior to change of shift. What statement requires a follow-up discussion to ensure the RN understands the role (aligned with the NPA) of the LPN?

a. The LPN/LVNs assignment will focus on the clients with chronic but stable conditions.
b. The LPN can assist with the new admissions by orienting them to the unit and providing data to the RN facilitating the initiation of a care plan.
c. The LPN/LVN can focus on the care for the high-acuity client who needs hourly monitoring due to his exacerbation of chronic obstructive pulmonary disease (COPD).
d. The LPN/LVN is a critical member of the health care team supervised by a RN or health care provider.

2. What statement best describes team nursing as a method of delivering nursing care?

a. The method is based on the level of staff skill and client need.
b. Task-oriented efficiency is divided among staff across all shifts.
c. The RN plans and is accountable for total client care 24 hours a day.
d. This method uses scarce nursing resources in a cost-effective way.

3. What are appropriate job settings and matching roles of an LPN/LVN, working as a vital member of the interprofessional team? *(Select all that apply.)*

a. Community: Team member for a chronically ill pediatric client in their home
b. Long-term care: Charge nurse on the evening shift of a skilled care facility
c. Acute care: Charge nurse on a surgical unit
d. Community: Team member in a geriatric clinic
e. Long-term care: Director of Nursing supervising skilled care and personal care units

4. Indicate whether the following nursing roles are performed by the LPN/LVN and/or RN.

NURSE ROLE	LPN/LVN	RN
a. Formulation of nursing diagnoses		
b. Collaborative role in health teaching		
c. Charge/management position		
d. Performance of triage clients in an urgent care setting		
e. Collection of data while administering care		

5. Which of the following are possible methods of delivering nursing care in acute care agencies? *(Select all that apply.)*

a. Primary care
b. Case method
c. Team method
d. Functional method
e. Delegation method

6. Complete the following sentence by choosing from the list of options.

LPNs/LVNs can fulfill the role of a(n) _______, in the setting of a_______.

Assistive Personnel	home health agency
Chief Nursing Officer	urgent care facility
Nursing Supervisor	hospital
Nursing Director	long-term care facility

Critical Thinking Scenarios

Scenario 1

A student desires to work as an LPN/LVN in the role of being a charge nurse in a long-term care setting. The student knows that these jobs are highly competitive and often require a minimum of a year of experience as an LPN/LVN. Assist the student in creating a plan for success in meeting their goal. When should this plan be initiated? Why?

Scenario 2

During an SPN's/SVN's medical-surgical clinical rotation, an assigned client is preparing to go home after a 2-day hospitalization. The client shows the student a list of health care workers who cared for them during their hospitalization and marvels at the number of people involved in their care in only 2 days of hospitalization. The client asks the student to explain why there are all types of nurses, such as RNs, LPNs, and SPNs. What is the student's explanation?

15 Health Care Settings: Continuum of Care

Objectives

On completing this chapter, you will be able to do the following:

1. Compare the characteristics of public and private health care agencies.
2. Differentiate between official and voluntary (nonofficial) public health care agencies.
3. Differentiate between acute care agencies and nonacute care agencies
4. Describe characteristics of different types of hospitals.
5. Discuss the differences between the various ambulatory services, including the role of the licensed practical nurse/licensed vocational nurse (LPN/LVN).
6. Differentiate between community-based care facilities, including the role of the LPN/LVN.
7. Discuss the characteristics of the various facility-based care agencies, including the role of the LPN/LVN.

Key Terms

acute care
adult day care centers
ambulatory care clinics
ambulatory surgery centers
assisted care
board and care homes
community health nursing
continuing care retirement community (CCRC)
free clinics
freestanding
general hospitals
home health nursing
hospice care
long-term care (LTC)
long-term acute care (LTAC)
nonprofit community hospitals
official (governmental) health care agencies
outpatient clinic
palliative care
primary care
private health care agencies
proprietary hospitals (for profit)
public health care agencies
rehabilitation
residential care
skilled nursing facility (SNF)
specialized hospitals
teaching and research hospitals
United Nations (UN)
US Department of Health and Human Services (HHS)
US Public Health Service (USPHS)
voluntary or nonofficial health care agencies
wellness center
World Health Organization (WHO)

Darius and Hilary, two student practical nurses, are discussing what they learned in clinical today. Darius reports that he learned the value of documentation. He says, "I thought documentation was just to provide evidence of the care that I gave to the client, but today I learned that documentation is also valuable to show how acute the client's status is. If the documentation doesn't include all the symptoms the client has, then an inpatient status may not be approved, which could affect whether the client's insurance will pay for care at a skilled nursing facility after the hospitalization." Hilary states, "That is interesting. It is hard for us to see the continuation of care when we only care for our clients when they are at one clinical site. Not all clients are discharged home after the hospitalization. Today, my client was transferred to a rehabilitation facility. I was able to help with the transfer-of-care process so the client could continue to receive safe care at the next location." This chapter will focus on the health care settings and the value of the continuum of care, as well as the role of the licensed practical nurses/licensed vocational nurses (LPNs/LVNs).

Keep in Mind

Over the course of a normal lifetime, most clients will need all levels of care and effective transitions between health care settings. Understanding these settings along the continuum of care will assist student practical nurses/student vocational nurses (SPNs/SVNs) in guiding clients to resources as well as identifying the best "fit" for their future.

Not all health care agencies are the same. They differ in size, focus, quality of service, and how they are financed. SPNs/SVNs should consider doing research before making an application for a future job to make an informed choice about employment after graduation and passing the NCLEX-PN®. Composing questions to ask during an employment interview allows the applicant to obtain desired information. Refer to Chapter 18 for ideas.

Critical Thinking

Why is it important for the LPN/LVN to understand the various types of health care settings? How does this assist the client?

What is your vision for working as a nurse after you complete nursing school? What type of setting do you imagine yourself working?

PUBLIC VERSUS PRIVATE HEALTH CARE AGENCIES

Health care entities, which provide a vast array of services, are owned and operated today by public (government) and private entities. Private entities include both profit (proprietary) and nonprofit organizations. Table 15.1 outlines the major differences between public and **private health care agencies**. As you read about public and private health care agencies, think of them as potential sources of employment for LPNs/LVNs. Also consider how clients access these services, when they are needed, and how clients finance the services provided.

PUBLIC HEALTH CARE AGENCIES

There are two types of **public health care agencies**: official (government) and voluntary. Official (government) health care agencies have the following characteristics:

- Supported by tax money
- Accountable to the taxpayers and the government
- Focused on the delivery of disease prevention and wellness promotion programs
- Providers of direct health care services

Voluntary health care agencies have these characteristics:

- Supported by voluntary contributions
- Structured on a fee for services (often based on financial ability to pay)
- Generally aligned with public opinion but accountable to their supporters
- Organized with services determined by supporter interest, not legal mandate
- Focused on education and research
- Providers of direct health care services

Official and voluntary health care agencies can operate at the local, state, federal, and international levels.

Official (Government) Agencies

Official (government) health care agencies are established and supported by the local, state, federal (national), and international governments.

Local. The official health agency at the local level is the city or county health department. These agencies have the following characteristics:

- Funded by local tax money, as well as by subsidies from the state and federal levels of government
- Structured to carry out state laws (mandated) concerning community health
- Structured to carry out nonmandated programs, such as health promotion programs
- In collaboration with other government agencies, they respond to community health issues (e.g., outbreak of a contagious disease)

State. Each state has a state health department. This official health agency has the following characteristics:

- Funded by state tax money
- Funded by the federal government at times

Federal (National). The official health agency at the federal level in the United States is the US **Department of Health and Human Services (HHS)**.

- Managed by a person (appointed by the President of the United States) who advises the president on health matters
- Funded by federal taxes

HHS has 13 operating divisions, including 8 agencies in the **US Public Health Service (USPHS)**. Pertinent agencies to your studies include:

- *Administration for Children and Families.* Provides services to improve access to health care as a means of creating strong, healthy communities

Table 15.1 Comparison of Health Care Agencies in the Public and Private Sectors

	PUBLIC		
	OFFICIAL (GOVERNMENT)	**NONOFFICIAL (VOLUNTARY)**	**PRIVATE**
Support	Tax money	Voluntary contributions and fees for service	Fees for service
Primary service	Programs of disease prevention and wellness promotion	Research and education	Curing disease and illness
Additional services	Sometimes direct service of health care	Offer direct health services	Disease prevention and wellness promotion
Accountability	Taxpayers and government	Supporters, boards, and so forth	Owners
How programs determined	Mandated[a] and nonmandated	Supporter interest	Defined goals of the organization

[a]Some mandates can apply to all types of settings.

- *Administration for Community Living*. Aims at improving the lives of older adults and people with disabilities through services, research, and education while promoting community living instead of institutional living
- *Food and Drug Administration* (*FDA*). Ensures food, human and animal medications, biological products, medical devices, and electronic products that emit radiation are safe and, if applicable, effective
- *Centers for Disease Control and Prevention* (*CDC*). Provides leadership in health prevention and promotion programs and responds to public health emergencies
- *National Institutes of Health* (*NIH*). Funds biomedical research in its own laboratories and in universities, hospitals, private research institutions, and private industry; trains new researchers and promotes collecting and sharing of medical knowledge; consists of 27 institutes and centers, including the National Institute of Nursing Research (NINR)
- *Health Resources and Services Administration* (*HRSA*). Improves access to medical care by strengthening the health care workforce, which builds healthy communities and achieves health equity
- *Substance Abuse and Mental Health Services Administration* (*SAMHSA*). Improves the quality and availability of prevention, treatment, and rehabilitation services for individuals who are dealing with addictive and mental disorders, as well as supporting their families and communities
- *Agency for Healthcare Research and Quality* (*AHRQ*). Supports research aimed at improving the quality of care, reducing costs, broadening access, and improving client outcomes
- *Agency for Toxic Substance and Disease Registry* (*ATSDR*). Works to prevent exposure and to minimize adverse health effects associated with exposure to hazardous substances from waste sites, unplanned releases, and other sources of environmental pollution
- *Indian Health Services* (*IHS*). Provides comprehensive health services to American Indians and Alaskan Natives
- *Centers for Medicare and Medicaid Services* (*CMS*). Provides oversight of Medicare and Medicaid (federal level), Children's Health Insurance Programs, the Center for Consumer Information and Insurance Oversight, and related quality assurance activities

The preceding information was based on information retrieved from HHS.gov

International. Health activities take place at the international level through the **WHO**, an agency of the **United Nations (UN)**. WHO acts as a coordinating authority on international public health (WHO, 2024).

- WHO has their headquarters in Geneva, Switzerland.
- WHO collaborates to manage world-wide health emergencies, promote health, prevent illness, and extend health care access (https://www.who.int/about/who-we-are)
- WHO defines *health* as a state of complete physical, mental, and social well-being and not merely as the absence of disease or infirmity.
- WHO is funded through fees paid by member nations of the United Nations.

WHO coordinates international efforts to control outbreaks of infections such as coronavirus (COVID-19), ebola, severe acute respiratory syndrome (SARS), malaria, tuberculosis, influenza, and HIV/AIDS. WHO also sponsors programs to prevent and treat such diseases.

Voluntary or Nonofficial Health Care Agencies

Voluntary or nonofficial health care agencies (Table 15.2) are so named because they are nonprofit. The health services they provide are complementary to **official (government) health care agencies**. They often meet the needs of individuals with specific diseases (e.g., heart disease) and certain segments of the population (e.g., those with disabilities). Although paid personnel work in voluntary health agencies, volunteers support the agency. Voluntary organizations are sites for volunteer service and can provide clinical experience for SPNs/SVNs and LPNs/LVNs. (SPNs/SVNs can search the internet for additional names and numbers of voluntary health care agencies in their region.)

Try This

Local Health Care Agency

Identify an official and voluntary health care agency in your geographic area. What services does each agency provide locally?

PRIVATE HEALTH CARE AGENCIES

You may be most familiar with private health care agencies, which have the following characteristics:

- Entrances to the health care delivery system in the United States through private health care agencies, such as outpatient medical offices
- Private health care entities, both profit and nonprofit institutions
- Faith-based health care agencies that are nonprofit entities
- Corporations that often own a chain of health care facilities to achieve low-cost, high-quality outcomes
- Agencies owned by small groups of individuals (i.e., health care providers, community members), although this has been decreasing in number because of increasing health care costs
- Structured to offer a continuum of health care services (i.e., acute care, subacute, **long-term acute care [LTAC]**, long-term care [LTC], home care, and outpatient services)
- Supported by a fee for services (often based on financial ability to pay), health care insurance payment, or government-based payment (Medicare/Medicaid)

Table 15.2 **Examples of Voluntary or Nonofficial Agencies**

AGENCY	PURPOSE	CONTACT
American Cancer Society (ACS)	Cancer research, public information resources to clients, families, professionals	www.cancer.org
American Diabetes Association (ADA)	Resource for diabetic care and management including nutrition information, resources, and educational programs	www.diabetes.org
American Lung Association (ALA)	Research, professional education, resources for professionals and public	www.lung.org
American Heart Association (AHA)	Research and education on heart disease and stroke	www.heart.org
American Stroke Association	Research and education on stroke	www.strokeassociation.org
Alcoholics Anonymous	Rehabilitation and support to clients and families experiencing difficulty with alcohol addiction	www.aa.org
ALS Society of America	Collects data on individuals with amyotrophic lateral sclerosis (Lou Gehrig's disease) for research purposes; resource for public and professionals	www.alsa.org
Easter Seals National Headquarters	Research and rehabilitative services for disabled children and adults	www.easterseals.org
La Leche League	Information and support for breastfeeding mothers	https://llli.org
Narcotics Anonymous (NA)	Rehabilitation and support to clients and families experiencing difficulty with narcotic addiction	https://.na.org
United Ostomy Association of America (UOA)	Education, information, and advocacy for clients undergoing intestinal or urinary diversion procedures	www.ostomy.org
Volunteer of America	Ministry of service focused on assisting people to reach full potential	www.voa.org

- Focused on disease prevention and wellness promotion
- Mandated by government policies, such as the Affordable Care Act (ACA), in regard to health care access and client payment structures

The various types of private health care agencies, such as hospitals, community-based care agencies, and facility-based care agencies will be discussed later in this chapter.

ACUTE CARE AGENCIES VERSUS NONACUTE CARE AGENCIES

ACUTE CARE AGENCIES

Hospitals

According to the American Hospital Association (AHA) 2024 Annual Survey, there are 6210 registered hospitals and 400 health care systems in the United States (AHA, 2024). Both federal government hospitals and community hospitals may be teaching and research hospitals. A discussion on community hospitals, federal or state (government) hospitals, teaching and research hospitals, and critical access hospital follows.

Community hospitals. AHA defines community hospitals as "including nonfederal, short-term general, and specialty hospitals" (AHA, 2019). Many registered community hospitals are short-term general hospitals, providing a diverse range of medical services. This setting for health care is often called **acute care**.

For most conditions, **general hospitals** can accommodate a client's needs. However, a general hospital may not have specialists with expertise in treating serious or unusual medical conditions. They also may not have the equipment, laboratory facilities, or other resources necessary to treat a serious or unusual medical condition. The client may need care from a hospital center that has highly skilled specialists with advanced knowledge of the condition. **Specialized hospitals** offer services related to a particular disease or condition, such as trauma; obstetrics and gynecology; eye, ear, nose, and throat; rehabilitation; and orthopedics.

Community associations and religious organizations operate nonprofit community hospitals. These nonprofit hospitals provide short-term inpatient care for clients with acute illnesses and injuries. **Nonprofit community hospitals** are dependent on gifts and donations to supplement sources of revenue. Ultimate responsibility for the hospital rests with the board of trustees, usually chosen from the community's business and professional individuals, serving without pay. The board of trustees appoints a paid administrator to manage the hospital.

For-profit community hospitals, sometimes referred to as **proprietary hospitals**, operate for the financial benefit of the owner of the hospital and investors. The owner may be an individual, a partnership, or a corporation. With good management techniques, the hospital runs efficiently, and a profit can be made.

Federal or state government hospitals (public hospitals). Public hospitals include Veterans' Health Administration (VHA), state, county, and municipally owned and operated nonprofit hospitals. Hospitals for people with serious mental illness are funded by federal, state, or county funds.

Teaching and research hospitals. Both community hospitals and federal government hospitals can be **teaching and research hospitals**. These hospitals have a variety of goals, including the following:

- Treating clients, especially those with serious or unusual conditions
- Providing training sites for health care providers, nurses, and other health professionals
- Researching and developing treatments for disease conditions, health promotion, and strategies to deliver low-cost, high-quality care

These hospitals are mostly affiliated with medical schools and have access to highly skilled practitioners.

Critical access hospitals. HRSA has provided specific Medicare Conditions of Participation for hospitals located in rural settings who meet certain criteria. According to CMS (2021), certain requirements for the critical access hospital (CAH) certification include:

- no more than 25 inpatient beds
- an annual average length of stay of no more than 96 hours for acute inpatient care
- emergency care offered 24 hours, 7 days a week
- location within a rural area, at least 35 miles away from any other hospital or CAH

CAH provides care for common conditions and outpatient care, while stabilizing and referring more complex conditions to larger health systems.

Try This

Hospitals

What kind of hospitals do you have in your area? Do they currently employ LPNs/LVNs? If so, which nursing units employ LPNs/LVNs?

Ambulatory Care Agencies

In recent years, accelerated by the implementation of the ACA, less client care services occur in acute care and specialty hospitals. Clients are more likely to receive care in **ambulatory care agencies**, such as subacute or community-based settings, receiving complete care within the same day. Care delivered in an ambulatory care-based or community-based setting, instead of an acute care setting, results in cost savings for the insurance company. Lower copays and deductible payments incentivize clients to receive care in these settings.

The continual rise in the cost of inpatient care has resulted in the rapid development of a variety of ambulatory services. Consequently, the number of inpatient days and the length of stay in acute care facilities have decreased. Ambulatory services offer less expensive care because it avoids admission to an acute care facility. Clients come to these facilities for assessment, advice, monitoring, teaching, treatment, evaluation, and care coordination.

Private sector ambulatory settings are in the following places:

- University hospital outpatient departments
- Community hospital outpatient departments
- Health care provider group practices
- Health maintenance organizations (HMOs)
- Health care providers' offices
- Freestanding ambulatory centers
- Urgent care centers
- Nursing care centers

Public sector ambulatory settings are in the following:

- Community health clinics
- Indian Health Service
- Community and migrant worker health centers

Outpatient clinics or medical offices. **Outpatient clinics** or medical offices provide follow-up care to clients after hospitalization and have the following characteristics:

- Manage disease on an ambulatory basis for those who do not require hospitalization
- Are a part of health care facilities or are **freestanding** (i.e., not attached to a hospital)
- Operate with scheduled appointments
- Include specialty areas, such as family care, diabetes, neurology, allergy, and oncology
- Determine the number of specialized clinics or medical offices by the population in the area and the medical needs of the population
- Employ a diverse group of interprofessional health care team members
- Employ advanced practice registered nurses (APRNs) to provide care where the number of physicians cannot meet the needs of the community, usually in rural areas (APRNs function within the state NPA; see Chapter 7)

Ambulatory care clinics. Services are available in **ambulatory care clinics** for walk-in clients who do not have an appointment when they are unable to see a **primary care** provider. These facilities have the following characteristics:

- Make primary health care available as an alternative to care from a family health care provider or a more expensive emergency department
- Are used by people who do not have a family health care provider
- Are used by clients who desire more convenient services outside of regular office hours
- Are named according to the type of care provided (e.g., convenience clinics, express care, quick care, urgent care)

One-day (or same day) surgical care centers. One-day (or same day) surgical care centers (**ambulatory surgery centers**) perform surgery at a scheduled date and time. Clients receive discharge orders after they recover from anesthesia and are in stable condition, which will be by the end of the same day, due to no overnight services. These surgery centers have the following characteristics:

- Eliminate the need and monetary charge for overnight hospitalizations
- Offer services that are also known as outpatient surgery within an established hospital
- Provide outpatient surgery services with or without affiliation to hospitals
- Offer most types of surgeries, except to those clients who have a complex history or require complex surgical procedures

Free clinics. Some communities have established **free clinics** or reduced-fee clinics as an alternative means of providing primary health care. These free clinics have the following characteristics:

- Offer services to clients who cannot afford traditional health services or are reluctant to use more traditional services; cost is based on income
- May limit care to age and/or income
- Are generally staffed with one salaried administrator, volunteer health care providers, and nurses
- Make policy decisions for the clinic as a volunteer board

> **Try This**
>
> **Ambulatory Care Services**
>
> What ambulatory care agencies do you have in your area? Do any of them employ LPNs/LVNs? If so, what skills will the LPN/LVN perform under the registered nurse (RN)/health care provider supervision?

NONACUTE CARE AGENCIES

Community-Based Care Agencies

Many older adults live at home and utilize community services as well as home care services to meet their health care needs. Independent and assisted-living facilities can provide services that allow the older adult to age in place (stay at home while aging).

Community health nursing agencies. Nurses have always been at the forefront of **community health nursing** activity. The major focus of community health nursing is to improve the health status of communities or groups of people through public education, to screen for early detection of disease, and to provide services to people who need care outside the acute care setting.

Community health nurses collaborate with different people and groups on the prevention and modification of health issues. Among the possible roles are advocate, caregiver, case manager, health planner, occupational health nurse, school nurse, and teacher. Community health nursing services may exist as a part of an outpatient clinic service, a service attached to an HMO, or a freestanding private service.

Home health nursing agencies. Home health agencies are public or private agencies that provide home health services that are supervised by a licensed health professional in the client's home, either directly or through arrangements with other agencies. Several types of home health agencies include the following:

- Public, nonprofit (e.g., visiting nurse association)
- Public, nonprofit, freestanding (e.g., city, county, including county visiting nurse associations, and state health departments)
- Private or nonprofit hospital-based (e.g., hospital home health agency)
- Private, for-profit, freestanding (e.g., home health care owned by a person or corporation)

Home health nursing differs from hospital and long-term care with an increased focus on relationship-centered care (i.e., family and the client's environment). The purpose of home health nursing is to promote, maintain, or restore health or minimize the effects of illness or disability. A significant role is to teach the client and the client's family self-care. Skilled services in home health care include the following:

- Skilled nursing
- Physical therapy
- Speech-language therapy
- Occupational therapy
- Medical-social services
- Health aide services
- Other therapy services (e.g., respiratory, nutritional, podiatry)
- Hospice services

RNs provide skilled nursing services and direct the nursing staff. LPNs/LVNs provide basic nursing services under the supervision of an RN. *Depending on state regulations and agency policy*, LPNs/LVNs can provide home health services. Coordinated care focuses on the goal of achieving the highest level of function for the client. The plan of care for all disciplines requires an ordered and recertified treatment plan by a health care provider according to current regulations. Examples could include the following:

- Teaching, supervising, administering, or preparing medications for self-administration
- Administering injections
- Blood glucose testing
- Assisting in creating a safe environment
- Treatments
- Ostomy care
- Wound care and dressings
- Bowel and bladder retraining
- Oxygenation and respiratory care

Try This

Community Health and Home Health Nursing Services

Are there community health nursing services or home health nursing services available where you live? What services do they offer? Do they employ LPNs/LVNs? What skills are the LPNs/LVNs expected to perform under RN supervision?

Adult day care centers. Hospital-based and freestanding **adult day care centers** provide services for individuals who need supervision because of physical or safety needs but are not candidates for residing in a long-term care facility. Clients with families who can assist the individual during evening hours and on weekends may prefer adult day care centers instead of an admission to a long-term care facility.

The purpose of adult day care is to provide mental stimulation, socialization, assistance with activities of daily living (ADL), basic observation, and a safe environment. The typical services include transportation, meals, therapeutic activities, nursing interventions, and rehabilitation activities. The supervisor is often a social worker or RN. Certified nursing assistants (CNAs) and personal care assistants who meet state requirements assist with ADLs. Volunteers play a significant role at adult day care centers. Large adult care centers employ LPNs, working in collaboration with an RN.

Try This

Adult Day Care Services

Is adult day care available in your area? Where are the centers located, what services are offered, and who staffs them? Do they employ LPNs/LVNs? If so, what are the LPNs'/LVNs' responsibilities?

Wellness Centers

The emphasis on promoting wellness continues to result in a multitude of services offered in this area of health care services. Hospitals develop programs to detect disease in early stages but also develop programs to promote wellness. **Wellness center** programs include nutritional counseling, exercise programs, stress reduction, and weight control. The private sector continues to be active in the wellness area. People have developed an interest in exercise and fitness clubs, weight-reduction programs such as Weight Watchers, smoking cessation classes, stress control, and parenting classes. LPNs/LVNs are often employed to work in collaboration with an RN or an APRN.

Try This

Wellness Programs

Choose one wellness program in your area. Find out what services it offers and the qualifications of the staff that provide services. Which programs employ LPNs/LVNs?

Facility-based Care Agencies

Continuing care retirement communities. **Continuing care retirement communities (CCRC)** provide a continuum of living options from independent living, assisted living, and skilled nursing care, all on one campus. Residents can move from one level of care to another to accommodate their changing needs because the facility provides a complete range of housing and health care services. Residents who enter when they are healthy can transition to care as needed. Short-term skilled care is also often available for residents who have had surgical procedures or medical complications and require rehabilitation. Financial payment options can be complex; clients and families should evaluate their needs carefully.

Options that exist include a life-care or life extended contract, modified contract, or fee-for-service contract. The life-care contract has a high entrance fee; however, it offers unlimited assisted living and skilled care as needs arise. Applicants can have admissions denied because of their health history. The fee-for-service contract requires assisted living and skilled care that are charged at market rates. Variations exist, and the "fit" is critical from both a financial and quality-of-life aspect. Visit the site aarp.org for more details.

Independent living facilities. Independent living apartments are not licensed entities nor are they regulated for health care delivery. People living in these facilities are not there for personal or medical care, but they like to live with seniors who share their interests. Facilities schedule planned activities, including trips and bus services for shopping.

Assisted living programs. Assisted living programs (ALPs) provide "a home with services" (**assisted care**) that emphasizes a resident's privacy and choice. Living quarters are available to older adults who want to remain as independent as possible but cannot manage all their ADLs. Residents typically have private, locking rooms and bathrooms (or apartments), which are managed by the resident. Living quarters are handicapped accessible to accommodate the changing needs of aging. Help with ADLs is available but not 24-hour basic care. These services can include bathing, dressing, daily activities, and health maintenance. Care management and skilled nursing services, when needed, come from an outside agency. ALPs may accept private pay, as well as Medicaid and Social Security Supplemental Income (SSI) recipients.

The facilities are family oriented, provide activities, and assist the residents with transportation for outside appointments. The fee for one- or two-bedroom apartments typically includes utilities, weekly housecleaning, and linen changes. An additional fee exists for meals, assistance with medication administration, and assistance with ADLs. However, if needed and desired, the resident may request a transition to a skilled nursing facility (SNF) if that level of care becomes necessary. Some institutions offer a full continuum of living options, including independent living, assisted living, and skilled care, called CCRCs. Dementia care units may also be available.

Board and care homes. **Board and care homes** are also known as adult care homes, group homes, or family-type homes. The facilities offer temporary or long-term **residential care**, housekeeping, and personal care for adults unrelated to the operator. The owner or manager will provide and supervise assistance with ADLs, self-administration of medication, preparation of meals, special diets, and transportation. The residence, typically a single-family home, has a license as an adult family home or adult group home. The Department of Social Services oversees the operation.

Skilled nursing facilities. In an **SNF**, skilled or licensed nursing personnel provide services and supplies. Skilled nursing care is nursing care that is medically necessary to improve the quality of the client's health or to maintain or to slow decompensation of a client's condition, including palliative treatment. See www.longtermcarelink.net/ for more details.

- RNs and collaborating LPNs/LVNs plan the care of the clients, including wound care after major surgery, administering medications, including administering/monitoring intravenous medications for a severe infection or other health issues.
- Physical therapists (PTs) help improve strength and balance problems that have caused a client to have difficulty walking or getting on and off the bed, toilet, or chairs. PTs help clients improve their functional ability and safety.
- Occupational therapists (OTs) can provide care on a long-term basis if clients require adaptive assistance using the upper body. Examples of therapy may include assistance in learning how to dress or feed themselves. In addition, OTs assess the environment for adaptive equipment needs or room redesign to enhance functional ability and safety.
- Speech therapists help regain the ability to communicate after medical conditions, such as a stroke.

Monitoring vital signs, administering medications, performing wound care, and other procedures are normally associated with skilled nursing care. The delivery of skilled nursing care is based on a written care plan. Residents who meet Medicare requirements and skilled care requirements receive payment from Medicare and private sources. There are many specific requirements that must be met for Medicare to cover skilled nursing care after a hospitalization, including an inpatient hospital admission of at least 3 days. Observation hospital admissions at an acute care hospital do not qualify for skilled nursing care after the hospitalization. It may be confusing to clients as to whether they are hospitalized as an observation status or an inpatient status, because they may reside on the same unit and receive similar care. It is the role of LPNs/LVNs to be an advocate for clients as they encourage clients and families to seek understanding regarding the client's admission status. The impact can be thousands of dollars. Visit www.medicare.gov/coverage/skilled-nursing-facility-care.html for details.

Try This

Inpatient Status

When you have clinical in a hospital setting, determine if your client is currently receiving care as inpatient or outpatient (observation) status. Try to determine if the status has changed since admission. The status is determined daily. Keep in mind that if the client has Medicare or a Medicare Advantage plan, skilled nursing services after the hospitalization may only apply if the client requires the care and the client has been hospitalized for at least 3 days as an inpatient stay.

Rehabilitation facilities. After a client remains stabilized following an acute illness or injury, a **rehabilitation** phase, lasting from days to years, may follow. These services help the client return to their pre-injury/pre-illness function or highest level of functioning possible. Rehabilitation may take place in the following areas:

- Rehabilitation centers
- LTAC facilities
- LTC facilities
- Outpatient facilities
- Group residential homes
- Client's home

The focus, regardless of the setting, is the return of function and prevention of further disability.

Try This

Rehabilitation Services

Where are the rehabilitation health services available in your area? What kind of rehabilitation is available? Do they hire LPNs/LVNs? If so, what skills will LPNs/LVNs perform with RN supervision?

Long-term care facilities. Various diverse elder living models exist today that focus on deinstitutionalizing **LTCs** by eliminating large nursing facilities and creating smaller units that mirror more closely a typical home environment. A newer agency under the US Department of Health and Human Services, the Administration for Community Living, focuses on ways to promote community living instead of institutional living for elderly clients. The relationship between staff, management, residents, and families is valued, including introducing pets, gardens, and children to the long-term care facility. These models focus on allowing residents to have more autonomy and choices like they did when they lived in their own home. Choices could include when to get up in the morning and the timing for meals and activities. Social interaction is important and is promoted by the design of the unit and surrounding environment. Defined resident space exists with small collaborative space, creating an environment that encourages interaction. Small dining rooms, encouraging a family-like atmosphere, exist instead of a large dining hall.

LTCs include a range of medical services designed to help people who have disabilities or chronic care needs. Common reasons why clients live in LTCs can include having chronic disease (i.e., diabetes and high blood pressure), disability, poor diet, and lack of exercise. All long-term facilities focus on promoting independence, maintaining function, and supporting autonomy as much as possible. Medicare, Medicaid, and the VHA/Veterans Benefit Administration (VBA) will cover the cost of LTC under certain conditions. For more details, visit https://www.longtermcarelink.net/.

Try This

Long-term Care Facilities

What LTC facilities are in your area? What level of care do they offer? Do they hire LPNs/LVNs? If so, what skills do LPNs/LVNs perform?

Hospice care centers. Hospice, or end-of-life, services are available to people who have been certified as terminally ill. The philosophy of **hospice care** is to maintain comfort as death approaches, while supporting family needs in the process. Hospice care is offered in a hospital or a freestanding agency if pain and symptom management are necessary, if the family caring for the person needs respite, or if terminal care is needed. Hospice home care is also available to those who wish to pass in their own home. Because RNs, LPNs/LVNs, home health aides, CNAs, and volunteers can provide hospice care, home care tailors to the individual's needs.

Palliative care provides comfort care to optimize the client's quality of life when experiencing a chronic condition. Palliative care can begin at the onset of treatment and continue at any stage of illness, whether terminal or not—from diagnosis to cure. While receiving palliative care, the client may still choose to receive life-saving measures (National Institute on Aging, 2021). Visit https://www.nia.nih.gov/health/hospice-and-palliative-care/what-are-palliative-care-and-hospice-care to further understand the difference between palliative and hospice care.

Try This

Develop Your Own Style

Using clustering (concept mapping) as shown in Chapter 2 as your guide, develop your own creative tool to summarize the health care settings described in this chapter.

Critical Thinking

Has My Vision Changed?

Throughout your course of study, you will find that your interest in a particular area of nursing may change. Based on what you have learned from reading this chapter, what kind of health care setting is most appealing to you at this time?

Critical Thinking

Client Care Transitions

Given the diverse array of client care settings, how will you support the client's understanding of the continuum of care that will best meet his or her needs, to achieve the highest level of client independence?

Get Ready for the Next-Generation NCLEX® Examination

Key Points

- Health care services exist in public and private sectors.
- Public health care agencies have classifications of official and voluntary.
- Official public health care agencies receive support from taxes.
- Official public health agencies are local, state, and federal agencies.
- The official health agency at the federal level in the United States is the US Department of Health and Human Services (HHS).
- The public health care agency of the United Nations is WHO.
- Voluntary health care agencies receive support from voluntary contributions and provide complementary services to official health care agencies.
- Private health care agencies are proprietary (for profit).
- Most hospitals are comprised of four types: community hospitals, federal government hospitals, teaching and research hospitals, and critical access hospitals.
- Primary care describes the point at which people usually enter the health care system.
- General hospitals deal with a full range of medical and surgical conditions.
- Specialized hospitals provide care to clients with specific diseases or health care needs.
- Teaching and research hospitals offer treatment for serious or unusual conditions and usually are a training site for health professionals.
- Ambulatory health care services are available in both private and public sectors.
- Free clinics provide primary care to individuals who cannot afford traditional health care services.

- Short-term care, also known as subacute care or transitional care, provides rehabilitation services and specialized care as a transition between hospital and home.
- Board and care homes, also known as adult care homes, group homes, or family-type homes, offer housing and personal care.
- Long-term care facilities provide a range of services for people living with severe disabilities and chronic care needs.
- Multiple elderly living models exist and continue to emerge, providing an innovative approach different from traditional skilled care and assisted living facilities, aimed at improving the resident experience and community living.
- Continuing care retirement communities provide a continuum of living options as needs change.
- Community health, public health, and home health services share many responsibilities. A major difference in home health is providing direct client care in the home setting.
- Adult day care centers provide socialization, mental stimulation, assistance with ADLs, basic observation, and health referrals.
- Wellness centers provide nutritional counseling, exercise programs, stress reduction, weight control, and other services.
- Hospice staff maintain the comfort of the client as death approaches and support to the family.
- Palliative care staff maintain the comfort of the client at any point in their disease process, as needed.
- Responsibilities of care agencies continue to be modified because of changes in the health care system.

Additional Learning Resources

Go to your Evolve website (http://evolve.elsevier.com/Carroll/success/) for the following FREE learning resources:

- Answers to Critical Thinking Review Scenarios
- Additional learning activities
- Additional Review Questions for the NCLEX-PN® examination
- Helpful phrases for communicating in Spanish and more!

Clinical Judgment Questions

1. What health agency is most likely to be a major resource if you have a measles outbreak at your health care institution?

a. WHO
b. CDC
c. NIH
d. FDA

2. Which statement best describes how official and voluntary agencies differ?

a. Official agencies are proprietary.
b. Voluntary agencies are tax supported.
c. Official agencies are accountable to the government.
d. Voluntary agencies emphasize research.

3. What quality/skill set described below would indicate a need for staff training when working with hospice?

a. Knowledge of the physiologic process occurring as death approaches
b. An ability to sit without the need for dialogue, if desired by the individual
c. Feeling the need to tell a client about personal beliefs on life after death
d. Willingness to honor the person's request for food, conversation, and visitors

4. Indicate which statement accurately describes community health nursing agencies or home health agencies.

NURSING SERVICE	COMMUNITY HEALTH	HOME HEALTH
a. Provides direct nursing services to people in their homes		
b. Nursing services focus on prevention and case finding		
c. Focus on population health vs. individual health		
d. Assists with creating a safe home environment		
e. Promotion of antismoking programs		

5. How do new elder living models differ from traditional long-term care facilities? *(Select all that apply.)*

a. Traditional homes provide personal care by assigning an LPN/LVN to give total care to the residents.
b. New elder living models follow strict schedules for eating, bathing, to provide a sense of security.
c. In new elder living models, elders have flexibility when they get up, eat, bathe, go outdoors, and receive visitors.
d. New elder-living-modeled home designs could minimize the need for wheelchairs.
e. Traditional homes establish times for meals that meet the needs of most of the residents.

6. How should a nurse explain the different levels of long-term health care to someone planning to seek placement for elderly relatives? *(Select all that apply.)*

a. Personal care assists with basic care needs and supervision, to maintain a safe environment.
b. Assisted care facilities offer 24-hour supervision and support the elderly to "age in place," providing flexible service options.
c. Specialty hospitals can provide rehabilitation services following a major neurological event (i.e., stroke).
d. Skilled care facilities can provide 24-hour supervision and access to many health care services, including dementia care.
e. Assisted living facilities can provide total nursing care for immobile clients.

7. Complete the following sentence by filling in the blanks.

The official health agency at the _____ level in the United States is the _____.

local	Public Health Services
state	World Safety Agency
federal	The Food and Drug Administration
international	Department of Health and Human Services

Critical Thinking Scenario

Scenario 1

An SPN/SVN is graduating soon and is thinking about where to work. While working in a long-term care facility, the nursing student developed an interest in working with elderly clients. How might this student find information about what is available in the area and what the LPN/LVN responsibilities will be in each facility?

The Health Care System: Financing, Issues, and Trends

16

Objectives

On completing this chapter, you will be able to do the following:

1. Discuss key characteristics of the current US health care system.
2. Differentiate the different health care service payment options for clients, such as personal payment, private health insurance, and public health insurance.
3. Discuss the nurse's role in containing health care costs in the workplace.
4. Describe issues facing the health care system and ways licensed practical nurse/licensed vocational nurses (LPNs/LVNs) can promote change.
5. Discuss the benefits of the current trends in the health care system and the role of LPNs/LVNs.
6. Examine strategies for how nurses can effectively respond to changes in the health care system.

Key Terms

coinsurance
copayment
cost containment
deductible
diagnostic-related group (DRG)
entitlement program
fee-for-service
Health and Medicine Division of the National Academies (HMD)
health care provider
health maintenance organization (HMO)
managed care organization (MCO)
Medicaid
Medicare
National Patient Safety Goals
preferred provider organizations (PPOs)
premium
private pay
prospective payment system (PPS)

Keep in Mind

Do you pay federal or state taxes? If you do, then you help pay for health care for others. Do you have health insurance? If you do not, who pays for your health care?

A group of practical nursing/vocational nursing students were chatting during lunch regarding health insurance coverage, particularly the Affordable Care Act. A student commented, "It is very difficult to assist the client in understanding their benefits and the possible advantage of the Affordable Care Act. There are so many rules; it's easy to misinterpret something. Most people know some basic principles, such as you cannot be denied coverage because of a preexisting illness. But beyond these basics . . . it is very complicated." Another student states, "I know what you mean. It is scary for clients if they do not fully understand their benefits. Last week, I had a client who was admitted to the hospital for pneumonia for 3 days. Following this admission, the client was transferred to a skilled care facility for rehabilitation before returning home. Luckily, the client realized the day he was being transferred that he had been on observation status during the hospitalization instead of in-patient status and thus would not meet the criteria for Medicare payment for the skilled care facility. The client opted for home care instead, to avoid the large out-of-pocket payment." It is an important role of the nurse to assist clients in understanding their benefits, as well as assisting them in finding the correct information. The licensed practical nurse/licensed vocational nurse (LPN/LVN) plays a lead role in helping clients understand their benefits, particularly in the nursing home setting. Consider this as you learn the finances of health care.

THE UNITED STATES HEALTH CARE SYSTEM

OVERVIEW

The US health care system has been described as a poorly organized and complicated maze of services that lacks preventive care, wastes resources, and is very expensive. Historical trends assist in understanding how this evolution occurred.

- In the early 1960s, the **health care provider's** key role in health care decision-making, combined with a **fee-for-service** payment model, contributed to spiraling health care costs and a lack of attention to cost

Box 16.1 Health Insurance Terms

Premium: The monthly fee a person must pay for health insurance coverage.
Deductible: The yearly amount an insured person must spend out of pocket for health care services before a health insurance policy begins to pay its share.
Copayment: The amount an insured person must pay at the time of an office visit, when picking up a prescription, or before a hospital service.
Coinsurance: Once a deductible is met, the percentage of the total bill the insured person must pay. The insurance company pays the remainder.
Health care provider: A licensed health care person, such as a health care provider, dentist, or nurse practitioner, whose health care services are covered by a health insurance plan.

containment (Cherry and Jacob, 2022). See Box 16.1 for health insurance terms.

- Multiple procedures were ordered, which increased costs. This process resulted in the unfolding of a very expensive, inefficient health care system. As a result, in the early 1980s, Medicare changed from a fee-for-service payment model, in which health care facilities charged for each service, to a **prospective payment system (PPS)** based on **diagnostic-related group (DRG)**, in which health care facilities charged one fee for a group of services. The hospital was paid for client services based on the DRG. During this time frame, the health care team was focused on minimizing the client's length of stay, through what became known as utilization management. In most cases, the shorter the stay, the more likely the hospital would make money.
- As time evolved, this payment system extended to include health care provider payments. Private insurers soon followed Medicare's lead by creating **managed care organizations (MCOs)**. MCOs include **health maintenance organizations (HMOs)**, **preferred provider organizations (PPOs)**, point-of-service plans (POS), and open access plans. A managed care organization is a type of health care delivery in which health care organizations negotiate with each insurance company for an overall payment for management of health care services for clients over a designated time frame. A focus on health care prevention is utilized to minimize costs of services for the health care organization.
- Despite these changes, only a small overall cost improvement was realized, followed by continuing increased costs and inequities in health care access. Some Americans did not have access to health care, particularly the underemployed. In addition, low-income individuals struggled with accessing care, despite health care coverage. Even though most people had access to health care through some type of health insurance plan, problems of quality, service, and cost remained an issue. Because fee-for-service payments, DRG payments, and MCOs continue to remain, many viewed the American health care system as complex, broken, and a drain on the overall economy of the nation.

? Critical Thinking

Who Deserves Health Care?

1. Should all individuals in our society have access to health care?
2. Do you think health care is a right or a privilege?

HEALTH CARE REFORM: THE AFFORDABLE CARE ACT

In 2010, the Affordable Care Act (ACA) was signed into law by President Obama. As a national health care initiative, it was the first sweeping piece of legislation to address health care reform in the United States since 1965, when Medicare was added to the Social Security Act.

- The ACA was designed to enhance the access and affordability of health care, particularly to all citizens with financial need. Although controversial, this law has decreased the number of uninsured in the United States. The Agency for Healthcare Research and Quality (AHRQ) concludes that the proportion of uninsured adults under 65 fell from a high of 22% in 2010 to 16% in the second quarter of 2014, after the implementation of the ACA. In 2023, the downward trend continued to be lower than 8% (CDC, 2024).
- The ACA established a Health Insurance Marketplace. This is a resource, found at https://www.healthcare.gov, where individuals, families, and small businesses learn about health care coverage options (including cost-effective, competitive health insurance plans), choose a plan, and enroll in coverage. The marketplace also provides information on programs that help people with low to moderate income receive a discount on the cost of health insurance coverage.
- On May 4, 2017 the American Health Care Act was approved by the House of Representatives (Library of Congress, n.d.). This would have replaced the ACA. However, this Act was never enacted. Thus the ACA remains in place except for the individual mandate penalty, which was repealed as part of a 2017 tax bill.

Try This

Health Care Reform: The Affordable Care Act

How well do you understand how this law affects you and your clients? Answer True or False to the following questions about the law.

1. The law allows a government panel to make decisions about end-of-life care for people on Medicare.
2. The law cuts health care benefits that were previously provided to all people on Medicare.

3. The law expands the existing Medicaid program and will cover more low-income, uninsured adults regardless of whether they have children.
4. The law will provide health insurance to undocumented immigrants.
5. The law increases Medicare payroll tax for Americans making more than $200,000/individual and $250,000/couple.
6. The law requires employers with more than 50 employees to provide health insurance.
7. The law cuts the health care benefits for people receiving Medicare before the implementation of the law.
8. The law will assist Americans (up to 400% of the federal poverty level) in purchasing health care benefits if they are not covered by their employer.
9. The law prohibits insurance companies from denying coverage if an individual has a preexisting condition.

ANSWERS

1: F; 2: F; 3: T; 4: F; 5: T; 6: F; 7: F; 8: T, 9: T

Modified from The Henry J: Kaiser Family Foundation, *Health Reform Quiz*, 2015. http://kff.org/quiz/health-reform-quiz.
Explanations for the answers in the quiz and additional information that applies to the ACA can be found at http://kff.org/quiz/health-reform-quiz. A timeline for implication of the ACA can be found at www.healthcare.gov. *Content in italics, contained in this chapter, further explains the ACA.*

FINANCING THE HEALTH CARE SYSTEM

HOW CLIENTS PAY FOR HEALTH CARE SERVICES

Personal Payment

In the past, clients paid health care providers directly (i.e. **private pay**) as the primary method of payment for health care services. Presently, most clients use health insurance to pay for health care services. Private pay is an option for clients who do not have health insurance. The high cost of health care services discourages those who do not have health insurance from seeking health care services or making personal payments, which can be problematic.

The uninsured. According to the US Census Bureau, the percentage of people without health insurance coverage in 2023 was 8% (Keisler-Starkey and Bunch, 2024). The percentage of children under the age of 19 was 5.8% in 2023.

- The uninsured often includes:
- **Low-wage employees**. This group of people is employed in low-wage jobs that are less likely to offer insurance benefits.
- **The middle class**. Some of these workers are unemployed. Those employed may be priced out of the health insurance market by the rapidly rising health insurance **premium**.
- In 2014, because of the ACA, citizens and legal residents were required to obtain health insurance or pay a penalty. However, a tax bill passed by Congress in 2017 eliminated this mandated penalty as of 2019. This has been the only major change in the ACA since 2019.
- Unemployment and a downturned economy increase the number of uninsured who seek treatment in emergency rooms.
- Emergency room treatment is expensive and is intended for seriously ill or injured people and not for less serious illnesses.
- Lack of access to health care prevents individuals from receiving preventive care and seeking treatment when a health problem develops.
- Individuals may seek treatment during the later stages of illness, resulting in a greater expense. Cancer is an example of a disease that is best treated and possibly cured when diagnosed in its early stage.
- Many people rely on emergency departments for all levels of health care because of a lack of insurance.
- Consider the case of a sinus infection. The most cost-effective means of diagnosing and treating a sinus infection is an assessment by a primary health care provider. However, this solution is not realistic if the individual does not have health insurance or does not have the money to pay for the **deductible**, **copayment**, or **coinsurance** of the individual's insurance plan. When the sinus infection reaches an acute stage, the individual might seek treatment at the local emergency department, a more expensive, preventable option.

Critical Thinking

Who Pays the Health Care Bill?

If a client does not have health insurance or the ability to pay the emergency room fee, who pays the bill?

Private Health Insurance (Commercial Insurance)

Health insurance, like any insurance, spreads risk. The premise is that the risk is spread over all the insured individuals, which means the young and the healthy generally subsidize (financially support) the sick and older individuals in the health insurance group.

- Individuals can purchase private health insurance from the Health Insurance Marketplace at https://www.healthcare.gov. *The ACA prohibits discriminating against people with preexisting conditions; insurance companies are prohibited from refusing coverage to anyone based on their medical history or health status. The ACA also prohibits individual and group health plans from placing lifetime limits on the dollar value of coverage and prohibits insurance companies from rescinding coverage of standard treatments, such as approved chemotherapy.*
- Employers may offer private group insurance to their employees. *The ACA does not require all employers to provide health benefits. However, it imposes penalties on larger employers (those with 50 or more workers) that do not provide insurance to their workers or that provide coverage that is unaffordable. Small businesses that offer health insurance receive a tax credit.* Blue Cross

and Blue Shield, available in 50 states, is an example of private group health insurance. Health insurance protects individuals from bills for unexpected illness.

Public Health Insurance (Government Insurance)

Veterans health administration. The United States has provided comprehensive health care services to all veterans since the 1800s. Today, the Veterans Health Administration (VHA) continues to meet the health care needs of our veterans inclusive of hospitals, outpatient clinics, nursing home care units, and domiciliaries. See www.va.gov for details.

Medicare. In 1965, **Medicare** was added to the Social Security Act.

- This federally sponsored **entitlement program** and public health insurance plan helps finance health care for all individuals age 65 and older who are citizens or permanent residents of the United States and who have at least a 10-year record in Medicare-covered employment.
- Coverage is also given to certain younger individuals with disabilities, individuals with end-stage renal disease, and individuals with Lou Gehrig's disease.
- No person is denied coverage based on past medical history.
- In 2023, there were over 65 million Medicare beneficiaries in the United States (Center for Medicare Advocacy, 2023).
- Approximately 10,000 American citizens turn 65 every day and become eligible for retirement benefits, placing huge demands on Social Security, including Medicare (AARP International, 2024).
- In 2023, Medicare spending totaled over $944 billion, which is a significant increase over the past decade (CMS, 2024; Kaiser Family Foundation, 2019).
- An inpatient hospitalization under Medicare Part A is reimbursed using the DRG system. Medicare pays a set fee based on the billed DRG for the entire hospitalization. If the acute care facility can provide treatment at a cost lower than the reimbursed amount, it can retain the difference as profit, creating an incentive to deliver high-quality care to Medicare beneficiaries. Visit www.medicare.gov for more details.

Medicare health care plans (www.medicare.gov). Medicare Part A (Box 16.2)

- Referred to as hospital insurance
- Covers *inpatient* hospital stays, limited care in a skilled nursing facility, hospice care, and some home health care
- Hospitalizations are covered under Part A if the client maintains *inpatient* status (requiring more than observation), supported by medical necessity, after two midnights (referred to as the Medicare Two Midnight Rule); the insurance is billed using DRGs, described above.

Box 16.2 Medicare Part A Provisions

Medicare Part A helps pay for inpatient hospital care after the deductible has been met ($1676 in 2025) and is funded by a payroll tax; a coinsurance fee starts on day 61 of the hospitalization. In 2025, Medicare Part A helps pay for the following types of situations:

- Inpatient hospital care (e.g., a semiprivate room, meals, medications, supplies, lab tests, radiology, and intensive care units).
- A total of 20 days of skilled nursing facility care for rehabilitation services (full cost), if this follows 3 days of inpatient status hospitalization. The next 80 days are paid after a daily coinsurance ($209 each day in 2025).
- Under certain conditions, home health care services with coinsurance charges for medical equipment and hospice care for terminally ill beneficiaries.
- Part A does *not* pay for long-term care custodial services (e.g., clients who need help only with activities of daily living [including feeding]), private duty nursing, private rooms, telephones, or televisions provided by hospitals, personal care items, and skilled nursing facilities.

Data from www.medicare.gov.

Medicare Part B (Box 16.3)

- Referred to as medical insurance
- Covers certain health care provider's services, outpatient care, medical supplies, and preventive services
- Hospitalizations are covered under Part B if the client is admitted with an *outpatient* status (only observation needed), due to a lack of medical necessity for inpatient status; the insurance is billed as fee for service (itemized billing), which typically requires more out-of-pocket costs to the client than Part A hospitalizations.

Medicare Part C (Medicare advantage)

- Offered by a private company that contracts with Medicare
- Can include HMOs, PPOs, fee-for-service plans, special needs plans, and Medicare Medical Savings Account Plans
- Also offers prescription drug, dental, and vision coverage
- Substitutes for Medicare Part A and Part B

Medicare Part D

- Prescription drug coverage
- Medicare drug legislation, passed in 2003, provided prescription drug coverage that helps pay for brand-name medications at participating pharmacies
- Offered by insurance companies and other private companies approved by Medicare

Medicare supplement insurance. Because of the items Medicare does not cover, beneficiaries are encouraged to purchase private supplemental insurance in addition to Medicare or Medicare advantage plans to cover copayments, deductibles, coinsurance, and

Box 16.3 Medicare Part B Provisions

Medicare Part B is like a major medical insurance plan. Part B is funded by monthly premiums that are income related. Most people pay a standard monthly premium. However, if a person's modified adjusted gross income is above a set amount, the person may pay an extra premium. In 2025, Medicare Part B helps pay for health care services that are medically necessary (needed for diagnosis and treatment of a medical condition) or preventive, such as the following:

- Health care provider visits and other medical services
- Outpatient hospital services (including emergency room visits)
- Mental health services
- Second opinion prior to surgery
- Clinical laboratory services and diagnostic tests (x-rays, MRI, CT scans, electrocardiograms [EKGs])
- Ambulance transportation
- Durable medical equipment (wheelchairs, walkers, oxygen, hospital beds)
- Kidney supplies and services
- Some diabetic supplies
- Physical, occupational, and speech therapy in a hospital outpatient department or a client who resides in a Medicare-certified bed in a rehabilitation agency
- Preventive services: "Welcome to Medicare" physical examination in the first 12 months after enrolling in Plan B and yearly health visits. A diverse array of health screenings and vaccinations are covered.
- There is a maximum payment of $35 per month for insulin prescriptions.
- Part B does *not* pay for most prescription medications, services not related to treatment of illness or injury, dental care, dentures, cosmetic surgery, routine foot care, hearing aids, routine eye examinations, or routine glasses.

Data from www.medicare.gov.

limited-coverage situations that exist with Medicare coverage. These plans are sold by private insurance companies.

? Critical Thinking

What Services Should Medicare Offer?

1. Should Medicare pay for new technological procedures that are developed to treat common medical problems of the elderly?
2. Should cost effectiveness enter the picture for treating Medicare clients?

Medicaid or medical assistance. The **Medicaid** or Medical Assistance program (Title XIX) was added to the Social Security Act in 1965. This program provides medical assistance for eligible families and individuals with low incomes and resources.

- Medicaid is a cooperative venture jointly funded by the federal and state governments. Table 16.1 provides a comparison of Medicare and Medicaid.
- The federal government establishes broad, national guidelines for Medicaid.
- Each state establishes its own program services and requirements, including eligibility. For this reason, when eligible for Medicaid in one state, an individual is not eligible in another state. Thus clients with Medicaid must obtain medical services in the state in which they have coverage.

Under the ACA, Medicaid improvements continue to take full effect. The Centers for Medicare and Medicaid Services (CMS) continues to work with states to base their Medicaid and Children's Health Insurance Program (CHIP) on modified adjusted gross income (MAGI). See www.medicaid.gov for details. As a result, the ACA creates a uniform Medicaid eligibility level and income definition across all states. Undocumented immigrants and legal immigrants who have resided in the United States for less than 5 years are not eligible for Medicaid.

IMPROVING THE COST OF HEALTH CARE

According to CMS (2024), the United States spent over $4.5 trillion on health care in 2022. Some reasons for the high cost of health care are the costs of prescription medications, medical malpractice lawsuits, and continual development and use of medical technology. The United States has the highest health care spending of industrialized countries but has lower life expectancy and the highest infant and maternal mortality than other industrialized countries of the world (Gunja et al., 2023; Petrullo, 2023). For all the money spent on health care, all clients are not experiencing quality and safety in their health care.

A driving force today in health care agencies is **cost containment** (the need to hold costs to within fixed limits) while remaining competitive in the health care marketplace. LPNs/LVNs need to remember that health care agencies are interested in improving their agency's financial status by reducing waste and inefficiency. LPNs/LVNs who identify wasteful practices and inefficient routines in their work settings while maintaining quality may in fact be saving their own jobs. The following are the LPNs'/LVNs' roles in containing health care costs in the work setting:

- Follow facility policy for charging clients for all supplies used in their care.
- Follow facility policy for documenting client care for reimbursement.
- Organize client care for effective and efficient use of the nurse's time.
- Be efficient and effective in delivering client care. If some aspect of care needs to be "redone," it may mean the nurse could have done it right the first time.
- Ensure reimbursement and decrease the client's length of stay by implementing nursing care to help prevent complications.
- Meet the clients' needs, not the nurse's needs.
- Provide client-centered (relationship-centered) care.

Table 16.1 Comparison of Medicare and Medicaid

	MEDICARE	MEDICAID
Purpose of program	Health care for people 65 years and older who are eligible for Social Security, younger people with disabilities, and people with end-stage renal disease and Lou Gehrig's disease.	Medical and health-related services for people with decreased income and resources that meet eligibility requirements.
Source of funding	Federal government (i.e., your tax money). An entitlement health care program. Congress must fund Medicare each year, as opposed to a discretionary program, in which funding must be approved yearly.	An entitlement program jointly financed by the federal and state governments (your tax money). Medicaid is a major expenditure in federal and state budgets.
Who administers the program?	The federal government.	Individual states. Variability relative to the Affordable Care Act.
Enrollment Costs	Part A: Hospital insurance for inpatient care. No cost for individuals who meet eligibility requirements for Social Security. Part B: Medical insurance covering health care providers' fees and outpatient services; deductible, copay, or coinsurance payments may be required. A premium or monthly fee is taken out of the monthly Social Security check when a person registers for program.	No fee. Must meet income eligibility requirements.

- Remember that quality outcomes (pay-for-performance) and *never events* (events that never should have happened) impact the institution's bottom line. Ask questions and seek guidance to fully understand factors impacting revenue.

Nurses are an essential factor when it comes to addressing quality, safety, and cost in health care. These attributes of health care need to be understood and brought to all clinical situations by all nurses, regardless of educational preparation.

Professional Pointer

Remember to consider cost in your practice. It is no longer good enough to simply provide quality care. High-quality, safety-focused, cost-effective care is the goal.

ISSUES OF THE HEALTH CARE SYSTEM

Although the high cost of health care is a concern, there are other issues affecting the efficiency of the health care system. LPNs/LVNs should stay aware of present issues so they can provide comprehensive care to clients.

SAFETY AND QUALITY OF HEALTH CARE

Strategies for improving the safety and quality of health care services are ongoing as health care professionals aim to do good (benevolence) and prevent harm (nonmaleficence). Many initiatives promote advancing the safety and quality of health care.

- *To Err Is Human: Building a Safer Health Care System* was an extensive report created in 1999 by the Institute of Medicine (IOM) that showed up to 98,000 people die each year from preventable medical errors and presented a comprehensive strategy to prevent such errors. A reevaluation completed over a decade later showed minimal improvements (Pellegrini, 2020).
- The **Health and Medicine Division of the National Academies (HMD)**, previously IOM, provides a major influence in promoting health policies on the federal level, by testifying before Congress, and on the state and local levels as well. HMD influenced policy changes concerning childhood poverty, COVID-19 vaccination distribution, regulation of e-cigarette usage, and the importance of testing CPR to children (HMD, 2024). The National Committee for Quality Assurance (NCQA) promotes high-quality health care by ensuring appropriate management of medical conditions. NCQA utilizes the Healthcare Effectiveness Data and Information Set (HEDIS) as a performance improvement tool to evaluate the effectiveness and access of health care.
- The Joint Commission (TJC) reviews studies done on adverse incidents that cause serious harm and death to clients. The **National Patient Safety Goals**, created by TJC, provide key health care aims for improving patient safety based on these findings (TJC, 2025). Medication errors are a primary cause of preventable patient injuries. Improper client identification is often a problem in giving medication, as well as doing wrong-site surgery. Nurses are often involved in client preparation for surgery and marking the site, so no confusion exists during the surgical process. Additional information is available at https://www.jointcommission.org/standards/national-patient-safety-goals/. Box 16.4 provides a list of TJC (2025) Client Safety Goals for hospitals and nursing care centers.

Critical Thinking

Patient Safety Goals

Discuss how you implemented TJC Patient Safety Goals in your last clinical experience.

Box 16.4 The Joint Commission 2025 National Client Safety Goals

HOSPITAL

- Identify patients correctly (two identifiers)
- Improve staff communication
- Use medicines safely
- Use alarms safely
- Prevent infection
- Identify patient safety risks
- Improve health care equity
- Prevent mistakes in surgery

NURSING CARE CENTER

- Identify patients and residents correctly
- Use medicines safely
- Prevent infection
- Prevent patients and residents from falling
- Prevent bed sores

Modified from The Joint Commission (TJC): 2025 National patient safety goals, simplified version, 2025. Available at. https://www.jointcommission.org/standards/national-patient-safety-goals/.

- Transition to Practice is an initiative of the National Council of State Boards of Nursing (NCSBN) that aims at improving the quality and safety of health care by improving the new graduates' transition to work. In collaboration with more than 35 nursing organizations, NCSBN developed an evidence-based Transition to Practice model. The model for acute care settings recommends a 9- to 12-month program to aid in the transition to the clinical setting. Details can be found at https://www.ncsbn.org/transition-to-practice.htm.
- Continued competency of health care professionals is an important component of high-quality health care. Current nursing licensure considers nurses, from all levels of educational preparation, to be minimally competent upon receiving the initial license. Continued competence is assumed throughout a career and is the responsibility of each nurse. Clients, lawmakers, employers, and professional organizations question this assumption. As this matter is debated and a method is devised to assure clients that their health care providers are competent and qualified, LPNs/LVNs need to update themselves continually in their area of practice.
- Quality health care should be consistent when client transitions to a different health care facility. A readmission reduction program has been implemented by CMS, resulting in reduced payment when clients are readmitted to an acute care hospital within 30 days of discharge. The applicable diagnosis includes acute myocardial infarction, heart failure, pneumonia, chronic obstructive pulmonary disease and total knee, hip arthroplasty, and coronary artery bypass graft (CABG) surgery. This readmission reduction program triggered a strategic effort to improve transitions in care, including intensive education and follow-up services. The LPN/LVN has an instrumental role in identifying early complications and immediately intervening, thus preventing a hospital readmission.

Try This

Licensed Practical Nurse/Licensed Vocational Nurse Role in Decreasing Hospital Readmissions

Discuss how an LPN/LVN in a long-term care setting can effectively decrease a client's readmission to the hospital.

ACCESS TO HEALTH CARE

Access to health care is a growing concern. Many people experience barriers to receiving health care, such as the high cost of services or medications, the lack of insurance, limited availability of services in the local area, disparities in care based on language, race, culture, ethnicity, and socioeconomic status, and social determinants of health (education, health care, housing, social environment, and income). When individuals are prevented from getting the health care they need, their health outcomes are diminished. Access to health care is a problem in many countries around the world. LPNs/LVNs should be client advocates to help reduce barriers so clients can receive high-quality health care.

Try This

Social Determinants of Health

Evaluate your own social determinants of health by reviewing them at: https://www.cdc.gov/public-health-gateway/php/about/social-determinants-of-health.html.

What changes do you need to make for improved health?

OTHER ISSUES

There are many other issues facing the health care system. LPNs/LVNs should stay abreast of the needs of clients and promote change through their professional development.

- Workforce shortages continue to exist in nursing as well as other medical professions, especially in the rural communities. A reduced workforce in health care can lead to a reduced quality of care and long wait times for clients to receive care.
- Mental health issues are increasingly recognized as being an essential component to wellness. These services are often difficult to attain due to professional shortages and underfunding of resources.
- The increased aging population provides an increased demand on health care services, which raises health care costs and increases the need for geriatric care and long-term care options.
- Increased numbers of infectious diseases affect health care systems nationally and globally. Pandemics—such as COVID-19 that started in 2019—antibiotic resistance, and newly formed infectious diseases present burdens on the health care system worldwide.

TRENDS IN THE HEALTH CARE SYSTEM

The issues that face the health care system bring about trends that are required to meet the needs of clients and communities. Current trends include the following:

- Telehealth and technology: The COVID-19 pandemic provided a boost in the implementation of technology in health care as a means of staying connected to clients. Remote connection through video consultations and mobile apps promoted health care access during the pandemic and beyond. Telenursing is a new trend in acute care settings that reduces the workload of staff nurses by allowing other nurses to remotely manages admission and discharge processes (Schwartz et al., 2024). The electronic health record (EHR) is instrumental in promoting accessibility to client information. Although this has improved health care delivery, errors with the EHR are problematic. LPNs/LVNs need to have adequate technology skills to efficiently document in the EHR. The use of artificial intelligence (AI) in health care helps advance diagnostics, predict patient outcomes, and optimize resource allocation. Digital health tools, like wearable devices, aid in the continuous monitoring of health conditions.
- Personalized Medicine: Advances in genomics, biotechnology, and data analysis allow health care services to be more personalized with treatments and medications. This advancement is especially helpful to clinical practices in oncology.
- Value-based care: Client outcomes have become the focus on the evaluation of valuable health care. The focus of value-based care is on providing high-quality care while reducing costs. LPNs/LVNs focus on client outcomes using the nursing process.
- Health care prevention and wellness: There is an increased focus on health promotion, lifestyle changes, and early detections of chronic health conditions to improve population wellness.
- Mental health integration: Primary care providers are focusing not only on physical health but on mental health as well (Muller et al., 2024). This emphasis is helping lower the stigma of mental health conditions and improve access to mental health resources. LPNs/LVNs should focus on the mental health as well as the physical health when performing client care.
- Alternative and complementary medicine: Alternative medicine practices, such as acupuncture, chiropractic care, and herbal medicine, are gaining popularity as complementary options with conventional treatments. LPNs/LVNs should consider the client's use of over-the-counter medications as well as prescription medications.
- Federal government involvement: In 2023, the Inflation Reduction Act allowed individuals with Medicare coverage to pay only $35 per month for insulin prescriptions. If this cost cap would have been in effect in 2020, the 1.5 million Medicare beneficiaries would have saved over $760 million that year (Sayed et al., 2023).
- Online services: There is a growth in online services that provide reduced pricing for costly medications. Prescription coupons provide a deduction in medication costs, such as those provided by GoodRx at goodrx.com. Online companies provide medications at a significantly lower cost than the local pharmacy, such as the option at costplusdrugs.com.

Try This

The Role of the LPN/LVN With Health Care Trends

Identify health care trends and consider how the LPN/LVN can assist with these trends to improve the issues affecting the health care system.

Do the health care facilities where you have clinical implement any of these trends?

How do LPNs/LVNs participate?

THE NURSE'S RESPONSE: DEALING WITH CHANGE

Current trends bring about changes. Changes will continue to occur in the health care setting. It is important for nurses to consider their personal response to change. Nurses need to remember that they have choices in their response to changes. An individual can be a victim, a survivor, or a navigator of change.

- **Victims** look at change in a negative way. They fear that the worst will happen because of the proposed change and feel helpless in the situation. They do not willingly participate in the change process; they allow change to control them.
- **Survivors** resist change but go along with the process. They claim the change will never work, and if their prediction comes true, they say, "I told you so!"
- **Navigators** of change feel in control of the situation. They feel confident and excited about the possibility of being part of the solution to a problem. Navigators believe they have some control over change rather than being controlled by the change.

Professional Pointer

Be a self-directed, self-motivated, problem-solving employee. Strive to be a navigator when change occurs.

In the 21st century, LPNs/LVNs need to define their role as more than just the nursing tasks and duties they perform. Less-trained, unlicensed individuals in the health care team are also performing these related nursing tasks and duties. *LPNs/LVNs need to define their role as assisting with the nursing process.* LPNs/LVNs are effective at noting new client problems and collaborating with registered nurses (RNs), setting client goals, performing nursing interventions, and evaluating the results of planning. It is these problem-solving and critical-thinking aspects of nursing that make LPNs/LVNs valuable members of the health care team. LPNs/LVNs need to be viewed as "thinkers" and not just "doers." LPNs/LVNs need to present themselves in clinical situations as being very valuable to the health care agency.

LPNs/LVNs should:

- Be self-directed, self-motivated, positive, and a problem solver in your daily work.
- Avoid being known as the person who always asks what needs to be done next.
- Identify what needs to be done, prioritize, and do it, collaborating when necessary.
- Respond flexibly to changes that are presented.
- Identify tasks or protocols that could be done more efficiently.
- Use the critical thinking skills learned in their nursing program to devise innovative suggestions to make client care more efficient, safe, and cost effective.
- Ensure colleagues and the community understand the role of the LPN/LVN and their unique contribution to advancing the health of the nation by providing high-quality, safety-focused, cost-effective care.

? Critical Thinking

LPNs/LVNs: Change Agents

Create a plan that you use when you are an LPN/LVN on how you can adjust to change in the workplace. There is a consistency in health care: There will always be change. What are your strategies for coping with change?

Get Ready for the Next-Generation NCLEX® Examination

Key Points

- The quality, safety, cost, and access to health care are major concerns in today's health care system.
- Reports of the IOM (now called the Health and Medicine Division of the National Academies) highlight concern for the quality, safety, and cost of health care.
- The number of uninsured individuals is a major concern in health care. The ACA is aimed at addressing this issue.
- CQI, aims of the IOM (now called the Health and Medicine Division), continued competency, TJC National Client Safety Goals, the National Council of State Boards of Nursing's Transition to Practice Model, and the LPN/LVN role in containing health care costs address the issues of quality, service, and cost of health care.
- Issues in health care create health care trends for improving client outcomes.
- Changes in health care delivery include client-centered (relationship-centered) care, HMOs, PPOs, POSs, open access plans, and health care alliances. LPNs/LVNs need to be self-directed, self-motivated, and positive problem solvers in their areas of employment.
- Changes in health care need to be approached with flexibility and a vision of the opportunity to improve quality, safety, cost effectiveness, and access to client care.
- LPNs/LVNs need to ensure quality and safety of client care by keeping updated and current in their areas of employment.

Additional Learning Resources

Go to your Evolve website (http://evolve.elsevier.com/Carroll/success/) for the following FREE learning resources:

- Answers to Critical Thinking Review Scenarios
- Additional learning activities
- Additional Review Questions for the NCLEX-PN® examination
- Helpful phrases for communicating in Spanish and more!

Clinical Judgment Questions

1. Student nurses are discussing the major driving forces in delivering health care today. What statement indicates the student nurse's need for additional knowledge?

a. Technology has almost eliminated the concern for client safety.
b. Clients' access to knowledge and understanding of their health needs contributes to safe care.
c. The technological explosion has improved the efficiency of the delivery of health care; however, safety risks remain.
d. Family members and the community may be important factors in creating a safe environment.

2. A new nurse is asking questions of their supervisor regarding Medicare coverage. What statement indicates that the nurse understands how Medicare impacts the prospective payment system (PPS)?

a. Hospitals have increased revenue because of the PPS.
b. When the client is discharged, the hospital calculates the bill and sends it to the federal government.
c. The hospital is paid based on diagnostic-related groups (DRGs).
d. Health care provider office visits cannot be covered by Medicare funding.

3. A client is discussing the Affordable Care Act (ACA) with a nurse. What statement indicates the client understands the ACA?

a. The ACA was implemented to expand health insurance coverage at no cost to the client.
b. The ACA mandates that all employers provide health insurance to all employees.
c. The ACA replaces Medicare coverage.
d. The law prohibits insurance companies from denying coverage if the client has a preexisting condition.

4. Indicate which insurance the following statements accurately describe the benefits of Medicare or Medicaid.

DESCRIPTION	MEDICARE	MEDICAID
Funded by the federal government		
Provides health care coverage for those 65 years and older		
Administered by individual states		
Provides health care coverage for those with decreased financial resources		
Covers hospitalization costs for insured individuals		

5. A client is discussing Medicare coverage with a nurse. Highlight or underline the sentence within the client's statement below that indicates more teaching is needed by the nurse.

"Medicare offers various coverage options for people who are 65 or older, as well as those with disabilities, end-stage renal disease, or ALS (Lou Gehrig's disease). Part A covers inpatient hospital stays, skilled nursing care, and hospice care. Part B covers outpatient care, including hospital services and medical office visits. Part C or Medicare Advantage plans provides Medicare coverage from private insurance companies. Part D covers the cost of over-the-counter medications."

6. Complete the following sentence by filling in the blanks.

All health care professionals should strive to improve the access, quality, _____, and cost of _____.

Structure	health care
appeal	food
safety	ethics
judgment	education

Critical Thinking Scenario

A group of practical/vocational nursing students are discussing new health reform legislation. One student is upset because the ACA is socialized medicine. Another student tells the group their grandfather told them the new law makes it necessary to have death panels evaluate care for Medicare clients. Another student shares that he heard that the new law rations care. How would you address these statements?

Collaboration: Leading and Managing

17

Objectives

On completing this chapter, you will be able to do the following:

1. Discuss the various roles of the licensed practical nurse/licensed vocational nurse (LPN/LVN).
2. Summarize the skills needed for a leadership and management role, including the difference between the two.
3. Discuss various forms of leadership, leadership styles, and approaches to leadership.
4. Describe core leadership knowledge and skills.
5. Discuss approaches to stress management.
6. Describe specific leadership knowledge and skills needed by the LPN/LVN.
7. Describe key aspects of the role of the charge nurse and strategies for preparing to undertake this role.
8. Summarize the responsibilities and knowledge needed by the LPN/LVN charge nurse to include various policies and regulations.
9. Discuss the steps of collecting data and data collection considerations for the charge nurse.
10. Summarize common problems that the charge nurse must manage.
11. Describe key aspects of assignment and delegation in nursing. Apply key aspect of using the nursing process as a guide for assigning tasks and delegating duties.
12. Give examples of how leadership skills may be used by the charge nurse in the nursing process.
13. Demonstrate an end of shift report, including all essential components.

Key Terms

assigning (assignment)
accountability
autocratic leadership
Centers for Medicare and Medicaid Services (CMS)
change-of-shift report
conflict resolution
continuum
delegating
goals (outcomes)
Howlett hierarchy
irrational thinking
leadership
management
mission statement
Omnibus Budget Reconciliation Act of 1987 (OBRA)
patient outcomes
performance evaluation
Quality Improvement Organization (QIO)
scope of practice
situational leadership
stress management
The Joint Commission
time management

Keep in Mind

"The manager does things right. The leader does the right things."
—Warren Bennis, On Becoming a Leader *(2003)*

Ishi and Marcielo, nursing assistants, collapsed in their chairs in the lunchroom. "I had forgotten how hectic mornings can be," said Ishi. "I am exhausted." This was the first day back on the day shift on the Evergreen Wing for both nursing assistants. Both had substituted for a week for vacationing nursing assistants, Ishi on nights and Marcielo on the evening shift.

"I don't care how tired I am, I sure am glad to be back with our charge nurse," said Ishi. "I missed Duke's way of running things." Ishi continued, "On nights, being with LVN Gina was like working with mass confusion. Anything you wanted to do was fine. It seemed the most important thing was the happiness of the nursing assistants, not the residents' care. Anything we wanted to do was hunky-dory. Duke listens to my suggestions but also offers input when I need it."

"That sure is different from my experience," said Marcielo. "Being with RN Regina taught me the real meaning of RN initials: 'real nasty.' We were commanded to do everything; nothing was ever suggested. Never a 'thank you' or 'good job.' We had a task list and a time sequence to follow, and, no matter what cropped up, heaven help us if we didn't stick to it precisely. We couldn't even ask questions about our assignments. The only time I appreciated Regina barking orders was the evening we had a code. I was

shaking in my boots, but Regina knew exactly what to do. And the resident pulled through."

"I'm glad we didn't have a code with Gina in charge," said Ishi. "We have so few codes around here. That is a situation in which I would appreciate having some direction."

"I liked the way Duke handled the situation this morning in the lounge when a resident complained of chest pain," Ishi added. "Duke gave us each something to do STAT. After the situation was over, we all discussed the emergency as a team. Duke listened to our suggestions on how to make things go more smoothly in the next emergency situation. Duke makes me feel like a real team member and not a slave!"

Ishi and Marcielo finished their lunches. As they went back to Evergreen Wing, they both agreed that LVN Duke had a way that gets the job done, makes you feel comfortable about expressing a concern or question, and makes you want to come back to work for the next shift. You feel good about your contributions to the team. Both agreed Duke is a good role model for the nurses and nursing assistants.

ROLES OF THE LICENSED PRACTICAL NURSE/ LICENSED VOCATIONAL NURSE (LPN/LVN)

LPN/LVN AS FIRST-LINE LEADER

Have you ever experienced employment situations similar to the ones just described by Ishi and Marcielo? Perhaps you received directions as a nursing assistant or in another job capacity and did not like the way you were approached by your supervisor.

Nurses at all levels need to manage client care. Some nurses will also be leaders. LPNs/LVNs have proved themselves effective as first-line leaders. First-line leaders are responsible for supervising nursing assistants who deliver care in long-term care units or community settings. Such positions are referred to as charge nurse positions. If you are a manager of client care and a leader, you will be more effective in this expanded role in LPN/LVN nursing.

LPN/LVNs need to develop leadership and management skills so they can direct and supervise others in a manner that will effectively meet the goals of the employing agency. In your nursing program, you started building a strong, solid base in these skills. This chapter will help you continue to develop skills to lead and manage. It focuses on the leadership and management role and provides interactive and reflective exercises to assist you in becoming an effective charge nurse and emerging as a leader. These roles are critical to both client and employee satisfaction. As you can see from the story above, the leader's role is critical to client and employee positive outcomes. In addition, this chapter will be a useful resource if you accept an LPN/LVN charge nurse position. Understanding the definition of a mission statement is a good starting point on your journey to being an informal or formal leader.

Mission Statements

All organizations have a **mission statement** or vision statement that defines their purpose (goals) and states their values, culture, and norms, thus providing the foundation for collaborative decision-making. Core values and/or beliefs can flow from a mission statement and often include topics such as customer service, teamwork, respect, trust, honesty, excellence, client-centered care, cost-effective, and safe care.

The LPN/LVN charge nurse needs to be aware of the mission statement of their employer. An example of a mission statement follows: "This nonprofit, consumer-oriented institution aims to provide relationship-centered, low-cost, high-quality, safe care in a supportive environment of compassion, trust and respect, resulting in positive client and institutional outcomes." All staff are required to understand and live the mission statement. It will be your role as a charge nurse to embrace the mission of the institution and ensure all members of the team are committed to the mission.

In a long-term care facility, a unit may focus on specific aspects of the mission statement that require a renewed team approach. For example, if your unit has a decrease in their client satisfaction surveys, specifically related to compassionate care, the unit may collaboratively develop a goal to improve in this area, thus contributing directly to the overall mission of the institution. As a charge nurse you will be instrumental in creating a climate of the work environment that motivates staff to meet this goal. Types of leadership styles and the four "I"s of transformational leadership will be presented in this chapter to assist you in building a solid team ready and willing to meet individual unit and institutional goals. Even if you are not in a formal leadership role as an LPN/LVN, this chapter will assist you in your professional and personal growth.

THE DIVERSE ROLE OF THE NEWLY LICENSED PRACTICAL NURSE/LICENSED VOCATIONAL NURSE

The LPN/LVN job role can differ significantly based on the setting in which you are employed and the acuity level of the clients. In a long-term care setting and in some community settings, the LPN/LVN, even as a new graduate, can be hired as a first-line leader. The organizational chart of an institution is a tool that can assist you in understanding your role in the hierarchy of the organization. The organizational chart is a picture of responsibility in an employment situation. In the traditional organizational chart, individuals who are lower on the organizational chart report to

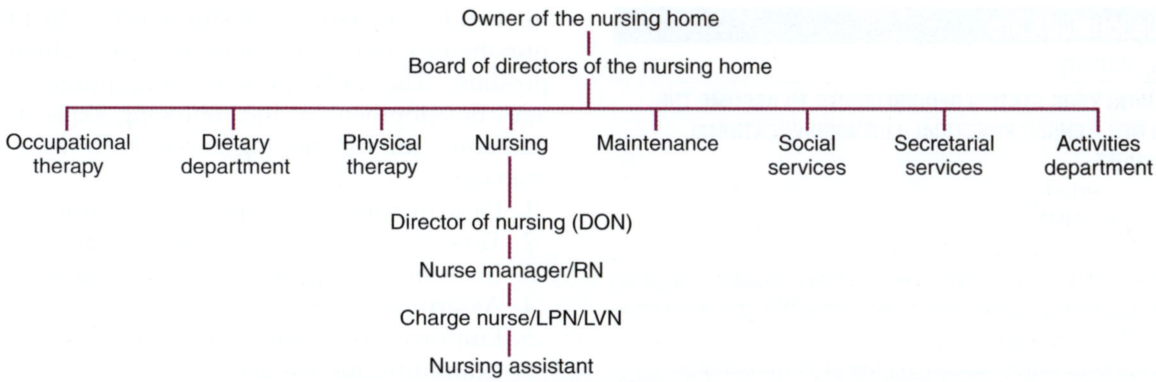

Fig. 17.1 Sample traditional organizational chart for the licensed practical nurse/licensed vocational nurse in the charge nurse role.

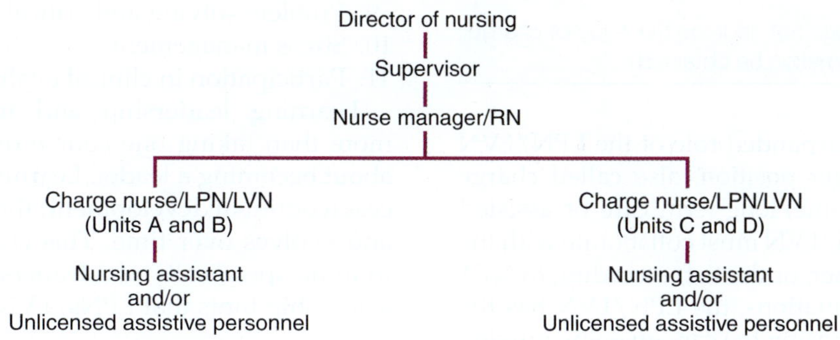

Fig. 17.2 Sample contemporary organizational chart for the licensed practical nurse/licensed vocational nurse in the charge nurse role.

the person directly above them on the chart. Fig. 17.1 shows where the LPN/LVN fits into the traditional organizational chart as a first-line leader. In Fig. 17.1, the LPN/LVN reports to the nurse manager, who is a registered nurse (RN). Nursing assistants and other assistive personnels (UAPs) report to the LPN/LVN. To whom does the nurse manager report?

Because of changes in the structure of organizations, organizational charts have become more horizontal than vertical in appearance. Fig. 17.2 provides an example of a contemporary organizational chart. This "flattening out" has eliminated some of the middle manager positions. As a result, the remaining middle managers have taken on more responsibilities and can be spread thin. Middle managers in this system have more persons reporting to them and depend on the people who report to them, such as the LPN/LVN charge nurse, to think critically and problem solve. Middle managers expect to be contacted only after you have tried and are unable to solve your own problems. However, always remember that LPN/LVNs are expected to collaborate with RNs as stated in their state's Nurse Practice Act (NPA). Understand the impact of your state NPA when in a leadership role. It is easy to step outside the boundaries in an attempt to "get the job done." This can result in disciplinary action by the state, particularly if an adverse client event occurs, such as a fall with injury.

Collaborative Care

Leadership Activity

EXAMINING ORGANIZATIONAL CHARTS

Resources needed:

- Organizational charts from clinical sites used by students in your practical/vocational nursing program
- Organizational charts may differ by region of the United States. Obtain organizational charts of long-term care facilities in your area. Clarify specific levels of responsibility of the LPN/LVN. Identify whether these charts reflect a traditional or contemporary style of organization.

EXPANDED ROLE OF LICENSED PRACTICAL/ LICENSED VOCATIONAL NURSING

Review the Current Nurse Practice Act of Your State

This law legally defines the exact role and boundaries for practical/vocational nurses. Also review the National Association for Practical Nurse Education and Service (NAPNES) standards of practice and educational competencies of graduates of LPN/LVN nursing programs (NAPNES, 2007) (www.napnes.org) and the National Association Licensed Practical Nurse (NALPN) nursing practice standards for the LPN/LVN (NALPN, 2003) (www.nalpn.org). See the Collaborative Care, Leadership Activity Box: Determining Your State's Requirements to Assume the Position of Licensed Practical/Licensed Vocational Charge Nurse box.

Collaborative Care

Leadership Activity

DETERMINING YOUR STATE'S REQUIREMENTS TO ASSUME THE POSITION OF LICENSED PRACTICAL/LICENSED VOCATIONAL CHARGE NURSE

Resources needed:

- Your state's NPA

Obtain a current copy of your state's NPA. Identify the part of the act that addresses your state's position on the practical/vocational nurse who is assuming the charge nurse position in the following areas:

1. Requirements before assuming the LPN/LVN charge nurse position
2. Site of employment
3. Scope of practice

If your state's NPA does not address the issue of charge nurse, how can this information be obtained?

An example of the expanded role of the LPN/LVN is the first-line manager position, also called charge nurse, in a nursing home/long-term care or assisted living facility. The LPN/LVN must collaborate with the RN, health care provider, or dentist, according to NPA guidelines. In these situations, the LPN/LVN has the responsibility of supervising the care given by nursing assistants and other nursing assistive personnel (AP). The LPN/LVN will direct, guide, and supervise these health care workers as they strive to meet the goals of the resident's plan of care.

Practice Analysis of Entry Level LPN/LVNs

The most recent practice analysis of entry-level LPN/LVNs by the National Council of State Boards of Nursing (NCSBN, 2025) occurred in 2024. The next practice analysis will occur in 2027. This survey identified that 40.1% of LPN/LVNs responding to the survey reported they had administrative responsibilities, lower than the previous two practice analyses. The percentages reported included three primary settings: long-term care (58.4%), community based (32.5%), and hospital based (14.5%). Administrative duties in a primary position occurred in community-based care (19.5%), long-term care (13.7%), and hospitals (10.3%). To effectively succeed as a first-line manager/charge nurse role, you will need the abilities found in both a leader and a manager. The 2024 LPN/LVN practice analysis can be obtained at https://www.ncsbn.org/public-files/24_NCLEX_PN_PA.pdf.

PREPARING FOR A LEADERSHIP AND MANAGEMENT ROLE

NURSING MANAGEMENT AND LEADERSHIP SKILLS

The topic of leadership and management for the LPN/LVN is vast. All LPNs/LVNs are already managers in the sense that they consistently need to direct, handle, and organize care for assigned clients. It is worthwhile for you to review the ways in which your LPN/LVN nursing program helps prepare you for a management position. The LPN/LVN nursing program encourages development of the following skills, which are necessary for functioning successfully as a first-line manager:

1. Basic nursing skills, including the nursing process
2. Time-management skills for home and clinical time
3. Decision-making skills—using evidence
4. Assertiveness skills
5. Empowerment/self-confidence skills
6. Communication skills
7. Ethical aspects of health care
8. Legal aspects of health care
9. Problem solving and critical thinking
10. Stress management
11. Participation in clinical evaluation

Learning leadership and management involves more than taking one course or reading one chapter about becoming a leader. Learning leadership is a process (continual development) that includes many skills and evolves over time. This chapter encourages you to think specifically of a leadership role and provides leadership hints that LPNs/LVNs need.

DIFFERENCE BETWEEN MANAGEMENT AND LEADERSHIP

Management is the organization of care required of clients in a health care setting for a specific period.

- The focus of management is planning and directing to meet client and institutional outcomes.
- The manager asks how and when and has an eye on the bottom line (day-to-day operation).
- Managers can value control but should focus on collaboration.
- Management is a formal role given to a person by the employer.
- Managers are appointed by their employers.
- The tools needed for management could be written in a step-by-step manner to follow.
- Following the directions for using the management skills would possibly get the job done in an efficient manner.

Leadership is how a person empowers and develops a team to meet and exceed client and institutional outcomes.

- The focus of leadership is to produce changes in the workplace that will meet the goals of the employing agency.
- The leader asks what and why and keeps an eye on the future.
- Leaders inspire trust.
- Leaders work "in" and "on" the business.
- Leadership can be an informal role that is given to a person by a group of workers. You become a leader when your team members decide to follow you.
- Leaders, if appointed, will fail quickly if no one follows.

- The leader needs to influence others in the work setting to want to implement desired change.
- Directions for leadership skills can also be learned, but it is through experience that leadership skills are truly developed.

The LPN/LVN who has the skills of both management and leadership will get the job done in the most efficient and effective manner, and the LPN/LVN manager and coworkers will experience greater job satisfaction. A manager is not automatically an effective leader, and a leader is not automatically an effective manager. Your goal will be to develop skills of management and leadership.

WHAT KIND OF LEADER ARE YOU?

You can lead in several different ways. What is your predominant leadership style? Each of the statements given in the Collaborative Care, Leadership Activity: Discovering Your Personal Leadership Style box is an extreme. The responses are not positive or negative. One answer does not have value over another answer.

Collaborative Care

Leadership Activity

DISCOVERING YOUR PERSONAL LEADERSHIP STYLE

Put a checkmark next to the statement that *best* describes the way you *might* be at work, not how you *want* to be.

A SHORT TEST OF LEADERSHIP STYLE

1. My primary goal at work is to:
   a. Get the job done
   b. Get along with the people with whom I work
   c. Do the job correctly
   d. Hope the work I do is noticed
2. My clinical coworkers would say I am:
   a. Domineering in my relationships
   b. Friendly and personable in my relationships
   c. Likely to attend to details of the resident care plan
   d. Creative and energetic in giving care
3. At work, I feel like I have to be:
   a. In control of the resident situation
   b. Liked by my coworkers
   c. Correct in giving care
   d. Recognized and praised for my care
4. When I communicate on the nursing unit:
   a. I am usually direct and to the point.
   b. I am more considerate of the person to whom I am talking rather than strongly getting my point across.
   c. I usually give detailed information.
   d. I usually elaborate on the point at hand.
5. My coworkers would say I am a person who:
   a. Gets the job done regardless of what shift I work
   b. Is very likable and client
   c. Is precise and accurate in giving nursing care
   d. Is optimistic and has good verbal skills
6. My charge nurse might describe my behavior while on my shift by saying that:
   a. Sometimes I alienate people.
   b. Sometimes I waste time and fall for excuses others may give.
   c. Sometimes I can be stubborn with coworkers.
   d. Sometimes I appear consistent to my coworkers.
7. I react to a stressful incident on the nursing unit:
   a. By being rude, blaming other departments, and yelling at coworkers
   b. By being accommodating to the person in charge and by passive behavior
   c. By becoming silent and withdrawing from the situation
   d. By talking faster and louder
8. When I deal with my coworkers on the nursing unit regarding client matters, I like them to:
   a. Get to the point and be businesslike in their behavior
   b. Be casual and sincere in their behavior
   c. Use the facts of the matter and go step-by-step when explaining a resident-care situation
   d. Be enthusiastic about the situation and use demonstrations to explain their points

Add up your "a" and "c" answers. These answers are more characteristic of a task-oriented person. In leadership terms, this person is called an *autocratic* leader. Add up your "b" and "d" responses. These are more characteristic of a people-oriented person. In leadership terms, this person is called a *laissez-faire* leader. Your score can give you a rough estimate of the tendency of your leadership style.

LEADERSHIP STYLES

The literature abounds with examples of leadership styles. Fig. 17.3 illustrates a **continuum** (a line with extreme opposites at each end) of leadership styles. Box 17.1 compares and contrasts the leadership styles found on this continuum.

Benefits and Disadvantages of Leadership Styles

A purely task-centered leadership style (called **autocratic leadership**) thrives on power. It involves telling

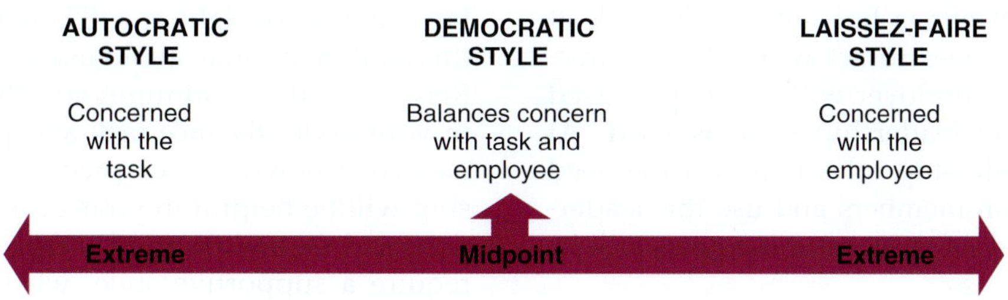

Fig. 17.3 Extremes of leadership styles on a continuum.

Box 17.1 Comparing Autocratic, Democratic, and Laissez-Faire Styles of Leadership

GENERAL DESCRIPTION

Autocratic: Does not share responsibility and authority with employees
Democratic: Shares responsibility and authority with employees
Laissez-faire: Gives away responsibility and authority to employees

IMPORTANCE OF AGENCY'S POLICIES

Autocratic: Emphasis is on policies
Democratic: Enforces policies but with concern for employees
Laissez-faire: Puts employees before policies

HOW LEADER GETS THE JOB DONE

Autocratic: Tells employees what tasks to do; does not seek input from employees
Democratic: Seeks input from employees and encourages problem solving
Laissez-faire: Tries to please everyone

WHAT GETS DONE

Autocratic: May reach goals
Democratic: Because of involvement of employees, goals may be achieved with positive staff feelings
Laissez-faire: May reach goals or possibly achieve nothing, but at least staff feels good

WHEN STYLE CAN BE USED

Autocratic: Crisis situations, code situations, emergencies
Democratic: Daily nursing care situations, meetings, committees, review of care plans
Laissez-faire: When agency goals/policies are not a consideration, or when staff are highly autonomous/goal oriented in function

someone what to do, with little regard for the employee as a person who may have ideas about how to improve resident care or reach the goals of the employer. Adopting the autocratic or laissez-faire style in Box 17.1 to use consistently as a leadership style is unrealistic. Its consistent use could be disastrous. However, there are opportunities when an autocratic leadership style is necessary; for example, in times of emergency. On the following lines, list two additional examples of situations that might require the autocratic style of leadership.

1. ______________________________
2. ______________________________

A purely people-oriented style (laissez-faire) focuses on people's feelings but ignores the task at hand. It allows employees to act without any direction. The goals of the employer will be compromised when the laissez-faire leadership style is used. At times, persons in leadership roles may feel the need to be liked by all team members and use this leadership style, but the task of accomplishing goals will be compromised.

Focusing on both the task and the employee is characteristic of the democratic style of leadership. In this style, the LPN/LVN charge nurse displays concern for the work that needs to be done, as well as for the team performing the work. When using this leadership style, the LPN/LVN charge nurse encourages supervised nursing assistants to discuss resident care, make decisions, and problem solve improvements in care. It may take longer than the autocratic style for work to be accomplished, but client goals (outcomes) will be achieved, with staff having positive feelings about their leadership team and the experience. Examples of situations in which the democratic style of leadership is useful include daily nursing care situations, unit meetings, and reviews of client care plans.

Situational leadership. A popular system of leadership for the 21st century is called situational leadership. **Situational leadership** involves varying your leadership style to meet the demands of the situation in the work environment. According to this system, the LPN/LVN needs to use a leadership style that fits the work situation at hand.

USING THE LEADERSHIP CONTINUUM AS A GUIDE

The value of a continuum, as shown in Fig. 17.3, is that as you move along the continuum from each extreme toward the center or midpoint, the two extremes begin to blend together. You have some of each style, depending on where you are on the continuum. A blend, to some degree, of the two extremes in the appropriate work situation would be the leadership style needed at the moment.

Empowerment

Leadership Activity

PLOTTING MY LEADERSHIP STYLE SCORE

Using your leadership style score from the Discovering Your Personal Leadership Style box, place an "X" on the continuum in Fig. 17.3 to indicate where you are at this point in general leadership style tendencies.

Does your leadership style change based on external factors? If so, what are they? How can your leadership style empower others on your team?

Do the exercise in the Collaborative Care, Leadership Activity: Plotting My Leadership Style Score box. Remember, this score is your tendency. If your "X" is far to the left or right, it will benefit you to be aware of this tendency and to avoid using this style consistently. Remember the continuum and the need to be flexible in your style. Balance task and people orientation as needed. Knowing your predominant style of leadership will be helpful in your evaluation of work situations and the style needed at that time. Some situations require a supportive style, whereas others require a more directive approach. Create a plan to avoid being rigid in your preferred leadership style—being open to change is empowering.

CORE KNOWLEDGE AND SKILLS NEEDED FOR LEADERSHIP

To function well in your expanded role as LPN/LVN charge nurse, you will strive to be a good leader. The scenario at the beginning of this chapter provides examples of what not to do as a nurse leader. Much research in learning about the business of leading others and theories, such as transformational leadership, is available in the literature (Bass, 1985, 2008). Core knowledge and skills lay the foundation for leadership. They will help you develop other necessary knowledge and skills for your leadership role. We identify five core areas of knowledge and skills that are necessary for the practical/vocational charge nurse to be an effective leader. These core areas include the ability to do the following:

1. Motivate team members to accomplish team goals.
2. Communicate clearly.
3. Problem solve effectively.
4. Collaborate effectively building team.
5. Manage stress effectively.

THE FOUR "I"S OF TRANSFORMATIONAL LEADERSHIP CAN HELP LEAD THE WAY

Transformational leaders are viewed as motivating their followers without a focus on their own personal power, elevating their team's needs through effective mentoring/coaching, and providing a clear vision to lead the way. Together as a team, this collective mission, coupled with intellectual stimulation and individualized consideration, results in heightened levels of overall effectiveness (Bass, 1985). Wong and Cummings (2007) conducted a systematic review of the literature, concluding that a significant association exists between transformational leadership style and increased client satisfaction and decreased adverse client events. Thus strong evidence supports the use of transformational leadership in health care settings. Bass (1985) identified four key behaviors of transformational leadership, commonly referred to as the four "I"s: idealized influence, inspirational motivation, intellectual stimulation, and individualized consideration.

An in-depth understanding of each of these key behaviors will assist in the journey of the LPN/LVN in becoming a highly effective leader. The information below describes how the leader exemplifies each of these key characteristics, and Box 17.2 provides

Box 17.2 Licensed Practical Nurse/Licensed Vocational Charge Nurse Behaviors/Actions That Use the Four "I"s of Transformational Leadership[a] to Improve the Work Environment

IDEALIZED INFLUENCE
- Model a high level of ethical and moral conduct
- Act confident and optimistic
- Lead by example
- Share and explain risks taken by the institution
- Avoid using power for personal gain
- Use teamwork language, such as "we" and "us." Convey the attitude "We have common goals, and together we will meet them"

INSPIRATIONAL MOTIVATION
- Review the mission statement of the facility and unit with your team
- Assist the team to see the value of their work
- Model and set high standards of care visible by the team
- Be optimistic and enthusiastic in the clinical area modeling this behavior for others on the team
- Highlight and reward positive outcomes
- Highlight the benefits of change

INDIVIDUALIZED CONSIDERATION
- Encourage politeness, cooperation, trust, and respect among nursing assistants
- Encourage honest feedback among nursing assistants
- Model active listening
- Be open to hear valid concerns and collaboratively identify solutions
- Provide an opportunity for sharing of ideas among nursing assistants
- Ask nursing assistants for ideas on how to do unit tasks more effectively
- Provide individual and group words of acknowledgment, praise, and thanks
- Be fair regarding who gets acknowledgment and thanks based on commitment and contribution as an individual and as a team
- Treat nursing assistants on your team as you would like to be treated
- Advocate for your entire team
- Provide occasions for the team to spend time together

INTELLECTUAL STIMULATION
- Provide opportunities for your assistive personnels (UAP) team to participate in training
- Provide opportunities for your UAP team to contribute to the client's plan of care
- Discuss how their job role impacts the client's, unit's, and institution's outcomes
- Encourage all to challenge the "status quo"
- Provide evidence for decision-making
- Empower the entire team to offer ideas to improve client care, before providing input
- Mentor UAP to advance in their job and the nursing profession
- Ensure fair workload distribution

[a]From Bass, B.M. Leadership and performance beyond expectations, New York, NY, 1985, Free Press.

examples of LPN/LVN behaviors based on the four "I"s of transformational leadership that will improve the work environment, resulting in improved client outcomes.

Idealized influence	The leader acts as a charismatic role model, promoting desirable behavior and establishing trust and respect of the team.
Inspirational motivation	The leader establishes a clear, focused vision and creates collective pursuit of this vision.
Intellectual stimulation	The leader encourages creative thinking and problem solving and is supportive of taking risks based on knowledge.
Individualized consideration	The leader communicates genuine concern for all followers, providing personal attention and individualized coaching and mentoring, supporting the development of followers.

Adapted from Knecht, P., Sosik, J.J. Transformational leadership of nurses in long-term care contexts: propositions and implications for research and practice. *Proceedings of the Institute of Behavioral and Applied Management*, Nashville, TN, 2012.

Empowerment

Huber and Schubert (2019) identified that attitudes about work engagement can be impacted by generational differences. For example, Generation Y was reported to attach less importance to work than do Generation X or Baby Boomers; however, professional ambition was more important to Generation Y than to Generation X or Baby Boomers. Huber and Schubert (2019) concluded, "Transformational leadership behavior represents an approach to guide employees of different generations individually and to harmonize different attitudes." As a charge nurse, how will you use transformational leadership concepts to effectively lead this age diverse workforce in harmony? How can transformational leadership skills empower your team and colleagues? Share your thoughts with a colleague.

UNDERSTANDING MOTIVATION AND HUMAN NEEDS

As a leader, you will have the task of getting your team members to meet goals set by your employer. Getting people to do what needs to be done is a complex task. What motivates one person does not necessarily motivate another. Understanding motivation and human needs coupled with the four "I"s of transformational leadership will assist you in becoming an effective leader.

Motivation

Motivation is a drive that causes individuals to set personal goals and behave in a way that will allow them to reach those goals. The motivation drive comes from within an individual and is intrinsic. Herzberg's two-factor theory (1959) states that intrinsic factors (also known as motivating factors or satisfiers) improve job satisfaction and extrinsic factors (also known as maintenance factors or dissatisfiers) decrease job dissatisfaction. Satisfiers (motivator factors) contribute to personal or psychological growth, increase job satisfaction, and arrive from intrinsic conditions of the job itself. Satisfiers include achievement, recognition, the value of the work itself, potential for growth and advancement, and responsibility. All of these intrinsic factors have to do with the job itself. In contrast, dissatisfiers are extrinsic to the work itself and include company policy and administration, supervision, salary, interpersonal relations, and work conditions. A good leader will address both intrinsic and extrinsic motivators in their workplace. Herzberg's theory parallels Maslow's theory of needs hierarchy, relevant to the human's need to engage in higher-order work.

Human Needs

All individuals have needs that must be filled to meet goals. Individuals are internally motivated to engage in various activities to meet these needs. The activity they engage in is called behavior and can be observed. Here are some facts about needs:

- Abraham Maslow, a psychologist, presented a pyramid of human needs that ranks those needs and can assist the learner in understanding self and others (see Fig. 13.1A).
- Meeting needs on one level of the pyramid acts as a motivator for meeting the needs on the next level.
- Progression through these levels is not clear-cut. In reality, as most of your needs are met on one level, you are already beginning to check out the next level.
- When faced with overwhelming difficulties, physical or emotional, some regression takes place; for example, physiologic needs become a priority if you have lost your job or housing.
- Safety and security needs become a major issue if you are facing a serious illness, move into an unsafe neighborhood, or are facing a divorce.
- Once these issues have been dealt with or resolved, higher needs will reemerge.

Motivating Nursing Assistants

Maslow's hierarchy of needs can be adapted to help the first-line LPN/LVN leader understand motivation of team members in a health care setting based on needs (Fig. 17.4). Remember, all behavior is internally motivated. Herzberg, like Maslow, noted that feelings of self-actualization and growth are true motivators. As an LPN/LVN manager, you can influence what nursing assistants might be motivated to do. If nursing assistants see that doing a good job helps them meet personal needs, they will also be meeting the goals of their employer. Providing for growth opportunities will further enhance their motivation.

All levels of the pyramid in Fig. 17.4 are considered to be needs of employees in an employment situation. As you go up the **Howlett hierarchy**, strategies could be used to encourage meeting needs of nursing assistants at each level. The opportunity to meet these needs can be encouraged or discouraged by the employer and/or the work environment, including the charge nurse (extrinsic motivators). If these needs are met, the

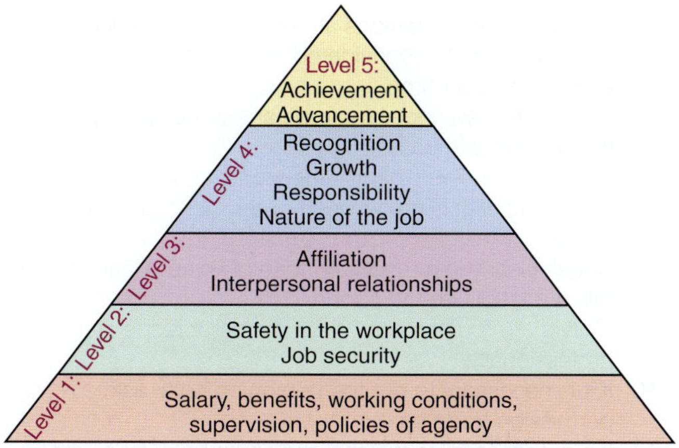

Fig. 17.4 Howlett hierarchy of work motivators. (From Hill SS, Howett HS: *Success in practical/vocational nursing*, ed 7, 2013, St. Louis: Elsevier.)

person can proceed to the next highest level of the pyramid. If these needs are not met, a person may become dissatisfied with the work situation. Strategies for levels 3 and 4 can play an important role in motivation for team members at any level of the Howlett hierarchy. Praise, recognition, and rewards are extremely important tools for leaders.

Empowerment at Work

Empowering employees goes beyond the daily tasks at hand and elevates the team to reach new levels of achievement. This can positively impact productivity, increase in job satisfaction, and commitment to the organization (Lee et al., 2018). Lee et al. (2018) found that empowerment influences employee creativity and helpful behaviors and increases a sense of trust in the leader. These outcomes are particularly important in the health care field. As costs increase, health care professionals are being challenged to develop new ways of providing high-quality, cost-effective care. Empowering others can be a key strategy to meeting overall outcomes, particularly when motivating and delegating to others.

Empowerment

What Motivates You as an Employee?

List what motivates you specifically in clinical situations to get your assignment completed.

Do you think these strategies will motivate others? How? Be specific and realistic, given time constraints and staffing patterns.

Empowerment

Motivating Nursing Assistants/Assistive Personnels

Resources needed:

Readings on motivation (i.e., Lee et al., 2018), the Howlett hierarchy, four I's of Transformational Leadership (described later in this chapter), and your creativity to find ways to meet the needs of nursing assistants.

This exercise inspires the charge nurse to be creative in finding ways to encourage motivation in nursing assistants. Examples of behaviors that encourage meeting needs at each level of the hierarchy are given; the person responsible for the behavior is listed in parentheses. Space is provided for you to fill in additional suggested behaviors at each level to encourage motivation of nursing assistants. Identify whether the employer needs to initiate the strategy or whether the strategy could be initiated by the first-line LPN/LVN nursing leader.

LEVEL 1 SALARY, BENEFITS, WORKING CONDITIONS, SUPERVISION, AND POLICIES OF AGENCY

Examples

- Explanation of policies that affect employees (employer)
- Cafeteria-style benefits; pick-and-choose benefits (employer)

LEVEL 2 SAFETY IN THE WORKPLACE AND JOB SECURITY

Examples

- Provision of adequate equipment to carry out standard precautions (employer and first-line LPN/LVN leader)
- Establish policy for hostile clients (employer and first-line LPN/LVN leader) and visitors

LEVEL 3 AFFILIATION AND INTERPERSONAL RELATIONSHIPS

Examples

- Plan monthly potluck dinners, pizza lunches, get-togethers (first-line LPN/LVN leader)

LEVEL 4 RECOGNITION, GROWTH, RESPONSIBILITY, AND NATURE OF THE JOB

Examples

- Encourage attendance at continuing education seminars, in-service training, and so on (employer and first-line LPN/LVN leader)
- Recognize employees when working short-staffed (employer and first-line LPN/LVN leader)

LEVEL 5 ACHIEVEMENT AND ADVANCEMENT

Examples

- Recognition of successful completion of class or seminar (employer and first-line LPN/LVN leader)
- Provide objective examples of how you can implement each of your suggested behaviors. For example, level 5 could be implemented by the following examples: a written account in the facility's newsletter
- Posting an announcement on a special section of the bulletin board
- Recognize employees complimented by clients/families or internal staff
- Send a personal note of congratulations from the charge nurse when applicable

APPLYING COMMUNICATION SKILLS AS AN LPN/LVN LEADER

One of the LPN/LVN leader's most productive tools is the effective use of verbal and nonverbal communication. The principles of communication in Chapters 8 and 9 are building blocks for the communication skills you will need as an LPN/LVN charge nurse. See the Collaborative Care, Leadership Hint: Communication of the Licensed Practical/Licensed Vocational Charge Nurse box and the Collaborative Care, Leadership Hint: Encouraging Verbal Communication from Nursing Assistants box.

Collaborative Care

Leadership Hint

COMMUNICATION OF THE LICENSED PRACTICAL/LICENSED VOCATIONAL CHARGE NURSE

Verbal

1. When talking to nursing assistants, deliver your message with clear, specific language. Spell out objectively what has to be done for residents. If you work with nursing assistants who do not speak English as a first language, determine their proficiency with English. Verify that intended messages were received by all.
2. As an LPN/LVN charge nurse, you are a role model for nursing assistants. Discourage profanity, personal criticisms, gossip, and rumors.
3. Use *I* instead of *you* messages. *I* messages indicate you take the responsibility for the message; for example, "I saw you tie the client's wrist restraint to the side rail. This could cause injury to the client when the side rail is lowered. I suggest you review the videotape on application of restraints. Also review the policy this facility has about the danger of restraint application." *You* messages imply that you are blaming the person to whom you are speaking; for example, "You did a poor job applying that wrist restraint." Take responsibility for your messages.
4. When talking with your supervisor, be valued for your input. Avoid being known as someone who just brings up problems. After objectively stating the problem, offer solutions, citing evidence when possible.

Nonverbal

1. Be sure your body language and message are consistent and professional. For example, avoid smiling when you are delivering a needed reprimand. Face the person to whom you are speaking. Be cognizant of personal space and related boundaries.
2. When delivering your message, appear confident. Have an attentive posture.

Written

1. Use language that all staff will understand.
2. Review your written messages before posting them to be sure the intent of the message is clear. Read them out loud to confirm clarity.
3. Provide written work assignments that do not require the nursing assistant to make judgments.
4. Provide written reports of all meetings. If information is not restricted, a report from a meeting with management can dispel/prevent rumors about what "they" are planning now. The reports can be placed in an area that is accessible for nursing assistants. Record staff meetings if permissible by policy.

Telephone

1. Gather your thoughts before you make a call. This includes the purpose for the call.
2. With a smile in your voice, greet the person by name, identify yourself, and offer a brief inquiry as to his or her well-being, if you know the person you called. For example, say, "Hello, Mrs. Kylie, this is Tricia Zak from the nursing home. How are you doing today?"
3. State the reason for the call: "I am calling to see if you can work at 3:00 pm today."
4. You initiated the conversation. Terminate it when your business is completed. The exception is when the person you called brings up a work-related question.
5. Avoid long conversations about non-work-related topics. This is what is considered allowing the telephone to extend into your time.
6. Arrange to have incoming calls answered quickly, by the second or third ring.
7. When you answer, identify the facility and give your name and title: "The nursing home, Tricia Zak, charge nurse."
8. Speak clearly in a moderate tone of voice. Most people talk too loudly on the phone.
9. Callers are "customers." Treat the caller respectfully and professionally.
10. If it is necessary to put the person on hold, ask permission to do so.
11. If it is necessary to put the person on hold, try to get back to her or him within 30 seconds. If you are still delayed, ask for a number so you can call back.
12. Provide any additional information requested.

Collaborative Care

Leadership Hint

ENCOURAGING VERBAL COMMUNICATION FROM NURSING ASSISTANTS

1. Actively listen to nursing assistants. Avoid distraction and inattention.
2. Stay focused on what the nursing assistant is saying.
3. Avoid forming a response while the nursing assistant is speaking.
4. Avoid judging the message or the nursing assistant.
5. Rephrase the message when the nursing assistant is done to verify that you understand the message.
6. Encourage comments. Your goal is to have the nursing assistant go back to the team and say, "That charge nurse really listened to me!"
7. Encourage constructive evaluation. Create an environment in which nursing assistants are encouraged to give their input, whether positive or negative.
8. Respect all opinions. Nursing assistants need to feel safe to speak up, ask questions, identify problems, and suggest solutions to those problems.

APPLYING PROBLEM SOLVING AS AN LPN/LVN LEADER

A hint for successful problem solving is to identify the real issue and solve it. What is the problem? Avoid spending precious time on finding solutions for what is not really the problem. Chapter 12 introduced you to the nursing process, an excellent problem-solving process. You have been using this problem-solving method throughout your nursing program. For problem solving, the nursing process can be used to solve resident problems as well as staff problems. The nursing process also works at home, as well as in the clinical area (Fig. 17.5).

Scenario: Late for Assigned Shift

A nursing assistant is assigned to the day shift in a long-term care facility. The shift begins at 6:45 am with a verbal report from the day LPN/LVN charge nurse

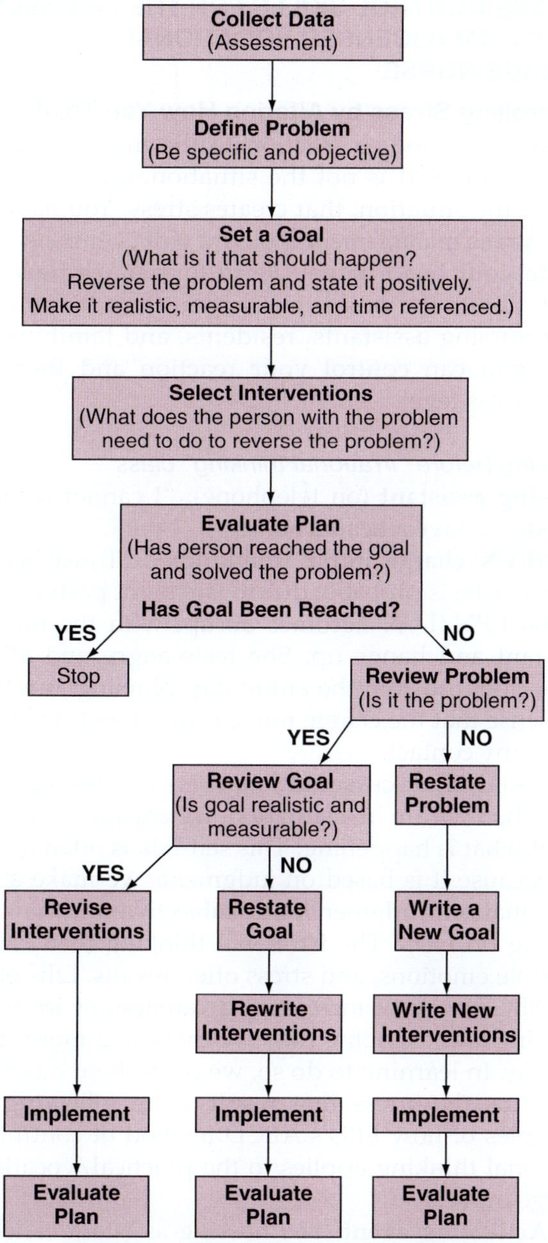

Fig. 17.5 Decision tree for problem solving.

for. All nursing assistants are expected to attend this report and receive their assignments at this time.

Data collection. On May 8, 10, 15, 16, 23, and 24, the nursing assistant (NA) arrived to work either during the charge nurse report or after the charge nurse had finished. When questioned about this behavior, the NA states "I am having problems getting my children up and ready for school."

Problem. A record of the NA's tardiness indicates this is a recurring problem and not an isolated incident. A pattern has been established in being late for report.

Goal. Starting immediately, the NA will be on time for the day charge nurse's report and will hear the entire report.

Intervention. As the charge nurse, it is your responsibility to talk to the NA about this tardiness. This includes the times and days of his or her tardiness. Select a private location for your discussion. Encourage the NA to think through why this behavior is inconvenient for the staff and residents. Review the long-term care unit's policy on punctuality. Inform the NA of the requirement to be on time. Encourage the NA to come up with ideas to be on time and set limits. Plan to meet in 1 week to discuss the NA's performance. At that time, if performance has not improved, a written reprimand will be given and included in the NA's personal file. At the end of the meeting, compliment the NA on an area of work that has been going well and summarize areas needing further development, including detailed next steps.

Evaluation. During the next week, continue to document the NA's arrival for the assigned shifts. If the NA complies, note and praise the change in performance.[a] If the NA continues to be late, issue a written reprimand. Place a copy in the NA's file, give a copy to your supervisor, and keep a copy in your file. Be sure the warning contains objective information, such as the following:

1. Days and times late for shift
2. Date of oral warning
3. Facts regarding impact of situation (related to policy as applicable)
4. Consequences/action plan

STRESS MANAGEMENT

STRESS AND ANXIETY IN A CLINICAL SETTING

Stress is a part of all work environments. The long-term care area has its fair share because of increased workloads (especially when a nursing assistant calls in sick) and potential conflicts with nursing assistants, health care providers, families, and residents. Stress and anxiety in the clinical area can result in dysfunctional behavior on the job. Examples of dysfunctional job behaviors include the following:

1. Decreased performance of nursing assistants
2. Negative interactions with nursing assistants
3. Ineffective communication
4. Inappropriate body cues, such as sharp tone of voice
5. High staff turnover
6. Unhappy residents, families, health care providers, and nursing assistants

As an LPN/LVN charge nurse, you have the responsibility to be a stress manager and role model for the team. Your goal will be to do the following:

[a]In the next week, the NA actually arrived a few minutes before the other nursing assistants. The LPN/LVN charge nurse allowed the NA to choose break and lunch times. The NA had never experienced this before and was very pleased.

1. Display the ability to cope with stress as it affects you.
2. Create a work environment with decreased stress levels.
3. Guide and support nursing assistants when they experience stress.

The LPN/LVN charge nurse needs to learn how to detect stress in the clinical environment. A good place to start is to be aware of your own stress level. See the Collaborative Care, Leadership Hint: Life Skills That Help Control Stress box and the Collaborative Care, Leadership Hint: Creating a Less Stressful Work Environment box.

Collaborative Care

Leadership Hint

LIFE SKILLS THAT HELP CONTROL STRESS

1. The actual stress reduction/relaxation technique you choose is personal. Whatever works for you is the skill to choose.
2. Massage.
3. Daily exercise: Walking is the easiest and least expensive form of exercise. No special equipment is required, except good walking shoes.
4. Listen to music.
5. Adequate nutrition.
6. Get the amount of rest/sleep you need to function at your best.
7. Take scheduled breaks when at work. You will be reenergized and increase your productivity.
8. Develop leisure activities you enjoy (or rediscover activities you put on the back burner during nursing school).

Collaborative Care

Leadership Hint

CREATING A LESS STRESSFUL WORK ENVIRONMENT

1. Your ability to organize your shift will help prevent some stressful situations.
2. Be sure adequate resources are available for nursing assistants to get their job done.
3. Encourage nursing assistants to take breaks as scheduled.
4. Create a calm environment.
5. Treat nursing assistants with respect. Remember your communication skills, especially "please," "thank you," and "I sure appreciate_______________."

Collaborative Care

Leadership Activity

IDENTIFYING SIGNS OF STRESS

Resources needed:

- Any textbook identifying physical and emotional signs of stress

The next time you feel yourself getting stressed, identify how you are feeling and what you are thinking. List the physical and emotional symptoms you experience.

STRESS CONTROL SKILLS FOR THE LICENSED PRACTICAL/LICENSED VOCATIONAL CHARGE NURSE

Controlling Stress by Altering How You Think

Stress is the body's reaction to the mind's analysis of a situation. It is not the situation, but your reaction to the situation, that creates stress. You have the only **stress management** tool you will ever need right inside your head. If you learn to manage how you think about the many interactions you have daily with nursing assistants, residents, and family members, you can control your reaction and therefore your stress level.

Thinking before "irrational thinking" class

Nursing assistant (on telephone): "I cannot come in today. I have a headache."

LPN/LVN charge nurse (thinking): "I'll just bet the headache is probably due to late night partying."

The LPN/LVN becomes abrupt with the nursing assistant and hangs up. She feels angry and allows the incident to ruin the entire day. Nursing assistants can sense that the charge nurse is upset and will try to avoid any contact.

Ellis (1994) discusses rational versus **irrational thinking**. When we are in a situation, we engage in self-talk about what is happening. This self-talk is often irrational because it is based on judgments we make about the situation. Judgments are subjective and have no bearing on facts. The irrational thinking then causes negative emotions, and stress often results. Ellis offers the ABCD way of increasing awareness of irrational thinking and changing how we think to a more rational way. In learning to do so, we control our emotions and thus the stress that results. The following are examples of how Ellis's ABCD method of controlling irrational thinking applies to the practical/vocational charge nurse.

A—Activating event: The nursing assistant called in sick with a headache.

B—Belief (self-talk) about the situation: The charge nurse thinks the nursing assistant must have been out partying.

C—Consequences: The LPN/LVN manager was abrupt with the nursing assistant on the telephone. She allowed herself to feel angry about the absence. She allowed it to ruin her whole day. Nursing assistants avoided her like the plague.

D—Dispute irrational thoughts: Choose a more rational, assertive response to the situation. Focus on the objective facts (nursing assistant has a headache). Avoid the subjective judgments that your beliefs (self-talk) call up (the nursing assistant was partying). You will avoid the anger over this incident and its effect on nursing assistants. Stress is avoided for all.

Thinking after "irrational thinking" class

Nursing assistant (on telephone): "I cannot come in today. I have a headache."

LPN/LVN charge nurse (tempted to use irrational thinking but remembers Ellis's ABCD instead): "I'm sorry to hear that. I hope you feel better after you get some rest."

See the Collaborative Care, Leadership Hint: Avoiding Irrational Thinking box.

Collaborative Care

Leadership Hint

AVOIDING IRRATIONAL THINKING

1. Be aware that beliefs about the situation are self-talk. Self-talk sometimes makes judgments. These judgments, if negative, can cause an emotional reaction. The emotional reaction leads to stress.
2. See situations objectively. Rational thinking is based on facts. Objective facts do not cause emotion. The situation "just is."
3. Avoid thinking that nursing assistants *should*, *must*, or *always* do something. This is another example of irrational thinking and can lead to anger. When you use these words for yourself, they can lead to anxiety and guilt.
4. We do not have the power to make nursing assistants do anything. We can encourage, prefer, or expect that nursing assistants do something. Realistic expectations are essential. Ask yourself, "How would I feel if asked a similar question or requested to complete a similar task?"
5. For you and team members, use the words *want*, *choose*, and *prefer* in your thinking.

SPECIFIC KNOWLEDGE AND SKILLS NEEDED FOR LEADERSHIP

To be a leader in long-term care, it is necessary to use the aforementioned core areas of knowledge as a base and to develop the following skills in three specific areas:

1. Occupational (clinical) skills: The knowledge and skills of nursing.
2. Organizational skills: Skills necessary to function in the organization that delivers health care.
3. Human relationship skills: The ability to get along with and relate to people.

OCCUPATIONAL SKILLS/KNOWLEDGE FOR FIRST-LINE LPN/LVN LEADERS

Nursing (Clinical) Skills, Including the Nursing Process

Proficient clinical skills are a must to be a good nursing leader. Visible expertise in clinical skills is a plus with the nursing assistants and gives you an informal power base. Get involved in the resident situation, assist in providing care, and demonstrate nursing skills to nursing assistants as needed. This attitude and action demonstrates that the facility mission statement, resident care comes first, and unit goals are the primary focus. It communicates that LPN/LVN charge nurses are there to support their staff.

Knowledge of your role in the nursing process is an important part of organizational skills. Your nursing program has started your development in organizational skills. You need to broaden and deepen these skills as you grow in your professional role. Refer to Chapters 9 and 12 for more about your role in the nursing process.

Documentation

Use the guidelines in nursing fundamentals for your charting. LPN/LVN charge nurses need to be aware of the documentation requirements of federal and state laws and accrediting agencies. Specific, objective documentation demonstrates whether or not the standard of care has been met. Effective nursing documentation is the basis for payment of resident fees or denial of payment by Medicare, insurance, and/or state programs. This is especially important when these agencies mandate client outcomes. Incomplete or questionable documentation could also result in a citation for the facility. It cannot be emphasized often enough that you must make sure all your charting is specific, objective, and complete. Avoid subjective comments and personal judgments in your charting. Students sometimes find this area of charting difficult, especially if they see examples of general and subjective entries on charts by other licensed staff.

Legal Aspects

The nursing assistants and you, the LPN/LVN charge nurse, are the people who have direct contact with residents and their families on a daily basis. You have the ability to ensure resident and family satisfaction with care. You are also in a position to voice concerns. These two roles are key in decreasing the need for legal action to resolve disputes. Chapter 7 provides you with information to legally protect yourself and your facility.

Be aware of your state's NPA, health care facility policies and procedures, state and federal regulations, and published standards of your nursing organizations and codes of conduct. These standards and codes are guidelines to evaluate safe practice. It is your responsibility as a licensed nurse to stay current and informed. The following regulations, legislation, and accreditation information are usually presented in an employment orientation.

Federal regulations. Your facility must be in compliance with federal, state, and local laws. The impact of federal regulations in your facility is affected by the **Omnibus Budget Reconciliation Act of 1987 (OBRA)** and the **Centers for Medicare and Medicaid Services or CMS** (https://www.cms.gov).

The Omnibus Budget Reconciliation Act of 1987. OBRA contains the Nursing Home Reform Act. The basic objective of the Nursing Home Reform Act is to ensure that residents of nursing homes receive quality care that will result in their achieving or maintaining their "highest practicable" (reasonable) physical, mental, and psychosocial well-being. The act also established a Resident's Bill of Rights. Collectively, the Affordable Care Act of 2010 and OBRA contribute to quality in nursing homes. See the Collaborative Care, Leadership Hint: OBRA Provisions That Deal Specifically with Nursing Assistants box.

Collaborative Care

Leadership Hint

OMNIBUS BUDGET RECONCILIATION ACT PROVISIONS THAT DEAL SPECIFICALLY WITH NURSING ASSISTANTS

1. Nursing assistants require a minimum of 75 hours of instruction before taking a state-approved written and skills competency evaluation. This establishes a baseline proficiency and competence of nursing assistants.
2. Each state must have a nursing assistant registry. This registry is an official list of individuals who have successfully completed nursing assistant training and competency evaluation. To be listed in a state directory, the history of the nursing assistant must be free of incidents of abuse, neglect, or dishonest use of property.
3. Your state's registry must be notified by the employer before employment of nursing assistants. The registry of some states is available online.
4. Nursing assistants' work must be evaluated "regularly."
5. Nursing assistants must complete in-service training hours per year. Number of hours can vary based on the state of registry.
6. If an extended period of time has passed without a person being employed as a nursing assistant, training and competency evaluation will need to be repeated.

Centers for medicare and medicaid services. This agency was formerly called the Health Care Financing Administration (HCFA). CMS, a federal agency of the Department of Health and Human Services (HHS), certifies nursing homes for Medicare and Medicaid reimbursement. To receive payment, facilities are required to meet conditions of participation. The long-term care unit will have the conditions of participation in its policies.

Your state's regulations. Long-term care units and nursing homes are licensed by the state in which they are located. Each state sets regulations that must be met to be licensed. Periodically, inspectors will conduct an inspection of the facility to identify compliance with the regulations. Noncompliance is identified as a deficiency. Being cited for deficiencies can affect licensing.

The Joint Commission. **The Joint Commission (TJC)** is an independent, not-for-profit organization. The purpose of this organization is to improve quality of care by creating a safe environment for clients through the accreditation process. TJC reviews organizations such as hospitals, long-term care facilities, and home health agencies. Accreditation is a voluntary activity. Detailed information about TJC and long-term care can be obtained at www.jointcommission.org.

ORGANIZATIONAL SKILLS FOR FIRST-LINE LPN/LVN LEADERS

Organizational skills are an essential ingredient for leaders as well as team members. The emphasis on the personal and professional issues/concepts course in your nursing program has given you the opportunity to learn and apply the principles of time management (see Chapter 2). Continuous quality improvement (see Chapter 16) and conflict management (see Chapter 8) are also necessary skills for the development of any nursing leader in today's health care organizations, including long-term care.

Time Management

Whether your dominance is on the left or right side of the brain, you have been given the opportunity this year to develop **time management** skills by applying the contents of Chapters 1 and 2. Your school year has certainly provided the need to use your time effectively (doing the right thing) and efficiently (doing it right the first time, and in the appropriate amount of time) for class, clinical, and personal life. The step-by-step procedures learned in the nursing skills lab helped you prioritize your care for efficiency and the safety and comfort of the client. You have experience organizing work for one or two clients in the clinical area. As an LPN/LVN charge nurse, you will direct the care of approximately 30 to 40 residents and supervise a team of possibly three to four nursing assistants.

Time management is more about management and less about time. Your ability to manage time will help you organize tasks and allow you to be successful as a charge nurse. Once again, the nursing process will be the tool to help you get organized. See the Collaborative Care, Leadership Hint: Applying the Nursing Process to Organize Your Shift box.

Collaborative Care

Leadership Hint

APPLYING THE NURSING PROCESS TO ORGANIZE YOUR SHIFT

Assessment (Data Collection) of Tasks

1. Make a *to-do* list that reflects unit routines and schedules. When new to the job, listing unit routines and schedules is helpful until you experience the actual routine. This list includes break times, staff meal times, resident meals and nourishments, scheduled health care provider rounds, tests scheduled outside of the facility requiring transport, physical/occupational therapy, and routine times for vital signs, blood glucose testing, medicine administration, and treatments.
2. Develop a *worksheet* to use during report. Use a style that meets your organizational style. Some examples

are lists according to a sequence of room numbers; residents that need special assessments; or by time of treatments, medication administration, and vital signs.
3. *Prioritize* the list. Use Maslow's hierarchy of needs to set priorities for residents. Remember physiologic needs must be met before other needs are considered. Using an A,B,C label, "As" are most important needs and must be done. They could be life threatening or urgent resident needs. "Bs" must be done, but there is flexibility in the exact time they are accomplished. Some "Cs" are necessary but not of urgent status. Some of the "Bs" and "Cs" can be assigned to assistive personnel (APs) or postponed if appropriate. Some "Cs" might not need to be listed at all.
Here are some examples:

Tasks	Examples	Comments
"A" tasks	STAT med, PRN med, q2h neuro check after resident's fall on prior shift	New "A" tasks always surface during the shift, requiring modification of the *to-do* list. These needs are unpredictable and cannot be planned in advance.
"B" tasks	Routine medicine administration, dressing changes, routine resident personal care, ambulation, activities, routine treatments, nourishments, meals	These needs are recurring and predictable but can have specific timelines.
"C" tasks	Mail and flower delivery, chitchat with family	Important but can be delayed.

Planning Use of Time (Goal Setting)

1. Plan tasks within a time frame of 2 to 3 hours. Arrange blocks of time according to unit routine. Planning allows you to feel you are in control of the situation. Take resident preferences into consideration. For example, one resident prefers to eat breakfast at 6 am, but breakfast is served at 8 am. Arrangements could be made for coffee and crackers at 6 am, if diet allows.
2. Use the same guidelines for setting goals for planning time as with care plans or personal goals. Focus on goals as outcomes (the results expected after a given period). Using action verbs, make sure goals are realistic and measurable. A measurable goal states specifically and objectively what results are expected after a specified period. Set mini-goals for timed tasks to keep you on task.
3. Planning involves having the equipment and supplies that the team needs for the shift and the shift that follows. As you collect data about residents when first starting your shift, check rooms and treatment closets for needed supplies. This includes linen, a well-stocked floor refrigerator, supplies for treatments, and supplies for medicine administration kept on a medication cart.
4. Make sure you have your personal tools for the shift: your watch (working), a pen that writes, bandage scissors, a stethoscope, and a small notebook. Use the notebook to jot down the equipment needed and the results of data collection.

Implementing Your Plan

1. Remember your plan is written in soft margarine, not hard marble. Be flexible.
2. As you carry out your plan for the shift, expect interruptions of your planned activities. You know they will occur, but not when. These include telephone calls, changes in residents' conditions, transfer of a resident, and staff injury/concerns.
3. When unexpected events occur, planning assists you to rearrange tasks. If you have a plan, you can return to the plan after interruptions. You can continue or revise the plan as needed.

Evaluating Your Use of Time

1. As nursing assistants give you reports for their assigned residents, seek input from them about the effectiveness and efficiency of the shift.
2. Ask for suggestions to improve staff and your use of time at the next shift you work.
3. Keep a log of your shift activities. Look for a pattern of inefficient use of time. Examples of time wasters are putting things off, allowing unnecessary interruptions, socializing with staff, inability to say "no," and allowing telephone calls to exceed needed time for business.
4. At the end of your shift, take a few minutes to plan for the next day. This will allow you to leave work-related activities at work and allow you to enjoy your much-needed leisure time.

PRN, pro re nata (as needed); *q2h*, quaque secunda hora (every 2 hours); *STAT*, statim (immediately).

Continuous Quality Improvement

Continuous quality improvement (CQI) is a program focused on quality of care and is found in all health care facilities. The principles of CQI found in health care are borrowed from those of the business world. Quality is indicated by client outcomes. **Client outcomes** are observable, measurable results of nursing activities. The CQI program involves all departments of health care facilities, including long-term care. You will receive information about the CQI program during orientation at your facility. See the box Collaborative Care, Leadership Hint: Continuous Quality Improvement Components That the Licensed Practical/Licensed Vocational Charge Nurse Needs to Incorporate into the Leadership Role.

The CMS is involved with quality improvement in nursing homes and long-term care facilities. The **Quality Improvement Organization (QIO)** program consists of a national network of experts, clinicians, and consumers working together to improve care to Medicare recipients. The core functions of QIO include the following (www.cms.gov):

- Improve quality of care for beneficiaries.
- Protect integrity of Medicare Trust Fund.
- Ensure beneficiaries receive appropriate care by expeditiously addressing individual complaints, notices, and appeals, such as noncoverage.

Collaborative Care

Leadership Hint

CONTINUOUS QUALITY IMPROVEMENT COMPONENTS THAT THE LICENSED PRACTICAL/LICENSED VOCATIONAL CHARGE NURSE NEEDS TO INCORPORATE INTO THE LEADERSHIP ROLE

1. Review job descriptions with your nursing assistants. Emphasize the role they have in achieving quality and safety in care and resident service for a reasonable price (do it right the first time).
2. Remember that CQI is a continuous, routine part of your unit.
3. Encourage nursing assistants to report safety issues in resident care and the work environment immediately.
4. Encourage nursing assistants to offer suggestions to solve safety issues stated in number 3 above.
5. When safety issues are noted, initiate a plan for improvement.
6. Consider volunteering for a CQI committee. Policies and nursing procedures are revised based on the input you and the nursing assistants provide regarding resident care and the functioning of the unit. It is personally rewarding to be included in policy and procedure revision because revisions improve resident care.
7. Document resident information in an objective and specific manner. Your documentation will be used to measure the effectiveness of CQI efforts.

Conflict Resolution

Conflict can occur whenever two or more persons interact. In long-term care, conflicts can arise with nursing assistants, staff, residents, families, and health care providers. Conflict is not always a bad thing; sometimes it is an opportunity for growth and learning. Other times, the presence of conflict can point out the need for change in an organization. When conflicts are out in the open, the opportunity exists to settle issues. This is preferable to leaving conflicts unsettled. Unsettled conflicts can act like cancer, slowly growing into something much larger that may be more difficult or impossible to resolve. Tools to reduce conflicts include clear communication and the ability to work well as a team. **Conflict resolution** involves people settling their differences. Resolution of the conflict is an exercise in problem solving. See the Collaborative Care, Leadership Hint: Applying the Nursing Process for Conflict Resolution box.

Collaborative Care

Leadership Hint

APPLYING THE NURSING PROCESS FOR CONFLICT RESOLUTION

Data Collection: Obtain All the Facts

1. When a conflict arises, avoid pursuing it on the spot. Plan your discussion and next steps based on facts, not emotions. Arrange for the involved parties to meet in an area that will provide privacy. First meet with each separately.
2. Separate the person from the problem. Attack the problem, not one another.
3. Each party has its own perception and strong emotions about what happened. Unclear communication may result. Clarify subjective statements and generalizations. You need to obtain objective and specific facts. For example, clarify what is meant by "she always does that" and "they."
4. Actively listen to the person presenting "the facts."
5. Avoid formulating your response while the other party is giving "the facts."

State the Problem: Identify the Specific Issue

1. After hearing all sides, state in your own words what you understand to be the conflict. Use *I* messages when presenting your perspective. For example, say, "Emma, I heard you say that Hannah always leaves the utility room in disarray and does not offer to help the other nursing assistants when she has completed her work and they are swamped."
2. Ask parties for feedback as to the accuracy of your understanding of the conflict: "Emma, am I clear about the nature of your complaint? Is there anything you would like to add or correct?" and "Hannah, is there anything you would like to add or correct about the situation?"

Interventions (Planning)

1. Convey the attitude of working side by side to settle the conflict. For example, sit side by side to work on the problem.
2. Involve all parties in identifying and discussing possible solutions to the conflict. The more alternatives, the better. The goal is a solution that will be agreeable to everyone's interests.
3. *Avoid* bargaining over *positions* (*what you want*). Egos are identified with positions. The parties involved will focus on defending their positions. In the end, all parties need to save face and be ready and able to take the next step.
4. *Focus* on *interests (why something is wanted)*. Behind a *position* is a *motivating interest*. Behind opposite *positions* lie shared and compatible *interests*. *Compromise* involves giving up aspects of an issue that are important to one of the parties involved. This is not a good intervention. *Collaborate* for a win/win solution that focuses on shared or compatible interests.

Implementation: Implement the Selected Solution

On a sunny, cool day in the fall, two residents are sitting in the sunroom of a long-term care facility. Resident A's *position* is that he wants a window open, and Resident B's *position* is that he wants the windows shut. The LPN/LVN charge nurse asks Resident A why he wants a window open. He replies, "So I can get some fresh air." The charge nurse asks Resident B why he wants the windows closed. He replies, "So it won't be drafty."

A solution built on *collaboration* would involve the charge nurse wrapping Resident B in a blanket and moving his wheelchair to the north end of the sunroom. She would move Resident A to the south end of the sunroom and open a window near him. This is a win/win solution. A solution built on *compromise* would involve the LPN/LVN charge nurse returning one of the residents to his room and accommodating the other in the sunroom. This is an "I win/you lose" solution.

Evaluation: Evaluate the Effectiveness of Interventions in Meeting the Goal

In the preceding situation, the LPN/LVN charge nurse returns 30 minutes later and finds both residents are comfortable and enjoying their quiet time.

Human Relationship Skills for First-Line LPN/LVN Leaders

LPN/LVN charge nurses can have excellent clinical skills, use the nursing process expertly, and document to the letter of the law. The LPN/LVN charge nurse can have a good understanding of federal and state laws and requirements of accrediting agencies. Charge nurses can get the job done efficiently, but human relationship skills are the most important skills for an LPN/LVN leader. Leaders with human relationship skills will get the job done with style and tact, without sacrificing quality. Nursing assistants will value their leader's style and be more effective in reaching the unit goals. Staff retention may also improve. Because success depends on what is accomplished through others, the ability to relate well to others is crucial.

Professional Pointer

Human relationship skills are important skills for an LPN/LVN to have in any clinical setting.

LPN/LVNs are well versed in clinical skills. Clinical problem-solving skills can support the development of leadership/management skills for the LPN/LVN charge nurse modeling the thought process inherent to problem solving.

Anger Management

Besides providing money on which to live, work provides people with the opportunity to be recognized for what they do, to belong to a group, and to display their competence. (Review the Howlett hierarchy of work motivators.) When any of these needs is threatened in the course of the workday, or when you feel like a victim in a workplace with lack of control, you may get angry. Anger is not automatically bad; it gives you a cue that something is wrong. If your anger is justified, it can help you get your needs met by stimulating you to action. Harassment and discrimination are examples of situations in which anger is justified. However, anger must always be displayed in a professional manner. If your anger is unjustified, or displayed inappropriately, it can get you and others in trouble. At all times, in all circumstances, behavior must be professional. See the Collaborative Care, Leadership Hint: Preventing Anger in Nursing Assistants box, the Collaborative Care, Leadership Hint: Personal Anger Management Techniques for the Practical/Vocational Charge Nurse box, and the Collaborative Care, Leadership Hint: Prevention of Workplace Violence box.

Collaborative Care

Leadership Hint

PREVENTING ANGER IN NURSING ASSISTANTS

1. Meet the needs above level 2 (e.g., belonging, affiliation, and recognition) on the Maslow and Howlett hierarchies.
2. Use assertive communication, especially *I* messages. This will prevent the LPN/LVN charge nurse from being perceived as a threat. In your *I* messages, remember to include what you observed, the possible result of that observation, and your recommendations.
3. Actively listen, using direct eye contact and alert body posture, to convey to nursing assistants that you are interested in understanding their point of view.
4. Successful team building helps nursing assistants feel like part of the group.
5. Seek input of nursing assistants to find solutions for unit problems. This provides a sense of control over one's work environment.
6. Use win/win strategies in conflict resolution to provide a feeling of having control over situations and being treated with respect.
7. Encourage nursing assistants to participate in objective evaluation of their clinical performance to maintain self-esteem, and give nursing assistants some control over what happens to them.
8. Facilitate self-evaluation/reflection when discussing a potentially volatile area, especially when areas for improvement are noted. It is best if the nursing assistant can identify the improvement needed through guided discussion.
9. Attempt to help nursing assistants become self-confident, reach their full potential, and achieve the higher levels of the Maslow and Howlett hierarchies. When needs are met at these higher levels, nursing assistants are more satisfied in their work environment.

Collaborative Care

Leadership Hint

PERSONAL ANGER MANAGEMENT TECHNIQUES FOR THE LICENSED PRACTICAL/LICENSED VOCATIONAL CHARGE NURSE

1. Learn your personal signs that communicate you are becoming angry. Pay attention to what you are thinking and feeling.
2. How you assess events can cause an anger response. Change irrational thoughts to rational thoughts.
3. If your heart is pounding, take deep breaths.
4. If you feel tension in a body area, rub the area for a few seconds.
5. When angry, take a time out, then speak slowly and in a lower tone of voice and acknowledge how you feel.
6. View a stimulus to anger as a problem. Use the problem-solving process to arrive at a solution.

Collaborative Care

Leadership Hint

PREVENTION OF WORKPLACE VIOLENCE

1. Suggest in-service education in anger management for all employees.
2. Create a work environment that is respectful and fun.
3. As an LPN/LVN charge nurse, be a positive role model for anger management.
4. Take conflicts in the work environment seriously.

5. Refer to/use your facility's employee assistance program (EAP).
6. If your facility does not have an EAP program, suggest that such a program be developed.

Performance Evaluation of Nursing Assistants

The thought of **performance evaluation** can send shivers up the spine or cause anxiety to the person doing the evaluating, as well as of the person being evaluated. Perhaps this goes back to bad evaluation experiences in prior situations. Perhaps it even goes as far back as grade school. Perhaps you and the nursing assistants have learned to associate evaluation with constructive criticism and weaknesses. Keep sight of the main purpose of evaluation, which is to encourage personal and career growth. Self-evaluation is critical to the evaluation process and can provide pertinent discussion points. Constructive evaluation gives you and your team members a profile of strong positive behaviors and behaviors for improvement, along with a plan to improve. Evaluation encourages the development of employees who will meet the facility's objectives and fulfill the mission statement. See the Collaborative Care, Leadership Hint: Providing Feedback to Nursing Assistants box.

Collaborative Care

Leadership Hint

PROVIDING FEEDBACK TO NURSING ASSISTANTS

Positive Feedback Identifies Strong Behaviors to Be Encouraged

1. Most nursing assistants know what it is like to be caught doing something "wrong." Catch them doing something "right." This encourages them to repeat the behavior.
2. Let nursing assistants know you notice their efforts, believe in them, and feel good about their contributions to the long-term care facility.
3. Praise people in measurable terms (specific and objective) so that the behavior can be repeated. For example, say, "When you disinfected the shower, I noticed that you paid special attention to the corners and the shower chair. Great job!"

Negative Feedback Identifies Behaviors That Need Improvement

1. Provide verbal feedback as close to the event as possible. The purpose of constructive feedback is to point out behaviors that need to be modified. Focus on the behavior as one needing improvement. Avoid addressing the behavior as a criticism.
2. Without emotion, objectively point out what is wrong with the behavior and its consequences. You want the nursing assistant to remember the message, not the manner in which it was delivered. You also want the team member to know it is performance that is being evaluated.
3. Negative feedback needs to be constructive to correct the behavior, including specific rationales. These suggestions need to be so specific that the nursing assistant will be able to correct the behavior by following them. For example, you might say, "I noticed that the ties of your isolation gown were untied while you were in the room with the client who has tuberculosis. Once you remove the gown, you risk spreading the bacteria to other clients, staff, and your family because the back of your uniform was not protected. When getting into an isolation gown, be sure to cover the back of your uniform and tie the gown at the waist."
4. Mention behaviors that need improvement first. Offer praise at the end of a reprimand. The message will be heard more clearly. The impact of the praising will not be ruined.

As a LPN/LVN charge nurse, your responsibilities in evaluating nursing assistants include the following:

1. Observing skill performance and attitudes of nursing assistants
2. Providing daily oral/written feedback, including suggestions for improvement
3. Documenting observations
4. Presenting a final evaluation form per institutional policy and procedure

Review the evaluation process and form for your facility. What you are evaluating is not subject to your personal judgment. You will be objectively evaluating the skills and attitudes of nursing assistants. These work-related activities are expected of nursing assistants and are found in their job description and the facility's policy manual. If a checklist format is used for daily observations, be sure you understand the scale used by the long-term care facility. In observing nursing skills, you will be evaluating the application of nursing assistant knowledge of a skill to actual skill performance. Attitudes are more difficult to evaluate. They are stated as observable behaviors and usually involve areas such as dress and grooming, attendance, functioning as a team member, and interpersonal skills. Concerns regarding attitudes should be discussed with your supervisor to facilitate a positive outcome.

The performance evaluation is written documentation of what you have been discussing and documenting throughout the period before the formal process of evaluation. Documentation is a time-consuming task. Familiarity with the system for the long-term care facility will result in completing it more quickly.

OBRA mandates regular evaluations for nursing assistants. In addition to scheduled performance evaluations, you will be giving spontaneous feedback to nursing assistants. Evaluation is the responsibility of the LPN/LVN charge nurse and the nursing assistant. No one needs to "give" another person an evaluation. Evaluation needs to be a joint process. Evaluation is not a secret that you surprise team members with at the end of the evaluation period. It is a tool for personal and career growth. A team member has the right to be able to correct areas for improvement as time goes by. It is unfair to have your discrepancies unloaded (i.e., dumped) on you during the final evaluation interview. See the Collaborative Care, Leadership Hint: Encouraging Nursing Assistants to Participate in the Evaluation Process box and the Collaborative Care, Leadership Hint: Meeting for the Final Evaluation Interview box.

Collaborative Care

Leadership Hint

ENCOURAGING NURSING ASSISTANTS TO PARTICIPATE IN THE EVALUATION PROCESS

1. Provide nursing assistants with their own copy of the evaluation form at the beginning of the evaluation experience. Tell them it contains the elements you will be evaluating. Encourage them to read it.
2. Encourage nursing assistants to evaluate themselves daily/weekly and record their evaluation on their copy of the form. This also gives them the opportunity to become familiar with the form.
3. Remind them to include their strengths. People are good at identifying areas for improvement but sometimes need reminders to acknowledge their strong points. Dispel the myth that doing so is egotistical or boastful. Their strengths can help other members of the team and vice versa.
4. Encourage nursing assistants to include a plan on the evaluation form for improving areas that need improvement.

Collaborative Care

Leadership Hint

MEETING FOR THE FINAL EVALUATION INTERVIEW

1. Remember that the goal of evaluation is to encourage personal and professional growth. In preparation for the evaluation, summarize positive behaviors of the nursing assistant and behaviors that need improvement on your copy of the evaluation form. Develop a suggested plan for improvement. Attach this summary to the front of the evaluation. Remind nursing assistants to do the same and to bring their copy of the completed evaluation form to the meeting.
2. Schedule the interview at a private location.
3. Allow 15 to 20 minutes for the interview.
4. Conduct the interview in a neutral manner. Be careful of both your verbal and nonverbal messages.
5. Use *I* messages when discussing the summary sheet. For example, say, "The following are the behaviors that I observed when you were working with residents and staff...."
6. Use the information on the 4 I's of Transformational Leadership learned in this chapter to guide your interaction.
7. Start with strong behaviors and compare them with the nursing assistant's list. This creates a good mood. The job description is a great guide if other documents are not available.
8. Compare behaviors for improvement.
   a. Similar behaviors appearing on both evaluation forms can indicate insight into the problem. Both the nursing assistant and the LPN/LVN charge nurse have noted similar behaviors in the clinical area.
   b. When the nursing assistant includes behaviors not noted by the LPN/LVN charge nurse, this can indicate the value of self-evaluation. The charge nurse cannot observe everything.
   c. If the LPN/LVN charge nurse includes behaviors not included by the nursing assistant, this can indicate lack of self-evaluation/self-reflection by the nursing assistant.
9. Finish the evaluation interview with the plan for improvement for any behaviors that need to be modified. The nursing assistant's plan is especially valuable because it indicates the ability to think through interventions needed for improvement and building strengths.
10. Check feedback throughout the interview to ensure clear communication. Have the nursing assistant rephrase feedback to see whether or not your intended message was heard. Some people may distort the message. Clarify messages given by the nursing assistant for information not understood. Encourage questions about any areas on the evaluation that are not understood. For example, say, "What did you understand me to say regarding your areas of strength I identified?"
11. Have the nursing assistant sign and date both evaluations. You do the same. The signature indicates that the forms were discussed and all questions were answered.

Your nonthreatening, objective approach to constructive evaluation will result in positive evaluation experiences for you and the nursing assistants on your team. Occasionally you may experience a situation in which a nursing assistant feels threatened and becomes defensive during evaluation. If the defensiveness begins to escalate or the person displays anger, terminate the meeting. Set a new time for another meeting. Have your supervisor and/or human resources present at this time. Such experiences are the exception, not the rule.

Empowering Team Members and Encouraging Personal Growth and Development of Confidence

It is rewarding to see the nursing assistants on your team increase their self-confidence and display career and personal growth. You can encourage personal growth in nursing assistants by demonstrating the leadership skills you have developed in your position as an LPN/LVN charge nurse. The nursing assistant must do the actual work to achieve confidence and grow. See the Collaborative Care, Empowerment: Strategies to Increase Self-Confidence in Nursing Assistants box and the Collaborative Care, Empowerment: Strategies to Encourage Personal Growth in Nursing Assistants box.

Collaborative Care

Empowerment

STRATEGIES TO INCREASE SELF-CONFIDENCE IN NURSING ASSISTANTS

1. Provide opportunities to be successful in new situations.
2. Praise beginning successes in new situations.
3. On clinical evaluation forms, include positive statements as well as negative statements.

4. With administration's support, plan educational opportunities for nursing assistants (e.g., seminars and in-service programs).
5. Include nursing assistants in planning meetings and in-service ideas.
6. Stand up for and support nursing assistants' contributions to the facility.
7. Actively listen to problems involving the clinical area.
8. Coach/mentor nursing assistants on a new skill and/or how to improve a one already known.
9. Provide challenging assignments that stimulate thinking.

Collaborative Care

Empowerment

STRATEGIES TO ENCOURAGE PERSONAL GROWTH IN NURSING ASSISTANTS

1. Display a balanced interest in the personal problems of nursing assistants.
2. Encourage nursing assistants to solve their own problems.
3. Suggest referral when nursing assistants are unable to solve personal problems. Follow facility policies.
4. Listen actively.
5. Be a mentor/coach.
6. Be a role model. Display a positive work ethic; demonstrate excellent clinical skills; make rounds frequently to see what residents; display professional grooming; give objective, specific feedback; address the problem, not people; and actively listen.

ADDITIONAL RESOURCES FOR THE LPN/LVN TO DEVELOP ORGANIZATIONAL, OCCUPATIONAL, AND HUMAN RELATIONSHIP SKILLS

There are many ways to develop occupational, organizational, and human relationship skills for survival in the workplace. Some of the following suggestions for additional learning offer continuing education credits. See the Collaborative Care, Empowerment: Sources of Learning Skills for the Licensed Practical/Licensed Vocational Charge Nurse Position box.

Collaborative Care

Empowerment

SOURCES OF LEARNING SKILLS FOR THE LICENSED PRACTICAL/ LICENSED VOCATIONAL CHARGE NURSE POSITION

1. Check with your local vocational/technical school for an LPN/LVN nursing leadership course.
2. Ask your supervisor to consider in-service programs on leadership techniques, including transformational leadership strategies and updates on nursing skills. Suggest cosponsoring in-services with the local technical college and making them available to a wide geographical area.
3. Form a network with other persons who fill first-line leadership positions. Be sure to go outside your institution, as well as the discipline of nursing. You will find that the leaders have similar problems regardless of the discipline.
4. Attend seminars relating to leadership topics as well as nursing topics.
5. Read books and articles that offer strategies for leaders. Be sure your personal nursing library is up to date.
6. Enroll for certification courses to enhance your knowledge and skills. See Chapter 18 for additional information.

Keep in Mind

"Effective leadership is putting first things first. Effective management is discipline, carrying it out."

—Stephen R. Covey

A reflection—The LPN/LVN was always a "saver," which several well-constructed scrapbooks and boxes of books and papers from nursing school verified. The LPN/LVN looked at the carefully preserved classified ad saved from 5 years ago, when first applying for the current nursing position. After 3 years' experience as an LPN/LVN in a nursing home, postgraduate courses in leadership at the local technical college, seminars, in-service programs, personal reading, and workshops, the LPN/LVN thought that this proved qualification for a charge nurse position.

The LPN/LVN smiled when imagining going in for the interview. That navy blue blazer and all the preparation for the interview paid off. What a sage the nursing instructor had been in the Transitions to Practice class to recommend that a job applicant read the facility's mission statement before the interview. Although not having LPN/LVN charge nurse experience, certainly knowledge of the facility's emphasis on and pride in providing quality care was a big plus in landing the job. And this was in addition to the enthusiasm and positive attitude displayed to the interviewer about a willingness to learn and having confidence to do the job. Also, following the textbook suggestion to obtain the respective state's NPA before employment provided the opportunity to learn how an LPN/LVN could delegate in the respective state and helped think of some supervision/delegation-related questions to ask at the interview.

Five years had passed since securing the job as LPN/LVN charge nurse. The LPN/LVN loved the job and smiled remembering many of the challenges faced early in the job as charge nurse. The LPN/LVN began to page through that old eighth edition of the textbook….

Licensed Practical Nurse/Licensed Vocational Nurse

Full-time position available for an experienced LPN/LVN to join our long-term care facility as a charge nurse on the evening shift. Must have excellent communication and customer service skills, needs to be team oriented, and must have a current state license. We offer a competitive salary and full benefits package. If you qualify, submit resume and cover letter to:

Before continuing with the LPN's/LVN's story, review the Collaborative Care, Leadership Activity: Determining Your State's Requirements to Assume the Position of Licensed Practical/Licensed Vocational Charge Nurse box in this chapter.

Looking at the job description the director of nurses gave at the job interview, it all seems such a routine and comfortable part of the job. However, the LPN/LVN remembers how overwhelming it was to read through the 12 areas of responsibility, along with the 15 duties of the charge nurse.

WHERE TO BEGIN? BECOMING A CHARGE NURSE

JOB DESCRIPTION FOR CHARGE NURSE

Read the Collaborative Care, Management Tool: Reviewing Licensed Practical/Licensed Vocational Charge Nurse Job Descriptions box. The charge nurse job description might seem overwhelming at first, but it illustrates the reason some state laws require that LPN/LVN charge nurses have education, training, or experience beyond the basic LPN/LVN nursing curriculum and documentation of such. It is difficult to prepare health care workers in 1 year or less to be able to function in this position immediately after graduation. After additional education, training, and experience, many LPNs/LVNs become charge nurses, also called first-line managers, in long-term care units and nursing homes. They are doing an excellent job in that role. The NCSBN (2025) 2024 job analysis survey identified that 40.1% of LPNs/LVNs responding to the survey reported they had administrative responsibilities (Box 17.3).

Box 17.3 Quality Care Licensed Practical/Licensed Vocational Charge Nurse: Job Description

QUALIFICATIONS

Licensed practical nurse/licensed vocational nurse (LPN/LVN) with a current license to practice in State XYZ. One-year experience as a charge nurse in a long-term care facility.

STANDARDS

The job of the LPN/LVN charge nurse is to ensure that residents receive high-quality, low-cost nursing care that has been ordered by their health care provider. The LPN/LVN charge nurse shall do the following:

- Collaborate with the RN and other team members to provide resident care services (e.g., health care providers, dietitian, activity director, physical therapist, and social worker).
- Assist the director of nurses in the orientation of new employees.
- Evaluate work performance of nursing assistants. Responsible For (Collaborating With The RN)
- Assessment and evaluation of residents' conditions at all times.
- Assigning actual nursing care tasks to nursing assistants.
- Providing nursing care according to health care providers' orders and in agreement with recognized nursing techniques and procedures, established standards of care as described in state statutes, and administrative policies of this long-term care facility.
- Recognizing symptoms: reporting residents' conditions, including changes, and assisting with remedial measures for adverse developments.
- Assisting health care provider in diagnostic and therapeutic measures.
- Administering medications and treatments as prescribed.
- Maintaining accurate and complete records of nursing data collection and interventions, including documentation on the electronic medical record (EMR) and Kardex.
- Efficiency in completing workload, including neatness and orderliness.
- Delegating duties, as appropriate, to nursing assistants.
- Maintaining a safe and hazard-free environment.
- Ensuring the residents' right to privacy.
- Maintaining the dignity of residents.

DUTIES (IN COLLABORATION WITH THE RN)

- Assesses, plans, implements, and evaluates client care per plan of care in collaboration with RN
- Observes and reports symptoms and conditions of residents.
- Administers medications safely and as prescribed by health care providers.
- Gathers data about therapeutic response and side effects of medications.
- Takes and records vital signs accurately when appropriate. Maintains charts and Kardexes, including residents' conditions and medications and treatments received.
- Notifies health care provider when necessary. Records phone/fax orders.
- Contacts pharmacist for prescription medications as needed.
- Assists in maintaining a physical, social, and psychological environment for residents that is conducive to their best interests and welfare.
- Receives report at beginning of shift from personnel on previous shift and assigns tasks to nursing assistants under the LPN/LVN charge nurse's supervision.
- Supervises, assists with, and evaluates delegated duties to nursing assistants.
- Evaluates the completion of nursing assistant assignments in a safe and timely manner.
- Provides report to oncoming shift.
- Evaluates nursing assistants in the performance of their job description and reports same to director of nursing.
- Attends client care meetings and supervisory staff meetings.
- Interprets state and federal guidelines to employees. Uses authority as LPN/LVN charge nurse to "follow code."
- Participates in orientation of all new employees assigned to LPN/LVN charge nurse.

Collaborative Care

Management Tool

REVIEWING LPN/LVN CHARGE NURSE JOB DESCRIPTIONS

Resources needed:

- Review LPN/LVN charge nurse job descriptions of long-term care facilities at sites at which you affiliate during your student year.

HOW LONG WILL IT TAKE ME TO PREPARE TO BE A CHARGE NURSE?

You are probably thinking, "How long will it take for me to get to this point in my practical/vocational nursing career?" The answer is individual to the person asking it. The law of some states specifically dictates that the LPN/LVN charge nurse functions in a nursing home and under the direct supervision of an RN. Also, the LPN/LVN could not function under general supervision until after passing the National Council Licensure Examination for Licensed Practical Nurses (NCLEX-PN®) examination. Be sure to check your state's NPA. Some LPN/LVN nursing programs offer a postgraduate course that prepares graduates for an expanded role. The answer to the question, "How long will it take for me to get to this point in my LPN/LVN nursing career?" depends on your state's NPA, additional education, prior related experience (including non-health care–related experience), your motivation to learn the manager role, your ability to be a risk taker, how you use your nursing experience, and the policy and procedures of the employing institution.

HOW THIS TEXT CAN HELP YOU PREPARE FOR A FUTURE CHARGE NURSE POSITION

This text is unable to provide you with a concise recipe of how to function in the role of charge nurse as an LPN/LVN. This chapter begins with a discussion of areas of responsibilities, problems, and concerns that affect the LPN/LVN charge nurse in a long-term care unit or nursing home. Through active learning and an interactive format, this chapter presents both management and leadership tools. These tools involve you with the many areas that need to be considered, understood, and investigated when assuming an LPN/LVN charge nurse position. In addition, critical-thinking exercises present the opportunity to apply learning in the area of assignment and delegation.

Scenarios for three residents are interspersed throughout the nursing process guide for leading, assigning, and delegating. You will be expected to be self-directed, to problem solve, and to think critically as you apply the information in this chapter. These are the very attributes employers expect of you as an LPN/LVN charge nurse. References to specific resources that you will need to work through the leadership and management tools are provided. You are encouraged to use the information from the entire text, your other classes, and your learning resource center. Your instructor is a valuable resource. Remember, also, the usefulness of peer group discussion.

At times we will flash back to the LPN/LVN reminiscing about the early days in the LPN/LVN charge nurse position. Initial experiences and adjustment to the charge nurse role will show you the challenges and opportunities the LPN/LVN charge nurse role provides.

The LPN/LVN thought back to the orientation phase of the job. It seemed so overwhelming at the time. The thought of going through those thick manuals of policies, regulations, and routines was enough to give the LPN/LVN a headache. However, they sure did contain valuable information. The nurse educator gave the class the following sample checklist as a guide when reviewing these manuals.

A CHECKLIST OF POLICIES, REGULATIONS, AND ROUTINES FOR THE LICENSED PRACTICAL/LICENSED VOCATIONAL CHARGE NURSE

Not all the areas included in this checklist are the responsibility of the LPN/LVN charge nurse in a nursing home/long-term care facility. However, LPN/LVN charge nurses need to have information for all the areas included so they can carry out their management duties. Because the LPN/LVN charge nurse has the responsibility to supervise nursing assistants, these personnel also need information about policies and routines. Orientation to your facility needs to include these items.

FACILITY ORGANIZATION/LEGAL ASPECTS

- Mission statement
- Organizational chart
- State statutes for all licensed persons on health care team
- Skills checklists for LPNs/LVNs and nursing assistants
- Skills checklists for all cross-trained personnel
- Job descriptions and duties of RNs and LPNs/LVNs
- Job descriptions and duties of unlicensed personnel and cross-trained personnel

FEDERAL, STATE, AND PRIVATE AGENCY REGULATIONS

- Inspection protocols/standards
- Current federal (including Health Insurance Portability and Accountability Act [HIPAA] regulations) and state regulations
- Regulations of the Omnibus Budget Reconciliation Act of 1987
- Regulations of the Centers for Medicare and Medicaid Services (CMS)
- Regulations of The Joint Commission (if facility seeks TJC accreditation)
- National Client Safety Standards
- Other related accreditation standards

PERSONNEL POLICIES

- Employee manual
- Time sheets: location and interpretation
- Vacation, holiday, sick leave policy
- Special request for time off, leave of absence
- Communication, reporting: on and off duty, sickness, absence, memos, bulletin board
- Meal and coffee break
- Smoking regulations
- Use of facility telephones, personal cell phones, and other electronic devices
- Uniform regulations
- Computer-related systems

RECORDS AND UNIT ROUTINES

- General shift routine for days, evenings, and nights
- Duties of each of the three shifts
- Methods of reporting
- Procedure manual
- Facility policy manual
- Procedures specific to each division of the facility
- Nursing care plan system
- Nursing Kardex and Pyxis systems
- Electronic medical record (EMR)
- Routine for care planning conferences
- Routine for health care providers' visits
- System of transcribing health care providers' orders
- Location of reference books

TECHNOLOGY

- Computer systems for documentation, medication administration, other
- Phone system
- IT support/contact
- Policies regarding acceptable use

UNIT ADMINISTRATION

- Admission, placement, transfer, and discharge of residents
- Care of clothing and valuables, including personal property list
- Procedure for caring for seriously ill residents
- Procedure for caring for a resident who has died
- Autopsy permit
- Authorization procedure and forms for diagnostic tests and surgery
- Visiting hours
- Notary public

SAFETY POLICIES

- Side rails
- Restraints and bed alarms
- Fire regulations: reporting, evacuation plan, fire exits, location and correct use of fire extinguishers, fire alarms, preventive measures, fire drill procedure
- Use of oxygen
- Transportation of residents by cart, wheelchair
- Body mechanics and back safety policy
- Door alarms
- Standard precautions
- Security policies
- Smoking policy

HOUSEKEEPING, MAINTENANCE, AND SUPPLIES

- Linen: how supplied, extra linen
- Care of contaminated linens and dressings
- Unit cleaning procedure and responsibilities
- How to obtain supplies: medications, sterile supplies, personal care items, kitchen items
- Maintenance and repairs requests
- Conservation of supplies, linen, and equipment

EQUIPMENT: HOW TO USE IT AND WHERE TO OBTAIN IT

- Oxygen
- Suction equipment
- Therapeutic beds
- Respiratory therapy equipment and services

FOOD SERVICE FOR RESIDENTS

- Ordering diets/diet changes
- Tray service
- Unit food stock items
- Special nourishments
- Policy for feeding residents
- Policy for dining room
- Policy for family trays

NURSING CARE PROCEDURES/ASSISTING HEALTH CARE PROVIDER

- Morning and evening care
- Bathing/showering, bed bath
- Mouth care
- Bed making
- Temperature (devices used), pulse, and respiration
- Blood pressure
- Catheterization
- Enemas
- Suppositories: rectal
- Recording intake and output
- Systems used for pressure ulcer care
- Collecting, delivering, and labeling specimens
- Assisting podiatrist with foot care
- Policies for sterile technique procedures
- Blood glucose monitoring
- Colostomy care
- Nasogastric and gastrostomy tubes: flushing, feeding, administration of medication
- Standard precautions
- Postmortem procedures

MEDICATIONS

- Medication system
- Policy for reordering
- Unit stock
- Ordering from pharmacy
- Review of metric system, proportions
- Drug errors: reporting, incident reports

- Narcotics count
- Sources of drug administration

DOCUMENTATION

- Method of documenting
- Electronic medical record
- Specific forms used
- Flow sheets used
- Policy for phone/fax/e-mail orders/software use
- Incident reports
- Lists for wanderers, hearing aid use, and so on
- Federal and state chart forms and requirements

SPECIAL AREAS

- Emergency supplies
- Central supply area
- Physical therapy
- Occupational therapy
- Laundry
- Maintenance
- Break room
- Dining room
- Kitchen
- Business offices
- Social services
- Director of nurses
- Chaplain services/chapel area
- Nurse educator
- Administrator of facility
- Conference rooms
- Recreational areas
- Activity department

MISCELLANEOUS

- Paging system
- Call light system
- Disaster plan, evacuation procedure
- Procedure for residents who desire cardiopulmonary resuscitation
- Volunteer services
- On-call schedule
- Handling of wanderers
- Procedure for signing resident in and out of facility
- Hair care services
- Podiatrist and dentist list
- Staff break room

See the Collaborative Care, Management Tool: Reviewing Policies and Routines box.

Collaborative Care

Management Tool

REVIEWING POLICIES AND ROUTINES

Resources needed:

- Aforementioned checklist of policies, regulations, and routines for the LPN/LVN
- Your opinion and reasons (rationale)

All policies, regulations, and routines of a health care facility are important. After reading the checklist, complete the following:

1. List the five items from records and unit routines that you think are most necessary for effective running of the resident wings of the long-term care unit. Provide the reason (rationale) for your choices.

ITEM	RATIONALE
a.	
b.	
c.	
d.	
e.	

2. List the five items from unit administration that you think are most necessary for management of the resident wings of the long-term care unit. Provide your reason (rationale) for your choices.

ITEM	RATIONALE
a.	
b.	
c.	
d.	
e.	

The LPN/LVN came across a data list. The Nurse Educator had stressed the importance of the LPN's/LVN's assisting role in collecting data and always said that what the LPN/LVN did with the data really separated the licensed nurse from unlicensed personnel. The nurse educator had provided a helpful list of signs and symptoms to be aware of in various client situations and stressed it would not be a complete list, but would be something to get us started. It had been some time since the LPN/LVN updated that list.

COLLECTING DATA AS A CHARGE NURSE

As LPN/LVN charge nurse, the change-of-shift report when coming on duty provides data for dividing the work of the shift among team members. Baseline data of residents for whom you are in charge must also be obtained. This involves a quick visit of each resident to compare the status of residents with the status reported at change of shift. You will also collect data periodically during your shift. The frequency of data collecting depends on client condition. Following is a list of signs and symptoms that may indicate illness, exacerbation of a previous disease condition, injury, or decline in prior functioning.

Be observant with each resident interaction. When nursing assistants report that "something does not seem right," visit the resident to collect your own data. Then record it on the proper form and report all abnormal observations according to agency policy. The actual data-collecting parameters given here are guidelines. Follow specific parameters given for the resident or dictated by institutional policy. Collaborate with the RN or health care provider as needed.

SIGNS AND SYMPTOMS

1. **Weight:** Increase or decrease of 5 to 10 lb in 1 week.
2. **Temperature:** Elevation over 100°F (37.7°C) orally or 100.6°F (38.1°C) rectally; temperature under 96.6°F (35.8°C) orally.

3. **Upper respiratory:** Head congestion, headache, sore throat, ear pain, runny nose, postnasal drip.
4. **Lower respiratory:** Acute onset or worsening of shortness of breath, dyspnea with exertion, orthopnea, cough (productive or nonproductive), wheezing, or other abnormal sounds on inhalation or exhalation.
5. **Cardiac:** Blood pressure over 135/85 (new symptom); blood pressure below 80/50; irregular pulse (new symptom); chest, neck, shoulder, or arm pain; fatigue; increased frequency of angina; shortness of breath; orthopnea; peripheral edema; sacral edema or distended neck veins.
6. **Breast:** Lump found on palpation, discharge from nipple.
7. **Abdomen:** Localized or generalized pain, especially of acute onset; epigastric burning or discomfort; constipation; diarrhea; nausea; vomiting; bloody or tarry stools; loss of appetite.
8. **Musculoskeletal:** Swollen and tender joints, loss of strength in limbs, pain, loss of motion, ecchymosis, edema.
9. **Reproductive system:** Vaginal discharge, abnormal vaginal bleeding.
10. **Genitourinary:** Urgency, frequency, dysuria, nocturia, hematuria, incontinence. Male: dribbling, inability to start or stop stream.
11. **Sleep and rest patterns:** Changes from normal routine, requirement of medication for sleep, nightmares or dreams.
12. **Appearance of skin:** Changes in color, turgor, contusions, abrasions, lacerations, rashes, lesions.
13. **Mobility and exercise:** Need for support in ambulation, changes in posture, weakness of extremities, changes in coordination, vertigo.
14. **Hygiene status:**
    a. Mouth: Condition of mucous membranes, gums, teeth, tongue, mouth odor.
    b. Body: Cleanliness, odor, especially of body creases and genital area.
    c. Hair: Grooming, distribution, scalp scaling, lesions.
    d. Nails: Color, texture, and grooming of fingernails and toenails.
15. **Communication:** Verbal, nonverbal, and affective, aphasia, level of understanding.
16. **Sensory-perceptual:** Ability to hear, and condition of hearing aid; ability to see, and condition of glasses; ability to feel in all extremities; ability to discriminate odors; ability to distinguish tastes.
17. **Cultural/religious:** Food preferences, wellness/illness beliefs, religious practices (e.g., rosary, prayer beads, Bible, Koran, Torah, religious readings, medals, icons, communion, clergy visits, confession, sacrament of the sick).
18. **Psychological status:** Level of consciousness, disorientation, intelligence, attention span, vocabulary level, interests, memory, affect.

The student remembered how the nurse educator stressed the importance of getting to a room and personally collecting client data, especially when there was a change of condition.

THE REPORT THAT WASN'T

An NA reported to the LPN/LVN charge nurse (CN) that the client "doesn't look too good to me." The charge nurse immediately called the health care provider (HCP).

Health Care Provider: What seems to be the trouble?
CN to NA: What seems to be the trouble?
NA to CN: I don't know. The client just doesn't look right.
CN to HCP: The client just doesn't look right.
HCP: How long has he looked like this?
CN: I don't know. We just noticed.
HCP: What's his temperature?
CN: Just a minute. I'll find out.
CN to NA: Take the client's temperature.
HCP: What are his other vital signs?
CN: I don't know. The nursing assistant is going to check them.
HCP: How much fluid has the client had?
CN: Just a minute. (CN puts the telephone down and goes to check the client's intravenous [IV] line.)
CN: The client is getting an IV now.
HCP (with sarcasm in his voice): Is the client breathing? Never mind, don't send anyone to check. I will be over to check myself. (The health care provider hangs up abruptly.)
CN to NA: I don't know why the HCP gets so upset every time I call. What am I supposed to do?

What do you think went wrong in this scenario?

See the Collaborative Care, Management Tool: Reporting Change of Condition to the Health care provider box.

Collaborative Care

Management Tool

REPORTING CHANGE OF CONDITION TO THE HEALTH CARE PROVIDER

Resources needed:

- A checklist of signs and symptoms (earlier in this chapter)
- SBAR (situation, background, assessment, and recommendation) information from Chapter 8
- A medical-surgical textbook or electronic access to evidence

List the data you would collect and any other pertinent information you would gather before notifying the health care provider of a "change of condition" in the following residents:

- Resident has history of compensated, left-sided congestive heart failure.
- Resident has cancer of the esophagus and uses a Duragesic patch for pain control.

The LPN/LVN began to think of the "people problems" that are continually experienced in the job as LPN/LVN charge nurse. With each day that passes, handling these problems becomes easier and easier. The nurse educator's basic advice to "treat people as you would like to be treated" has saved the day on many occasions. That was good advice even for reporting change of condition to the health care provider: "What information would I need if I was the health care provider and my client had a change of condition?" As for managing with health care providers, residents, staff, and families, I sure remember situations that arose as clearly as if they happened yesterday.

Professional Pointer

Treat others as you would like to be treated.

COMMON PROBLEMS OF LICENSED PRACTICAL/ LICENSED VOCATIONAL CHARGE NURSE

The LPN/LVN recalled one morning during the second week of work after orientation to the charge nurse position. The nursing assistants were upset. The babysitter for the three young children of one of the nursing assistants had quit the evening before. When the NA got up the next morning for work, the car would not start. All the nursing assistants were talking about the NA's problems from the time they hung up their coats, straight through lunch, and beyond. It was only the week before that the NA found out about the overdraw at the bank because of checks written before the NA's paycheck was deposited by Quality Care Home and cleared by the bank. It seemed as though "things always happened to the NA, despite being such a nice person. It just was not right." All the nursing assistants were feeling bad because these problems happened to the NA. Everyone got involved with how to get the NA out of the current mess. Several of the nursing assistants forgot to do some of their tasks/duties, and the NA needed a lot of assistance to get the assignment completed. The LPN/LVN then remembered when the nurse educator stood in the front of the class with a stuffed toy monkey on the instructor's back.

WHEN NURSING ASSISTANTS BRING PROBLEMS FROM HOME

As an LPN/LVN charge nurse, it is important that you do not fall into the "monkey trap," as described by Blanchard et al. (1991) in *The One-Minute Manager Meets the Monkey*. You fall into the trap each time you take on a responsibility (monkey) that belongs to an employee. Once monkeys are adopted, they take a lot of time in their care and upkeep. LPN/LVN charge nurses can help nursing assistants become aware of this trap and be a role model for avoiding it. Remember this thought, "This is not my monkey … this is not my circus."

Realize that you do not own any problems that nursing assistants experience. The nursing assistant owns the problem. Avoid feeling bad because you cannot solve the problems of team members. Be supportive and express genuine concern and empathy (individual consideration), but realize that you do not have a license to counsel nursing assistants. Team members need to solve their own problems. Follow facility policies when personal problems interfere with work performance. Report the situation to your supervisor. Professional counseling in the community may be necessary, and they may be able to access the employee assistance program (EAP). See the Collaborative Care, Management Tool: When Nursing Assistants Bring Problems From Home box.

Collaborative Care

Management Tool

WHEN NURSING ASSISTANTS BRING PROBLEMS FROM HOME

Resources needed:

- Reading: The section in this chapter "When Nursing Assistants Bring Problems From Home"
- Creative thinking
  Pretend you are the LPN/LVN charge nurse the morning NA comes to work with problems. Identify a way to handle the situation.

Simon, the LPN, remembered Betty, a nursing assistant who had been employed at Quality Care Home for 6 months. Chio told Aisha, a nursing assistant on the same wing, that she did not know how to use the new client-lifting device. Aisha stated she did not really have time, but Chio coaxed her to take the time to get the resident out of bed. Simon had suggested to Aisha a way of handling the situation that could be implemented in the future, a tip that would help Chio be more accountable.

ENCOURAGING PERSONAL RESPONSIBILITY IN NURSING ASSISTANTS

When nursing assistants cannot do something that is in their job description (e.g., transferring a resident by a lifting device), it is their problem. Staff persons need to avoid assuming it is a staff problem. Be sure to follow the policy of the facility. For safety reasons, encourage nursing assistants to report to the charge nurse when they are having problems carrying out their assignment. This gives the charge nurse the opportunity to determine what staff member is skilled and available to assist in the situation. Encourage the nursing assistant to offer suggestions for learning to do the part of their job that they do not know how to do. Praise them for coming up with a plan, and add to the plan, if necessary. Write a note to your supervisor explaining the situation objectively and how you proceeded to remedy the situation. If necessary, request additional training for the nursing assistant. Learning who owns problems will help you control a large part of the stress you experience as an LPN/LVN charge nurse and help ensure the safety of resident care. See the Collaborative Care, Management Tool: Encouraging Nursing Assistants to Be Accountable for Learning Skills box.

Collaborative Care

Management Tool

ENCOURAGING NURSING ASSISTANTS TO BE ACCOUNTABLE FOR LEARNING SKILLS

Resources needed:

- Reading: The section in this chapter "Encouraging Personal Responsibilities in Nursing Assistants"
  Develop a plan to encourage Betty to approach the lifting-device situation in a more accountable manner.

Estella remembered instances while a student and as an LPN when families had complained about care given to their relatives. These complaints troubled Estella, who had high standards and was prideful of the quality of nursing care. Complaints were taken seriously and each criticism investigated thoroughly. Sometimes nothing could be found out of order, and sometimes Estella began doubting and decided to self-evaluate. Once again, the nurse educator offered insight into this common problem, which Estella still uses today.

MANAGING DEMANDING/COMPLAINING FAMILIES

A common problem in the nursing home is managing complaints of family members regarding care of their relatives. A common complaint involves physical care. Sometimes the family members become verbally aggressive, express concerns in an angry manner, and are very critical of the charge nurse. Others will be nonassertive and sarcastic. Remember the problem-solving process. First, collect data to determine the real problem. If there is a problem with physical care, identify and correct it. Be honest and apologize as appropriate. Sometimes when the problem is identified and solved, the complaints continue. Sometimes when no problem with physical care is identified, the family may continue the attack. It is always important to try to identify the source of the anger and then proceed.

It is necessary to consider the situation in which the family finds itself. They are in a position of seeing their loved one progressively aging and decompensating. This is a time of loss for the family. They may feel guilty about placing a relative in a long-term care facility or about not being able to continue caregiving. They may be contending with grieving issues. Lashing out may be their attempt at relief. To avoid personal issues, family members may unconsciously project blame onto nursing assistants and other members of the nursing staff. It is similar to looking at skeletons in other people's closets so you do not have to look at those in your own closet. This behavior may make a family feel better. It is important for staff to understand these issues to avoid hurt feelings. Avoid personalizing the situation. Suggested interventions to manage the demanding or complaining family are included in the Collaborative Care, Management Tool: Interventions to Use When You Perceive the Family to Be Demanding/Complaining box. When family complaints surface, investigate them, but remember to keep broad shoulders. The exercise in the Critical Thinking: Interventions to Use When You Perceive the Family to Be Demanding/Complaining box can help you practice managing family members who you perceive to be demanding and complaining family.

Collaborative Care

Management Tool

INTERVENTIONS TO USE WHEN YOU PERCEIVE THE FAMILY TO BE DEMANDING/COMPLAINING

- Develop a sincere, nonpunitive relationship with the resident's family.
- Encourage the family to vent feelings about the resident's placement in a nursing home, aging, and behavior.
- Apologize if a mistake has been made or if care has not been of high quality as expected.
- Be specific regarding steps taken to remedy the adverse situation.
- Try to identify the unconscious issue (possible hidden bias) and address it.
- Determine the needs the family is trying to fulfill through their demands, criticism, and complaints.
- Spend time with the family when demands or complaints are not being made.
- Establish rapport with the family to provide emotional support during this difficult time.
- Explain the resident's disease and expected behavior.
- Assess the family's understanding of the client's condition. Clarify any misperceptions.
- Suggest joining a support group. These groups offer explanations for specific diseases, as well as a place to share feelings and frustrations.
- Encourage the family to stay involved with the resident and continue caregiving and visiting.

Critical Thinking

Interventions to Use When You Perceive the Family to Be Demanding/Complaining

Resources needed:

- Reading: Review the Decision-Making Tree for Problem Solving.

The client, age 82, was admitted 2 weeks ago to Quality Care Home. You are an LPN/LVN charge nurse on the evening shift. The client has osteoarthritis, short-term memory loss, and Parkinson disease. In the past few days the client's family has been complaining about hair care, mouth care, appearance, and missing items in the laundry.

- Develop a plan with specific interventions to investigate and alleviate these complaints.
- Despite modifications in the client's care plan, the complaints continue. Plan specific interventions to handle the continuing specific complaints.
- Inform and engage all members of the interdisciplinary care team to problem solve effectively.

ASSIGNMENT AND DELEGATION

Estella stopped at the topic of "Assigning Tasks and Delegating Duties to Nursing Assistants," remembering very well the confusion experienced in class in trying to understand the difference between "assigning" and "delegating" to nursing assistants. Like most of the students in the class, all of them thought assigning and delegating meant the same thing. They sure sounded the same. The fact that the school was in a state that did not allow delegation to nursing assistants compounded the confusion in understanding these concepts. The nurse educator, as usual, had the situation well under control. Although assigning and delegating had many similarities, there were differences that had legal consequences. The best place to start was to identify the boundaries, define and describe the terms, and then proceed. In case the students thought assigning and delegating were new concepts, read the following quote:

> *To be "in charge" is certainly not only to carry out the proper measures yourself but to see that everyone else does, too. It is neither to do everything yourself nor to appoint a number of people to each duty, but to ensure that each does that duty to which he is appointed.*
>
> *Florence Nightingale*
> *Notes on Nursing, 1859*

CHECKING YOUR NURSE PRACTICE ACT

At this time, not every state in the United States allows LPNs/LVNs to delegate in their charge nurse positions. It is crucial that you check your state's NPA to determine whether or not you may delegate as an LPN/LVN charge nurse in your state. If you cannot clearly find an answer, contact your state Board of Nursing (BON). Click on your state at the NCSBN website (https://www.ncsbn.org/contactbon.htm) for contact information. Unfortunately, some states are silent regarding delegation. This means that you will be unable to identify any clear direction. In this case, carefully follow the policy and procedure of your employer. See the Collaborative Care, Management Tool: Reviewing Your Nurse Practice Act for Authority to Delegate box.

Collaborative Care

Management Tool

REVIEWING YOUR NURSE PRACTICE ACT FOR AUTHORITY TO DELEGATE

Resources needed:

- Your state's NPA
  - Locate the section of your state's NPA that discusses your ability to delegate nursing duties as an LPN/LVN charge nurse.
  - In your own words, write that position.

Discuss with a colleague how the LPN/LVN charge nurse can delegate effectively at clinical sites.

If your state's NPA allows LPN/LVN charge nurses to delegate duties, you will have the authority to delegate duties to nursing assistants (unlicensed AP). States may differ in their interpretation of "delegation." This is one reason you need to check with the BON in your state for its interpretation. In addition to your state's NPA, be sure to review the following:

1. Rules and regulations of your state's BON
2. Interpretations, guidelines, and memorandums developed by your state's BON regarding delegation

A state's NPA usually presents information in a general manner. Rules and regulations and interpretations of your BON are more specific statements. They make clearer the intent of the NPA and provide more specific details that describe your nursing practice.

Your state may give you permission to delegate as an LPN/LVN, but to delegate in your place of employment, your facility must also give permission for that function by including it in its written policies. For this reason, check facility policy regarding delegation of nursing duties by the LPN/LVN charge nurse.

The standards of nursing organizations are not legal statements, but they provide support to the legal decisions of your state. Be sure to review the standards of your nursing organizations that apply to delegation by the LPN/LVN. See the Collaborative Care, Management Tool: Locating Positions of Nursing Groups and Employer on Delegation Function of Licensed Practical/Licensed Vocational Charge Nurse box.

Collaborative Care

Management Tool

LOCATING POSITIONS OF NURSING GROUPS AND EMPLOYER ON DELEGATION FUNCTION OF LICENSED PRACTICAL/LICENSED VOCATIONAL CHARGE NURSES

Resources needed:

- Rules, regulations, interpretations, guidelines, and memorandums regarding delegation of your state's BON
- NAPNES Standards of Practice and Educational Competencies of Graduates of Practical/Vocational Nursing Programs
- NALPN Nursing Practice Standards for the LPN/LVN
- Policies on delegation of employer
- Review the policies/rules and regulations/interpretations/guidelines/standards of the following agencies in regard to delegation:
- Board of Nursing
- National Association for Practical Nurse Education and Service, Inc.
- National Association of Licensed Practical Nurses
- National League for Nursing
- Health care facility

GENERAL CONSIDERATIONS

Assignment and *delegation* are terms used in reference to allocating client care activities to team members. Both terms refer to nursing actions or activities, but the terms do not have the same meaning. Think about and use assignment and delegation in the way they are legally intended. **To help improve your understanding and reduce confusion, the terms assignment (assigning) and delegation (delegating) are used in this chapter in the following way.**

- When discussing **assignment**, this topic will be used in reference to "tasks." **Tasks** are activities that are carried out by staff. Nursing assistants learn "how to" perform a task in their nursing assistant training, and these tasks are listed in their job description. According to the National Guidelines for Delegation (NCSBN and ANA, 2019), an **assignment** is defined as "the routine care, activities and procedures that are within the authorized scope of practice of the RN or LPN/LVN or part of the routine functions of the AP."
- When discussing **delegation**, this topic will be used in reference to "duties." **Duties** are functions that are performed by LPNs/LVNs because they successfully passed a licensing exam. The duties are included in the state's NPA. The duties are their

scope of practice. The LPN/LVN learns "why" a duty is performed and "what" could go wrong during performance of a "duty." According to the National Guidelines for Delegation (NCSBN and ANA, 2019), a delegated responsibility is defined as "a nursing activity, skill or procedure that is transferred from a licensed nurse to a delegatee." In the case of the LPN as the licensed individual, the delegatee is the AP (i.e., nursing assistant).

Resident circumstances can change a "task" for a nursing assistant into a "duty" requiring the LPN/LVN to use the nursing process.

Whenever the title "charge nurse" is used, it will be in the context of the LPN/LVN.

Differences Between Assigning and Delegating

Assigning. **Assigning** is the way that work is distributed among team members for the shift. Assigning is a skill that every LPN/LVN needs to develop if their state allows them to assume a charge nurse position. Distributing the workload by assignment is a routine part of the LPN/LVN charge nurse's job. Assignment occurs at the beginning of every shift and as the need arises during the shift.

When LPNs/LVNs give assignments to nursing assistants, they are **allotting tasks that are in the job description of these health care workers**. The assigned tasks are tasks that nursing assistants are trained, hired, and paid to perform. The tasks are in their job description. These unlicensed personnel have the responsibility to complete the assignment in a safe and timely manner. The LPN/LVN charge nurse shares responsibility with unlicensed personnel for the quality of the care delivered. In assigning situations, the LPN/LVN charge nurse needs to monitor the performance of the task and evaluate the quality and effectiveness of the care that was assigned. See the Collaborative Care, Management Hint: Assigning Tasks box for help in understanding assigning tasks.

Collaborative Care

Management Hint

ASSIGNING TASKS

- The need to assign can occur at any time during the shift but always occurs at the beginning of the shift.
- The assigning of tasks is part of the LPN/LVN charge nurse's job.
- The LPN/LVN charge nurse assigns tasks to nursing assistants that are in their job description.
- Nursing tasks are tasks that nursing assistants are trained, hired, and paid to perform. Refer to the subsection "Specific Tasks for Nursing Assistant Assignment" for more details.
- Because assignments involve allocating the tasks that are to be done by nursing assistants in their job description, these team members cannot refuse the assignment unless they do not feel qualified to perform the task.
- Nursing assistants assume responsibility for completing assigned tasks safely and in a timely manner.

Delegating. LPNs/LVNs receive the authority to provide nursing care from the nursing license they receive after successfully passing the NCLEX-PN® examination. When allowed by your state's NPA and facility policies, **delegating** duties in the long-term care unit or other appropriate settings involves **transferring the authority to perform nursing duties that are in the job description of the LPN/LVN charge nurse (the person doing the delegating)** to competent nursing assistants (unlicensed personnel, known as the delegatee) in selected situations. These nursing duties are in your job description and "emerge" from your nursing license. These duties are in your scope of practice. **Based on your scope of practice, one of the most important duties of LPNs/LVNs is their role in the nursing process Table 17.1**. presents a comparison of assigning tasks and delegating duties.

Delegating is a complex skill requiring sophisticated clinical judgment. Effective delegation protects the public when all three entities (employer/nurse leader, licensed

Table 17.1 Assigning Versus Delegating by the Licensed Practical/Licensed Vocational Charge Nurse

	ASSIGNING TASKS	DELEGATING DUTIES
To whom may tasks or duties be assigned or delegated?	Nursing assistants and other unlicensed personnel	Nursing assistants and other unlicensed personnel
Are tasks or duties in nursing assistant's job description?	Yes	No. The duties delegated are in the job description of the licensed practical nurse/licensed vocational nurse (LPN/VN). Specific duties are not listed. Delegated duties depend on the situation.
May nursing assistant refuse nursing task/duty?	No, unless nursing assistant thinks he or she is unqualified for the assignment.	Yes. In addition, the nursing assistant must voluntarily accept delegation function.
Who has accountability for nursing task/duty?	The nursing assistant is responsible for completing the task and in a safe manner. The supervisor (i.e., LPN/VN) also retains responsibility legally.	The LPN/VN is accountable for delegating the right duty to the right person.

Adapted from National Council of State Boards of Nursing Decision Tree for Delegation to Nursing Assistive Personnel, App. B of 2006 Joint Statement on Delegation, American Nurses Association (ANA), and the National Council of State Boards of Nursing (NCSBN). Available at https://www.ncsbn.org/Delegation_joint_statement_NCSBN-ANA.pdf.

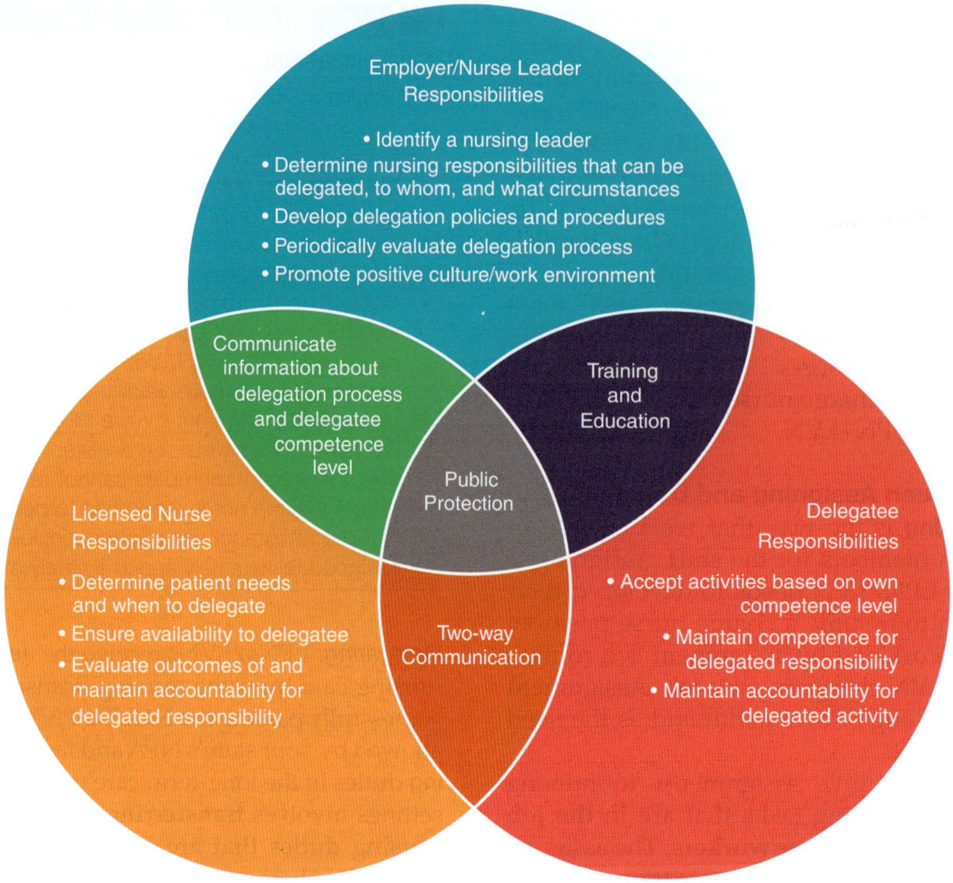

Fig. 17.6 The delegation process. (From the National Council of State Boards of Nursing (NCSBN) and the American Nurses Association [ANA]: *National Guidelines for Nursing Delegation*, 2019. Available at https://www.ncsbn.org/public-files/NCSBN_Delegation_Guidelines.pdf.)

nurse, and delegatee) understand their key responsibilities in the delegation process (Fig. 17.6). Delegation information, including scenarios, might be included in theory classes in your LPN/LVN nursing program, but opportunities to apply the information on clinical may be limited. To be effective, delegation is a skill that needs to be developed with a licensed nurse as a mentor after graduation (Grumet, 2005).

Delegating duties and assigning tasks are written in the job description of the LPN/LVN charge nurse at Quality Care Home. When allowed by your state's NPA and your facility, **delegating is a voluntary function**. You do not have to delegate because the facility allows it. The Collaborative Care, Management Hint: Delegating Duties box contains helpful information for delegating duties.

Collaborative Care

Management Hint

DELEGATING DUTIES

- When delegating duties, you are allowing a delegatee to perform a specific nursing activity, skill, or procedure that is beyond the delegatee's traditional role and not routinely performed (NCSBN and ANA, 2019).
- Delegation is *not* asking nursing assistants to do duties that the LPN/LVN dislikes doing.
- As LPN/LVN charge nurse, you are asking nursing assistants to help you perform some of *your* job description so that you may perform other prioritized job responsibilities, with the ultimate goal of improving resident care and meeting resident goals (outcomes).
- Because you are delegating part of *your* job as charge nurse, nursing assistants must give approval to the assignment. Nursing assistants must voluntarily accept the delegation; they cannot be forced to accept the delegated duty.
- When delegating duties, the LPN/LVN charge nurse needs to provide the nursing assistant with the necessary information, assistance, and equipment to safely carry out the delegated duty.
- Employers may suggest that certain duties can be delegated, but the LPN/LVN is ultimately responsible for the following:
    - Deciding to delegate a duty
    - Deciding what duty to delegate
    - Deciding to whom to delegate a duty
    - Deciding under what circumstances to delegate a duty
    - Retaining the ultimate responsibility for the delegated duty

Why Delegating Is Important

When allowed by your NPA and facility policies, learning to delegate some of the duties in your job description to nursing assistants can have many advantages. Delegating can do the following:

- Increase your effectiveness and efficiency as an LPN/LVN charge nurse

- Be instrumental in realizing client goals (outcomes) in a cost-effective manner
- Assist nursing assistants learn new job skills while collaborating with the licensed nurse

Legal Aspects of Delegating

In the long-term care facility, the LPN/LVN charge nurse, who is under the general supervision of an RN, is managing and directing the activities of nursing assistants. The RN might be in the building on days and evenings. On the night shift the RN might be at the other end of a cell phone. When the RN delegates a duty to the LPN/LVN charge nurse and the charge nurse then delegates to a nursing assistant, the RN is ultimately responsible for the supervision of nursing assistants. But the LPN/LVN charge nurse assists in the supervision of these health care workers, collaborating with the RN, and shares **accountability** with the RN for their actions.

Scope of practice for the LPN/LVN. Legal scope of practice, determined by your NPA, is what you are able to do because you are an LPN/LVN. Your scope of practice includes the assisting role in the nursing process. The LPN/LVN charge nurse can delegate to nursing assistants the duty of checking a resident's IV site for intactness and dryness of dressing. However, nursing assistants are not trained in the basics of collecting and analyzing data. If the resident complained of being cold at the site of the IV, nursing assistants might provide the client with another blanket, turn up the heat, or turn down the air conditioning. They may not automatically check to see if the infusion device had come out of the resident's vein and was infusing fluid onto the bed sheets.

Although unlicensed APs obtain data while caring for residents, they do not have the nursing education to make a judgment about or interpret those data. Therefore nursing judgment cannot be delegated to or expected of nursing assistants. The LPN/LVN charge nurse needs to use his or her knowledge and experience to interpret data gathered by these members of the team.

Your license is at stake in the matter of delegating nursing duties. To be legally sound when delegating duties, see the suggestions in the Collaborative Care, Management Hint: Suggestions for Legal Soundness When Delegating box.

Collaborative Care

Management Hint

SUGGESTIONS FOR LEGAL SOUNDNESS WHEN DELEGATING

- Delegate only if allowed by your state's NPA and facility policies.
- Determine stability of the client's condition.
- Delegate duties only for which nursing assistants have obtained additional education/training and demonstrated competence.
- Provide specific, objective, clear-cut directions to nursing assistants for delegated duties.
- Provide assistance and instruction to nursing assistants when you delegate a duty.
- Monitor the activities of nursing assistants when they carry out delegated duties. Depending on the nursing assistant and the situation, this monitoring can mean anything from being "right there" to a periodic check.
- Intervene if correction is needed to maintain safety.
- On completion of the delegated duty, evaluate the safety and effectiveness of duties delegated to nursing assistants.
- If you delegated improperly and a resident was harmed, you are liable. This could result in a disciplinary action against your license and/or a civil suit (see Chapter 7).
- If you delegated properly, including monitoring, and the client was injured, the nursing assistant is also liable.
- Delegation should always occur in collaboration with an RN.
- According to the American Nurses Association (ANA)/NCSBN, the RN should follow the five rights of delegation: the right task, under the right circumstances, to the right person, with the right directions and communication, and under the right supervision and evaluation.

Tricia continued paging through the textbook and notes used in school. What memories they brought back! All those shifts of taking report and focusing on important aspects of each client or resident on the clinical area had a purpose. Tricia remembered the first time taking report as an LPN/LVN charge nurse. The new position of responsibility gave a heightened sense of awareness of the data being given. Based on the data received in report, Tricia had to decide what to assign and what to delegate to nursing assistants for the shift.

USING THE NURSING PROCESS AS A GUIDE FOR ASSIGNING TASKS AND DELEGATING DUTIES

The nursing process will be used as the tool to cover the various aspects that need to be understood and used when assigning or delegating.

- Collecting data: Oncoming report, assessment of residents
- Planning: Establishing goals (outcomes) for the shift, setting priorities, and assigning/delegating
- Implementing: Monitoring, assisting, being available, and intervening
- Evaluating: Two-way feedback

COLLECTING DATA

Oncoming Report

National Client Safety Goals require a standardized approach to communications (e.g., change-of-shift report, which is sometimes called "handoff"), including an opportunity to ask and respond to questions during reports. If your facility has TJC accreditation, there may be a standardized form to use when receiving report. The National Client Safety Goals of TJC are in Chapter 16 and can also be accessed at www.jointcommission.org.

Change-of-shift report allows the LPN/LVN charge nurse to collect data to determine how the work of the shift will be divided. Always keeping in mind client goals (outcomes) for shift report helps guarantee continuity in resident care.

Report When Starting Your Shift

Reports in long-term care units and nursing homes, as in other health care facilities, are a way to communicate pertinent data to the oncoming shift. The report you receive when you are starting your shift will be your basis for collecting data about resident needs. This is legally necessary so you can safely distribute the work of the shift to nursing assistants to provide care for specific residents by keeping in mind client goals (outcomes). Report may be recorded, oral, or may be walking rounds at the client bedside, depending on TJC accreditation or agency policy.

When report is recorded, off-going personnel usually are still on duty. They answer call lights and attend to residents' needs while the oncoming shift listens to report. This enables the charge nurse to question unclear information after report. If facilities do not have a standardized report form, nurses develop personal ways of gathering data when they are taking report, including the use of symbols and abbreviations. See the Collaborative Care, Management Tool: Developing Your Personal Form for Collecting Data During Report box.

> **Collaborative Care**
>
> **Management Tool**
>
> **DEVELOPING YOUR PERSONAL FORM FOR COLLECTING DATA DURING REPORT**
>
> Resources needed:
>
> - Method of gathering data during report that you have developed during the clinical year
> - Sample of forms/method to gather information for report used by clinical sites where you have worked this year
> - Your creativity and organizational skills
>
> Develop a form that will help you gather the pertinent information needed to assume responsibility of taking charge of the residents on your wing/unit. Include format, symbols, and abbreviations you find helpful and that will allow you to quickly and accurately gather the information. Compare your form with forms of classmates.

Assessment of Clients

Assignment/delegation of clients is usually done after report. Ideally, the LPN/LVN charge nurse makes rounds to personally assess each resident before making assignments. This baseline assessment allows the charge nurse to note any changes in condition of residents or discrepancies that may have occurred since report. If distribution of work for the shift is done before rounds and a change in assignment/delegation is required, the nursing assistant needs to be notified. In some states an initial assessment of clients can be completed by the LPN/LVN independently; however, in many states the LPN/LVN cannot complete an initial assessment, it is an RN's responsibility. Refer to your respective NPA for details.

PLANNING

"We may be very busy, we may be very efficient, but we will also be truly effective only when we begin with the end in mind."

—Stephen R. Covey

Planning involves deciding goals (outcomes) for the shift, setting priorities of care, and then using specific directions, assigning the appropriate task/duty to the nursing assistant who can safely and effectively complete the assignment.

Before Assigning Tasks/Delegating Duties to Nursing Assistants

Distributing the work to be done among nursing assistants follows change-of-shift report. Encourage nursing assistants to take notes and ask questions regarding the directions you give for assigned tasks/delegated duties. Resist the urge to think of work only as tasks to be completed and to just divide the work equally among team members. In other words, just because there are 32 clients and 4 nursing assistants, it does not mean that each assistant automatically gets 8 clients. Take time to plan how work will be distributed. At first this part may seem tedious and time consuming, but planning becomes easier with practice and experience. Level of client acuity and education and experience of team members should be considered when creating an assignment. This part of the nursing process is a good reason why the charge nurse position, by some state laws, can require experience beyond a new graduate.

Hansten and Jackson (2009) state, "Fail to plan—plan to fail." When nurses must decide what to assign/delegate, they should identify resident goals (outcomes) and set priorities.

Identifying resident goals. To be more effective when assigning/delegating and to make these functions more understandable, think in terms of resident **goals (outcomes)**. Goals are desired results in resident progress after nursing intervention. What should happen after nursing intervention by the nursing assistant? Why is the nursing activity being done? What is the goal (outcome) for each resident for the shift?

> **Critical Thinking**
>
> **Formulating Goals/Outcome for Residents**
>
> Formulate a goal (outcome) to be met at the end of the shift for each of the following residents:
>
> - Harold, an active 90-year-old with osteoarthritis, had a right total hip replacement and is completing his rehabilitation at Quality Care Home, with the goal to go back to his apartment in assisted living. He is to walk ×2 with stand-by assist and have one dry clean dressing change daily. His temp went to 100.4°F (38°C) last evening, but he is not displaying respiratory symptoms.
> - Goal (outcome) for Harold for day shift: Harold will maintain hip abduction when turning and getting out of bed

to prevent hip dislocation. Harold will have causes of his elevated temp investigated.

- Adelia, age 76, and a 2-year resident of Quality Care Home, has type 1 diabetes and receives an intermediate-acting insulin injection each morning and capillary blood glucose monitoring ½ hour before meals with sliding scale short-acting insulin coverage. Adelia can be up ad lib, and today is her shower day, which Adelia is looking forward to. The PM shift had trouble getting a blood sample and had to do *two* fingersticks to obtain a blood sample for testing.
- Goal (outcome) for Adelia for day shift: Adelia will have blood glucose monitoring done ×2 with only one fingerstick required for each test. Blood sugar will be monitored as ordered.
- Jose, age 82, has resided at Quality Care Home for 3 years. He has arteriosclerotic heart disease (ASHD). He recently was hospitalized with a cerebral vascular accident (CVA) and is back at Quality Care Home. Jose has weakness on the right side of his body, is allowed up with the assistance of one person, and uses a walker. He has dysphagia (difficulty swallowing).
- Goal (outcome) for Jose for day shift: Jose will eat breakfast and lunch without signs of aspirating. A safe environment will be maintained.

Setting priorities. Set priorities among the goals (outcomes) for the shift. The priority (most important) care to be done can be evaluated according to the following criteria:

1. Life-threatening situations: real or potential
   a. A resident who has unrelieved back pain that started on the last shift. (Goal/outcome: Resident will be pain free at end of shift or pain level will be decreased from the previous shift.) Rating the pain is effective.
   b. A resident who is dying. (Goal/outcome: Because of comfort measures provided and presence of family, resident will have a peaceful look on his face and lie still in bed without thrashing and picking at sheets.)
   c. A resident who is showing untoward effects to a newly ordered drug. (Goal/outcome: Resident will have stable blood pressure and respirations of 22 to 26 per minute. This requires frequent monitoring and reporting PRN [as needed] to health care provider.)
   d. A resident attempted to flee the building several times on the last shift. (Goal/outcome: Resident will be present in the building at the end of the shift, secondary to constant supervision.)
2. *Essential to safety*. This criterion pertains to residents and the nursing team.
   a. Which residents, because of their weight, require two persons to turn and position?
   b. Which residents, because of poor balance, need assistance to get out of bed and/or ambulate?
   c. Who is going to check special equipment (e.g., the stock of supplies used in emergencies) for shift?
   d. Does a resident require standard precautions that infrequently need to be used in the facility? Instruction may need to be given to nursing assistants.
3. *Essential to the medical/nursing plan of care*. Criteria include ordered treatments, facility routines for care, and interventions listed on the nursing plan of care; for example, dressing changes, administration of medications, measuring vital signs, turning, transferring, ambulating, feeding and encouraging fluids, and monitoring of capillary blood glucose levels.

Criteria for Assigning/Delegating to Nursing Assistants

In 2016, the NCSBN and the ANA issued a joint statement on delegation to assist licensed nurses to delegate safely and effectively in clinical settings. Table 17.2 adapts the NCSBN's decision tree for delegation to nursing AP. National Guidelines for Nursing Delegation were jointly adopted by NCSBN and ANA in 2019. These guidelines build on previous work of the NCSBN and ANA are applicable to all levels of nursing licensure, including LPNs/LVNs. These guidelines are particularly critical when the NPA is silent to delegation.

The joint statement provides a list of five areas to assist RNs (LPN is working in collaboration with the RN) in making decisions about delegation. When discussing delegation, the joint statement uses the term "task." Remember, to help differentiate and understand assigning versus delegating, we use "task" to apply to assigning and "duty" to apply to delegating those functions that require the knowledge and judgment of your nursing license and experience.

1. Right task (duty)
2. Right circumstance
3. Right person
4. Right directions and communication
5. Right supervision and evaluation (some states use the term monitor instead of supervision when the LPN/LVN performs this function.)

Right task. A crucial legal consideration in dividing work among nursing assistants is nursing judgment. The LPN/LVN charge nurse needs to avoid real and potential harm to residents when allocating workload to nursing assistants. You are legally liable for improper assigning/delegating. **Change-of-shift report** and rounds for beginning of shift resident data collection gave you the opportunity, as LPN/LVN charge nurse, to collect data about the specific nursing needs of the residents for your shift and the complexity of those needs. Actual tasks/duties allocated depend on the following criteria:

- Laws in your state
- Policies of the long-term care facility
- Needs and condition of the residents on your unit
- Training of nursing assistants

Table 17.2 Delegation Decision-Making Tree for the Licensed Practical/Vocational Nurse

Starting with question 1, if you answer "no" to a question, do not delegate. If you answer "yes," proceed to the next question.			
1. Does your Nurse Practice Act give the licensed practical nurse/licensed vocational nurse (LPN/LVN) permission to delegate?	No	Do not delegate	Yes
2. Does the employing agency give the LPN/LVN permission to delegate?	No	Do not delegate	Yes
3. Is the duty to be delegated within the scope of practice of the LPN/LVN?	No	Do not delegate	Yes
4. Does the LPN/LVN have the education necessary to delegate nursing duties?	No	Do not delegate	Yes
5. Has the LPN/LVN collected data of the client's needs and condition?	No	Collect data and continue	Yes
6. Is the nursing assistant to whom a duty is being delegated competent to accept the delegation? (See later in chapter for suggestions to determine competency.)	No	Do not delegate	Yes
7. Is the delegated duty performed according to a sequence of steps?	No	Do not delegate	Yes
8. Does the delegated duty occur repeatedly in the daily care of clients?	No	Do not delegate	Yes
9. Does the delegated duty involve little or no modification from one client situation to another?	No	Do not delegate	Yes
10. Can the delegated duty be performed with a predictable outcome?	No	Do not delegate	Yes
11. Is there danger of affecting the client's life or well-being if the nursing duty is carried out?	No	Do not delegate	Yes
12. Is the delegated duty in the nursing assistant's job description?	No	Do not delegate	Yes
13. Does the nursing assistant accept the delegated duty?	No	Do not delegate	Yes
14. Does the nursing assistant have the knowledge, skills, and abilities to accept the delegated duty?	No	Do not delegate	Yes
15. Does the nursing assistant's ability match the client's needs?	No	Do not delegate	Yes
16. Can the delegated nursing duty be performed without requiring nursing judgment?	No	Do not delegate	Yes
17. Are the results of the delegated duty reasonably predictable?	No	Do not delegate	Yes
18. Can the delegated duty be safely performed according to exact, unchanging directions?	No	Do not delegate	Yes
19. Can the delegated duty be safely performed without constant data collection, interpretation of that data, and the need for decisions based on that data?	No	Do not delegate	Yes
20. Does the agency have a written policy, procedure, and/or protocol for the delegated duty?	No	Do not delegate	Yes
21. Is the LPN/LVN who delegated the duty available for monitoring the nursing assistant?	No	Do not delegate	Yes/May delegate

Assigning tasks. Assigning tasks involves dividing work that is in the job description of nursing assistants. The Collaborative Care, Management Hint: Specific Tasks for Nursing Assistant Assignment box lists specific tasks that could be assigned to nursing assistants.

Collaborative Care

Management Hint

SPECIFIC TASKS FOR NURSING ASSISTANT ASSIGNMENT

Routine:

- Personal care, including hygiene, dressing, toileting, grooming, and skin care
- Feeding and hydration
- *Basic restorative skills*, including transfer, positioning, ambulation, and maintaining range of motion
- Measuring and recording vital signs, height and weight, and intake and output
- Assistance with elimination, including catheter care and enemas
- Maintaining safety factors, including fall prevention, application of heat and cold, and infection prevention
- Collecting specimens of urine and stool
- Nursing assistants who have displayed an excellent work ethic, job performance, and skills may be offered additional, specialized training to become restorative aides. Additional training occurs for positioning, transferring, performing range of motion, using assistive devices, and preventing pressure ulcers.

Delegating duties. Remember, delegating involves transferring the authority (the right) to perform a selected nursing duty (a duty your license gives you the right to do after attending a practical/vocational nursing program and passing a licensing exam given nationally). Delegation generally involves selected activities in client care. A nursing assistant can receive an assignment, and within that assignment might be activities that need to be delegated. Avoid assuming that simpler duties may be automatically delegated. According to the National Guidelines for Nursing Delegation (NCSBN and ANA, 2019), decisions to delegate a nursing responsibility are made based on the following:

- the needs of the client or population
- the stability and predictability of the client's condition
- the documented training and competence of the delegatee
- the ability of the licensed nurse to supervise the delegated responsibility and its outcome, with special consideration to the available staff mix and client acuity

Collaborative Care, Management Tool: Criteria for Delegating Duties box lists criteria for delegating duties to nursing assistants.

Collaborative Care

Management Tool

CRITERIA FOR DELEGATING DUTIES

The following are criteria for nursing duties that can be delegated for residents whose conditions are stable:

- The delegated duty must apply to an unchanging situation. (If there is a chance for a change in the client during a procedure, do not delegate.)
- The results of the delegated duty must be predictable.
- The potential for risk during performance of the delegated duty must be minimal (e.g., the client with difficulty swallowing is a risk).
- The delegated duty should be necessary and routine in daily care.
- The delegated duty should not require nursing judgment (e.g., "I think the blood glucose level is normal").
- The delegated duty should not require frequent, repeated collection of data during performance of the duty.

The following suggestions include information to help decide what duty can be delegated.

- A question that can help the LPN/LVN make a decision as to what to delegate is "What is the intended outcome (goal/desired result) of the nursing care in question?" In their article, "Delegating to APs—Making It Work," Hansten and Washburn (2001) use a bath given for several different reasons (goals/outcomes) as an example.
  - If the bath of a client in long-term care who is recuperating from total hip replacement is being used as a teaching situation for family members to learn how to observe for signs of skin breakdown, then a licensed nurse needs to be part of the procedure.
  - If a resident who is recuperating from a stroke has a mobility issue, then a physical therapy assistant may be involved with range-of-motion training for the family during the bath.
  - The aforementioned two baths could be given as a team, with the nursing assistant bathing the resident, while the licensed nurse points out pressure points susceptible to skin breakdown or the physical therapy assistant gives range-of-motion training.
  - If the desired goal of a bath is to have a long-term care resident bathed before being discharged, then the nursing assistant would be assigned.
- Given specific directions, nursing assistants can assist to collect, report, and document simple data, but not interpret that data. All this occurs in collaboration with the LPN and RN.
- More complex skills to delegate depend on the following:
  - What is allowed by law in your state
  - Resident needs of your unit
  - Further training of nursing assistants; for example, electronic blood glucose monitoring

A concise, across-the-board list of what nursing duties to delegate and what not to delegate does not exist. The Collaborative Care, Management Hint: Why Lists of Duties to Delegate Do Not Exist box contains the drawbacks of such lists.

Collaborative Care

Management Hint

WHY LISTS OF DUTIES TO DELEGATE DO NOT EXIST

- A duty list for nursing assistants eliminates the need for collecting data of the needs of each client.
- A duty could be on a list of acceptable duties to delegate to a nursing assistant, but the client situation might indicate the duty would be dangerous or inappropriate for a nursing assistant; for example, feeding a client with dysphagia (difficulty swallowing).
- The BON has the responsibility to protect the client. Licensed nursing personnel carry out this responsibility.
- A duty list for nursing assistants puts the control of nursing care into the hands of unlicensed persons who have had minimal training for client care.
- The exact duties delegated to nursing assistants are interpreted by each state's BON and by each client situation.

It is somewhat easier to list what duties of the LPN/LVN/RN should not be delegated to unlicensed staff. The Collaborative Care, Management Hint: Examples of Duties Not to Delegate box contains examples.

Collaborative Care

Management Hint

EXAMPLES OF DUTIES NOT TO DELEGATE

- Complex sterile technique procedures: Nursing assistants do not have in-depth training in sterile technique.
- Crisis situations (you must be there): An example of a crisis situation is a resident who develops chest pain.
- Initial client education by an RN: In most states, LPNs/LVNs may reinforce initial client teaching given by the RN.

- Although nursing assistants can collect simple data, they have not been trained to make decisions about or interpret those data. For example, nursing assistants cannot evaluate results of capillary blood glucose monitoring or determine when vital signs need to be rechecked.
- When delegating to a licensed nurse, the delegated responsibility must be within the delegatee's authorized scope of practice under the NPA.

Critical Thinking

Delegating Duties

You practice in a health care facility that allows the LPN/LVN charge nurse to delegate nursing duties to nursing assistants. List two additional items to consider before actually delegating:

1.
2.

Right circumstance. NCSBN emphasizes that the setting and client situation must be considered when delegating. The same criteria must be considered when assigning tasks. Assignment/delegation of duties would not occur if the following is true:

- Resident is unstable. For example, the LPN/LVN would probably work as part of "pair caring" with the nursing assistant when a client has difficulty swallowing, needs to be fed, and has a history of choking. The LPN/LVN would feed the resident and could use the situation as an opportunity to teach the nursing assistant techniques to use to avoid choking.
- The unit does not have equipment or supplies needed to safely carry out the procedure. The procedure would not be attempted until equipment and supplies were obtained.
- There are safety issues for the nursing assistant, including infection control issues.
- The staffing level is so limited that:
  - Supervision (monitoring) of assigned/delegated duties would not be adequate.
  - Assistance from the LPN/LVN/RN might not be available when needed; for example, assistance when the nursing assistant has questions or needs directions.

Right person. The National Council's guidelines describe delegation as transferring the authority to perform a "selected nursing task" to a competent person. These guidelines also apply to assigning tasks to nursing assistants. According to NCSBN interpretation (2005), a competent nursing assistant should be capable of the following in addition to basic care:

- Communicate effectively
- Collect basic subjective and objective data
- Perform noncomplex nursing activities safely, accurately, and according to standard procedures
- Seek guidance and direction when appropriate

The following suggestions will help you determine competence of nursing assistants.

Review job descriptions. Legally, you need to know the job descriptions of nursing assistants to whom you assign tasks. Check these job descriptions of the facility in which you are employed or on clinical affiliation as a student. See the Collaborative Care, Management Tool: Reviewing Nursing Assistant Job Descriptions box.

Collaborative Care

Management Tool

REVIEWING NURSING ASSISTANT JOB DESCRIPTIONS

Resources needed:

- Job descriptions of nursing assistants
- Make a list of the tasks nursing assistants can perform in various health care facilities.

Know level of competence. Know the level of clinical competence of nursing assistants you supervise. The following questions can help you determine the competency of nursing assistants on your team:

- Is the nursing assistant certified?
- How much nursing assistant training have they had?
- What skills are taught in their nursing assistant program?
- What is the nursing assistant's job description?
- Does the facility conduct yearly skills list updates? (Some LPNs/LVNs keep a laminated copy of nursing assistant job descriptions and skills lists on their clipboards.)
- What clinical strengths have you observed?
- Have the nursing assistants demonstrated previous competency when performing the activity?
- What clinical weaknesses have you observed?
- Is orientation to your unit completed?
- What activities do nursing assistants say they feel qualified doing?
- What activities do nursing assistants feel unsure doing?
- Ask nursing assistants to describe what they would do in a specific situation; for example, "Tell me how you would get this resident with a total hip replacement out of bed." If the nursing assistant hesitates or looks baffled, suggest that you will assist the nursing assistant when she gets the client out of bed for the first time and use it as a teaching situation.
- Ask what the nursing assistant would do if a deviation from the normal procedure should develop. For example, you might say, "While getting this resident to stand up, what would you do if he got dizzy when attempting to stand?"
- Ask if the nursing assistant has done the procedure before. If nursing assistants misrepresent themselves by saying they know how to perform a nursing activity when they do not know how to perform the activity, they could be liable in a court of law. For example,

if a nursing assistant tells you that he or she can do a fingerstick test and then does it incorrectly, causing injury to the resident, he or she could be liable. The LPN/LVN/RN can still be named in the suit.

Refusing assignment. If a nursing assistant does not feel qualified to safely perform an assigned task and refuses the assignment, the team member is then reassigned. It is a fine art distinguishing between "I don't want to" and "I don't know how to." If there is a training problem, follow the suggestion in the Collaborative Care, Management Tool: Reviewing Nursing Assistant Job Descriptions box. Make arrangements with the staff educator of your facility for this team member to receive the training necessary to safely perform the task(s). Also see the Collaborative Care, Management Tool: Handling Refusal of Assignment by Nursing Assistants box.

> **Collaborative Care**
> **Management Tool**
>
> **HANDLING REFUSAL OF ASSIGNMENT BY NURSING ASSISTANTS**
> Resource needed:
> - Reading: The "Refusing Assignment" section in this chapter.
>
> A nursing assistant on the team has refused your assignment to give a resident a whirlpool bath because he does not feel qualified to do the job safely. Write a brief note to the nurse educator of the facility regarding this situation to facilitate training and achieve the nursing assistants' competence in this skill. (In a real situation, also send a copy of the note to your supervisor.)

Once you work consistently with nursing assistants, they will prove their dependability and ability to pursue assigned tasks. Nursing assistants have the right to refuse a delegated duty. The LPN/LVN charge nurse, collaborating with the RN, then uses questioning to determine if the team member feels unqualified or simply does not want to do the activity. Feeling unqualified is a training problem; not wanting to do an activity is an attitude problem. Problems in attitude can interfere with a nursing assistant's growth as a member of the health care team.

Rina reflected, thinking about the time asking a nursing assistant to force fluids for a resident with an elevated temperature. When the nursing assistant was approached during the shift, the NA kept reporting that this task of forcing fluid was getting done. At the end of the shift, when asked for the volume of fluid taken by the resident during the shift, the nursing assistant replied that although forcing fluids every hour, the resident took only 80 cc for the entire shift. Upon self-reflection, Rina realized that discussion with the nursing assistant was not adequate regarding the client expectations for fluid intake and what parameters required an immediate report to the LPN/LVN.

Right directions and communication. Using effective communication techniques is an excellent example of the leadership skills that are needed by LPN/LVN charge nurses. The LPN/LVN charge nurse's ability to communicate assignments effectively to nursing assistants for reaching client goals depends on these skills.

As with all communication, assigning/delegating is a two-way process. The communication skills of LPNs/LVNs and their management styles are crucial for establishing a positive working relationship between charge nurse and nursing assistant. It is not only what you say as LPN/LVN charge nurse but also how you say it. *Inadequate communication is the most common reason assigned/delegated duties are not completed as required.* The communication guidelines for delegating duties also apply to communication for assigning tasks. Communication skills need to be learned by studying and using the techniques. Communication must be a two-way process, inclusive of feedback regarding the client from the delegate. Review Chapter 8 regarding straightforward communication.

Do not just tell a nursing assistant what to do. A discussion is more effective, unless it is an emergency situation. Be sure to give the rationale for duties assigned or delegated. Explain why an assigned or delegated duty must be done first or at a specific time. Explain *why* you need the results at a specific time. Nursing assistants become frustrated and feel unsafe when expected to complete an activity when too little information is given. Most importantly, be sure you are available to collaborate as needed. See the Collaborative Care, Management Hint: Communication/Direction Responsibilities of the Licensed Practical/Licensed Vocational Charge Nurse When Assigning or Delegating box for communication guidelines that apply to assigning and delegating.

> **Collaborative Care**
> **Management Hint**
>
> **COMMUNICATION/DIRECTION RESPONSIBILITIES OF THE LICENSED PRACTICAL/LICENSED VOCATIONAL CHARGE NURSE WHEN ASSIGNING OR DELEGATING**
> When assigning tasks or delegating duties, be sure to provide nursing assistants with the following information:
> - Give objective, detailed, clear-cut verbal and written directions. Get to the point!
> - Consider writing assignments in a concise, objective manner on a master assignment sheet.
> - Clarify if the nursing assistant has performed delegated duty in the past.
> - Explain what is expected at the nursing assistant's level of understanding.
> - Be specific about the results you are expecting and when to report. Do not ask nursing assistants to "find out how the client is." Instead, ask a client who has been itching because of a rash if the rash still itches.
> - Provide guidelines for reporting after the delegated duty is completed. Provide the time you expect to be informed and why.
> - Make sure your directions are specific and complete. Provide all the necessary information, including time, to get the task or duty done correctly and safely. For example, say, "Please report the numbers immediately

after you measure Mr. Chen's blood pressure, pulse, and respirations. I need to know the numbers before his 9:00 am blood pressure medicine can be given."

- Given specific directions, nursing assistants can collect, report, and document simple data. However, they are unable to make judgments based on those data. For example, say, "Please report the results of Mr. Ali's fingerstick immediately after you perform it so I can determine if he needs insulin."
- Instruct nursing assistants when to consult with the charge nurse during the performance of an assigned/delegated duty. For example, say, "Let me know immediately if you are having trouble getting the specimen."
- Clarify all messages by asking nursing assistants to tell you what it is you expect them to do and when to report. Listen attentively to any feedback.
- A "please" and "thank you" are in order as part of common courtesy.
- Be sure to recognize outstanding work.

Inform nursing assistants when you expect a report/rundown on activities. A suggested "routine" for reporting back to the charge nurse is before and after breaks and meals and before going off duty. The exact number of reports depends on your familiarity with how the nursing assistant functions, the condition of the residents, and the nature of the assigned/delegated duty. Examples of delegated duties that need priority or more frequent reporting are blood pressure numbers when the resident is to receive blood pressure medicine and blood glucose monitoring with sliding scale insulin coverage. State when you expect to be informed and why you need to be informed.

? Critical Thinking

Identifying Resident Goals/Outcomes

Using the information in the "Identifying Resident Goals/Outcomes" section, the "Signs and Symptoms" list, and a medical/surgical text, write the following activities/observations to be assigned/delegated to nursing assistants in specific, objective, clear-cut terms. The directions need to be realistic, measurable, and time referenced.

1. Be sure to clean up Client A.
2. Make sure Client B drinks today.
3. Client C must get up today.
4. If Client D does not pass any urine, let me know.
5. Have Client E ready for her health care provider's appointment.

? Critical Thinking Exercise

Communicating Objectively to Nursing Assistants

This is your first month as charge nurse at Quality Care Home. Provide specific, objective, clear-cut data for the nursing assistant to be aware of while giving care in the following resident situations:

1. Resident has compensated right-sided congestive heart failure.
2. Resident is a poorly controlled diabetic who receives an intermediate-acting insulin each morning.
3. Resident has lost 5 pounds in the past 2 weeks.
4. Resident has an order for a catheterized urine for residual.

Remember. When delegating, clarify that the nursing assistant has accepted the delegation. The nursing assistant's responsibility in delegation includes accepting the delegated duty, as well as safe performance in carrying out the duty.

Tricia Makes Assignments for the Nursing Assistants

See the resident goals on p. 269.

- **Harold:** Tricia has worked with Margarita, certified nursing assistant (CNA), for several years and assigns Margarita to Harold for personal care and assistance with ambulation because Margarita has had training as a restorative aid. Margarita verbally explains understanding to make sure Harold gets up from the right side of the bed, does not cross legs, and does not lean forward while getting up or sitting in the chair. Tricia assigns Margarita to care for Harold and set up for the dressing change. Although Margarita is allowed to change clean dressings, Tricia must be notified before the nursing assistant begins so Tricia can observe the surgical site because of Harold's temperature.
- **Adelia:** Lenore, CNA, has had training for capillary blood testing. Tricia has worked with Lenore for several months and thinks Lenore has demonstrated proficiency in safely and accurately obtaining samples for glucose testing. Tricia assigns Lenore to Adelia and delegates capillary blood testing. When given information of the need for two fingersticks on the evening shift, Lenore explains understanding to identify the finger to be used for the fingerstick, warm Adelia's finger under warm water at the sink in the bathroom, and keep that hand down after Adelia sits before attempting to get the sample. Tricia reminds Lenore that the sample is needed at 6:30 am before breakfast and 11:30 am before lunch trays to can determine if Adelia's sliding scale insulin coverage is needed ½ hour before meals. Adelia is to report the result immediately following collection.
- **Blake:** Sergio is a nursing assistant with 7 years' experience, but he is new to Quality Care Home. Sergio has had restorative nursing training and does well with range of motion (ROM), positioning, and transfers. Sergio has generally been doing well feeding residents. However, last week Tricia saw a resident almost choke on a grapefruit segment while being fed by Sergio. Tricia assigns Sergio for the following care of Blake: Assist with morning care in bed, range of motion, positioning, and assist with transfer from bed to chair. Tricia decides to be with Sergio and "care pair" for meals. Tricia will feed Blake and use this as an opportunity to review with Sergio hints and safety techniques for feeding residents with dysphagia.

IMPLEMENTATION

Right Supervision, Feedback, and Evaluation

The National Guidelines for Nursing Delegation (NCSBN and ANA, 2019) emphasizes the need of the licensed nurse to supervise the delegated task, considering staff mix and client acuity. This supervision includes appropriate monitoring, intervention, and evaluation of the nursing assistant, as needed, while providing the delegated duty and feedback after the delegated duty is completed. The following suggestions also apply to assigning tasks. To comply with the National Guidelines for Nursing Delegation, the LPN/LVN charge nurse needs to carry out the suggestions found in the Collaborative Care, Management Hint: Supervision and Feedback box for nursing assistants regarding assigned tasks/delegated duties.

Collaborative Care

Management Hint

SUPERVISION AND FEEDBACK

- How often or closely the charge nurse monitors the nursing assistant carrying out the assigned task or delegated duty depends on the resident condition and status and the nursing assistant.
- The LPN/LVN/RN needs to make himself or herself available for questions or concerns as they arise and to provide guidance and assistance when needed. Ask the nursing assistant if assistance is needed.
- Determine if the assigned tasks or delegated duties are being completed. If not, determine the reason for this (e.g., change of condition).
- If necessary, intervene in the situation to ensure carrying out the assigned task or delegated duty safely.

If you fail to supervise adequately and the resident is harmed, the situation could result in a civil suit in a court of law or disciplinary action against your license. See Chapter 7 for information about nursing and the law.

Assessment of residents and functioning of the team by the LPN/LVN charge nurse occurs periodically during the shift. Although clear communication with nursing assistants during assignment helps ensure that helpful information about residents will be collected during the shift, nothing can replace the charge nurse's contact with residents and judgment based on knowledge and experience.

Collaborative Care

Management Hint

TRICIA SUPERVISES THE NURSING ASSISTANTS

At 7:30 am and 11:30 am, Lenore reports, without reminder, Adelia's blood glucose levels. Lenore states there was no trouble getting the samples with one fingerstick. Tricia interprets that no sliding scale insulin is required.

Tricia sees Margarita and Harold as they walk to the dining room for breakfast, and Margarita reports that Harold is very careful about getting up. Harold informed Margarita that "I need to keep that new hip in its socket," so the resident always gets up on the right side of the bed and never crosses legs. Margarita notified Tricia after setting up for the clean dressing change, and Tricia assessed the incisional line. There was no redness or edema at the area. The wound was well approximated. Harold's lung sounds are clear, and he denied coughing or congestion. Tricia asks Margarita to check Harold's temperature again at noon.

Sergio sets up Blake for breakfast and notifies Tricia when the tray arrives. When Tricia enters Blake's room, noting that Blake is sitting up in bed. Tricia suggests that they have Blake sit in the chair for meals. When seated, Tricia reminds Blake to keep his head straight, slightly flexed forward, and not tilt it back while swallowing. Tricia turns Blake's head to the left (the unaffected side) and starts with a couple of spoonfuls of thickened liquids and explains this will moisten the membranes of Blake's mouth and throat to make swallowing easier. Tricia feeds one-third of a teaspoon at a time of Cream of Wheat and scrambled eggs. Sergio is attentive as Tricia continues with thickened liquids periodically. When done, Tricia arranges with Sergio to be present while setting Blake up and assisting with feeding lunch.

EVALUATION

You discovered in this chapter that clinical evaluation is a two-way process. The information applies to this part of the assignment/delegation process. See the Collaborative Care, Management Hint: Evaluation and Feedback box.

Collaborative Care

Management Hint

EVALUATION AND FEEDBACK

Evaluation

- Check the completed duty that was assigned/delegated. Was the task/duty completed? Was the task/duty performed safely and correctly?
- Legally, the LPN/LVN charge nurse may not delegate a duty without checking the outcome of that delegation. Have resident goals (outcomes) been met?
- Has something unusual, undesirable, or unexpected occurred? Does the nursing assistant have suggestions to improve carrying out the delegated duty? What went well and what was challenging?
- Did the nursing assistant report as requested?
- Has the nursing assistant documented the activity?

Feedback

- Encourage the nursing assistant to offer input about the assignment/delegation. For example, you might say, "Harper, what problems did you have while assisting Mr. Paul with his shower?" or "Carlos, what suggestions do you have that would make things flow more smoothly during the shift?"
- The LPN's/LVN's leadership skills again come into importance during evaluation and feedback. Provide feedback as needed by the nursing assistant.
- Review communication strategies important for performance evaluation from Chapter 8.
- Did the LPN/LVN thank the nursing assistants for their team work during the shift?

Tricia's Evaluation of and Feedback From Nursing Assistants

Tricia thanks Margarita, Lenore, and Sergio for their help and for getting back to her with information and notifying her as quickly as they did. She asks each aide how they thought the day went. Margarita and Lenore say the day went fine and that Tricia was available when they needed to report. Sergio says the hints for Blake's feeding, especially getting up to eat and giving thickened liquids first to moisten membranes, were very helpful. All three say they hope to get the same assignment tomorrow, and Lenore asks to watch Sergio feed Blake, to pick up some hints to use with clients with dysphagia.

PUTTING IT ALL TOGETHER

See the exercise in the Critical Thinking: Assigning Residents in Long-Term Care box.

Critical Thinking

Assigning Residents in Long-Term Care

Resource needed:

- As the LPN/LVN charge nurse, and with available staff, make assignments for the day shift for wing 1 of the nursing home. Include the rationale (reason) for your assignment decisions. Assign and delegate as you feel is appropriate.

STAFF AVAILABLE FOR THE TEAM

- Two student practical/vocational nurses who have completed half of their nursing program. Instructor makes assignments and is present on the clinical area.
- One nursing assistant who has worked at the facility for 10 years (on state registry). One nursing assistant who has 7 years' experience and has worked at your facility for 6 months (on state registry).
- One nursing assistant who was sent from a temporary agency to fill the position of a nursing assistant who has the flu. She completed a nursing assistant advanced course 2 months ago (on state registry).

TASKS FOR DAY SHIFT OF WING 1

- *Four showers*. Each of these residents transfers with the help of two nursing assistants. Each of these residents needs to be weighed, have blood pressure checked, and have a complete linen change on shower day. One resident scheduled for a shower says she feels dizzy and has a congested-sounding cough.
- *Sixteen AM cares*. Ten residents are able to wash their own face and hands when set up. Of the remaining six, one has developed a rash over his entire body, one needs electronic glucose monitoring ½ hour before breakfast and lunch on day shift, and four are confused and incontinent of urine and feces. Each of these residents needs one assistant to transfer and ambulate.
- *One complex dressing change for a resident on a Clinitron bed*. (This resident is transferred by a client-lifting device and requires total care.)
- *One percutaneous endoscopic gastrostomy (PEG) tube intermittent feeding with commercial tube feeding formula and drug administration at 8:00 am and 12:00 noon on day shift*. (This resident is confused and requires two persons to ambulate.)

You have just completed assigning team members, when one of the nursing assistants states that she feels warm and then faints. As it turns out, she has a temperature of 102.2°F (39°C) and will not be able to engage in resident care. Reassign the residents on wing 1.

Critical Thinking

Delegating to Nursing Assistants

Resources needed:

- Descriptions of recent clinical assignments for students in your clinical group
- Critical thinking

If your state allows LPNs/LVNs to delegate, use Table 17.2 and the nursing process format in this chapter to practice assigning/delegating recent clinical duties for your clinical group to nursing assistants.

REPORTING AT THE END OF YOUR SHIFT

Giving report at the end of your shift requires planning. As the LPN/LVN charge nurse, you need reports from the nursing assistants before you can tape or give report. This is where the concise, clear directions that you gave to these team members during assignment/delegation will pay off. You will need to set priorities in deciding pertinent information to give to the next shift. Be sure to personally assess residents who have the following:

- Changes in condition
- Current ongoing problems
- New orders (and resident response to new orders)
- Suspected side effects to medications/treatments

Use the same sequence of data for each resident. This will make it easier for the oncoming charge nurse to take notes from your report. An example of a suggested sequence of data for reporting to oncoming shift for residents in a long-term care unit can be found in the Collaborative Care, Management Hint: Reporting to Oncoming Shift box.

Collaborative Care

Management Hint

REPORTING TO ONCOMING SHIFT

Things To Report

Resident name, room number, and health care provider

1. New problems/concerns (i.e., change in diagnosis, medication side effect)
2. Contact with health care provider and new orders
3. Progress of current, established problems
4. PRN medication: name of drug, time given, and reason for PRN medication; time follow-up is required
5. *Briefly* describe resident's behavior during shift; include any changes in resident's physical and mental status
6. Resident's voiding, bowel movement (continent versus incontinent), intake/output

7. Follow up with residents, family, or team members still needed
8. Highlight and update key client goals

THINGS TO AVOID DURING REPORT

1. Meaningless chatter that has nothing to do with residents' nursing care and goals/outcomes
2. Routine nursing care, unless it is related to a current nursing problem
3. Personal opinions about residents' conditions
4. Value judgments, gossip about residents' lifestyles, behavior, or families

Tricia was very tired and began to put away the textbooks and scrapbook. The review of delegation in the old text proved demanding for Tricia, but it also had been very pleasant reminiscing about being in school and the early years as an LPN/LVN. Tricia felt good with the great improvements made since feeling insecure in those beginning days, now knowing what to question and where to find the answers. It felt good to have a grasp of the LPN/LVN charge nurse position, especially the fine points of assignment and delegation of duties. Later, as Tricia was relaxing, she starting smiling, a really big smile. Tomorrow would be a big day in her life. The nurse educator had strongly recommended membership in professional organizations. Tricia had been a member of the National Association of Licensed Practical Nurses at the national, state, and local levels since graduation. Over the years, Tricia had assumed various committee assignments and officer positions at the local level of the organization. Tomorrow, Tricia would be installed as the president of the organization at the state level, being the first one from the local district! Tricia was proud to be of service to the nursing profession and looked forward to promoting and having a say in the direction practical/vocational nursing would take in the 21st century.

Get Ready for the Next-Generation NCLEX® Examination

Key Points

- When the state's NPA allows, LPNs/LVNs are used as first-line leaders and or managers (charge nurse) in the nursing home/long-term care unit.
- The basic student practical/vocational nursing program offers students the opportunity to develop skills in nursing procedures, the nursing process, critical thinking, communication, time management, assertiveness, and stress control. These are skills needed for everyday practice, as well as leadership and management positions.
- Development of a leadership style is important in guiding nursing assistants to meet the goals of the long-term care facility.
- Established leadership styles range from the extreme of autocratic, with a pure emphasis on the task, to laissez-faire, which emphasizes concern with the employee.
- Situational leadership adapts a leadership style to the environment and situation at hand. It is the suggested way of leading in the 21st century.
- No one chapter or course can teach you how to become a leader. The development of leadership skills is a process and evolves over time.
- Understanding and applying the four "I"s of transformational leadership (idealized influence, inspirational motivation, individualized consideration, and intellectual stimulation) can assist the LPN/LVN in becoming a successful leader.
- The five core skills of leadership involve the ability to (1) motivate team members, (2) communicate assertively, (3) problem solve effectively, (4) build a team of cooperative workers, and (5) manage stress effectively. These core skills lay the foundation for the development of other specific skills for leadership.
- Specific skill areas for nursing leadership include occupational skills, organizational skills, and human relationship skills.
- In addition to training given by the institution, first-line practical/vocational nursing leaders need to educate and update themselves continually in the five core and three specific skill areas noted.
- Herzberg's two-factor theory indicates that managers/leaders should implement strategies to support intrinsic and extrinsic motivators in the work setting, thereby increasing job satisfaction and decreasing job dissatisfaction.
- Common charge nurse challenges include nursing assistants who bring personal problems to work, the need for nursing assistants to be accountable for learning new job skills, and managing with the residents and family members' concerns.
- Oncoming shift report gives the charge nurse the opportunity to collect data about resident needs, identify resident goals (outcomes) for the shift, and assign nursing tasks to nursing assistants for resident care from their job description.
- Assessment of each resident after assignment/delegation identifies changes in condition/circumstances that may require a change in assignment/delegation.
- The charge nurse shares responsibility with nursing assistants for the quality of care that is given.
- LPN/LVN charge nurses routinely assign care to nursing assistants.
- Charge nurses, as part of their jobs, evaluate the thoroughness and safety of all tasks they assign.
- If allowed in your state's NPA, included in facility policies, and having additional training, the LPN/LVN charge nurse may elect to delegate duties from the LPN/LVN job description to nursing assistants.
- Delegation gives the charge nurse time to focus on duties that cannot be delegated.
- Duties can be delegated, but the accountability that goes with those duties remains with the RN, with whom the charge nurse functions under general supervision. The LPN/LVN shares accountability and collaborates in these situations.
- The charge nurse position is a complex role for LPNs/LVNs. With additional education and experience, many

practical/vocational nurses are doing an excellent job in this expanded role position.

Additional Learning Resources

Go to your Evolve website (http://evolve.elsevier.com/Carroll/success/) for the following FREE learning resources:

- Answers to Critical Thinking and Scenario
- Additional learning activities
- Additional Review Questions for the NCLEX-PN® examination
- Helpful phrases for communicating in Spanish and more!

Clinical Judgment and Next-Generation NCLEX® Examination-Style Questions

1. A family member is continually finding fault (no evidence available) and criticizing the care given to a relative by nursing assistants. Which of the following best describes the coping mechanism utilized by the family member?

a. Projection
b. Validation
c. Introversion
d. Conversion

2. A group of LPNs/LVNs are discussing key elements to safe delegation. Which of the following statements indicate the best understanding of concept of safe delegation?

a. "Nursing assistants cannot refuse a duty delegated to them by the practical/vocational nurse for any reason."
b. "Delegating duties depends on state law, facility policies, resident condition, and the need of the LPNs/LVNs to delegate based on the situation."
c. "Any LPN/LVN may delegate his or her role to a qualified, dependable nursing assistant."
d. "LPNs/LVNs delegate duties routinely to nursing assistants that are in the facility job description of the nursing assistant."

3. An LPN/LVN is charge nurse on the evening shift at a nursing home. Which of the following priority actions best contribute to safe client assignment to nursing assistants?

a. The nurse obtains feedback from the nursing assistants as to the type of procedures for which they feel comfortable.
b. The nurse distributes the nursing tasks to be completed on the evening shift equally among the nursing assistants on the team.
c. After report, the nurse asks the clients who they would like to care for them that evening.
d. The nurse checks job descriptions and skills checklist for nursing assistants to clarify who is competent to perform selected duties.

4. A nursing assistant has been absent four times this month, each absence occurring on the weekend. Which of the following LPN/LVN charge nurses is using problem solving to handle this situation?

a. Focuses feedback on the nursing assistant's frequent absences and explains the related discipline measures according to policy.
b. Downplays the importance of absences to make the nursing assistant feel better.
c. Provides the nursing assistant with all the suggestions needed to correct the problem.
d. Assumes being present for assigned shift is something the nursing assistant cannot do.

5. A nursing assistant, with a history of minimal absences, is attending a practical nursing program. Before the staffing schedule is posted, the nursing assistant requests to be off the night before two final exams. As the LPN/LVN who has the responsibility for the scheduling process, you comply. Which of the following best describes this leadership approach?

a. Individualized consideration
b. Intellectual stimulation
c. Idealized influence
d. Inspirational motivation

6. Which of the following are an important resource regarding legal authorization for the LPN/LVN to delegate in long-term care? *(Select all that apply.)*

a. BON
b. NCSBN
c. NALPN
d. NLN
e. NAPNES

7. Which of the following best describes an LPN/LVN charge nurse in a long-term care facility assigning in a legally sound manner? (*Select all that apply.*)

a. The LPN/LVN assigns clients primarily based on geographic location to enhance timeliness of the response to client inquiries.
b. The LPN/LVN clarifies skill levels of nursing assistants by reviewing skill competency records.
c. The LPN/LVN makes rounds after report to gather data on actual resident conditions to develop shift outcomes for residents before making assignments.
d. The LPN/LVN provides specific, concrete information for what nursing assistants should do while engaging in resident care and follows up appropriately.
e. The LPN/LVN asks the CNAs which clients they prefer to care for and assigns accordingly.

8. A work-related conflict has surfaced between two nursing assistants on their shift at the long-term care facility, where an LPN/LVN is charge nurse. Which of the following intervention strategies should the charge nurse use to resolve the conflict? (*Select all that apply.*)

a. Develop a collaborative solution to solve the conflict so the two parties are satisfied with the solution.
b. Limit the number of possible solutions offered to solve the conflict, thus saving time.
c. Instead of focusing on what solution each assistant wants, focus on why they want that specific solution.
d. Actively listen while each nursing assistant presents his or her side of the conflict and solutions.
e. Request that the nursing assistants stay away from each other for a week to encourage time for self-reflection.

9.

The nurse received a change of shift report and has prepared the assignments for the nursing assistants. As an LPN/LVN, the need to collect date on a client's condition cannot be delegated. Residents of concern from the report are of concern. Resident A: 62-year-old resident is on hospice palliative care. Respirations were last reported at 8 breaths/min. Resident B: 58-year-old resident fell about 30 minutes ago and is now experiencing a severe headache and is disoriented. Becoming combative to caregivers. The resident is usually ambulatory, steady gait, and alert/oriented. Resident C: 82-year-old resident with chronic obstructive pulmonary disease is having increased breathing difficulty. Resp rate of 22, on 1 L of oxygen via nasal cannula. Last O_2 Sat was 88%. Resident D: 78-year-old resident with oral temperature of 100.7°F (38.167°C), having three episodes of incontinence in the past 8 hours, recent stent insertion after lithotripsy (kidney stone crushing). Also complaining of pain level if 6 with no relief from pain medication.	The nurse is organizing the plan to see all residents on the unit at the beginning of the shift. Prioritize the order of the residents to be seen to gather additional data and complete a focused assessment. List the residents in the order of priority Resident______ Resident______ Resident______ Resident______

Critical Thinking Scenarios

Scenario 1

A nursing assistant has accepted a delegated duty to complete for several evenings. There have been three new admissions to the unit in the last 24 hours. This evening, the LPN/LVN charge nurse says the duty that has been delegated on prior shifts will no longer be delegated to the nursing assistants. The nursing assistant complains to the other nursing assistants that the charge nurse isn't trusting. Comment about this situation.

Scenario 2

The LPN/LVN is the new charge nurse on the evening shift at the local nursing home. The nursing assistants on the evening shift are complaining to the nursing assistants on the day shift about the way the LPN/LVN gives them directions about their assignments. They indicate that the LPN/LVN micromanages them and does not respect them for the knowledge that they have regarding the clients. They also never have an opportunity to leave the floor for continuing education. The LPN/LVN always states that their unit is too busy to attend. As a result, recently they were unable to be certified in dementia care. Provide advice for the LPN/LVN based on the four "*I*"s of transformational leadership.

18 Workforce Trends and Preparing for Employment: How to Find a First Job You Will Love

Objectives

On completing this chapter, you will be able to do the following:

1. Based on workforce trends, list employment opportunities available to licensed practical nurses/licensed vocational nurses (LPNs/LVNs).
2. Differentiate workforce settings for the LPN/LVN.
3. Give examples of interpersonal styles and how to use them to improve your interview and networking skills.
4. Describe how to effectively participate in an information interview.
5. Discuss strategies for completing various aspects of the job application process.
6. Describe role-play for an interview, preparing for complex interview questions.
7. Give examples of factors to focus on prior to the interview to leave a lasting good first impression.
8. Discuss how to address pregnancy in an interview.
9. Discuss components of a preemployment physical examination and background checks.
10. Describe the composition of an effective resignation letter.
11. Discuss how Transition to Practice or residency programs can decrease reality shock during your first year of employment as an LPN/LVN.
12. Discuss the advantages of belonging to professional organizations.
13. Give examples of ways to fulfill continuing education requirements.
14. Discuss organizations that provide certifications and continuing education opportunities, after initial licensure, for nurses.
15. Describe your postlicensure education career goals
16. Develop a nursing career pathway and a plan for ongoing review.

Key Terms

Certified Managed Care Nurse (CMCN) certification
conditional job offer
follow-up illusion
hidden job market
illegal questions
informational interviews
interpersonal styles
Long-Term Care Certification (CLTC)
mobility program
National Association for Practical Nurse Education and Service, Inc. (NAPNES)
National Certification in Gerontology
National IV Therapy Certification
National Federation of Licensed Practical Nurses (NFLPN)
National League for Nursing (NLN)
networking
NAPNES Pharmacology Certification (NCP)
pharmacology certification
podcast
preceptor
reference hierarchy
residency
resignation courtesy
resume
silence
Transition to Practice model
voice control

Keep in Mind

You've decided what you want to be when you grow up; now get out there and do it!

Duke and Kamy, students at the Success Practical Nursing Program, are chatting as they leave their clinical experience on Monday afternoon. They had a great day, learned immensely, and felt like an integral part of the health care team. Duke had interacted with a wellness nurse in a continuing care facility, and Kamy had participated in a pediatric home care experience. During the clinical day, the mom stated to Kamy, "You are going to be a great nurse. My son really connected with you today and performed all his exercises well. It is often a struggle. You have a gift." In addition, they are excited about their upcoming graduation in 4 weeks. Despite this positive clinical experience, fellow student Kwan enters the conversation, sensing frustration as the conversation tone changes. Duke and Kamy are sharing comments made by friends and community members at a holiday event this past weekend. They were asked by two different people the following question: "Why are you wasting your time in LPN school? I hear there are no jobs available for LPNs; all nurses must soon be an RN who graduated from a university." They share that they felt at a loss for words. Duke recalls becoming quiet, and Kamy changed the topic of conversation. Kamy states to Kwan, "I know in my heart this has been a great step on the nursing career pathway for me, but I just did not know what to say, and to be honest it makes me worry a bit. I hope this is not true." Kwan, unsure of what to say, stated, "Well, you know that it is not true," and walked away frustrated.

As you read through this chapter, write down ideas that could have been a great response. Remember, often the public is misinformed. Licensed practical nurses/licensed vocational nurses (LPNs/LVNs) and all nurses need to be their own advocates ensuring the public knows the facts. In the future, if you were in a situation similar to Kwan, how could you help ease you peers' anxiety and spread the word about a great career as an LPN/LVN? Likewise, if you were Duke or Kamy, how could you communicate effectively the strong and diverse job market for LPNs/LVNs? As you read the chapter, you will see LPNs/LVNs are important members of the health care team and that the job opportunities are countless.

LICENSED PRACTICAL NURSE/LICENSED VOCATIONAL NURSE (LPN/LVN) DEMOGRAPHICS AND EMPLOYMENT OPPORTUNITIES

LPN/LVN DEMOGRAPHICS

The LPN/LVN workforce trends identify a lead role in diversifying the nursing workforce and in building a diverse health care workforce. According to the National Council of State Boards of Nursing (NCSBN) 2024 LPN Practice Analysis reveals the changing demographics of the newly licensed LPN/LVN workforce (see Box 18.1). According to the 2022 National Nursing Workforce Study (Smiley et al., 2023), the nursing workforce has undergone a dramatic shift, with many older nurses leaving during the COVID-19 pandemic. The workforce is more demographically diverse, with the proportion of men increasing steadily since 2015. The LPN/LVN workforce is 66% white, 17.6% Black, 12% Hispanic or Latino (an increase of 6% since 2020), and 6.3% Asian, the total minority representation increasing by 3.6% since the last study in 2020. According to the National League for Nursing (NLN, 2014) statement, "A Vision for Recognition of the Role of the Licensed Practical/Vocational Nurses in Advancing the Nation's Health," LPN/LVN graduates are a critical pipeline to building a diverse nursing workforce, playing a vital role in the delivery of culturally sensitive health care in a variety of settings to vulnerable populations (NLN, 2014).

Box 18.1 LPN/LVN Demographics

AGE (AVERAGE) 34.6 YEARS (SLIGHT INCREASE FROM 2021'S 33.2 YEARS OLD)	
Gender	
Female	89.5% (no change from 2021's 90.2%)
Male	No change
RACIAL/ETHNIC BACKGROUND	
White	41% (decrease from 2021's 48.8%)
Black or African American	34.9% (increase from 2021's 28.8%)
Hispanic	12.1% (no change from 2021's 12.2%)
Asian	7.1% (increase from 2021's 5.8%)

From National Council of State Boards of Nursing: 2024 PN Practice Analysis: Linking the NCLEX-PN® to Practice, 2024. Available at: https://www.ncsbn.org/public-files/24_NCLEX-PA_PA.pdf.

NURSING: THE LPN/LVN ROLE, OPPORTUNITIES FOR COUNTLESS WORKFORCE OPTIONS, AND LIFELONG LEARNING

Nursing opens the door to an entirely different world, with countless opportunities. Not only will you have access to a financially secure job; you will also experience many intrinsic rewards. Every day, you enter and touch the lives of many individuals and families. Clients trust you without having to prove yourself. They feel safe in the knowledge that you have pledged to do your best in providing care without passing judgment. Some clients and families will let you know their appreciation for your skill in providing nursing care, but some will never tell you how deeply you touched their life and the lives of their loved ones.

Unfortunately, approximately one-third (36%) of those who enter an LPN/LVN nursing program do not complete the program (ACEN, 2024), for any number of reasons. A major reason is that the course of study demands a great deal of personal discipline, time management, and prioritization of needs (knowing the difference between "I want to" and "I need to") and support systems to be able to focus on studying. So how does your enrollment in the nursing program affect you?

Nursing changes you; you see and hear more in a short period than you ever imagined. Because of confidentiality, most of what you see and hear cannot be shared with anyone out of the immediate setting.

Nursing is a maturing experience, often beyond your years. Both self-confidence and the ability to say, "I don't know, but I will find out," grow as your professional honesty is tested.

Nursing provides opportunities for you in traditional and atypical careers and provides a lifelong career pathway. Be proud of choosing nursing as a career and become an advocate for nurses, particularly LPNs/LVNs. Seize opportunities to educate colleagues and community members regarding the critical role of the LPN/LVN.

Nursing challenges you throughout your career. As a student, you are expected to learn and use an entirely new language and yet always explain to a client what you are doing in terms he or she can understand. The challenge continues when you graduate because you have only scratched the surface of knowledge in nursing. Every day will provide at least one answer to your question, "What did I learn today?"

Lifelong learning is a must to stay current in your career. You will participate in in-services, workshops, and collaboration with other health care providers. To renew your license your state may require completion of a minimum number of continuing education units (CEUs). You may also decide to pursue a formal education route resulting in achievement of various certifications and/or the pursuit of a degree to become a registered nurse (RN). Being a lifelong learner is a strong quality and contributes to job satisfaction and financial security in the United States.

According to the NCSBN 2024 LPN practice analysis, approximately 25% of responders reported enrollment in an RN educational program broken down as follows: 78% were in associate degree programs, 15.5% were in baccalaureate programs, and 4.7% were in diploma programs. It was anticipated that the percentage of LPNs enrolled in baccalaureate RN programs would increase; however, this is not the case.

The response to the Institute of Medicine (IOM) report to increase baccalaureate-prepared nurses to 80% of the workforce by 2020 has not resulted in a major increase of baccalaureate-prepared RNs. In the recent 2024 RN Practice Analysis (2025), of the number of new RNs, 45.3% graduated with baccalaureate degrees in nursing, whereas 45.3% graduated with an associate degree in nursing.

Given the continued nursing shortage, fueled by the aging nursing workforce, aging Baby Boomers, and the COVID-19 pandemic, your selection of a career in nursing and particularly a career as an LPN/LVN is a great one! Projected job growth for LPNs/LVNs is predicted to be 3% (2023–2033), which is as fast as the average rate for all occupations, and for RNs it is 6% (faster than average) (Bureau of Labor Statistics Occupational Outlook Handbook, 2025). In addition, the average age of LPNs/LVNs was 50 years, decreasing from 2020 (2024 National Nursing Workforce Study) (Smiley et al., 2025). This average age of the LPN workforce coupled with predominance of the LPN as the licensed nurse working in long-term care settings and the prediction by the Department of Health and Human Services that 56% of people turning 65 between 2021 and 2025 will need long-term services and support in their lifetime (Dept. of HHS, 2021) intensifies the predicted shortage of LPNs. Recruitment and retention of LPNs/LVNs will remain a focus for the future. Meeting the job satisfaction needs of LPNs/LVNs will be critical to maintain a robust workforce.

The US workforce consists of 3,300,100 RN jobs and 657,800 LPN jobs according to the Occupational Outlook Handbook (2025). Thus LPN/LVN jobs represent approximately 19.9% of the total nursing jobs in the United States. National entities support the role of the LPN as noted in the NLN report "Recognizing the Vital Contributions of Licensed Practical/Licensed Vocational Nurse" (2011) and the IOM reports "Retooling for an Aging America: Building the Health Care Workforce" (2008) and "Future of Nursing" (2010). The IOM (2021) report recognizes the unique contribution of LPNs in long-term care. The report states that LPNs/LVNs are important because they "provide health care to mostly racially and ethnically diverse populations both in the community and in health care organizations. They also add meaningfully to the pipeline for RN and advance practice registered nurse (APRN) roles, and importantly, allow RNs to concentrate on care for medically complex patients" (p. 70).

According to the NCSBN LPN/LVN 2024 practice analysis, the majority of new LPNs continue to be employed in long-term care settings (48.3%), whereas 25.6% work in hospitals. Additionally, 26.6% work in community-based or ambulatory care facilities. This represents a significant increase in hospital settings compared to 2021. Also, 40.1% of newly LPNs indicated that they have administrative duties, with 15% having a primary administrative position. LPNs working in long-term care facilities were more likely to have administrative responsibilities than LPNs working in a hospital (58.4% vs. 14.5%, respectively) (NCSBN, 2025). In community-based settings 32.5% reported having administrative responsibilities. This represents a trend in lesser responsibilities than in past practice analyses. The NCSBN survey indicates that LPNs/LVNs care for a diverse array of clients in need of chronic care in the community. This includes caring for the chronic pediatric client who is ventilator dependent, caring for clients with mental health and dependency issues, and providing care in correctional settings, clinic, and urgent care settings.

There have been several workforce trends noted in the newly graduated LPN/LVN workforce, representing a shift from long-term care to acute care and/or community-based care. See the NCSBN 2024 LPN practice analysis for specific details: https://www.ncsbn.org/public-files/24_NCLEX_PN_PA.pdf. This aligns with changes in client access to health care fueled by the Affordable Care Act, positioning the LPN/LVN for a continued strong presence as a member of the health care workforce team. What does this mean to you? A strong future for continued stable employment despite swings in the economy. The LPN/LVN is a low-cost, high-quality health care team member.

Try This

Consider the following questions:

1. What type of environment do I want to work in: direct health care, state/federal government, private duty, insurance related, sales, industry, or other?

   ____

2. What population (i.e., type of client) do I find most rewarding to work with?

   ____

3. What kinds of nursing skills do I find most challenging and rewarding? What new areas would I like to be involved in? How can I become immersed in these areas?

   ____

4. What workforce trends impact positively on my practice setting preferences for employment?

   ____

COUNTLESS WORKFORCE SETTINGS EXIST: FINDING THE RIGHT FIT IS A REWARDING CHALLENGE

While you are in your educational program, carefully evaluate each unique clinical or volunteer experience. Be proactive, introducing yourself to staff and the human resource department. Be sure to communicate directly if you are interested in a particular specialty area or practice setting. Then, note whether your area of interest is reported as a likely employment setting for new nursing graduates in the PN practice analysis. Consider taking additional coursework or obtaining certifications to enhance your employability in the areas of basic life support, intravenous (IV) therapy, phlebotomy, advanced cardiac life support, behavioral management, and rehabilitation as available. See the NCSBN 2024 LPN practice analysis for specific details (https://www.ncsbn.org/public-files/24_NCLEX_PN_PA.pdf). Lastly, focus on increasing your knowledge of the diverse health care settings where LPNs/LVNs are employed. Identify your passion, understand the usual role of the LPN/LVN in this setting, and evaluate the future LPN/LVN workforce trend for this setting. The information below provides details of many possible workplace settings for LPNs/LVNs to guide your decision.

LONG-TERM CARE FACILITIES (INCLUDING SUBACUTE UNITS)

The Congressional Budget Office (2025) reports that by 2055, the US population of 65-and-older residents will grow from 350 million to 372 million and is expected to grow more quickly than younger groups. This reflects the ongoing aging of the Baby Boomer generation born after World War II. This has a positive impact on the job demand for LPNs/LVNs. The long-term care population is made up of residents who are:

1. In need of transitional care upon discharge from the acute care hospital, allowing time to recover from surgery or trauma before returning home.
2. Elderly people who are unable to care for themselves because of medical or mental impairment.
3. Young to middle-aged people with chronic debilitating disease or injuries from accidents.
4. Young, chronically mentally ill persons who need continual supervision and are not candidates for independent living or group homes.

LPNs/LVNs who are hired for direct care measure vital signs, collect data, provide physical care and comfort measures, and administer medications. LPNs/LVNs often have administrative responsibilities in long-term care settings. Some state Nurse Practice Acts (NPAs) permit more extensive use of LPN/LVN skills in nursing homes. Other state regulations are more restrictive.

There are some inconsistencies in the NPAs for LPNs and RNs. Some inconsistencies are noted for terms such as assessment, delegation, and decision-making. The difference in the terms assessment and data collection (the preferred term for LPNs/LVNs) is difficult to define. Some NPAs use the term focused assessment for the LPN/LVN. Because critical thinking and clinical judgment has been incorporated into the National Council Licensure Examination for Practical Nurses (NCLEX-PN®), critical thinking is promoted in the PN/VN school curriculum. As noted in the 2024 Practice Analysis, many LPNs/LVNs in long-term care facilities have administrative duties. These LPNs/LVNs often function as the charge nurse. Clinical judgment and critical thinking are necessary components of their job performance. The LPN/LVN must collect data and determine which are most important to apply to the client's plan of care.

Many states and organizations offer courses and certifications. The **National Association for Practical Nurse Education and Service (NAPNES)** offers certification programs in pharmacology, IV therapy, and long-term care (www.napnes.org). The National Association of Licensed Practical Nurses (NALPN) offers certifications in pharmacology, long-term care, IV therapy, rehabilitation, and palliative care (www.nalpn.org). The American Board of Managed Care Nursing (ABMCN) offers certification in managed care nursing (www.abmcn.org). Other certifications such as wound care, dementia care, and end-of-life care can be obtained, which are valuable assets in a variety of work settings. Some technical colleges offer post-licensure courses in management and leadership. Some states recognize post-licensure courses and certifications and permit the LPN/LVN to use the skills they have learned in providing care. A major benefit of post-licensure information is knowledge gained for more effective client outcomes and job satisfaction.

Long-term care as an employment option may be available to you if you possess the following characteristics:

- Use solid nursing process skills in gathering data and use the care plan as a guide.
- Use critical thinking/clinical judgment.
- Use therapeutic communication skills; differentiate between therapeutic and personal.
- Enjoy longer-term contact with people. (High turnover rates of staff have been associated with lower quality of care in some extended care facilities.)
- Provide quality nursing care with collaboration but without immediate, direct supervision of an RN or health care provider (i.e., health care provider, advanced practice nurse or APRN).
- Seek assistance or additional instruction as needed to provide safe, quality, cost-effective care.
- Apply information about growth and development changes during illness.
- Seek to learn new skills through continuing education (CE) and certification courses to take care of a diverse population and age group.

- Listen to clients regarding what they see as their needs for care.
- Treat clients of all ages and levels of growth and development with respect.

Other special qualities needed include the following:

- Patience
- Ability to understand a person's behavior and thinking process
- Strong listening skills
- Maturity
- Understand the significance of the work you are doing
- Ability to determine priorities
- Ability to set limits
- Interest in working with people with disabilities
- Willingness to collaborate and problem solve with other health care givers, residents, significant others, and family members
- Self-understanding your personal value system
- The ability or willingness to learn to manage and lead a team effectively

Experience on a medical/surgical unit, including student clinical experiences, is helpful before working in a long-term care facility.

The level of responsibility in long-term care is significant. LPNs/LVNs who work in long-term care are challenged to create a homelike atmosphere while working with residents with chronic, long-term, and terminal health problems. The LPN/LVN often works in a charge nurse role, and although supervision must be available from an RN or health care provider, during some periods of the day supervision may be virtual (i.e., at the other end of a cell phone). Consequently, solid knowledge and skills are essential to understanding when to seek help and from whom. The nursing process and critical thinking provide the basis for skilled, compassionate care.

The charge nurse role also means that the LPN/LVN is responsible for managing care given by other LPNs/LVNs, certified nursing assistants (CNAs), and other direct care workers (DCWs). (Refer to Chapter 17 for more details on leadership and charge nurse skills.)

Working as an LPN/LVN in a long-term care facility, much of your work ultimately relates to assisting the residents to achieve their highest level of health and independence possible. Through your efforts, residents who are recuperating from surgery or trauma will realize their goal for recovery and discharge. For other residents, your role includes supporting them through the final step of the growth process: a dignified death.

ASSISTED LIVING FACILITY

Adults who live in assisted living facilities do not need 24-hour skilled nursing care; however, they benefit from an LPN/LVN using strong nursing processes and critical-thinking skills. The LPN/LVN is constantly gathering data on the medical and psychological condition of the client. A skilled LPN/LVN, for example, will note early signs of exacerbations of chronic conditions or an impending acute issue, such as an early cough before it progresses to pneumonia. Assisted living facilities are often a part of a continuing care retirement community (CCRC). The RN in charge evaluates the needs of the resident at the time of admission and assigns specific duties to the LPN/LVN. The RN also identifies the chain of command for the LPN/LVN should there be an emergency. If you like the human connection and you function well with less supervision, this may be an area to consider. The LPN/LVN is often in a supervisory position.

INDEPENDENT LIVING FACILITY

As the geriatric population continues to grow, the practical nurse continues to excel in various settings. Some independent living centers assign LPNs/LVNs to provide wellness services and health teaching to the residents, in collaboration with the RN.

SCHOOL-RELATED POSITIONS

Although the LPN/LVN cannot be certified as a school nurse (Post RN Bachelor of Science in Nursing [BSN] certificate required), current trends are to hire the LPN/LVN to join the school nurse team. This has been a cost-effective and successful implementation for many school districts. In addition, LPNs/LVNs are often hired to meet the needs of students with special needs attending regular education or special education classes. A newer trend for LPNs also is finding employment in specialty day care centers.

HOME HEALTH NURSING

According to the US Bureau of Labor Statistics Occupational Outlook Handbook (2025), faster-than-average growth is expected in home health services. Home health and personal care aide job growth is projected at 21% (2023–2033). This is in response to the number of older persons (aging Baby Boomers) with functional disabilities, preference for home care, implementation of the Affordable Care Act, and technological advances that make it possible to do more complicated treatments/care in the home.

Because of shorter hospital stays, clients are receiving an increased amount of care in the home. The actual initial care given is under the supervision of an RN, who uses nursing process steps to finalize a plan of care approved by the client. Data from the LPN/LVN involved with care is essential to complete and implement the plan of care. LPNs'/LVNs' observations of physical and mental changes update ongoing data collection and evaluation of the plan of care. Because of difficulty in receiving payment from nonprivate sources, some home health agencies use LPNs/LVNs for private-pay clients only. However, the increase in home health care needs has improved the employment of LPNs/LVNs in home care. In recent years,

LPNs have been obtaining positions caring for stable, chronic, complex pediatric clients at home, in addition to elderly clients. The LPN/LVN may travel to a school setting with the pediatric client.

Helpful Qualities for Home Health Nurses

- **Flexibility:** You will have to improvise in the home yet practice sound nursing principles, for example, improvising when equipment is not available, determining how to clean the equipment, and using it to attain desired results. Flexibility is also needed when the client assignment changes because of the client's needs. Collaborating with the RN or other health care providers is essential.
- **Communication skills:** You are working in the client's domain. You need the client's trust to develop a cooperative nurse-client relationship. Implementing communication principles and techniques to ensure understanding between you and the client is essential. You must understand the client's expression of needs and make sure you express yourself clearly and tactfully. For example, you may need to use words in the client's vocabulary, speak slowly, and explain procedures in detail.

  Self-confidence: Present yourself in a confident manner to gain the client's trust. The client will notice insecurity or uncertainty, resulting in lack of confidence in you. You should not fake confidence. You know you have the knowledge and nursing skills to perform tasks efficiently. Be adequately prepared prior to arrival in the home. It may be difficult to find the reference needed once in the client's home. Make phone calls or consults with the RN or health care provider outside of the client's home. Do not ask for reassurance from the client when performing basic skills. Ask questions outside of the client's room, unless an emergency exists. For example, you may be tempted to tell the client, "This is only the second time I have changed a dressing on a foot, and I'm kind of nervous about it." Do not make a comment like this. It will worry the client.
- **Sensitivity to physical and emotional changes:** Once the initial assessment is completed by the RN, you will alert the RN to any changes in client status. The RN depends on your observational skills to assist the client to meet their health outcomes while providing a safe environment. For example, be tuned in to the person's affective, verbal, and nonverbal communication. If the client or family is beginning to show signs of agitation, diffuse the situation before continuing your assigned work.
- **Managing emergencies:** Staying calm and following agency protocol are essential. For example, the client may start to bleed from the wound you are dressing. Remembering what you learned in nursing fundamentals and first aid class is more effective than panicking and yelling for a family member to call 911. Initiate emergency help (911) when appropriate; however, do so in a calm manner and communicate clearly. In an emergency, your motto is, "Function now, and shake later."
- **Nonjudgmental attitude:** This is important because you are in the client's home providing a service. If you are comfortable with your own values, different values are not personally threatening. For example, the home may not meet your standards in cleanliness but is a safe environment for the client. Be aware of your hidden biases and reflect often to avoid stereotyping clients.

MENTAL HEALTH NURSING

Mental health nursing facilities include psychiatric hospitals, community mental health centers, day treatment centers, and group homes for the recovering mentally ill. Many community mental health centers and group homes are staffed primarily with LPNs/LVNs and nursing assistants, with RNs in a supervisory role. The LPN/LVN may also function in a supervisory role collaborating with the RN. The workforce trend has remained relatively constant over the last decade.

In mental health nursing, LPNs/LVNs are involved in the following:

- Performing treatments
- Administering medications
- Supervising activities of daily living
- Observing clients
- Assisting with group meetings and activities

Furthermore, LPNs/LVNs perform a significant role in developing a therapeutic relationship with the client and following through with appropriate interventions, according to the client's care plan. Mental health facilities practice a team concept in which everyone is expected to contribute to the client's care plan, know the therapeutic guidelines in a client care plan, and carry out the plan. A solid knowledge of mental health concepts and nursing process is essential.

Specific beneficial qualities for working in a mental health unit include the following:

Professional Pointer

Desirable Qualities in a Mental Health Setting

- Basic knowledge of managing psychiatric behaviors
- Keen observational skills regarding behavioral change
- Staying calm and be able to make quick decisions
- Empathetic rather than sympathetic
- Therapeutic communication skills
- Separates personal and professional life
- Nonjudgmental and respectful
- Stable mental health
- Excellent nursing process and critical-thinking skills
- Sets client-centered limits assertively
- Knowledge of basic self-defense
- Does not take unnecessary risks with a client who is acting out, knows when to seek assistance
- Experience with medical/surgical clients before working in a mental health unit

MILITARY SERVICES

As an LPN/LVN, you initially attend basic training if you volunteer for military service in the reserves or for active duty. Contact recruiters for all branches of the military services, including the National Guard. Compare the differences in available nursing careers to determine which branch best fits your needs. The US Army, for example, cross-trains LPNs/LVNs to work in any area of the hospital as well as out in the field on military maneuvers. The benefits of military service include financial educational benefits to continue education, and some LPNs/LVNs have taken advantage of this benefit to become an RN and an officer. Others have gone on to get advanced degrees in nursing.

Professional Pointer

Desirable Qualities in Military Service Nursing

- Interest in teamwork
- Strong ego
- Ability to cope with changing situations
- Emotional stability
- Good communication skills
- Desire for adventure
- Flexible and adaptable
- Empathetic (rather than sympathetic) with clients
- Self-directed, but knows when to seek help
- Healthy personal stress-relieving habits
- A desire for a challenging career and an ability to adjust quickly to new situations

HOSPITAL NURSING

The acute care experience in most LPN/LVN nursing programs is complete in hospital medical and surgical units. The percentage of LPNs/LVNs working on medical surgical units has trended positively in the last 5 years due to an increasing shortage of RNs and the commitment of the hospital to utilize the LPN/LVN in their full scope of practice. Additional trends include health care systems employing LPNs/LVNs to work in their specialty and medical surgical clinics. Sometimes the LPN/LVN is underused in the hospital setting because the RN is not familiar with what the LPN/LVN is permitted to do legally. Your responsibility is to know your state's NPA (scope of practice). Provide this information and information on CE (including certifications you have earned) to your RN supervisor. Some RNs do not trust LPNs/LVNs primarily because they have never worked with them. Do your nursing care with skillful professionalism and help pave the way for other LPNs/LVNs to be a collaborative care partner in this important hospital nursing role.

If you consider working in a specialty area, it is helpful to have both theory class and clinical experience, or additional education. Areas with complex nursing duties mean that additional post-licensure education such as in-service, workshops, or courses related specifically to the area are required. Previous nursing experience may also be listed as a requirement. Refer to your state's NPA to see how performance of nursing acts beyond basic nursing care is handled. These acts are referred to as the expanded role of the practical/vocational nurse or performance of acts in complex client situations. Always review the facility policy and procedure book to ensure the hospital allows the LPN/LVN to proceed.

Professional Pointer

Desirable Qualities in Hospital Nursing

- Strong technical skills
- Organizational skills
- Nursing process and critical-thinking/clinical judgment skills
- Strong ego
- Copes well during emergencies
- Teamwork: knows own and others' scope of practice
- Knows own limits and asks for help as needed
- Self-motivated and self-directed learner

AMBULATORY CARE: OUTPATIENT CLINICS, HEALTH CARE PROVIDERS' OFFICES, URGENT CARE CENTERS, AND CHIROPRACTIC OFFICES

Outpatient clinics and health care providers' offices continue to provide jobs for many LPNs/LVNs. According to the NCSBN 2024 LPN job analysis, 26.6% of newly LPNs/LVNs work in a community or ambulatory care facility indicating a continued use of LPNs/LVNs in this market.

Most clinics and offices are open Monday to Friday, although extended and weekend hours are quickly becoming the norm. Assigned work varies, but generally includes the following:

- Data collection
- Measuring vital signs/weighing clients
- Venipuncture
- Treatments
- Administering medications/vaccinations
- Preparing the client for an examination
- Assisting the health care provider, nurse practitioner, or RN with the examination
- Performing additional duties delegated by the health care provider
- Maintaining and ordering supplies
- Data entry and insurance processing
- Managing client flow and team communication
- Office tasks and management

Cross-training (learning to do jobs other than nursing) is expected in some facilities. For example, you might be expected to do clerical work, including answering telephones and making appointments, basic lab tests, and assist with x-rays and other diagnostic tests.

If you are working as a private nurse for a health care provider, you can also expect to assist with examinations and treatments as needed. When clients remain with the same health care provider, these nurses develop rapport with the clients, which is an asset to both the client and the health care provider.

Professional Pointer

Desirable Qualities in Ambulatory Care Nursing

- Strong communication skills
- Attention to detail
- Enjoys routine
- Excellent organizational skills
- Applies nursing process and critical-thinking skills, demonstrates clinical judgment
- Flexible, adaptable, self-directed as client load changes
- Treats all clients and their families with respect and empathy
- Practices confidentiality and respects client's right to privacy
- Uses a well-modulated voice throughout the work period
- Willing to learn

Previous work experience in a medical-surgical unit is advised to prepare you for data collection, administering medications, doing select treatments as assigned by the health care provider, and keeping records, as required.

SURGICAL OR PERIOPERATIVE NURSING

LPNs/LVNs who have worked in surgical nursing in the operating room (OR) for years describe their work as assisting the surgeon with instruments and equipment, collecting data, doing preoperative and postoperative client care, and supporting postoperative education. They strongly urge that if interested in this line of work to provide details to your future employer about your education and clinical skills to reflect readiness for this type of position as an LPN/LVN.

The employment options as an LPN/LVN in the OR are limited. In some states, LPNs/LVNs can become trained to become a surgical technician. There is the combined value in being an LPN/LVN and a surgical technician. If surgical nursing is your passion, it will be worth researching the possibility.

VETERANS HEALTH ADMINISTRATION NURSING CAREERS

Working with the nation's veterans in Veterans Health Administration (VHA) hospitals. long-term care, or community-based facilities is an option for LPNs/LVNs. You do not have to be a veteran to apply for employment. More LPNs/LVNs are hired in veteran's long-term care facilities and community settings than in acute care veteran's facilities.

Facilities generally provide new nurses with an extensive orientation during duty hours regardless of the shift you are assigned. Veteran's care includes medicine, surgery, spinal cord injury, alcohol/drug treatment, psychiatry, intensive care, hemodialysis, ambulatory care, and long-term care. Minimum qualifications include US citizenship, graduation (or pending graduation from a state-approved or an accredited nursing school), English language proficiency, and passing an employment physical. Benefits are usually generous and based on civil service grades. If interested, go to the "Job Search" section of the VA Careers website at https://vacareers.va.gov/.

HOSPICE AND PALLIATIVE CARE

Hospice care is for medical care for terminally ill clients of any age (expected to live 6 months or less) and is in an institutional setting or client's home. The nurse's role is to maximize client comfort by managing symptoms while supporting their quality of life and addressing the client's physical, psychosocial, and spiritual needs. The same personal and professional nurse's qualities that are important in a long-term care facility are important in a hospice setting. According to the Hospice Foundation of America (2025), hospice provides an interdisciplinary team of professionals trained to address the patient's medical, physical, spiritual, and psychosocial needs. The focus is on the person, not the illness, and tailors care to the client's needs and wishes. Hospice focuses on caring, not curing.

Palliative care focuses on providing relief from pain and physical, mental, and spiritual stress for any type of disease or illness. It can be provided with a curative approach. See Chapter 11 for more information.

Critical Thinking

Pain Medication for the Terminally Ill Client

Think about the statement, "You should withhold pain medication from a terminally ill client so he or she does not become addicted." Does that statement make sense to you? Explain your response.

OTHER WORKFORCE SETTINGS

Private Duty Nursing

LPNs/LVNs have been employed for years as private duty nurses. This is frequently a long-term commitment on the part of an LPN/LVN. The most common responsibility is for elderly, ill individuals who wish to be cared for in their home. Some private duty nurses accompany the person on extended trips. Private duty nursing can also involve a child or adult with a long-term chronic illness. The LPN/LVN may be part of an around-the-clock care system with RNs on opposing shifts. Responsibilities vary according to the shift involved and includes basic nursing skills and varied procedures/medication administration. The LPN/LVN works under the general supervision of the client's health care provider, collaborating with the RN.

Health Insurance Companies

Health insurance companies provide in-depth orientation. This work generally includes less direct care. It can include venipuncture and data collection related to a physical exam by visiting a client's home, a wellness nurse or health coach, or managing a workman's compensation case.

Travel Nursing

Travel nursing can be an exciting way to experience many different types of care settings in various geographic locations. The cost of the nurse's lodging is generally provided.

To learn about travel nursing, using a computer and any search engine, type in "travel nurse" or "travel nursing career." Research licensure requirements and the state's NPA to work within your legal responsibilities.

Veterinary Clinics and Hospitals

This is an opportunity to combine a love of nursing with a love of animals. In some states you may work as a veterinarian assistant in the care and treatment of animals. Other states, such as California, require a special training program and a passing grade in a state test to assist veterinarians.

Pharmaceutical/Medical Equipment Sales

Usually a role more likely for a BSN-prepared RN, some pharmaceutical and medical device companies may select LPNs/LVNs to work in a particular area of the company.

Forensic Nursing: Coroner's Office

Usually requiring a RN license with a BSN degree, there may be a role for you if you have an interest in this type of nursing. A former student practical nurse (SPN) working with a coroner commented, "I never saw myself as doing this, but it is so interesting. I've learned a lot about people, pain, compassion, and myself. The health care provider I work with is a born teacher and is always respectful of the person on whom he is doing the autopsy. He has helped me accept the life cycle."

Parish Nursing

Some church parishes employ their own nurse to take care of the basic health needs of the congregation. The work includes basic nursing skills such as measuring vital signs, medication education, and contacting a health care provider as needed. Health education and making healthy choices is also a focus. The LPN can work collaboratively with the RN or nurse practitioner in this role. See Chapter 11 for more information.

Staffing Agency

Staffing agencies supply nurses when requested by a health facility. Some provide temporary help exclusively for certain kinds of health facilities (e.g., long-term care). The need for help may be related to a shortage or nonavailability of nurses and need for temporary coverage. Assignments are intended to be short term, though sometimes the facility decides to hire the temporary nurse. Nurses who work for staffing agencies must be ready to "hit the floor running." Consequently, the agency rarely hires a newly licensed nurse. A nurse with at least 1 year of experience in a clinical setting is preferred. The nurse must be competent in required procedures. The staffing agency handles the contract for the health facility and for the nurse. Because of the immediate need for a nurse, the temporary agency usually pays the nurse at a higher salary than the facility nurse. A former student used this method of nursing employment to pay for CE to become an RN. The ability to grasp information quickly, good nursing process skills, and good critical-thinking skills are essential. Some staffing agencies hire nurses for other countries and states.

Less Common Employment Opportunities

Countless other possibilities for LPN/LVN employment exist. Consider the following:

- Residential treatment centers
- Medical management companies
- State, federal, or private correctional systems
- Corporate short-term or long-term disability benefit administration case manager
- Day care centers for adults and children
- Weight loss clinics
- Social service agencies
- Entertainment complexes (i.e., amusement park)
- Ambulance and emergency medicine staff
- Dentist office
- Blood bank
- Substance abuse clinics
- Welfare and religious organization
- Specialized mobile units (e.g., bloodmobile)
- Fitness centers
- VISTA (Volunteers in Service to America) or the Peace Corps
- School nurse
- Industrial/occupational health
- Camp nursing
- Your own other areas of interest. Dare to apply!

Try This

Area Job Opportunities

Investigate nursing job opportunities in your area. Add ideas to the listed job choices.

PREPARATION FOR EMPLOYMENT—BUILDING YOUR RESOURCES

HELPFUL PERSONAL ATTRIBUTES

LPNs/LVNs must be caring, empathetic (not sympathetic), and have a genuine concern for the welfare of their clients. Emotional stability is essential because work with sick and injured clients can be stressful. You also need keen observational, critical-thinking, and decision-making skills and be able to communicate at a client's level to be understood. A comfort level in doing basic nursing skills is absolute. If you have been taught advanced skills, compliant with the state board's scope of practice for LPNs, then perfect them. The condition of a client may quickly change from stable to acute, and you will have to respond to the situation without panic.

- LPNs/LVNs work as part of a team and are accountable for their own actions while working under supervision of an RN or health care provider.
- Assertiveness and client advocacy are other important attributes.
- Confidentiality is a must because the LPN/LVN will often hear or see things that cannot be discussed with someone outside of the immediate area.
- The LPN/LVN must also find healthy ways to relieve stress at the end of the shift that will not contribute to his or her personal health problems.

Try This

Personal Skills and Characteristics

Name some additional nursing skills and personal characteristics you have that enhance your ability to work in an area that currently appeals to you.

INTERPERSONAL STYLES

Tony Beshara (2008) suggests that by recognizing your personality type and that of your interviewer, it may be easier to answer questions as well as pose your own. With that, it was noted that in 370 BC, Hippocrates defined four basic personality types:

1. The *analytical* type is highly detail oriented, can make difficult decisions without all the facts, is perceptive, and may tend to be pessimistic.
2. The *driver* type tends to be blunt, is objective focused, is a hard worker, makes quick decisions, is independent, and is considered a can-do person. There is a tendency to be assertive, distrusting, impatient, high energy, and motivated by external recognition.
3. The *amiable* type likes to be liked, is easy going, and is not a big risk taker. They like to blend in, are highly sensitive, have difficulty making firm decisions, and can be quiet and soft-spoken.
4. The *expressive* type is a natural salesperson and storyteller. This type is gregarious, a good motivator, tends to exaggerate, leaves out facts and details, and is relationship oriented.

An easier way to remember the four types is to associate them with characters from Charles Schultz's *Peanuts* comic strip: Linus, who is the analytical type; Lucy, who is the driver type; Charlie Brown, who is the amiable type; and Snoopy, who is the expressive type (Personality Types, 2011).

Being able to recognize different personality types around you is a plus. It is recommended that you practice this identification skill with other students and friends, so that recognizing personality type comes quickly to you. Some examples of conversation responses to individuals with these types of **interpersonal styles** can be found in Box 18.2.

POTENTIAL REFERENCES

Take a moment to consider who has seen you work and might be willing to confirm in writing and verbally that you are someone employers should hire. Instructors, unit managers, supervisors, team leaders, staff RNs, and LPNs/LVNs are potential sources of references and job opportunities. Ask the person for permission to use their name as a reference. Do not assume an instructor or anyone will give you a positive reference. Specifically ask, "May I list your name for a positive reference?" If yes, write down the nurse's name (spelled correctly), job title, work address, and work telephone number. Take the initiative to ask for a letter of recommendation. Be sure to acknowledge their busy schedule and ask if they'd prefer you to draft a possible letter for their use (Boxes 18.3 and 18.4). Also consider using managers and employees with whom you have worked as a volunteer or health care worker. Lastly, clients and families can also serve as references, especially if you were a consistent caregiver.

NETWORKING YOUR WAY TO SUCCESS

Networking with influential people can lead to finding new jobs, better pay, faster promotions, and greater job satisfaction (Fig. 18.1).

- **Placement personnel** are good sources to find job opportunities. Register with your school's career service center (if available) and local or state Career/Job Workforce Centers Plan to attend job fairs or professional association conferences. Talk to clinical facility nurse recruiters, learn about job opportunities, provide your resume, and obtain their business cards. Visit your local employment center and use free services such as job-seeking workshop series and access to job postings. This can augment services received at your school and strengthen your ability to secure a first job. Many states have a website that

Box 18.2 Responding to Individuals Through the Four Major Interpersonal Styles

Analytical type: Tell me how the client is. (Speak rapidly and to the point about the client's status.)
Driver type: How is your day going? (Speak slowly and deliberately, hitting the highlights of the shift.)
Amiable type: How are we doing today? (Start off with small talk, such as, "The day has been going good," and then go on to highlights of the shift. If there is a problem, present it to them with a solution and ask if they agree.)
Expressive type: Did Mr. Jones get his dinner yet? (Start off with small talk and leave an opening in the conversation for her to fill, such as, "Yeah, but I don't think he was so happy about the peas on his plate.")

Box 18.3 Sample Letter to Reference Writer

May 12, 2025
Ms. Valerie George
Surgical Care Charge Nurse
Veterans Hospital
1000 Veterans Lane
Minneapolis, MN 55402

Dear Ms. George,

Thank you again for agreeing to be a work reference. My experiences on the medical-surgical unit were both challenging and rewarding. I am pleased to have the opportunity to use the skills you taught me.

I am actively seeking employment in medical-surgical units at hospitals within the metro area. A letter of recommendation from you is an asset to my job search.

Knowing your busy schedule, I have enclosed a draft letter of recommendation for your review, edit, and signature. However, if you prefer to write your own letter, per your observation, you may wish to mention my ability to work under pressure, ability to administer medication on time, communication skills with staff and clients, computer proficiency, and willingness to take on new assignments. Your assistance in helping me secure employment is greatly appreciated. I plan to give you a call next week to let you know how my job search is going and answer any questions you may have regarding the letter. I look forward to talking with you soon.

Cordially,
Katelyn Bieser

2001 Putt Drive
Cottage Grove, MN 55016
612-555-2728 or ktbieser@star.com
ENC: Reference letter

Box 18.4 Sample Letter for Reference Writer to Complete and Place on Facility Letterhead

Dear Employer:

Please accept this as a letter of recommendation for Ms. Katelyn Bieser, whom I supervised during her medical-surgical rotation. Katelyn was enjoyable to work with and displayed a high degree of skill as a student practical nurse.

Specifically, she learned new tasks quickly, measured client vital signs accurately, was proficient in computer charting, provided nutritional care, and administered medication safely and promptly. Ms. Bieser was able to follow both health care provider orders and RN instructions and had a keen sense of knowing when to ask for help.

I believe that Katelyn will make a positive contribution as an employee. Should you have further questions about Katelyn's skills and abilities as a nursing professional, please feel free to contact me.

Cordially,
Valerie George, RN
Surgical Care Charge Nurse

lists current job postings by specific county or city location. PA Career Link is an example (https://www.pacareerlink.pa.gov/jponline/).

- **Family and friends with nursing contacts**. Ask anyone you know for job leads and contact names. Follow up with the contact every 2 weeks until you get the job. And remember to thank these people for their help once you get it! You never know if you might need their help in the future.
- **Social media**. Your presence on social media creates your own personal brand. For example: What passion/interest do you pursue? Who do you chat with? What groups do you join? Social media is now an essential job-seeking tool. Be careful to post appropriately to reflect your professionalism and quality of character. Stories abound about individuals who have had successful job interviews, only to lose their opportunity when the employer saw what was on their personal web page or social network site. Discussions about partying, recreational drug use, religion, and views about certain classes of people or past employers should be avoided. Once you have a job, this is not the time to relax and feel you can post anything you'd like. Often teachers are highlighted in the news for being fired for posting negative comments about their students and community members on social media (i.e., Facebook). Never forget that others, not just true friends, are reading and developing opinions about what you've written for the world to see. Always act as a professional! NCSBN (2024) provides guidance in their publication *A Nurse's Guide to the Use of Social Media* (www.ncsbn.org).
- **Professional Social Media**. LinkedIn (www.linkedin.com) is a professional social media site that can help you find mentors, stay in touch with favorite teachers, and find hiring managers and recruiters in your chosen career. Some people refer to LinkedIn as Facebook with a tie. The advantage of LinkedIn is that it allows you to look at others' networks and reach out to them for suggestions and recommendations. The goal is to make a second connection in hopes that this may be a person with hiring authority. LinkedIn has more than 1.2 billion members (about.linkedin.com, 2025) from 200 countries. It is considered the must-have tool for ambitious professionals, whether looking for a job now or in the future. Consider LinkedIn as an investment site like a 401(k) retirement plan. What you do to invest in the plan now will help you later in your career when you are looking for new, higher-paying opportunities. Consider following strategies to increase views of your LinkedIn profile. Add a profile picture; fully complete your profile; and add LPNs/LVNs, RNs, nurse managers, recruiters, other health care team members, and any contacts made through active networking with health care and insurance company staff. You may be contacted by recruiters who

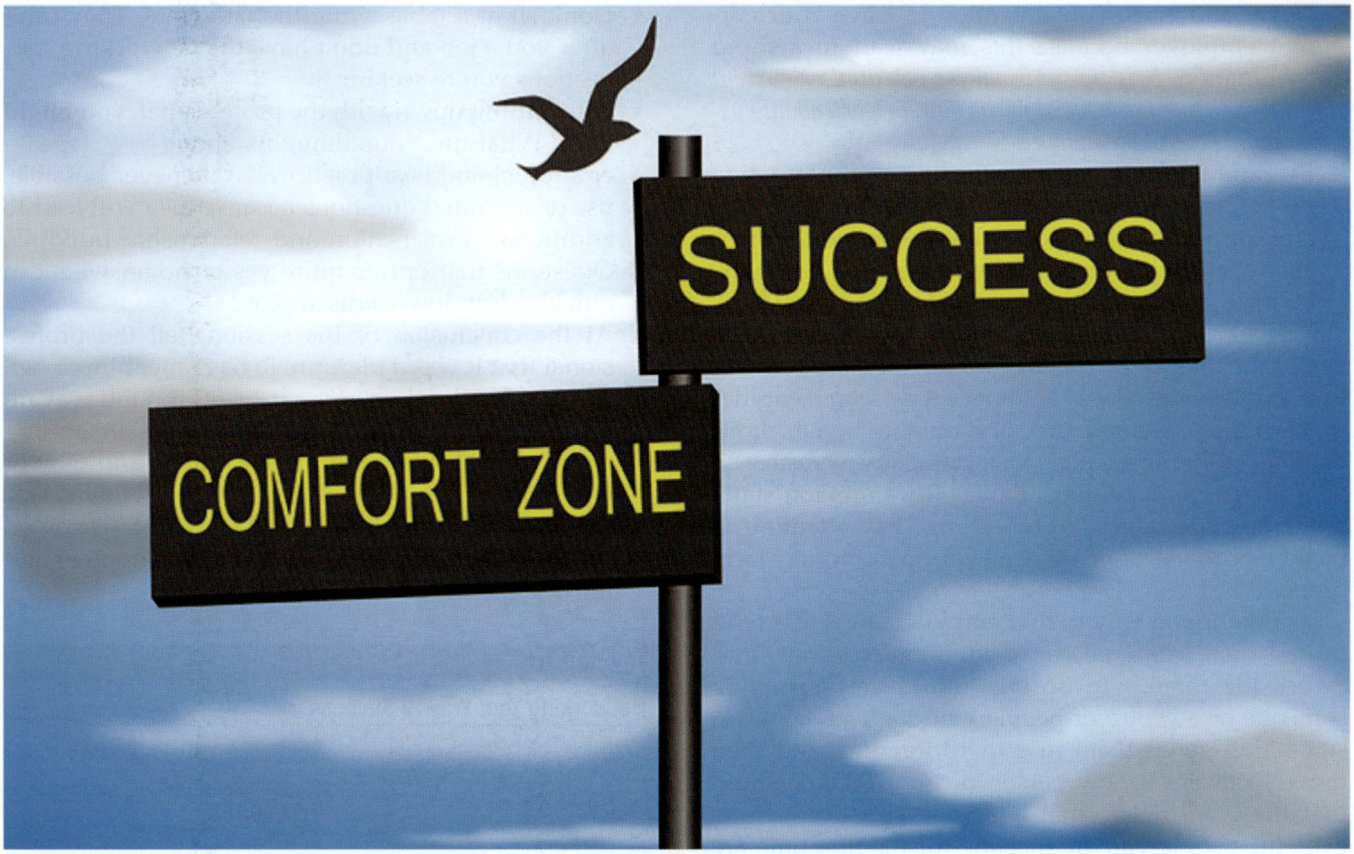

Fig. 18.1 Get out of your comfort zone to succeed in your career. (Copyright Maria Stavreva/iStock.)

use LinkedIn as part of their regular scouting for candidates. Reach out to alumni, creating a common bond and a new network.

- **Job boards**. Countless job boards exist today. Typing in "LPN," "LVN," "licensed nurse," "nurse," or "long-term care" will yield some job listings through search engines such as Simply Hired (www.simplyhired.com) or Indeed (www.indeed.com). Today, hospitals, facilities, and government agencies are increasingly using job boards. According to the Society for Human Resource Management (SHRM, 2017), 84% of companies currently recruit through social media. This continues to be a current practice. See www.shrm.org for more detail. As you search through the website, you will discover recruiters, companies, and other health care professionals. Box 18.5 lists multiple job board websites.
- **X** (formerly Twitter) (x.com) and **Facebook** (www.facebook.com) can be used to expand your job search network. For an X profile, list basic information because your online "biography" is limited to 160 characters. X will load your address book and show you which of your contacts are using the site. X will give you the option of inviting people in your address book who are not yet registered to join X. Through Facebook you can access the Simply Hired (www.simplyhired.com) and CareerBuilder (www.careerbuilder.com) for job listings.

Box 18.5 Common Internet Sites for Job Sites

Job site suggestions include typing "practical nurse jobs" into your Internet search engine or visiting the following job boards: Indeed.com; careerbuilder.com; jobcentral.com; monster.com; and simplyhired.com. Other sites such as glassdoor.com can provide employment data such as average wage and information regarding employee satisfaction. This is important for salary negotiation, if you are offered the job.

Also, for a quick reference on the median wage in the state you are researching, go to www.bls.gov/oes/current/oessrcst.htm. Find the blue map of the United Stated titled "Annual Median Wage," and highlight the state. If looking for nursing statistics in Canada, check out the Canadian Nurses Association website (https://www.cna-aiic.ca/en/nursing/regulated-nursing-in-canada/nursing-statistics).

Here are some tips when using professional or social media sites:

1. Do not add your current employer/supervisor to your network of contacts.
2. Be selective about adding coworkers.
3. Add only people that you know to your "friends list."
4. Never post opinions about any of your employers.
5. Do not post any nonmainstream beliefs, hobbies, or recreational activities.
6. Never let anyone post items on your "wall."

7. Never announce your intention to leave your current employer because this may lead to a rapid termination. *It is not unusual for potential or current employers to browse social media sites to learn about current and potential employees.*
8. Be careful about extra costs: For example, using LinkedIn's "InMail" system to contact people who are not part of your network can cost you money. Try contacting these individuals via Facebook because you can do that free of charge.

Preparation is essential in your job search, even before the interview. You are looking for a job you will love and become a loyal employee. Use search engines to learn the name and URL of a nursing home, clinic, or assisted-living facility. Visit company websites to find current job openings, the facility's mission statement, any specialties, and locations. Pay attention to facility locations, depending on your plans to stay local or move.

Another good way to find employment is to attend professional conferences or training sessions and "work the room." To do this, introduce yourself to someone or a group of people you don't know, learn something about them in 5 to 10 minutes, and then move to the next new person or group. Understand that these are not formal interview situations; however, the people you are meeting for the first time are "sizing you up," just as you are doing to them. Wear clothing you would wear to an interview. Ask for business cards, and send a follow-up e-mail. Thank them for the conversation and request that they keep you in mind for future job opportunities. Your e-mail may arrive just as they have received two resignations and a medical leave of absence. Great timing can result in a quick hire!

Professional Pointer

First impressions count, and you may be talking with the person who does the hiring, has the boss's ear, or knows of job openings.

Here are some more tips for job hunting:

- Don't bring your "significant other" to the conference. Conscientiously or not, he or she will impose on your time during and after the session. You want to be able to focus on the people you are talking to.
- Plan to arrive early, obtain your name badge, and ask the registration people to point out the key representatives conducting the conference. These individuals may know who may be hiring.
- Strike up conversations with the key representatives. If not available, look for individuals who are professionally dressed. A good way to start a conversation is saying, "Hi, I am___ [your first name]. Are you part of the conference?" and/or "What part of the session are you attending/attended?" As people sit down for the conference, ask if you might join them.
- Don't sit at a table with other students. They can't offer you a job and don't have the networking connections you're seeking.
- After sitting down with the professional, you might ask, "What are your thoughts about_____ [speaker's topic] and best practices?" Whenever possible, use open-ended questions because they will lead to additional conversation and relationship building. Questions that only require yes or no answers can quickly shut down a discussion.
- At the conclusion of the session, tell the professional that it was a pleasure to have met him or her. Request his/her business card, and if none is available, ask where he/she works. If you are feeling brave, ask, "Is it a good place to work, and why or why not?" Then be prepared to listen. Finally, ask, "Would it be okay to call you at work to check on job openings?" If yes, ask for the phone number and the best time to call.

Try This

Networking Your Way to Success

Who are potential individuals I haven't yet contacted? List them in the spaces provided.

NAME	TELEPHONE
______________________	______________________
______________________	______________________
______________________	______________________

Voice control is important as you will be judged on how you sound to others on the telephone and at the interview. It is important to understand that spoken English is broken down into five areas:

- *Low-pitched:* Can sound more mature and truthful
- *Nasal:* Can grate on the listener's ears
- *Monotone:* Can sound boring or disinterested and puts people to sleep
- *Loud:* Can be viewed as dynamic or nonprofessional
- *Whiny:* Can imply a lack of self-confidence—annoying to the receiver

Networking should be a never-ending process whether you are happily employed or looking for employment. The successful person makes a goal to meet someone new each day, always planning for the future for continuing your career path. Always look for opportunities to increase earnings, advance positions, and develop professionally. Identify potential mentors. These mentors can be formal, by asking them directly to be your mentor, or indirectly, someone you watch as they develop their career path. In your professional and personal lives you will have countless mentors with unique skill sets. Seek out mentors and willingly mentor others by focusing on the following:

- Display a positive attitude with everyone you meet (i.e., facility staff, clients and their families, technical vendors, professionals at conferences, etc.).

- Seek the input of your supervisor and other experienced LPNs/LVNs and RNs about how to build your career. Ask them to be your mentor.
- Try to build relationships with key people where you work.
- Be willing to lend a hand **without** being asked. Mentor others.
- Ask about facility committees to join.
- Join professional and community organizations; members often know about job openings before they are posted.

INFORMATIONAL INTERVIEWS TO CREATE FUTURE EXPECTATIONS

OBJECTIVES AND INTERVIEW STRATEGIES

When on a clinical assignment at community health facilities, complete the learning objectives given by your instructor. Additionally, focus your own job exploration objectives to include:

- Mission
- Days/hours of operation; types of employee shifts
- Staffing patterns
- Facility specialty
- The identities of the training staff and their expertise
- Newest technologies being used
- LPN/LVN job assignments and duties

Viewing this clinical assignment also as an information interview allows you to find out how the facility works firsthand, assists you in determining whether you would want to work there, and allows you to meet the employer before you actually seek a job.

If you want to talk to a person in a leadership role, practice with another individual before making that telephone call. It may be tempting to use the example script without practicing in advance, but if you do, remember that this is exactly how you will sound: as though you are reading a script! The following is an example of a telephone request:

1. "Hello, my name is__________ [first and last name]."
2. "Who is the manager for the______ [specialty floor or area you are interested in]?" (Emphasis is on first learning the name of the right person. Do *not* begin by asking, "May I speak to the manager for_____?") You can also try to bypass human resources and talk directly to the decision-maker (i.e., long-term care nurse manager).
3. "Please connect me with Mr./Ms.__________."
4. "Hello, Mr./Ms.__________. My name is __________ [first and last name]."
5. "I am a student practical/vocational nurse at [school's name]."
6. "As a part of my learning experience, I would like to visit your facility and meet with you."
7. "Would it be possible to set up an information interview tomorrow at ______ [give several time options]?"
   - *If the answer is yes:* "Great! I'll see you on__________ [day]. Thank you!"
   - *If the answer is no:* "Is there someone else you can recommend that I contact there for follow up?"

Your friends can help you gain control over your voice by modulating with you, or you can find voice self-help books and/or companies that can help you speak more clearly and pleasantly.

Try This

Practicing and Getting a Critique of Mock Interviews

With a peer, make a digital recording of you making information interview requests, using the telephone script in this chapter. Ask them to play the part of the employer on the other end of the telephone line. Then, debrief with your peer. Evaluate the ease with which you present yourself, how your voice sounds, and the pitch and fluency of your speech. Listen to the recording while they give you feedback. Continue to practice with them until your voice sounds right with minimal effort on your part.

You should not encounter any difficulties when you speak directly to senior nursing management to request an information interview. Management wants to "get the word out" about their facility and will often give tours and let you meet the training staff. However, do not make the mistake of turning this into a job interview. No one likes to be tricked, and management tends to have a long memory about such things. Respect that they are extremely busy people and be very flexible with your time and understanding if they need to cancel. Reschedule as soon as possible.

Arrive looking sharp! This is not a T-shirt, shorts, jeans, and sandals casual meeting. Wearing your uniform is acceptable if you are coming directly from a clinical rotation. However, share this information immediately, making it clear that you are not here on a clinical rotation. Consider the interview as an opportunity to get insider information about what employers are looking for in potential employees. Keep a copy of the information you obtained with the name, address, and phone number in a safe place (ask for their business card) for the time when your job search begins. Creating a file on your computer or phone will ensure you can retrieve this information in the near future. Follow up the information interview with a thank you letter and mention the staff you met by name. Employers will sometimes share letters like this with their staff, which will bring a smile to their face. Who knows; this may gain you allies should you apply for a job there (Box 18.6).

SEARCHING FOR EMPLOYMENT OPENINGS

If you expect to work shortly after graduation, apply for employment approximately 2 months before that date. Use your cell phone or a landline messaging system so you do not miss any calls from potential employers. Be sure your voicemail is not full and is

Box 18.6 Follow-Up Letter After Informational Interview

January 22, 2026

Ms. Elizabeth Ekholm
Director of Nursing
Lyngblomsten Health Care Facilities
1415 Almond Avenue
St. Paul, MN 55118

Re: Informational Interview

Dear Ms. Ekholm:

Thank you so much for meeting with me yesterday. The information you provided was both valuable and interesting. I found that the variety of programs offered was progressive and individualized to meet the needs of the resident and their families. The tour that followed supported your comments about the positive interactions between staff and clients. I was pleased to have the opportunity to meet staff trainers Ms. Abbinante and Ms. Wexler, who certainly inspire confidence.

Your suggestions about strategies to improve my competitiveness through certification were appreciated. I have already registered for an applicable preparation course. Thanks for your time. This visit confirmed my hope to be fortunate enough to work at such a center after my graduation this June.

Sincerely yours,
Katelyn Bieser

2001 Putt Drive
Cottage Grove, MN 55016
612-555-2728 or ktbieser@star.com

able to accept messages. Record a professional-sounding message, such as the following:

> *"Hi, this is___________ [first name], and I am not available right now. Please leave your name, telephone number, and the reason for your call. I will return your call as soon as possible." (Be sure you have caller ID enabled on your phone.)*

LPN/LVN employers are often familiar with the unusual graduating times of LPN/LVN programs; however, it can become confusing to them. Share this information frequently, during casual conversation throughout the last level/semester of your classes. Employers have immediate unexpected needs and are also planning staffing patterns for the fiscal new year. Be responsive to both situations.

Do your homework in preparation for seeking employment. Learn about the facility where you would like to work. Facilities have websites and may have information pamphlets. Look for the facility's "mission statement"; determine the number of people they employ and annual profits earned.

Use the Internet to search for news stories/releases so you can work current events into your interview and talk about how your skills relate. A good site is www.healthcarefinancenews.com, which addresses health care business issues of interest to employers. If considering a move to another community, research the local chamber of commerce and economic development organizations. If applying to a specialty health care setting, visit related associations websites.

Not all available jobs are advertised. Do not wait for an ad to appear before seeking employment. Here are some ways to tap the "**hidden job market**":

- Get assistance from family and friends.
- Get employee/staff recommendations from your school's clinical site(s).
- Submit direct applications to employers.
- Do internal job searches. For example, depending on your skills, you could obtain less-skilled employment with a health care provider in a different job that would allow you to post for jobs internally before they are released to the public. Jobs might include sterile service technician (process/package surgical instruments), CNA, and health care coder (ICD-10). Search company websites, using terms such as "careers," "employment," and "jobs."
- Use State Job Service/Workforce Centers.
- Use Internet job sites (i.e., Careerbuilder.com, Indeed.com).
- Find out about your school's social alumni network sites, or if they don't have one, try X.com or Facebook to see who may be alumni and contact them by asking a school-related question (i.e., "What dorm did you live in the first year?" or "Was instructor_____ there when you were there, and what did you think about her class?").
- Use private employment or recruiter companies (i.e., type "practical nurse recruiters" into your search engine).
- Search state or federal government websites.
- Read school placement office postings/e-newsletters.
- Do volunteer work and read professional association newsletters.
- Contact the state's nurses' union and ask about employers who are hiring.
- Use recruiting services. The three types of staffing services are temporary or contract, in which employees work for a specified period of time; temp-to-hire, which allows employees to work with an employer on a trial basis, and if it is a "good fit," they may be offered a permanent job; and direct hire, where the employee is recruited by a staffing service and then hired by the client. Determine which service will best meet your needs.
- Job fairs are typically advertised 2 to 3 weeks before the event. Visit the companies' websites to learn about the companies. Forward your resume to the fair producers both before and after the event. The producers frequently forward resumes to participating employers at no cost to you. If you attend a job fair, go prepared with a high-energy, **30-second pitch or elevator speech** that covers your key skills, your passion for that type of work, and how it's related to the needs and goals of the recruiter's company. Because most applicants don't have a

prepared speech, your presentation will make you stand out.

- Participate in virtual job fairs by searching the internet. Beware of scam job ads. If it looks too good to be true—it probably is! People's eagerness to find any job until the right one comes along sometimes overrules their common sense. Avoid these jobs if they try to convince you to pay money or send money to an address prior to being hired, ask for personal information such as bank account/credit card information, or promise access to federal or state jobs for a fee or promises of high salaries for "simple" work. You may become a victim of identity theft. See the Federal Trade Commission website for more details: https://www.ftc.gov/about-ftc/bureaus-offices/bureau-consumer-protection/our-divisions/division-privacy-and-identity. It is standard practice to apply directly to employers using website job applications, e-mails, or cover letters and **resumes**. Often, a traditional brief, to-the-point cover letter, accompanied by a resume addressed to the director of nursing or nursing recruiter at the facility is best. Box 18.7 provides an example cover letter. Do not include a personal reference list or a photograph of yourself with it. Retain the reference list for your interview and provide it on request.

It is best to use Sundays and Mondays to research job opportunities and then contact employers from Tuesday forward. Try to call employers to schedule interviews or make follow-up contacts after 9 am. This gives them time upon arrival to plan their days and review e-mails. As a rule, most employers don't have the luxury of contacting every prospective job candidate, owing to time constraints and demands of their own jobs. Candidates who are waiting to hear from employers should not hold their breath or be disappointed when employers do not call.

Once you identify an applicable job posting, follow the directions provided, which can include e-mailing or uploading a cover letter and resume, completing an online application, reporting to an open interview session, or calling for an interview. Don't forget that many other people are also reading the job posting. The candidate who hesitates is lost. If you call the employer, your conversation needs to reflect the following example:

1. "Hello, my name is____________ [first and last name]."
2. "Can you share the name of the person in charge of hiring?"
3. "May I please speak with Ms.____________?"
4. "Hello, Ms.______________. My name is__________________ [first and last name]."
5. "Do you have any practical/vocational nursing positions open now or projected in the near future?"
   a. *If hiring:* "Would it be possible to set up an interview on . . . (give a choice of two upcoming dates and time) [pause for a moment]" *If no:* "What would be a better time and date? [Offered time and date.] Great! I will see you then."
   b. If they are not hiring or are under a hiring freeze, catch your breath and don't be put off. An acceptable reply then would be:
      - "Oh, I hadn't heard that. Your facility sounds like a great place to work. Would it be possible to meet with you anyway? I would like to be the first person you consider when an opening occurs or the freeze ends." *If yes*, see 5a. *If no:* "Do you know of anyone who might be hiring?"
      - *If yes*: "Would you also know the contact person and/or have a telephone number?"
      - *If no:* "I appreciate your time. Thank you." Or *if no:* "Thank you for trying. Would it be possible for me to come in for an informational interview?" *If yes*, see 5a. *If no:* "Well, thank you again. Good-bye."

Deflect the employer's interview type of questions until the actual interview. Often when employers do not have an opening, they feel it is kinder to applicants to ask some questions and then tell the applicant that he/she is not what they are looking for. Also, you do not want to be "washed out" by a telephone conversation if the employer does have a job.

Box 18.7 Sample Cover Letter for Employment

April 14, 2026
Cheryl Krutchen
Human Resources Director
Columbus Hospital & Clinics
2031 Lakeside Drive
Columbus, MN 55025

Re: LPN Staff Nurse Position

Dear Ms. Krutchen:

I will graduate from the Rainy Lakes Technical College practical nursing program this June. While completing a medical nursing clinical rotation at your hospital, I was impressed by the quality of client care, staff professionalism, and learning opportunities.

In addition to this rotation, my work experiences have included a focus on electronic client documentation, care coordination using a multidisciplinary approach, follow-through on individualized client/family plans, working with a diverse population, client advocacy, and participation in the evaluation process toward achievement of client and institutional outcomes.

I am interested in obtaining employment at your hospital and being able to work with your staff again. I will contact you on Tuesday, April 21 to see whether you have received my resume and to determine when we might arrange an interview. Should you wish to contact me before then, I can be reached weekdays after 3:30 pm. I look forward to speaking with you.

Cordially,
Katelyn Bieser

2001 Putt Drive

Cottage Grove, MN 55016
612-555-2728 or ktbieser@star.com

If the employer begins to ask you questions about your background, education, or work experience, you might respond, "I have completed an accredited practical/vocational nursing program, passed the NCLEX-PN® examination, obtained my license, and have the necessary work experience. I would like the opportunity to discuss my qualifications during our interview." The tone of your voice can make a significant difference on the telephone. If you smile while you are talking, you will project a positive tone. Consider looking at a picture that will make you smile. Practice the preceding format several times in advance with a friend so there are no hesitations in your presentation and you're prepared for the challenging questions.

Leaving a Voicemail Message

At some point you may have to leave a phone message for the employer. Here is a script you can practice beforehand:

> *"Ms./Mr.____, my name is_____, and I am calling about a licensed practical nurse position. I have strong clinical and interpersonal skills and am willing to work all shifts. I would like to meet with you and can be reached at______ [phone number]. Again, this is_____ [name] at________ [phone number]. I look forward to talking with you."*

APPLYING FOR A JOB—JOB APPLICATION, COVER LETTER, RESUME

REFERENCES: A TIMELESS TREASURE

Prospective employers will be more interested in certain types of work references than others. There is a **reference hierarchy** of individuals who act as references. References ranging from most to least important are current or former nursing instructors, clinical staff from your clinical rotations, and supervisors from past nursing-related work or volunteer experiences; past employers or supervisors from non–nursing-related jobs; and personal references or friends. (Employers rarely contact personal references because their opinions are likely to be biased.)

Try This

Pick Your References

List the people in your reference hierarchy, including the person's name, job title, work address, and telephone number. Most employers request three references. Pick and choose from your list of resources for maximum impression.

The statement "References available on request" does not need to be placed on your resume. Letters of recommendation (preferred) or a reference list should be given to the interviewer if requested, so bring them to the interview. References, however, are a "treasure." Avoid requesting references unless you are interested in a job. People's time is a valuable commodity. Do not abuse their willingness to help and/or mentor you.

RESUMES: THE CONTRIBUTIONS YOU WILL MAKE

Developing two versions of your resume is a must! First is the traditional *design-focused* document you mail and bring with you to the interview. The second is a scannable or *text-focused* resume, which is good for Internet applications and pasting onto e-mail.

Your resume is a painting of your life. Remember that a painting generally uses broad strokes to create an impression. This is your goal. Resumes are not a confession or "tell-all" script, nor should they include reasons for leaving past jobs, salary requirements, or personal photographs. Additionally, listing personal data, such as marital status, race, religion, height, weight, number or age of children, and other demographic/personal characteristics, is discouraged. Resumes can look different based on the professional discipline. A nursing resume looks very different than graphic designer's resume.

Resumes should include a "Summary" or "Profile" (keyword focus) section. Use short, bulleted sentences of no more than two to four words, which allow employers to compare resume key words to their job description. Remember that "white space" is your friend. An employer decides whether to interview in the first few minutes of reading a resume. Plan to modify your resume to contain the key words from the ads you apply to. This will enhance your chances of being contacted for an interview.

Essentially, all resumes have a format of heading, profile/summary, work and military experience, education, and licenses/professional memberships. With respect to the heading, list your e-mail address so employers can reach you any time of the day or night. Consider setting up a separate e-mail account when job searching. This account will be a time saver and ensures that you will not lose e-mails in your regular personal e-mail account.

It is recommended that you stop and think about what specific classes or jobs you have performed and record them in your resume. Spell out the job tasks, and do not assume an employer will understand a statement like "Performed nursing duties." It is recommended that military/work experience be listed in years. Do not list more than 10 years of work history, outdated training (i.e., 2019 CPR certification), or old versions of computer programs (i.e., Windows 2003). In addition, avoid listing job tasks that are very routine for the position. For example: If you were a nursing assistant, do not include a task such as bathing the client, but do include if you were responsible for obtaining vital signs or you mentored new staff.

Remember that your resume must be truthful. Human resource departments will look for inconsistencies such as work experiences that are too good to be true or resumes that appear purposely vague. Keep your resume consistent and well balanced. Communicate in your accompanying cover letter why there are gaps in employment, particularly when there is a logical explanation (i.e., child rearing or training).

Statements on "personal goals" or "health" are a waste of both time and valuable space on your resume. Many traditional resumes are never read because they are too cluttered, too wordy, or contain the aforementioned problems. The initial impression made by the resume is very important. Box 18.8 lists some basic factors to consider for scannable/personal and traditional resumes. Fig. 18.2 shows sample resumes.

COVER LETTERS: TAILORED TO FIT THE JOB YOU WANT

Try This

Cover Letters

Why do cover letters need to be sent in with resumes?

Include a cover letter with each resume, regardless of method of submission. Cover letters have three main components: an introduction, a short list of relevant work that highlights one or two positions or accomplishments, and a conclusion (Schrager, 2021). The cover letter should highlight unique skills that make you a good candidate for the job. It should also demonstrate that you have read about the position and the organization. Neatness, conciseness, correct spelling, and proper grammar are mandatory. The cover letter should be one page, an original, should be error free, and typed in block letter format. Address any specific experience listed in the job posting, even if the experiences are not listed on the resume. The cover letter should not be repetitive; however, it should highlight critical information from your resume. Each cover letter is unique to the specific job posting. Use key words from the job posting in your cover letter to highlight how you align with the job requirements.

Consider referring to a prior telephone conversation, including the name of the person who referred you. If the employer is located out of town, briefly discuss plans to relocate with a request to interview for the job virtually.

Box 18.8 Basic Resume Factors

SCANNABLE/ELECTRONIC/E-MAIL RESUME FACTORS

For a scannable resume, you do not want visual distractions to confuse the OCR (optical character recognition) scanner that reads the resume. As noted previously, a text-focused format is required when completing/submitting online applications or faxing your resume:

- **Length:** Two pages maximum; one page is preferred.
- **Paper:** *Quality bond*. Use colors such as white or off-white only (no designs, textures, or recycled paper). Use matching paper for the cover letter and envelope.
- **Type:** Arial or Times New Roman typeface (10- to 14-point type) is preferred; underlining, italics, or graphics should generally be omitted. Bolding is permitted. Avoid multiple columns, newspaper-style layouts, landscape printing, and designer fonts. Always place your name at the top of the page because scanners assume that whatever is at the top of the page is your name. As such, if your resume has a second page, place your name and a "page 2" designation at the top.
- **Spellcheck:** Use the computer's spellcheck feature and then proofread the resume from the bottom up so there are no extra marks or spelling or grammatical errors.
- **Printing:** If you don't have a computer, borrow a friend's or go to the library. Type the resume and save it onto a USB stick, which is inexpensive and fits in your pocket. For printing, use a laser printer, which is less likely to smudge, or take your USB stick to a quick print shop. Avoid standard copy machines because they often provide poor-quality copies.
- **Faxes (limited use):** Avoid faxing your resume unless it's specifically requested because faxing degrades the text; this would not be a common request
- **E-mails:** If asked to e-mail your resume as a nonattachment, use the scannable resume. Simply copy and paste it into an e-mail to the employer. However, before sending it to the employer, send a copy to yourself first to see what the recipient will see and then decide if you can use it or need to go with another option of getting the resume to the employer. An attachment generally preserves formatting.
- **Balanced space:** An uncluttered, balanced design is desirable, so the resume is easy to read. Also, because most managers don't have time to read, a "bulleted" style is recommended when listing your job skills and past duties.
- **Emphasis:** Whether you have a strong or limited work history, keep in mind that your use of key words will help answer the employer's question, "What can you do for me?"

TRADITIONAL RESUME FACTORS

- **Length:** Two pages maximum; one page is preferred.
- **Paper:** *Quality bond*. Use colors such as white or off-white only (no designs, textures, or recycled paper). Use matching paper for the cover letter and envelope.
- **Type:** Arial or Times New Roman typeface (10- to 14-point type) is preferred. Underlining, italics, graphics, and bolding can be used to draw the reader's eyes to points being made. Different resume formats may be used, with conservative design recommended. Multiple columns and newspaper-style layouts are permitted. Make a practice of using your computer's spellcheck feature, and then proofread the resume from the bottom up so there are no extra marks or spelling or grammatical errors. For printing, use a laser printer, or take your thumb drive to a quick print shop. Avoid standard copy machines because they provide poor-quality copies.
- **Faxes:** If specifically requested to fax your resume, use the scannable one (uncommon).
- **E-mails:** Use a scannable resume instead or send your traditional resume via US mail (snail mail).
- **Balanced space:** Use an uncluttered, balanced design with a "bulleted" list of job skills.
- **Emphasis:** Whether you have a strong or limited work history, key words are important.

If sending your resume via e-mail, it is recommended that you "paste" your resume to the end of the electronic cover letter and send out as a whole unit rather than an attachment. Box 18.9 shows sample cover letters to employers through an unsolicited telephone call and Internet advertisement.

Try This

Resume

Develop a resume and include a cover letter.

Access resources on the Internet and Microsoft Word to assist you in writing a resume.

Microsoft Word has a template that can be used found by clicking on file, new from template and resume (may vary based on version of Microsoft Word). A simple or block resume is appropriate.

Helpful Internet resources: www.resumehelp.com, https://www.myperfectresume.com/

Purdue Owl: https://owl.purdue.edu/owl/

ANSWERS TO APPLICATION QUESTIONS

You complete an application either before or after an interview. Answer the questions truthfully. If you have had three or more jobs in the past 3 years, the employer will be concerned and expect an explanation for the change in jobs. Reasons for leaving might include work interfered with school, a layoff, a relocation, career exploration, and no potential for job growth. Employment gaps might be explained by responses such as laid off, job hunting, returned to school, or family responsibilities.

If there are questions you wish to defer until the face-to-face interview, write "N/A" (for not applicable) or "Will discuss," or leave the space blank. However, do this sparingly. One such area might include expected wage and wages from former jobs. For current wage expected, write "Open" or "Prevailing wage"; do not specify a dollar amount. With wages in former employment, leave the spaces blank if you know you were underpaid, or tell the truth if the wage was fair. Be factual—not emotional.

Katelyn Bieser
2012 Putt Drive
Cottage Grove, MN 55301
Phone: (651) 555-2728
E-mail: ktbieser@star.com

SUMMARY OF QUALIFICATIONS

Cardiac-oriented Licensed Practical Nurse with rudimentary Spanish who is patient oriented, has working knowledge of sterile techniques, possesses strong clinical judgment, and is hardworking. Available night shift.

EXPERIENCE

St. Michael Hospital– Minneapolis, MN
Cardiac Unit – Practical Nurse School Rotation (Spring 2016)
- Worked with interdisciplinary health care team including patients, physicians, nursing staff, patient families, and social workers.
- Performed basic data collection, utilized time management, and infection control.
- Medication administration, measured vital signs, quality assurance, and charting.
- Patient/family education, positive attitude, and positive learning attitude.

Forest View Nursing Home – Hastings, MN
Certified Nursing Assistant (2014 – present)
- Served on memory unit, health care intervention, and provided direct patient care.
- Promoted daily living skills, resident feeding/hygiene, and room sanitizing.
- Measured/charted vital signs, worked with staff of 10, monitored patients with confusion.
- Positive family interactions, assisted with patient turning/lifting, and duties as assigned.

The Small Town Café– Bloomington, MN
Waitress (2012 – 2014)
- Strong focus on customer service, promotion of specials, and cashiering.
- Grew café customer base by 20%, participated in marketing strategies, and assisted with food preparation so food served hot.
- Worked full time, including holidays, and welcomed customers by name.

LICENSE/CERTIFICATION

State of Minnesota Board of Nursing – LPN License (2016 to present)
American Red Cross - CPR Certification (2011 to present)
Hmong Cultural Awareness Class – School District 916 (Spring 2014)

EDUCATION

Rainy Lakes Technical College – Practical Nursing Diploma

A

Fig. 18.2 **(A)** Sample typed resume scannable/electronic plain text/fax.

Katelyn Bieser
2012 Putt Drive, Cottage Grove, MN 55301 (651) 555-2728 • ktbieser@star.com

PROFESSIONAL SUMMARY

Key Strengths

• Cardiac-oriented LPN	• Rudimentary Spanish	• Patient oriented
• Sterile Tech knowledge	• Strong clinical judgment	• Available night shift
• Willing to move	• Quality assurance	• Hardworking

PROFESSIONAL EXPERIENCE

St. Michael Hospital, Minneapolis, MN
Spring 2016
PN School Rotation; Cardiac Unit

• Interdisciplinary H.C. Team	• Basic data collection
• Time management	• Facilitated Sterile Tech's
• Medication administration	• Vital sign measurement
• Quality assurance	• Patient/family education
• Charted data	• Positive attitude
• Solicited Sup. feedback	• Assisted staff as needed

Forest View Nursing Home, Hastings, MN June 2012 – present
Certified Nursing Assistant; Memory Unit

• Health care intervention	• Direct patient care
• Resident feeding/hygiene	• Promoted ADLs
• Charted vital signs	• Room sanitization
• Coordinated with 10 staff	• Monitored patient activity
• Positive communications	• Patient turning/lifting, etc.
• Duties as assigned	

The Small Town Café, Bloomington, MN May 2010 – May 2012
Waitress; Full Time

• Active customer service	• Promotion of specials
• 20% Sales increase	• Cashiering/Inventory
• Time mgmt./memory dev.	• Assisted food preparation
• Worked holidays, etc.	• Cleaned restaurant
• Duties as assigned	

LICENSE/CERTIFICATION

State of Minnesota Board of Nursing, St. Paul, MN 2014 to present
Practical Nursing
License (LPN)

American Red Cross, St. Paul, MN 2011 to present
Cardiopulmonary Resuscitation
Certification

School District 916, White Bear Lake, MN Spring 2014
Hmong Cultural Awareness Class

EDUCATION

Rainy Lakes Technical College, International Falls, MN Diploma
Practical Nursing 2014

B

Fig. 18.2 cont'd **(B)** Sample typed traditional resume.

If applying via the Internet, several companies use software job application programs that are set to reject applicants if all the requested data are not provided. Some job experts recommend listing a midrange salary to position you to get the interview. Lying or falsifying information on any application is typically grounds for termination. Be aware that you do not have to answer questions about age, religion, marital status, children, physical data (unless they are specific requirements for the job), or workers' compensation injuries. However, recognize the risk in refusing to answer questions either on the application or during an interview. An employer's eyes will naturally gravitate toward any blank spaces. Therefore answer every question, even if it does not apply to you (i.e., for military experience, write "N/A" in the space if you did not serve). Some employers view blanks or "Will explain" as an automatic screen for someone they do not want to employ.

Box 18.9A Sample Cover Letter: Unsolicited Telephone Call

August 12, 2026

Ms. Jana Williams, RN
Director of Nursing
St. Helen General Hospital
8354 177th Lane
St. Paul, MN 55084

Re: LPN Staff Nurse Position

Dear Ms. Williams:

Thank you for taking the time to speak with me about the Practical Nurse position. As we discussed, I believe that my clinical work experiences and skills are a good match for the job.

In addition to two-plus years of Nursing Assistant experience, my education, job skills, and abilities also include direct client care, electronic charting of observations, verbal/written communications, strong interpersonal skills, being safety oriented, advocating client/family rights, and the ability to perform efficiently and effectively during emergencies.

I will contact you on Tuesday, August 18 to see if you have had an opportunity to review my resume and to determine when an interview may be arranged. I look forward to speaking with you soon.

Cordially,
Katelyn Bieser

2001 Putt Drive
Cottage Grove, MN 55016
612-555-2728 or ktbieser@star.com

ENC: Resume

Box 18.9B Cover Letter: Internet Ad Response With No Contact Person Listed

Please accept my resume as application for the Licensed Practical Nurse position advertised on Careerbuilder.com. I believe that my work experiences through the Rainy Lakes Technical College nursing program and clinical rotation at St. Michael Hospital are a good match for the position.

As a recent graduate, I will be taking my NCLEX-PN® examination on September 27. My clinical work experiences include a focus on electronic client documentation, care coordination under a multidisciplinary approach, follow-through on individualized client/family care plans, working with a diverse population, client advocacy, and participation in the evaluation process toward achievement of outcomes. Additionally, I have worked as a Certified Nursing Assistant, which honed a positive attitude when working with seniors.

I will contact your company on Tuesday, August 18 to confirm receipt of my resume and to determine when an interview may be arranged. I look forward to speaking with you soon.

Katelyn Bieser
612-555-2728 or ktbieser@star.com

Box 18.10 Sample Answers to Illegal Questions

HAVE YOU BEEN HOSPITALIZED WITHIN THE PAST 5 YEARS?
Answer: I do not have any health problems that would interfere with fulfilling the described position.

HAVE YOU EVER BEEN ON WORKERS' COMPENSATION?
Answer: N/A (not applicable) [Or] I am able to perform all of the described job duties.

DO YOU HAVE A CRIMINAL RECORD?
Answer: Be honest and factual. I have received a speeding ticket, but I have never been convicted of any misdemeanors or felonies. [Or] I have paid for that error in judgment, taken special classes, and am now wise enough not to repeat it. It was a misdemeanor when I was a young adult.

Should you choose to answer **illegal questions**, the examples in Box 18.10 will be helpful. The personnel department may contact your references, schools, former employers, licensing board, and others to verify the information on your job application and resume. The application is a legal document. The resume is your own painting, your own creation.

Try This

Job Application

Using the suggestions in the text, fill out a practice job application for a nursing position.

THE INTERVIEW

PREPARING FOR THE INTERVIEW

During an interview, you should also be interviewing the potential employer. It is important to find a "great first fit" job (Box 18.11). As Steve Jobs stated, "The only way to do great work is to love what you do." Invest time in finding this great first fit! If you have prepared adequately, you will be able to evaluate whether your job skills, physical abilities, and interests match the objectives of the facility. Bring a copy of your traditional resume; LPN/LVN license (if you have passed the NCLEX-PN® examination); current cardiopulmonary resuscitation (CPR) card; certification certificates; medical records documenting tuberculosis skin tests and hepatitis B and tetanus vaccinations; and letters of recommendation and/or awards received. Collecting these in a portfolio (can use a new three-ring binder) is always impressive.

If the interview is virtual, look into the camera to simulate looking into the interviewer's eyes. For those who have difficulty looking into a camera, tape a picture of someone onto the computer monitor to look at, at the same level as the camera. It will be as though you are speaking directly to the person and focusing on what is being said. Skype (www.skype.com),

Box 18.11 Sample Questions to Ask the Interviewer

Use four or five of the following questions:

- Can you explain the scheduling process?
- What types of clients will I work with?
- How big is the facility, and how many beds are in the unit?
- What is the nurse-to-client ratio?
- Do you have 8-, 10-, or 12-hour shifts?
- Will I be routinely floated to other units? If so, will I receive orientation?
- What type of electronic charting system is used?
- How long does orientation last, and what can I expect? Is there an opportunity to extend the orientation if needed? Do you have a nurse residency program for new graduates?
- Do you provide support or mentoring for new hires?
- In the last year, how often is overtime available or mandated?
- Is there a weekend commitment?
- Is competency testing required before going to the floors?
- Is this a new position, or am I replacing someone? If new, why was this position added?

If an existing position, why did they leave?

- Will I be required to do any on-call duty? If so, how often?
- Given my interests in the ___ unit, when is it possible to move there if an opening occurs?
- Are there annual or review-based bonuses available?
- What can you tell me about the culture and environment here?
- What opportunities does the facility offer for career development?
- Tell me about your background and why you joined this organization.
- What were the results from the last Department of Health or Accreditation survey? What actions needed to be taken? When is the next one scheduled?

Zoom (https://zoom.us), and Teams (https://teams.microsoft.com) are common virtual meeting computer software used in conjunction with a webcam. They are useful tools for interviewing when travel or associated costs are not practical to meet with the employer. Create an account so you are prepared if this type of interview is used. It is used often in the first round of interviews to save time and money for all participants.

Interviews are stressful not only for you but also for employers. They have to fit interviews into their regular work duties, justify why one job candidate should be hired rather than another, and be on constant guard not to discriminate in matters of age, gender, race, and so on. Knowing that there are concerns on both sides (yours and the interviewer's) will help you be less defensive and answer in an honest and reassuring way.

Part of your responsibility is to help the interviewer become comfortable with you and be convincing as to why you should be selected for the job. There are ways to manage cultural differences and age when encountered in an interview (Box 18.12).

Box 18.12 Tips for Handling Differences Between the Interviewer and You

Job seekers near or over the age of 50 may be vulnerable in interviews unless they adopt a vital, energetic, and positive approach. If the interviewer is younger than you and slights your age through a question, then a response like "I'm in excellent health, and as you can see by my resume, I have a solid work history and am not afraid to learn new things" would be appropriate. If the employer representative is older than you, an appropriate response is "I have always been surrounded by workers older than myself, which has taught me to work hard, listen, and collaborate with the team."

With respect to cultural background, when there are differences between you and the interviewer, you need to remember that different groups have different norms concerning eye contact, the loudness of your voice, personal distance, body language, joking/teasing, divulging too much information, and other subtle aspects of communication such as the use of metaphors, proverbs, and colloquialisms.

It is recommended you follow the interviewer's lead in the course of communication. Additionally, you can never go wrong by being polite, and if you are unclear about what was said, say, "Excuse me, I'm not quite following what you're asking. Could you ask it in another way?"

Also remember the need to be computer literate.

INTERVIEW QUESTIONS AND ANSWERS: A CHALLENGING OPPORTUNITY

Often the first interview question, "Tell me a little bit about yourself," is an icebreaker designed to make you comfortable and determine what is important to you. Take advantage of the question. Be positive and energetic, and speak briefly about your education, accomplishments, and life hurdles you have overcome. Maintain eye contact and remember to relax and smile. Do not talk about illegal job application questions, your dysfunctional family, the bad day you had because of a fight with your significant other, or why nursing can be stressful.

Prepare for your interview by practicing sample responses to typical interview questions (Box 18.13). Role-play with another person in the role of the interviewer. For better preparation, ask the person to mix up the order of the questions. Have them include so-called illegal questions. This will prepare you to handle these questions effectively and make you appear confident when the actual interview occurs.

By being prepared, you will not fall victim to the interviewer's most powerful tool: **silence**. Candidates will usually try to fill the void of silence by providing more information (often revealing details beyond their prepared answers) than they should. If this should happen to you, smile at the interviewer and wait for the next question. An example of "too much information" is:

Question: Why did you leave your last job?

Answer: As you know, I am a recent graduate and am looking for employment in my field of study, *and I have never done anything before but work as a babysitter*. (The italicized portion constitutes "too much information.")

Box 18.13 Sample Interview Questions and Answers

TELL ME ABOUT YOURSELF

Answer: Would you like to know about my work history or personal life? *If work history*, discuss your passion to help care for and treat people. Then provide a brief description of your education, past jobs, and goals to work as a staff/long-term care (or whatever) LPN. *For personal*, you might say, I have lived in this area all my life, (or) my plans are to make this area my home. I recently graduated from (your school name) and am looking for a career in which I can grow and advance.

HAVE YOU EVER DONE THIS TYPE OF WORK BEFORE?

Answer: Yes, in fact some of my experiences include direct client care during clinical rotations, volunteer work as a hospital volunteer, experiences as a mother, and ....

WHY DO YOU WANT TO WORK HERE?

Answer: Your company has an excellent reputation in the community and has job opportunities that align with my training. Additionally, this company's mission statement of______ reflects my views on______.

WHAT MOTIVATES YOU?

As a nurse I am motivated by work and its challenge of my skills on a daily basis. I know with the right employer, I will continue to learn new skills as nursing changes. (Consider giving an example of a recent achievement.)

WHY DID YOU LEAVE YOUR LAST JOB?

Answer: As you know, I am a recent graduate and am looking for employment in my field of study. *Note:* If you have worked as an LPN/LVN: I am looking for a new position to expand my work skills, keep the job interesting, and provide more opportunities for advancement.

TELL ME ABOUT YOUR LAST EMPLOYER

Answer: I really enjoyed my work at______, which has an excellent reputation for______. I learned______. However, now it is time to move on to new opportunities.

WHAT HAVE YOU DONE TO KEEP YOUR CLINICAL SKILLS CURRENT?

Answer: Well, in addition to participating in several clinical rotations during school, I recently joined the______ (LPN professional organization) to keep abreast of new developments in nursing.

HOW DO YOU COMPARE YOUR VERBAL SKILLS WITH YOUR WRITING SKILLS?

Answer: Organizations are more dependent than ever on their employees' communicating well both verbally and in writing. I am constantly taking advantage of opportunities to develop in both areas by asking for feedback and then putting the suggestions into practice.

WHY SHOULD I HIRE YOU INSTEAD OF SOMEONE ELSE?

Answer: I think my references can best answer that question. I am sure when you contact them they will agree I am hardworking and dependable and get the job done correctly. In addition, I am flexible, adaptable, and work well with a team.

WHEN ARE YOU AVAILABLE FOR WORK?

Answer: Right away. [Or] I would need to give my employer 2 weeks' notice. It will provide me time to tie up loose ends and give my employer time to find a replacement. *Note:* If the interviewer insists you terminate your job immediately, you are witnessing a power play. You need to ask yourself if you really want to work for this individual. This could be the tip of the iceberg for future power plays.

HOW IS YOUR HEALTH? ARE THERE ANY PARTS OF THE JOB YOU CAN'T PERFORM?

Answer: I have always been in good health. I see myself being able to perform all parts. I think the best approach to any job is to use common sense. If I need help, I am not afraid to ask for it.

WHAT ARE YOUR GREATEST STRENGTHS?

Answer: I would have to say that my strengths include (1)______, (2)______, (3)______, (4)______, and (5)______. *Note:* Your responses should be consistent with what your references say about you.

WHAT IS YOUR GREATEST WEAKNESS?

Answer: As you know, everyone has weaknesses. My greatest weakness right now is my "driven" personality. It has certainly assisted me in getting the job done efficiently and effectively. However, at times, some colleagues will request that we slow down and have a break. I have learned to assess and carefully listen to the team to avoid "burnout."

WHAT ARE YOUR LONG-TERM GOALS?

Answer: Eventually, I would like to work as a Charge Nurse at this facility. My goal is to learn all I can. This will help me develop skills to manage and lead a team, ultimately contributing to the mission of the institution, to advance the health of the residents.

HAS AN EMPLOYER EVER FIRED YOU?

Answer: Before going to nursing school and getting my priorities straight, an employer fired me for attendance problems. It was a valuable lesson that I learned from and will never repeat. My attendance was excellent in nursing school. I only missed one day due to illness. *Note:* Do not start your response with "Yes"; address the issue.

HOW DO YOU APPROACH DOING THINGS THAT YOU DON'T LIKE TO DO?

Answer: I tell myself, "Let's get it done, and done right." There is nothing worse than having to go back and redo work that was done incorrectly the first time.

CAN YOU WORK UNDER PRESSURE?

Answer: Yes, I have experienced working under pressure for many years. This has meant meeting deadlines, dealing with challenging people, and developing employer confidence that the job will be done right.

WILL CHILD CARE BE AN ISSUE?

Answer: No, I have found a good day care setting for my children. If they cannot go to day care, I have worked out a system of alternating days with another provider or relative to take care of them so that work is minimally affected. *Note:* Although some individuals believe this is an illegal question, it is important for the employer to anticipate any staffing issues. A stable staffing pattern is needed to maintain quality client care.

WOULD YOU BE WILLING TO WORK OVERTIME?

Answer: Yes, if it will help the unit. I am sure your requests of your staff are reasonable focused on client safety.

Box 18.13 Sample Interview Questions and Answers—cont'd

MAY WE CONTACT YOUR CURRENT EMPLOYER?
Answer: Yes, but only after a firm job offer has been made. I would appreciate it if before you contact my employer you will allow me to talk with my supervisor first as a courtesy.

AREN'T YOU OVERQUALIFIED FOR THIS JOB?
Answer: I may be more qualified than other individuals you are considering, but this simply means that I will be able to make an immediate contribution. After learning your system, I hope to be eligible for advancement opportunities within the organization.

IS YOUR SPOUSE EMPLOYED? WILL THERE BE A CONFLICT?
Answer: Yes, my spouse has a job. No, I do not see that there would be a conflict. We are both looking forward to my working for you.

WHAT KIND OF SALARY OR WAGE DO YOU EXPECT?
Answer: What would a person with my background and qualifications typically earn in this position with your company? [Or] I am ready to consider your best offer. *Note:* If an employer insists you give a wage quote, give a range using your bottom dollar and a realistic top wage.

Answer: I would think we could agree on a salary between $00.00 per hour and $00.00 per hour. (Note that an hourly wage, not an annual salary, is stated.)

Salary resources include the Internet and labor market sites through your local Job Service/Workforce Centers. Right now, you can use the average median wage because you are new to the profession. Visit the following site for more details: www.glassdoor.com/Salaries/licensed-practical-nurse-salary-SRCH_KO0,24.htm. For an idea about the national average median wage, check www.bls.gov or your local state workforce web site

DO YOU HAVE ANY QUESTIONS?
Answer: See Box 18.11 for questions to ask the interviewer. After your questions, ask if it would be possible to take a tour of the facility and meet a staff member.

HOW DO YOU MANAGE CRITICISM? DESCRIBE A TIME YOU WERE CRITICIZED FOR POOR PERFORMANCE
Answer: A person who does not make mistakes will never grow. Most recently, in school, I had problems with time management. Because of this, I did not do very well on a couple of tests, and my teachers let me know they were disappointed because I had not done my best work. I agreed they were right and asked for assistance. One of my teachers then showed me how to improve my time management so the problem would not happen again. And it didn't.

HOW DO YOU VENT ANGER OR FRUSTRATION IF YOUR DAY HAS BEEN CHALLENGING OR STRESSFUL?
Answer: I am a walker and a talker. My first choice is to burn off the stress by walking/biking/going to the gym/whatever. I always feel better after exercising. If that is not available, I will go outside on my break alone or with one trusted peer and talk out the problem and associated emotion. It is amazing what talking for 10 minutes will do for getting perspective back. Of course, I would not violate Health Insurance Portability and Accountability Act (HIPAA) and respect the rights of all team members.

DO YOU HAVE A VALID DRIVER'S LICENSE?
Answer: I will use the city bus system to get to work. If the buses aren't running, there is always a taxicab/Uber/Lyft available, plus I have a network of friends who can help me in a pinch. I have never been late to work.

IS THERE ANY TIME WHEN IT IS OKAY TO BREAK COMPANY RULES?
Answer: Yes, if someone's life is in danger or if there is a natural disaster. Even in these cases I would collaborate with the RN or health care provider, if possible, to confirm my decision-making.

HOW DO YOU HANDLE CHANGE?
Answer: It is all about attitude! If you go in with the thought that the proposed change will help you do your job better and improve client care, it is easy to embrace it. I also know that creating champions can work. I would try to identify a nurse aide who could be a champion for the proposed change.

ILLEGAL QUESTIONS/RESPONSES
You do not have to answer these questions. However, it is recommended that you have considered a response, if asked.

WHAT RELIGIOUS FAITH ARE YOU?
Answer: Religion certainly is a part of this great country of ours, but I prefer to separate religion from work. (You can still choose to state your religion.)

THAT'S A NICE NAME. IS IT JEWISH/MUSLIM/IRISH/OTHER NATIONALITY?
Answer: America is a melting pot. That is why it is the greatest country on earth. I feel we are all Americans first and foremost, and that's the most important issue here. Don't you agree?

HAVE YOU EVER BEEN TESTED FOR HIV?
Answer: No, I have never had a reason to test for HIV, nor do I anticipate a reason to do so.

[MALE NURSE] THE SUPERVISOR IS JANET SMITH, WHO, ALTHOUGH BEING VERY GOOD, IS ALSO VERY TOUGH AND CAN'T SEEM TO KEEP MALE STAFF ON HER UNIT. WHY DO YOU THINK YOU WOULD BE DIFFERENT?
Answer: First off, I work well with both male and female bosses. They, like me, have a job to do, want it done right, and want to go home at the end of the day feeling like something was accomplished. So, if there is a better or faster way to accomplish job tasks and to communicate with everyone, it is her job to see that it is done that way.

CLIENTS AND THEIR FAMILIES CAN BE PRETTY MEAN. ARE YOU SENSITIVE ABOUT YOUR WEIGHT?
Answer: In my younger days, it was a problem, but now I like who I am and the profession I have chosen. Insults are like emptying bedpans. You flush them away and move on. I'm healthy and agile—ready to do this job well!

TELL ME A PERSONAL OR WORK STORY ABOUT SOMETHING THAT WENT WRONG AND WHAT YOU DID ABOUT IT
Answer: Years ago, a friend of mine was celebrating her birthday on a weeknight at one of the local bars. There were folks there I had not seen in a long time, which meant staying longer to get caught up with them. The next thing I knew, it was 3:00 am, and I had to be at work by 8:00 am. Needless to say, I was pretty tired and useless that day at work. Never again did I stay out excessively late on a work night. It just was not worth it and can be unsafe.

Continued

Box 18.13 Sample Interview Questions and Answers—cont'd

IT'S YOUR LUNCH BREAK, AND YOU SEE A RESIDENT FALL. WHAT WOULD YOU DO?

Answer: I would stop eating, notify another staff member to let the charge nurse know, and then assist the resident as needed. Like CPR, we want help on the way in case the fall is more serious.

PLEASE DISCUSS HOW YOU HANDLED A SITUATION WHEN AN IRATE HEALTH CARE PROVIDER, COWORKER, CLIENT, OR CLIENT'S FAMILY MEMBER WAS INVOLVED

Answer: There was a day at the nursing home when we were short-staffed, had a new resident moving in, and had to remove the belongings of one who had recently passed away. An out-of-town daughter of one resident turned on the call light and began yelling in the hallway that her father needed a drink of water. Upon entering the room, the daughter continued to yell about how her father was being neglected and that she would be making a complaint to the state.

The first thing I did was smile and thank her, in a quiet voice, for letting us know that her father needed assistance. I then went to her father, poured him a glass of water, and asked him how he was doing. When she began to yell again I asked her to lower her voice, so I could hear what her father had to say. This was repeated twice more until her voice level dropped. After it was determined that her father was fine and in no distress, I smiled and asked the daughter her name and then introduced myself. Calling the daughter by name, I let her know that her father's care was very important to us, as were all the residents at the facility whose families expected the same. Also, at this point, I reminded her that in the future, if she needed assistance in a similar situation to come to the nurse's station and to ask for me rather than to yell down the hallway, which upsets the other residents. She agreed to this, and I then left, letting her know that I needed to care for some other residents and would be back in one hour to check on her father. Following this, I updated my supervisor about the incident.

Also, never be afraid to ask the interviewer to repeat the question or clarify the question. This is a critical approach to ensure you understand the intent of the interviewer.

MAKING A LASTING IMPRESSION

Try This

Impression Counts

The kind of person you are is an additional concern to the interviewer. The impression you make includes everything that has been previously discussed plus your appearance and habits during the interview.

PERSONAL HYGIENE

- Good hygiene is essential the day of the interview.
- Make sure your hair is clean, dry, and arranged in a moderate style.
- Age can be a hidden bias. Methods to give a more youthful appearance may be helpful but should not be extreme.
- Men's hair, mustaches, and beards should be neatly trimmed.
- Keep nails short, clean, and conservatively manicured, with clear nail polish. Research has identified long fingernails and fake nails as sites for infection, which subjected some health facilities to litigation.
- If you are a smoker, remove yellow finger stains. A dilute solution with bleach and water may help.
- Use an unscented or very lightly scented deodorant.
- Brush your teeth, tongue, and palate, and floss. Do not consume any food, candy, or drink with a heavy, unpleasant odor or that will stain your teeth or tongue near THE time of the interview. Use breath fresheners before you walk into the building. Do not chew gum.
- It is best to use lightly scented or no scent aftershave or perfume. Don't sprinkle fragrance on your clothing.
- Smell your clothes; don't go into an interview smelling like you have come from a smoke-filled bar.

CLOTHING

Interview clothing should be conservative. You will always look your best in conservative clothes that are clean and ironed, with polished shoes. Go to thrift stores and consignment shops to find a suit/dress/outfit that fits you well; they are resources waiting to be discovered. Additionally, check out www.dressforsuccess.org or research the web using "clothes closet" for possible sources. When selecting clothing, consider the following points:

Men: Wear a long-sleeved white dress shirt, a solid or pinstripe navy blue or gray suit, and a conservative tie. Wear dark-colored shoes, "long" dark socks, and a belt that matches the color of your shoes. A jacket may not be necessary, but dress pants are essential. Cargo pants and jeans are not dress pants.

Women: Choose solid or conservative prints in black, navy, gray, or blue dresses, suits, or a skirt and appropriate blouse or pantsuit. Look for simple, straight, or pleated skirts that reach at least knee level and are comfortable to sit in. (Save short skirts for other occasions.) If wearing a dark skirt or suit, consider wearing a white, off-white, or light blue cotton or silk blouse with a conservative neckline and buttons. For women with prominent cleavage, a camisole under the blouse is recommended to keep the focus on your face. No visible cleavage is acceptable for an interview. Wear dark, polished, low to moderate heeled shoes with primarily closed toes.

MAKEUP

Conservative makeup is always appropriate. Wearing too much makeup is a common mistake; try to keep it at a minimum. Remember: It is the confidence you display in the interview that makes you an attractive hire to the interviewer.

ACCESSORIES

Wear simple jewelry or none at all. Simple necklaces such as a single strand of pearls, colored beads, or a silver or gold chain work well. Avoid large drop, dangle, or chandelier-type earrings and noisy charm bracelets that clank. Remove any piercings in the nose, tongue, or lips, and cover tattoos, particularly based on the culture of the institution. Also, limit yourself to a small portfolio that is large enough to hold any papers, resumes, and so on. If you have a coat or umbrella, leave it in the car or politely ask where you can hang or lay it. The main point is to avoid holding items or balancing them on your lap. The fewer distractions, the calmer and more focused you will be on the interview.

EYEWEAR

If you usually wear eyewear, do not wear the latest craze in eyeglasses because they will only serve to distract the interviewer. Wear contact lenses or glasses that contrast the shape of your face and do not make a "statement."

POSTURE

Walk tall, and sit erect in the middle of the chair. Both feet should rest on the floor, and your head should be upright. Arms and hands should be in an open position and not crossed. (Remember, you have nothing to hide.) Keep your hands inactive, or if you habitually fidget, consider bringing a paper clip to hold in your hands during the interview. Some people may even need to slightly sit on their hands to prevent fidgeting.

MANNER

Your manner should be assured. Do not interrupt the interviewer or rush the interview. Pause to think as needed, and then answer without hesitating. Ask for an explanation or repetition of any questions you do not understand. Eye contact is essential, especially when answering questions. If you are uncomfortable with making eye contact, two techniques can be used to correct this: look at the person's nose, or look at the space between the interviewer's eyebrows. Both techniques give the illusion of eye contact. Remember to look away periodically so you do not appear to be staring. Avoid making negative statements about your school, former bosses, jobs, current finances, and personal problems. No one likes a whiner! Be positive!

COURTESY

Arrive for the interview 5 minutes early and remember to **shut off your cell phone** or leave it in the car; don't switch it to mute/vibrate because the interviewer may still be able to hear it. When the employer enters the room, stand, smile, and extend your hand for a firm handshake. Do not use a limp, "dead fish" handshake or "bone-crusher" grip. To get the handshake right, find someone to practice with before the interview. Additionally, if your palms tend to sweat, slide your hands along the top of your thighs, toward your knees, when standing up. It will remove the moisture while appearing very natural.

With a handshake, say, "Hi, Mr. [Ms.] Smith, I am_____ [your name]. I'm pleased to meet you." Wait until you are asked to be seated. If this does not occur, ask if you may be seated. When the interview is over, stand up, look the person in the eyes, and offer your hand for a firm handshake. Address the employer by surname: "Mr. [Ms.] Smith, thank you for the opportunity to interview with you. I am very interested in the job. Would it be all right if I call you next week to learn if you have made a decision?" If you want the job, give the employer your work references or letters of recommendation. Last, ask the interviewer for his or her business card. The card will help you when sending your thank you letter (e.g., correct title, name, etc.).

HABITS

Make it a habit to go to bed early the night before so there are no dark circles under your eyes and you appear more energetic. Wear under eye concealer if needed. Upon arriving at the interview location, do not chew gum while in the waiting room or during the interview. Also, do not smoke outside the building and then come in for the interview. Although the nicotine may make you feel calmer, you will be bringing in the fresh smell of smoke, which is often offensive to nonsmokers. Politely refuse an offer of a beverage. In addition, do not attempt to read any materials on the employer's desk or computer screen.

DISCUSSING PREGNANCY ISSUES

? Critical Thinking

Pregnancy

If you are pregnant, what do you need to consider before discussing it with an employer? When should you tell a new employer that you are pregnant? When should you discuss the pregnancy so it doesn't interfere with career advancement?

Even if the Pregnancy Discrimination Act and/or Family and Medical Leave Act will protect your job (FMLA applies if the company has 50 or more employees), pregnancy can lead to some tough questions. Consider disclosing your pregnancy when it is noticeable, before being asked.

Be prepared to discuss how long you plan to work, how long you intend to be on leave, and possibly how your work will be covered while you are away. Consider sharing your plan A and B for childcare. Although this is not necessary, this proactive approach can be viewed positively.

Try This

Mock Interview

Enlist a peer to practice traditional and virtual webcam interviews (if planning to move). Take turns in the role of a nurse seeking a job and the employer. Practice asking and answering anticipated questions for an interview. Use the suggestions in this chapter, including appropriate dress and behavior, and stage a mock interview. Have a friend record the interview on their smartphone or on the practice virtual interview. Review the interview and ask your peers to evaluate your performance. Keep an open mind to any criticism given because the goal is to refine your techniques and get a job.

PREEMPLOYMENT PHYSICAL EXAMINATION, DRUG SCREENING, AND BACKGROUND CHECKS

More employers are requiring preemployment physical examinations as part of conditional job offers. A **conditional job offer** states that you have been offered the job contingent on your passing a physical examination, drug screening/urine analysis, and/or background check. If you fail, the job offer is withdrawn.

PHYSICAL EXAMINATION

Do not be surprised if you are required to meet with an employer-specified health care provider who will perform an examination and can legally ask you about your past medical history. Think about any past surgeries, workers' compensation injuries, allergies, and family history, including cancer and heart trouble. Be prepared to provide the dates of these occurrences and the names of the health care providers who provided treatment. If you have any personal concerns about the answers your health care provider might provide, call the health care provider before the preemployment physical examination to discuss the prospective job and obtain their opinion.

DRUG SCREENING

If you are taking medications, be sure to notify the prospective employer before the screening, although they may state that the outside vendor performing the tests will be your point of contact. You will want to reaffirm in the employer's mind that your health care provider prescribed the medication and its effects will not interfere with your work. You may need to provide a copy of your prescription to the employer testing vendor as verification. This is often called a medical officer review. Once the medical officer reviews your prescriptions and ensures that they are an exact match for the substance identified, your employer should receive a negative drug screening.

Although drug screening accuracy is improving, it is not 100% accurate. Most drug screenings used by employers today are legally binding. Some false-positive drug results may occur if medical conditions such as kidney infection/disease, liver disease, or diabetes exist. Common foods such as poppy seeds, riboflavin in food (vitamin B_2 and hemp seed oil), or vitamin B_2 tablets may trigger false-positive results. False-positive reactions can occur with some prescription medications and over-the-counter medications. If you are taking a prescribed or over-the-counter medication, **call your pharmacist** and ask if the medication could trigger a positive drug result.

Do not drink excessive amounts of liquids before drug screening as this can trigger a "dilute" result. Some employers will view a second dilute as a positive drug test and will not hire you. Avoid this possibility by drinking normal volumes of fluid before your drug screening appointment. Do not overhydrate.

BACKGROUND CHECKS

According to a 2024 HR.com report, 92% of surveyed employers indicated that they use one or more types of employment background screening (SHRM, 2024). This is common in health care settings, potentially preventing strong candidates from obtaining a position. Following the issuing of your nursing license, you must notify the State Board of Nursing (SBON) if you are arrested or convicted of a crime. Visit your respective SBON website for details.

There are many state and federal laws (i.e., SBON nursing assistant requirements and/or school law) that list prohibitive offenses for employment in health care. In most cases, these requirements were also necessary to participate in clinical assignments while enrolled in nursing school. Thus there are minimal surprises when beginning your job search unless the charge and/or conviction occurred while enrolled in the nursing program and you did not disclose it. This can be viewed as a violation of school policy and could result in dismissal. It will also cause issues as you seek licensure and employment. Honesty and integrity are integral to a successful health career.

AFTER THE INTERVIEW

Following up after a job interview is essential. It is a source of amazement to employers that often people who interview never follow up to see if they got the job. Recent graduates and even nurses who have been working in the field for some time are under the **follow-up illusion** that it is the employer's responsibility to contact *them*. If you are not interested enough to follow up after the interview, why did you bother to interview in the first place?

Write a handwritten or e-mail thank you letter to the interviewer the same day you were interviewed. Write it while the information is fresh in your mind and before you become distracted by other projects. Remember, the more often the employer sees or hears your name, the better your chances are of being hired. Do not be the person left waiting for a telephone call. A thank you letter may be as simple as the one provided in Box 18.14. Be sure the letter is well written, legible, and free of grammatical and spelling errors.

Box 18.14 Letter: Thank You for the Interview

August 12, 2026

Ms. Irene Fedun, RN
Director of Nursing
St. Helen General Hospital
8354 177th Lane
St. Paul, MN 55084

Re: LPN Staff Nurse Position

Dear Ms. Fedun:

Thank you for meeting with me today to discuss the LPN staff position. After our conversation about the job duties and the tour of the hospital floor, I feel that my work experiences and education are a great match for the job. I am especially interested in working on the Memory Unit because this is a special interest of mine. Through our work together, the clients will receive timely, quality care.

I remain very interested in the position. I will contact you on Thursday, August 18 to see whether you have made a decision or whether a second interview will be arranged. I look forward to speaking with you soon.

Katelyn Bieser
2001 Putt Drive
Cottage Grove, MN 55016
612-555-2728 or ktbieser@star.com

Remember to follow up with the employer! Call the employer on the date stated in your letter. Make it a practice not to make follow-up contacts on Mondays, which are traditionally full of staff meetings, weekend concerns, staff discipline, paperwork catch-up, and other duties. The best time to make follow-up calls is after 9:00 am. The key to a successful follow-up call is to be courteous but firm with the assistant. Ask to speak with the person who interviewed you.

The following is a sample follow-up contact to an employer:

Assistant: Good morning, Human Resources [do not be surprised if no name is given].

You: Hi, I'm________ [your name]. Is Ms. George available? I am following up on our meeting.

Assistant: One minute, please. [Although the employer might be away from the office or on another line, the assistant will probably check whether he or she wants to take your call.]

Assistant: I am sorry. Ms. George is away from her desk/on another line/in a meeting. May I take a message, or would you like to leave a message on her voice mail?

You: Yes, thank you. Also, when is the best time to typically reach her?

You: [message if transferred to voicemail] Hi, Ms. George, this is______ [your name], and I am following up on our interview for the LPN staff position to see if you have made a decision. I remain very interested in the job and can be reached at_____ [telephone number]. Again, that number is____________ [say each number of the phone number slowly and clearly].

You: [If the employer takes your call] Hi, Ms. George, this is_______ [your name], and I am following up on our interview for the LPN staff position. I was wondering if you have made a decision yet? Oh, you have not. Would it be okay to call you next Tuesday to see if you have made a decision? Great! I will call you then. [Or] Oh, you've decided on someone else? Is there any other position available that my qualifications meet? [If the answer is no, add] Can you please keep me in mind if any other positions become available, and I will continue to monitor your job postings. Thank you for your time. I hope our paths cross again soon.

Try This

Thank You Letter

Compose a thank you letter after an employment interview for a nursing position.

RESIGNATION WITH STYLE

Try This

Keep the Connections

Is there a difference between "burning bridges" and "untying the connection"? What is the value of recapping your accomplishments with a resignation letter?

If you are contemplating a change in employment or career pathway, it is recommended that you work a minimum of 1 year to obtain experience and demonstrate job stability. If you have made the decision to leave your employer, leave the job with a positive reputation. Perhaps the best expression is "Untie, don't sever, the connection." You never know who may call your former employer for follow-up. The nursing community, particularly a similar setting (i.e., nursing home), is like a small town. Everyone knows everyone. This can be helpful or harmful to your career. Continually take steps to ensure it is helpful. Always leave sharing a positive message.

It is strongly recommended that you have a position secured before leaving. Many employers today have what is called **"at will" employment**. Simply put, you or the employer can terminate your employment at any time for any reason without advance notice. As such, an employer may terminate your job the day you give notice.

Some "at will" employers have personnel policies requiring that a 2-week notice be given when resigning. The policies typically indicate that if a 2o-week notice is given, the employee will be eligible for future rehire and may be eligible for a reference.

It is **resignation courtesy** to give 2 weeks' notice whether or not a policy is in place. This is a courtesy to your coworkers and to the employer so a new person might be hired and oriented before you leave.

Use a business letter format and plain paper and type the letter of resignation. Even if you are leaving because of unhappy circumstances on the job, do not vent these feelings in the letter. As mentioned before, you may need this employer as a work reference in the future. Additionally, your current supervisor may also leave in the future, and all there is to remind the employer about you is your personnel file.

Because resignation is part of your permanent record, it provides you with an opportunity to recap your accomplishments or special recognition. The employer may refer to the letter when employers with whom you are seeking employment make contact. See the sample resignation letter in Box 18.15.

Try This

Letter of Resignation

Compose a letter of resignation from a nursing position.

NATIONAL COUNCIL OF STATE BOARDS OF NURSING TRANSITION TO PRACTICE MODEL

In an effort to help new RN and LPN/LVN graduates transition to the work environment from their nursing educational programs, increase retention in their employment, and improve client outcomes, the NCSBN developed the **Transition to Practice model**. This model, similar to a **residency**, is an additional program in tandem with orientation to a clinical facility. The primary parts of the model include:

- A trained nurse (**preceptor**) to assist the new graduate apply theory to practice, develop clinical reasoning, improve safety, and decrease practice errors in the care of clients.
- Five online modules of study: communication and teamwork, client-centered care, evidence-based practice, quality improvement, and informatics.

The IOM (2010) called for the implementation and evaluation of nursing residency programs. In collaboration with 35 nursing organizations, the evidence-based Transition to Practice model was developed. Phase I took place in hospitals with RNs, Phase II was conducted in public health, home health, and nursing home settings with RNs and LPNs. Residency programs are aimed at improving nursing staff retention and creating/maintaining a safe care environment. According to American Nurses Association (2024), approximately 18% of new nurses leave a position within their first year of practice. A full description of the model and study can be found at www.ncsbn.org/transition-to-practice.htm.

In 2015, the NCSBN released results of the initial transition to practice study in hospital settings with RNs, and later in the year it released the study results of the nonhospital settings that included both RNs and LPNs/LVNs (Spector et al., 2015). The studies concluded that more evidence is required before requiring transition programs.

In researching a possible facility for employment, ask about orientation for newly licensed nurses and if they have a residency program additionally.

Try This

Transitional Practice

Investigate if health care facilities in your area have a Transition to Practice model or Residency model for new employees.

Box 18.15 Sample Resignation Letter

September 24, 2025
Ms. Silvia Hinkkanen
Director of Nursing
George County Hospital
1515 Rodeo Lane
Minneapolis, MN 55401
Dear Ms. Hinkkanen:
Please accept my resignation as Charge Nurse on Unit 3, to be effective on October 1, 2025. My association with the George County Hospital has been rewarding professionally and personally. It is satisfying to have been able to contribute to the positive reputation of client care.

I am especially pleased to have been a member of the Quality Assurance Committee, which furthered my professional growth. In addition, I remain appreciative of having been honored as "Employee of the Month."

Please accept my thanks for the support you have provided me during the past one and a half years of employment. I wish the members of this hospital the very best.

Cordially,
Katelyn Bieser, LPN
Alzheimer's Unit

STAYING SATISFIED AT YOUR JOB

You have landed your first job as an LPN/LVN. Orientation was excellent, followed by a stressful first 3 months. You were proactive in asking for extended orientation as needed, have found a mentor, and have begun to love your job. It is now 2 years later, and you feel the spark is of working there is fading. You find yourself complaining more often about your job and joining others in finding continual fault with administration, clients, and families. Strong evidence exists supporting a relationship between nursing satisfaction, nursing retention, and client outcomes. In fact, the average turnover rate is 50% for nurses in long-term care (Mission Care Collective, 2025). Knecht's (2014) qualitative study of LPNs working in six diverse long-term care settings found there are four critical job satisfaction attributes: value, growth, real connection, and empowerment. In addition, one dissatisfier was identified: working conditions. Working conditions were impacted by the availability of working equipment and the LPN's perception of an unrealistic workload fueled by staffing issues and

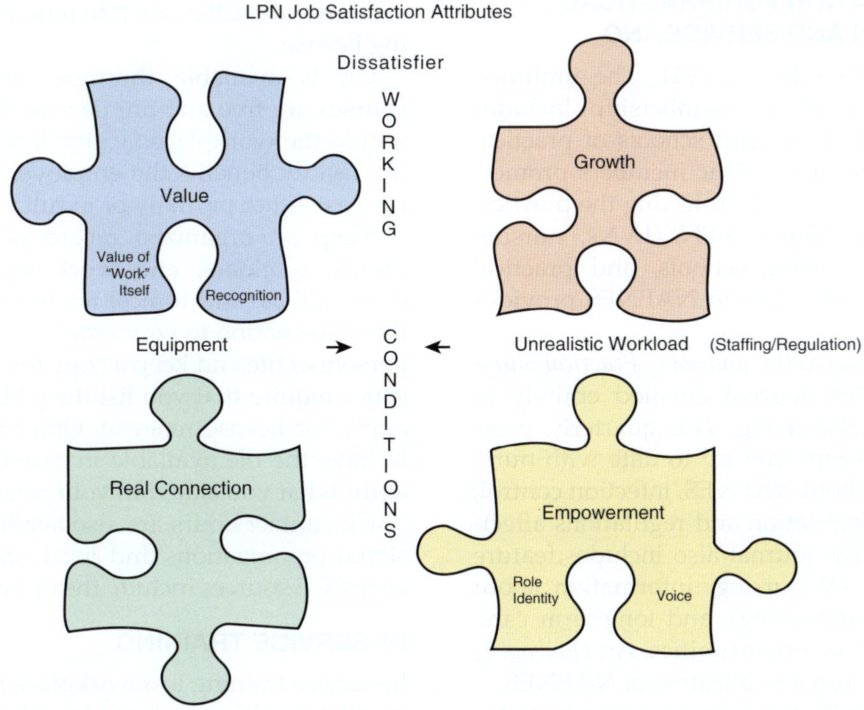

Fig. 18.3 Licensed practical nurse job satisfaction/dissatisfaction attributes in long-term care. (From Knecht P: *Demystifying job satisfaction in long-term care: The voices of licensed practical nurses [Doctoral dissertation]*, 2014, The Pennsylvania State University. Available at https://etda.libraries.psu.edu/catalog?utf8=%E2%9C%93&search_field=all_fields&q=knecht.)

regulatory demands (i.e., paperwork). It is critical for long-term care administrators and the LPN themselves to address these attributes, thus improving their job satisfaction and decreasing their job dissatisfaction (Fig. 18.3). Growth is an important attribute identified by the LPNs. A discussion follows describing professional organizations available to the LPN/LVN and nursing career pathways.

PROFESSIONAL ORGANIZATIONS

Joining and participating in at least one professional nursing organization is essential for career development. Becoming an active member permits you to have a voice in the future of nursing. It is an opportunity to meet nursing leaders, learn about current issues that affect your career, and take part in education opportunities, as well as serve on committees that influence nursing policy.

NATIONAL LEAGUE FOR NURSING

The **NLN** membership is open to all levels of nurses and is focused on meeting the particular needs of the nursing educator, ultimately advancing the health of the nation. One of the goals of the NLN is to lead in setting standards that advance excellence and innovation in nursing education. The NLN's "Excellence in Education Model" has relevance for all levels of nursing education programs, from LP/LV nursing to doctoral level nursing.

Because of changes in health care, the NLN (2010) developed a national model for nursing education that includes competencies that graduates of all levels of nursing programs should be able to meet needs of the workforce and an increasingly diverse population. The following are NLN competencies for graduates of LP/LV nursing programs:

- Promote the human dignity, integrity, self-determination, and personal growth of clients, oneself, and other members of the health care team.
- Provide a rationale for judgments used in the provision of safe, quality care and for decisions that promote the health of clients within a family context.
- Assess how one's personal strengths and values affect one's identity as a nurse and one's contributions as a member of the health care team.
- Question the basis for nursing actions, considering research, evidence, tradition, and client preferences (National League for Nursing, 2010).

In 2014, the NLN supported the importance of the role of the LPN in their vision statement, "A Vision for Recognition of the Role of the Licensed Practical/Vocational Nurses in Advancing the Nation's Health."

THE AMERICAN NURSES ASSOCIATION

The American Nurses Association (ANA) only represents RNs. Some state affiliates of the ANA allow LPNs/LVNs to join the association at the state level; however, because the LPN role is not recognized at the national level they may not have a voice or vote in the organization. The ANA does not represent LPNs/LVNs. Continued advocacy is needed to provide a unified nursing workforce.

NATIONAL ASSOCIATION FOR PRACTICAL NURSE EDUCATION AND SERVICE, INC

The **NAPNES** was founded in 1941. The multidisciplinary composition of its membership includes LPNs/LVNs, RNs, students, and schools of practical nursing, organizations, and public members promoting the ideals of NAPNES and protecting the practice, education, and regulation of LPNs/LVNs, nursing educators, practical nursing schools, and practical nursing students. Membership in NAPNES provides the following benefits:

- A year's subscription to the *Journal of Practical Nursing* (*JPN*), the oldest journal devoted entirely to practical/vocational nursing. This quarterly, peer-reviewed journal keeps you up to date with nursing articles, news about NAPNES, infection control, nursing law, and legislation and regulations affecting LPNs/LVNs. The journal also includes feature articles about LP/LV nursing, information about certification in pharmacology and long-term care, and other educational opportunities. An *eJournal of Practical Nursing*is also a publication of NAPNES.
- The NAPNES website (www.napnes.org) includes information about certifications, regulation news and updates, clinical articles, CEUs, podcasts, webinars, blogs, and jobs.
- Networking with other LPNs/LVNs through the constituent state members throughout the United States.
- The NAPNES technology department has developed a tool for making nursing updates and education on line faster and easier.
- National representation and a voice for the future of nursing.
- NAPNES Standards of Practice for LPNs/LVNs (www.napnes.org).

NATIONAL ASSOCIATION OF LICENSED PRACTICAL NURSES

The **NALPN** is the professional organization for LPNs/LVNs and practical/vocational nursing students in the United States (www.nalpn.org). NALPN, formerly the **National Federation of Licensed Practical Nurses** (**NFLPN**), was formed by LPNs/LVNs who wanted an organization to work for and speak on their behalf. NALPN is made up of LPNs/LVNs, SPNs/SVNs, and affiliate members. The NALPN has established Nursing Practice Standards for the Licensed Practical/Vocational Nurse. In addition, the NALPN Educational Foundation provides certifications for LPNs/LVNs in IV therapy and gerontology.

CONTINUING EDUCATION

Because initial licensure is questioned as reflecting continued competency, your ongoing learning (remember you are a lifelong learner) keeps you up to date and ensures continued competency as an LPN/LVN. Some states require CEU or CE to renew your practical nursing license.

CE is available through varied sources. Some courses are free and are part of continuing education within the workplace facility. If the education outside the facility benefits the employer, they often will pay the cost either partially or in full.

Keep an organized record of all in-service programs, seminars, and workshops taken (including dates, CEUs, and topics) for future reference. Submit this information to your employer to be added to your personnel file and keep a copy for your own file. Many states require that you list the CEUs earned when you apply for license renewal. Other SBONs instruct you to have the file available in case the board decides to audit what you stated in your renewal application.

CE contact hours are also available through professional organizations and local/state/national conferences. CE sources include the options discussed below.

IN-SERVICE TRAINING

In-service training in a workplace is developed to meet specific needs or state/federal facility/staff licensing regulations. Attendance at some in-service programs is mandatory, such as annual bloodborne pathogen education. Usually a specified amount of time is required for in-service programs, such as 1 hour per month or three times per year, according to the agency policy and accreditation standards. Offer suggestions for training topics to your employer. CE credits may be available depending on the credentials of the instructor and the content.

WORKSHOPS

Workshops present content and opportunities to learn new skills. Workshop length varies. Workshops can be major sources of CE credits required by many states for nursing licensure renewal. Workshops may be available through local or state Health Care Industry Partnerships at reduced costs, aimed at building a robust workforce.

CONTINUING EDUCATION UNITS

Technical schools and community colleges may provide any course you request, if enough people are available to meet the required minimum enrollment. Many of these classes provide CEUs instead of course credit. Upon satisfactory completion, you receive a certificate. Classes are often taught involving complex nursing skills such as IV therapy, physical assessment, LP/LV charge nurse (leadership/management), mental health concepts, and the nursing process for LPNs/LVNs. One of the most valuable benefits of CE classes is the opportunity to network with other working LPNs/LVNs. You discover similarities in challenges and satisfactions. Ideas are shared on how to manage difficult situations in the work place.

NALPN provides LPN/LVN certification courses in IV therapy and gerontology.

INTERNET RESOURCES

Numerous sources are available online depending on what fits your needs:

- **Podcasts**. A podcast is a digital recording of audio and video information on the Internet that can be downloaded or streamed to a portable media player (e.g., an iPod), smartphone, or a computer. The term "pod" is derived from iPod of Apple Computer, Inc., but an iPod is not necessary to listen to a podcast. The term "cast" is derived from "broadcast," as many podcasts are radio-style shows. They may/may not be commercial free, are of interest to the listener, and can be listened to when convenient. There are many online resources that provide podcasts on nursing topics. Search for these on many streaming sources such as YouTube, Spotify, and Pandora for a wide selection of podcasts. Some examples of nursing topic podcasts include *Nursing School Week by Week; Straight A Nursing: Study for nursing school exams and NCLEX®; Calling all Nurses;* and *Shift Talk*. There may or may not be a cost or subscription requirement. Remember, anyone can upload anything to the Internet. Check podcasts for relevancy and accuracy, and check with your instructors for further suggestions. A good primer to understand podcasting is "Podcasting for Beginners: How it All Works, Easily Explained" at https://www.thepodcasthost.com/planning/podcasting-for-beginners/
- **Medscape** offers latest medical news and expert perspectives and podcasts by medical experts on health care changes, new care guidelines, emerging infectious diseases, sudden disasters, and daily summaries. Medscape offers partial CE hours through their Medscape Medical News service. Although the focus is primarily for RNs, there is useful information for all nurses on a daily basis. The membership subscription is free through www.Medscape.com.

CERTIFICATION OPPORTUNITIES

Knowledge is power! Knowledge is the basis for improved nursing skills and safety in client care. Take advantage of knowledge available during certification seminars and self-study courses. In some agencies, certification is also the basis for salary increases and advancement. Enhancing your competence as a nurse increases both personal and professional satisfaction. Use the extended title you have earned and wear your pin(s) proudly. See specific certifications discussed earlier in this chapter.

NAPNES CERTIFICATION PROGRAMS

NAPNES offers **Long-Term Care Certification** (LPN CLTC or LVN CLTC), **Pharmacology Certification** (LPN NPC or LVN NPC), and IV Therapy Certification (LPN IVT or LVN IVT), all of which are available online (www.napnes.org/). Visit the website for more information. After NAPNES notifies you of successful completion of the examinations, you may use the preceding title that applies in your signature/title.

NALPN CERTIFICATION PROGRAMS

NALPN offers **National Certification in Gerontology** (LPN GC or LVN GC) and **National IV Therapy Certification** (LPN IVC or LVN IVC). Visit the website at https://nalpn.org/.

Membership is required to learn about certification details. NALPN notifies you upon successful completion of the examination. You may use the appropriate initials as part of your signature/title.

Recertification is required every 2 years to maintain a valid certificate. Do not assume that requirements are the same for all certifications. Visit www.nalpn.org for full details.

> **Try This**
>
> **Availability of Leadership Course**
>
> Almost half of the newly LPNs/LVNs who participated in the 2024 NCSBN Job Analysis regularly assumed administrative responsibility, primarily in long-term care. Inquire whether a postgraduate LPN/LVN leadership/management course or certification is available. Ask for details about the course. This can increase your marketability as an LPN/LVN.

AMERICAN BOARD OF MANAGED CARE NURSING CERTIFICATION IN MANAGED CARE

ABMCN **Certified Managed Care Nurse (CMCN)** certification is available to LPNs/LVNs through a home study course. Order the course materials through ABMCN (www.abmcn.org).

The examination includes basic knowledge of managed care, health care economics, health care management, and client issues. Upon successful completion of the examination, the nurse is certified and may use the title Certification in Managed Care in Nursing. Certification is valid for 3 years and requires additional CE and a fee for renewal

REGISTERED NURSE CAREER PATHWAY

If you are an LPN/LVN who says, "I want to be an LPN/LVN, but I have no desire to be an RN," you have obviously given careful consideration to your personal goals. Being an LPN/LVN is an essential role on the health care team. Satisfaction in nursing, both for you and the clients you care for, is closely related to defined goals. If you decided you want to be an LPN/LVN, chances are you will be satisfied with your choice and will provide high-quality care to your clients. If, however, someone else decided you should be a nurse, chances are you will never be entirely satisfied with the choice. This lack of satisfaction will be mirrored in the care you give to clients. The same process is true in regard to deciding to become an RN.

If you do not want to become an RN, avoid letting anyone push you into it. Only when a goal is truly your own will you be motivated to do your best both in the educational process and in the care of clients. Consider the following: If you want to enter an RN program, learn what programs of study are available. There are numerous reasons (beyond personal choice) for considering additional nursing education, including:

- You have investigated job opportunities in the area in which you plan to live and find that jobs for LPNs/LVNs are limited.
- The salary difference will be a good return on your investment.
- Your current place of employment will assist you in paying for additional schooling.
- You will welcome the expanded responsibilities in the RN job role.

? Critical Thinking

What are some other reasons you can think of to pursue additional education and become an RN?

MOBILITY: PLANNING YOUR NURSING CAREER PATHWAY

In the past, a major problem in developing upward **mobility programs or seamless career progression in education** for LPNs/LVNs was the belief held by some educators that a practical nursing course was terminal in nature; that some SBON would not permit upward career progression education programs, nor would educational/work experience credit be given by some professional nursing programs. This has changed dramatically in the past few years. Much work has been done and is ongoing in many states to research best practices and to develop seamless education pathways. Although not yet fully successful, organizations such as the Robert Woods Johnson Foundation had collaborated with nursing leaders to develop a Campaign for Action to focus on multiple issues, including advancing nursing education (2025). See https://campaignforaction.org/.

Many institutions of higher learning have successfully negotiated with SBON to develop progressive LPN/LVN-to-RN or LPN/LVN-to-BSN programs.

Distance (Online) Learning Nursing Program

One example: Excelsior University. Excelsior College (previously known as Regents College), of Albany, New York, was the first in the United States to have a distance learning nursing program (online). The Associate Degree in Nursing program began in 1972 and has been continuously accredited by the Accreditation Commission for Education in Nursing (ACEN). The majority of courses are online with some requirements to travel for a Capstone course to demonstrate achievement of program outcomes. The student has flexibility to manage time to study and take examinations. Financing options are available.

LPNs/LVNs apply for admission and must be accepted to the School of Nursing before enrolling. Requirements are found on their website at www.excelsior.edu. LPNs/LVNs are eligible to apply (except for California residents). The university has generous credit acceptance practices; learners can transfer academic credits and can receive credit for military and workforce training, professional licenses, and certifications.

Nursing online programs proliferating to facilitate your career progression. Today there are many online nursing program options. Assess how the college/university and nursing program mission, philosophy, curriculum, and program outcomes align with your needs as a learner. Many LPN/LVN-to-RN, LPN/LVN-to-BSN and other in-person and on-line programs exist today. Flexibility and access are a benefit to students, with increasing, more seamless options to continue on your professional pathway.

Contact your SBON, or check out their website, for a list of available accredited nursing programs in your state. Talk to your current school counselor about available accredited nursing programs. Research how to apply and admission requirements; the education program costs; the availability of grants and financial aid; and their policy on transfer of credits. You can access accreditor websites such as acenursing.org, cnea.nln.org, and aacnnursing.org to find the accreditation status and location of nursing programs.

REGISTERED NURSE PROGRAMS: DO LPNS GET ADVANCED STANDING?

Turf issues continue to exist in all levels of nursing; CNA to LPN/LVN to Associate Degree in Nursing (and) to BSN to Master of Science in Nursing (MSN) to a Doctorate in Nursing (PhD vs. DNP). Slowly these barriers are diminishing. Plan to be a part of the solution, not the problem, especially when you are in a position to make a difference. This is an area where you, as a member of your professional nursing organization, can make your voice heard.

Although some RN programs continue to ignore the value of practical/vocational education, most programs have changed. Some programs require that LPNs/LVNs start from the beginning and repeat all previously covered theory and skills courses, including basic nursing skills. The good news is that there are many options available throughout the United States in which an LPN/LVN can become an RN, with credit given for being an LPN/LVN.

Box 18.16 **Possible Response to Critical Thinking Scenario**

From the day we are born until the day we die, we judge people and they judge us on how we look, act, talk, and respond to the environment. Based on this, decisions are made to like, dislike, or not care one way or the other about a person. For the Western culture there is a drive toward being youthful and fit, being a "man's man" or a "woman's woman," and having energy to burn. It is neither good nor bad; it just is! So, play the game, get the job, and, afterwards, when you get the job, decide what to let go. Below is a checklist for consideration:

1. There are always many tasks to juggle. Are you getting a good night's rest before the interview?
2. Use all available resources, including makeup, to avoid looking tired and improve youthful appearance.
3. Confirm you have a firm handshake and pleasant-sounding voice.
4. Practice quick responses to interview questions and project confidence. Use the power pose as described in Chapter 9 to build confidence prior to the interview.
5. Plan to highlight your ability to manage a household, school, and work effectively, emphasizing your time management skills.
6. Review key concepts in this chapter related to diverse job sources.
7. Check the health care business news and incorporate the information into a question for the employer to stand above the other candidates.

Lastly, contact references through LinkedIn, which will provide additional personal contacts within different companies. Those contacts will know if there are employment opportunities at their companies and may be used as a "name drop" to get an interview. The old adage is, "It is not what you know, but who you know," so use it.

Get Ready for the Next-Generation NCLEX® Examination

Key Points

- LPNs/LVNs are employed in a diverse array of settings, providing many career options.
- Workforce trends include an increase in LPNs/LVNs working in hospitals, whereas LPNs/LVNs working in long-term care are decreasing and increasing in the community.
- To be successful in your job search, begin your search with the first day of classes and continue throughout your enrollment.
- Opportunities present themselves to those who are willing to put forth effort and seek opportunity.
- The methods presented in this chapter have proved successful for graduates, people wishing to make career changes, or those wanting to institute a change in their work. Treat your job search like a job.
- Make contacts by telephone or e-mail, sending resumes and cover letters, or by physically going to the employer to apply and schedule an interview.
- Explore the hidden job market via networking and the Internet, and call employers, whether or not an ad has been placed.
- Dress for success for the job you want, not the job you have.
- Actively follow up on all interviews! Let the employer know you are interested. Remember, the more often the employer hears or sees your name, the better your chances of getting hired.
- If you are hired, send thank you notes to those who helped you. You may need them again someday. Remember, you are responsible for making your own luck.
- Start imagining your nursing career pathway and continue to update it often so you can get to where you want to be in your career.

Additional Learning Resources

Go to your Evolve website (http://evolve.elsevier.com/Carroll/success/) for the following FREE learning resources:

- Answers to Critical Thinking Scenarios
- Additional learning activities
- Additional Review Questions for the NCLEX-PN® examination
- Helpful phrases for communicating in Spanish and more!

Clinical Judgment Questions

1. A group of practical/vocational nursing students are discussing interpersonal styles. What interpersonal style is representative of being easygoing, likes to blend in, has difficulty making decisions, and tends to be quiet and soft-spoken?

a. Analytical type
b. Driver type
c. Amiable type
d. Expressive type

2. Your employer has an employment policy of at-will employment. Which of the following best reflects the meaning of this?

a. The employer expects a 2-week notice before you leave their employment.
b. The employer will determine the length or extension of probationary periods.
c. The employer may terminate your job immediately, without notice or reason.
d. The employer will continue your job indefinitely, provided job requirements are met.

3. An interviewer asks you a question for which you do not have an answer. Which of the following would be the best response?

a. Ask the interviewer to please rephrase the question.
b. Begin to answer and switch to a topic you know about.
c. Smile pleasantly and say you don't know the answer.
d. Take a key word from the question and make up a response.

4. Your peer is creating a personal resume. Which of the following statements would trigger you to suggest your peer seek out additional learning?

a. "You are legally bound to include every employer (even if it was only for one month)."
b. "Resumes are your own personal portrait inclusive of key elements that paint you in your best light."
c. "White space is beneficial."
d. "Most employers spend less than 3 to 5 minutes reviewing a resume to determine the next step: an interview."

5. A student is completing their nursing program. Which of the following uses of the Internet are helpful in job hunting? *(Select all that apply.)*

a. Identify salary range.
b. Complete job application.
c. Locate job opportunities.
d. Research facility information.
e. Professional and social networks.

6. A practical/vocational nursing student has completed an interview at a long-term care facility. Which of the following next steps should occur following the interview? *(Select all that apply.)*

a. Write down, on paper, information learned and points stressed by the interviewer.
b. Send a thank you letter to the interviewer noting some of the points discussed during the interview.
c. Contact your references immediately after the interview and let them know that they may be contacted. Then discuss points about the job the employer stressed as being important.
d. Follow up 4 weeks after the interview with the employer to see if there were additional questions to assist in making their hiring decision.
e. Continue an active job search until a job offer is made.

Critical Thinking Scenarios

Scenario 1

The student is in their late 40s, with graying hair, and recently divorced. There are three children at home, including a senior in high school who plans to go to college, a sophomore in high school, and a child in the eighth grade. The student's ex-spouse was paying alimony until losing a manufacturing job. Wanting the best for the family, the student returned to school and became an LPN. Unfortunately, the job interviews did not go well, and no job offers have been received. The former student, now a graduate, knows that there are ways to better represent oneself both on paper and in an interview. What would you recommend for a person in this situation? See Box 18.16 for possible responses.

Scenario 2

During clinical rotations, the PN/VN student was a "star," and the staff said they would provide references if needed when seeking a job after graduation from school. The student's passion was to help others and be the BEST nurse. Classmates described the student as a little nerdy, overweight, and a loud talker. The student graduated and is seeking employment. During interviews, the graduate noticed that the interviewers would have nonverbal reactions, which the graduate perceived as negative reactions, throughout the interview in response to the graduate's answers and conduct. No job offers were received. The new graduate felt the dream of being a nurse was slowly slipping away, until a friend offered some ideas. What suggestions would you make to the student after reading this chapter? See Box 18.15 for possible responses.

Licensure and Regulation: Becoming Licensed and Understanding Your State Nurse Practice Act

19

Objectives

On completing this chapter, you will be able to do the following:

1. Describe the role of states' Nurse Practice Acts and how they govern licensure for nurses.
2. Describe key aspects of the NCLEX-PN®.
3. Discuss the application process for the NCLEX-PN®.
4. Differentiate between applying for licensure and applying for examination.
5. Summarize key aspects of the administration of the NCLEX-PN®, including the reporting of results.
6. Discuss the confidentiality agreement and consequences for violating the agreement.
7. Recall considerations regarding preparation for the NCLEX-PN®.

Key Terms

Authorization to Test (ATT)
candidate
computerized adaptive testing (CAT)
confidentiality agreement
endorsement
NCLEX-PN® examination
Nurse Practice Act (NPA)
State Board of Nursing (SBON)

As graduation nears, it is natural for most practical/vocational nursing students to be focused on the licensure exam or National Council Licensing Examination for Practical Nurses (NCLEX-PN®) (sometimes referred to as state boards). However, the reality is that NCLEX-PN® preparation begins the day you apply to a nursing program. Most practical/vocational (LPN/LVN) nursing programs, whose graduates consistently achieve NCLEX-PN® pass rates above the state and national norm, know that it is imperative to implement NCLEX-PN® preparation from the first day of the program. Unfortunately, sometimes it is difficult to convince students that this strategy is essential. Instead, students often feel burdened by the "computer work" and find "shortcuts" to get the work done quickly, not realizing that this may haunt them in the near future. Trust in the program you have chosen. Accept the need to complete NCLEX-PN® preparation work as assigned. This will enhance your ability to successfully pass the NCLEX-PN® the first time and improve your overall achievement of program outcomes. When you pass the NCLEX-PN® and receive your license, you will want to keep it forever. A thorough understanding of your state ***Nurse Practice Act (NPA)*** *is essential to being a safe and effective caregiver. Because each state has a unique NPA, you must be knowledgeable of the NPA for each state in which you are licensed.*

STATE NURSE PRACTICE ACTS AND APPLYING FOR A NURSING LICENSE

WHAT IS THE STATE NURSE PRACTICE ACT?

The NPA exists to protect the public. Despite the intent of all nurses to provide competent, safe, high-quality nursing care and assist the client and communities to regain, maintain, or advance their health, there is inherent harm that can occur as you perform your duties. The vast array of unique health care needs, complicated by constant technological advances in a variety of health care settings, provides a constant challenge. The NPA provides a foundation to guide and govern nursing practice. It includes information regulating nursing education schools, the practice of nursing professionals, requirements for licensure, and grounds for disciplinary action and dismissal. The NCSBN New Nurses: Your License to Practice Video found at https://www.ncsbn.org/video/new-nurses-your-license-to-practice provides more details. Other related resources can be found at www.ncsbn.org, and see Chapter 7.

HOW DOES THE NURSE PRACTICE ACT GUIDE/GOVERN NURSING PRACTICE?

Decades ago, State Boards of Nursing (SBON) were established to enact the NPA and give the authority to provide ongoing development of administrative rules and regulations to govern/guide nursing practice. Each state has a specific NPA for all nurses, including licensed practical nurses/licensed vocational nurses (LPNs/LVNs), which is enacted by the state legislature. This information is often referred to as the nurse's "scope of practice." The SBON is responsible to the public, and as such, any proposed changes to regulation go through a vigorous process, vetted by various stakeholders and accessible for public comment. A licensed person is the responsible of LPNs/LVNs to know their state's NPA. Ignorance is not an excuse for noncompliance or substandard nursing care (Boehning and Haddad, 2025). Visit https://www.ncsbn.org/policy-gov/npa-toolkit.page to learn more details and find resources to access an NPA toolkit and a link to find your NPA.

VARIABILITY OF THE STATE'S NURSE PRACTICE ACT APPLICABLE TO LPN/LVN PRACTICE

Corazzini et al. (2013) concluded that states varied considerably regarding their NPA. In addition, several states were silent regarding key aspects of nursing care, such as assessment or delegation (Corazzini et al., 2013). This variability and lack of clarity of the state NPAs can contribute to confusion and variability in LPN/LVN job roles. Candon et al. (2023) also suggests that delegating tasks is more likely to affect the workload of LPNs and therefore points to a potential and unexplored element of explain the scope of practice for nurses to reduce turnover. Practice boundaries between the LPN and RN scope of practice can vary from facility to facility and state to state. A facility can limit, but never expand, the LPN scope of practice the LPN job description beyond the scope stated in the respective state's NPA. For example, it is possible as an LPN that you could be licensed and working in a facility in your home state where you are permitted to administer intravenous (IV) therapy via a central line device. However, you could travel across a state line to a neighboring state and work in a facility owned by the same corporation and this same act (IV therapy administration via a central line) could be prohibited.

You can see why this situation is complex and can be confusing to the LPN, other members of the health care team, the public, and the employer. If a situation arises where you are being directed to perform a prohibited act by your employer, it is your responsibility to educate your employer about the scope of practice or NPA of your state. The issue becomes more confusing when the state NPA is silent regarding an LPN/LVN job duty such as delegation. When this occurs, carefully review your institutional policy and procedure and discuss the situation with your supervisor. Have your evidence (state NPA) available. This state NPA is easily found if you web search for your state board of nursing or use this link from the NCSBN https://www.ncsbn.org/membership/us-members/contact-bon.page. The SBON staff can provide assistance; however, remember it is their role to regulate, not advise. They cannot advise regarding particular situations; however, their legal counsels can provide you with a recount of a similar situation and the outcome to guide you in your decision-making. Many states have a decision-making guide that is located on their website to assist nurses and employers.

? Critical Thinking: Nurse Practice Act

Locate the NPA for the state you anticipate obtaining a license. Review at least three other state sites and discuss the differences between each NPA related to the LPN's role in assessment, delegation, and IV therapy. Determine if your state has a decision-making model and review the model. How does this model guide your decision-making?

APPLYING FOR A PRACTICAL/VOCATIONAL NURSING LICENSE OR A TEMPORARY PRACTICE PERMIT

Your nursing school will provide information to assist you to obtain an application for a temporary practice permit to work as a graduate practical nurse/graduate vocational nurse (GPN or GVN) or for a practical/vocational nursing license to work as a LPN/LVN. Graduates must apply for a license to practice. However, some of you may wish to obtain a temporary permit. This is less of a necessity today because you can take the NCLEX-PN® within a month or two following graduation. If you decide to apply for a temporary permit, it is your responsibility to understand the restrictions with a temporary permit. For example, it may be required that a registered nurse (RN) is physically present on the unit where you work. In addition, once you have received results of the NCLEX-PN®, the temporary permit is automatically revoked if you do not successfully pass the examination. You will be required to surrender your temporary permit and no longer work as a GPN/GVN.

Scheduling the NCLEX-PN® as soon as possible, following execution of a well-developed study plan, is the best option. Passing the NCLEX-PN® means that you will work as an LPN or LVN. Research shows a correlation between delaying first-time completion of the NCLEX-PN® more than 3 months following program completion date and predicted probability of passing the examination. Obtaining a temporary permit and beginning work may cause you to delay taking the exam. Follow the guidelines carefully regarding the submission of the licensure application. Your school will submit the required documents indicating you have successfully completed all the requirements of a state-approved practical/vocational nursing program. Be attentive to the correct spelling of your name and use of a maiden, married, hyphenated, or middle name. This information must align exactly with the information submitted by your school or your application will be rejected, lengthening the time to receive your **Authorization to Test (ATT)** and sit for the NCLEX-PN®.

Keep in Mind

Almost without exception, when student nurses are asked about their goal for the year, they respond by saying they want to pass the "boards," meaning pass the NCLEX-PN® to become an LPN or LVN. They should also always respond by saying they want to deliver competent, safe, high-quality care adhering to the guidelines of their state NPA. However, reality is that you will never be licensed unless you pass the NCLEX-PN®. As mentioned many times throughout this book, NCLEX-PN® preparation begins the first day you enter a nursing program.

WHAT IS THE NATIONAL COUNCIL LICENSING EXAMINATION FOR PRACTICAL NURSING?

The NCLEX-PN® is the acronym for the National Council Licensing Examination for Practical/Vocational Nursing graduates. It is designed to assess the knowledge, skills, abilities, and clinical judgment needed to safely and effectively practice nursing as an entry-level LPN/LVN, in the first year of employment in the LPN/LVN role. The NCLEX-PN® results provide the basis for licenses granted to LPNs/LVNs by the **SBON**.

The National Council of State Boards of Nursing (NCSBN) developed a secure method of examination by computer in April 1994. This testing method is called **computerized adaptive testing (CAT)**. CAT is a method of delivering exams using computer technology and measurement theory. Each **candidate's** exam is unique because it is assembled as the exam proceeds matching the candidate's ability. The items (or questions) are stored in a large item pool classified by test plan category and level of difficulty, as well as clinical judgment steps. The exam is tailored to the candidate's knowledge and skills while fulfilling the NCLEX-PN® Test Plan requirements (NCSBN, 2025).

Candidates answer a minimum of 85 items and a maximum of 150 items in a 5-hour time period. The majority of the items come from the eight content areas, and a lesser number of items will comprise three clinical judgment case studies. Each case study is composed of six items that measure each of the six domains of the NCSBN Clinical Judgment Measurement Model (NCJMM). The case studies span any number of content areas and are counted independently of the content are specific items. Fifteen of the items are unscored pretest items (possible future test questions).

The time allotted includes the introductory screen, all breaks (scheduled and unscheduled), and the examination. Breaks are optional. There are three methods for scoring items for partial credit: plus/minus, zero/one, and rationale scoring. There is partial credit scoring for items for which more than one key exists. The computer continues with questions until it determines that the candidate passes or fails the examination. If the candidate runs out of time, the exam will be computed from the responses to all completed items. Those scoring above the passing range will pass; otherwise the exam will be scored as failed.

CAT administers items with difficulty levels so that each candidate will answer about half correctly. These items provide the most information. All candidates answer about 50% correctly because the computer presents them with questions to match their ability. The next item should not be too easy or too difficult. The computer goes down a "pathway" or "branch," and no candidate has exactly the same test. Items that follow are based on the candidate's previous answer. This is why you *must* answer every item presented on the computer screen You will not be able to go back and answer a previous question. The computer calculates each answer before it can choose the next item. Visit www.ncsbn.org for more details.

The NCLEX-PN® and the NCLEX-RN® changed in 2023. The reason for the change was to ask better questions to gauge critical thinking when providing care and make the right decisions (Next-Generation NCLEX® Project | NCSBN, 2021). The exam uses realistic case studies reflecting the kinds of critical decisions nurses make in a variety of health care settings. Much research and the 2018 LPN/LVN Practice Analysis determined that essential skills for LPNs/LVNs include recognizing cues, analyzing cues, and taking action. The new types of exam questions have been determined to be a valid and reliable measurement of LPN/LVN competence.

The NSCBN Clinical Judgment Measurement Model (or NCJMM) https://www.nclex.com/clinical-judgment-measurement-model.page is the model used by the NCSBN as an evidenced-based framework to develop, classify, and score test items (Fig. 19.1).

The NCSBN Board of Directors maintained the passing standard for the NCLEX-PN® effective April 1, 2023.

HOW THE NATIONAL COUNCIL LICENSING EXAMINATION FOR PRACTICAL NURSES IS KEPT UP TO DATE

The NCSBN has an ongoing process that reviews what LPNs/LVNs are doing in practice and seeks out expertise of a wide variation of nurses in practice, nursing education, and regulatory bodies to ensure that the licensure exam is reliable and valid in core content.

Currently, the April 2023 NCLEX-PN® Test Plan reflects the outcome of the *2021 LPN/LVN Practice Analysis: Linking the NCLEX-PN® Examination to Practice* (NCSBN, 2022). This test plan is valid through March 31, 2026. The Test Plan, updated every 3 years, serves a variety of purposes to include candidate preparation, direct item writers in the development of items, and facilitate classification of examination items. The document offers a comprehensive list of content for each Client Needs category and subcategory and provides

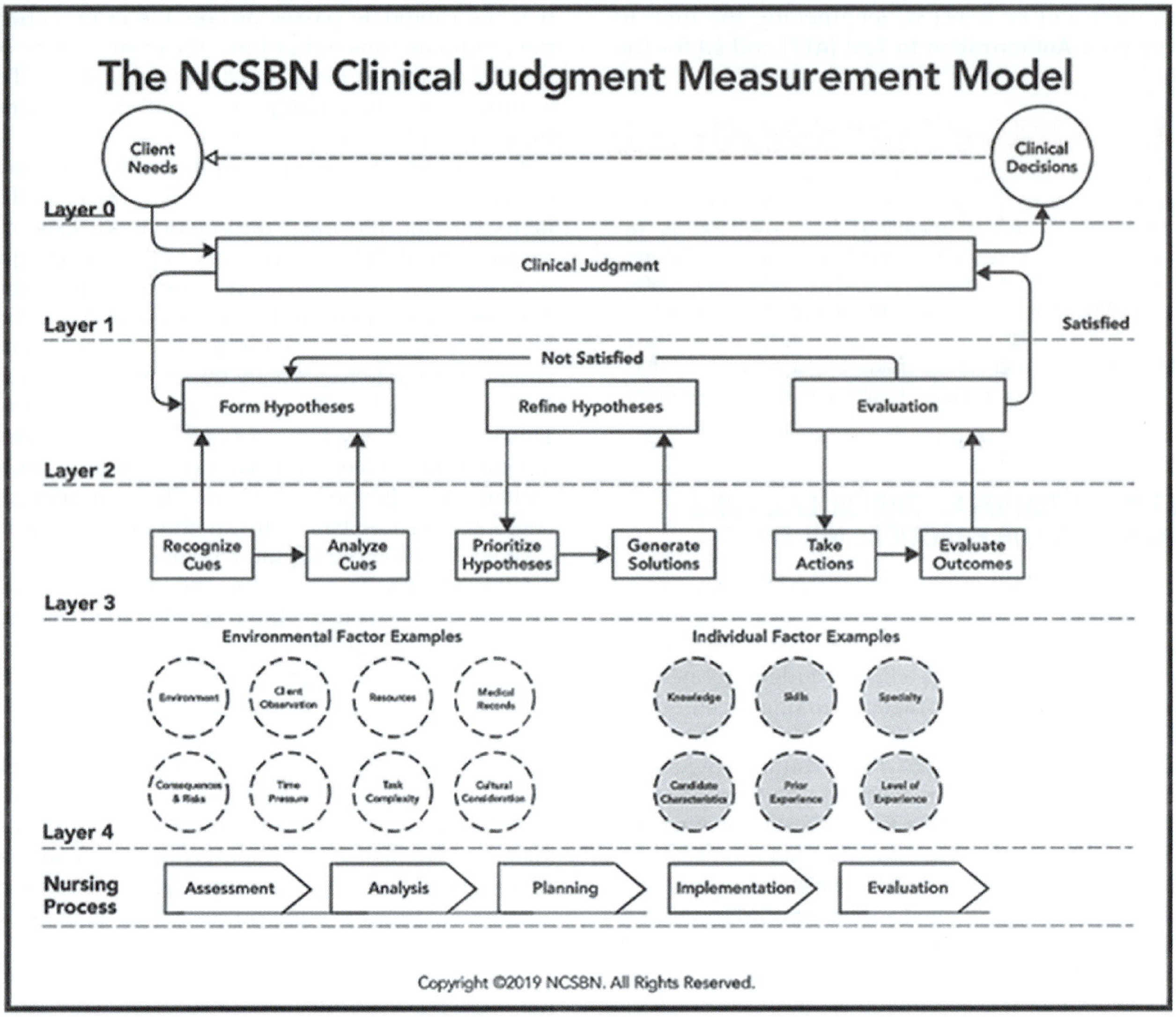

Fig. 19.1 The NCSBN Clinical Judgment Measurement Model (NCJMM). (From The National Council of State Board of Nursing, 2019. Retrieved from https://www.nclex.com/clinical-judgment-measurement-model.page.)

item writing tips for guidelines for nurse educators (NCSBN, 2023).

Every 3 years the Council sends out a practice analysis survey to a sample of newly licensed LPNs/LVNs. Of the 26,559 surveys sent in 2023 via e-mail, 5845 were returned. The analyzable response rate was 18.1%. The NCSBN (2025) explains that the practice analysis was developed using several methods to describe the practice of newly licensed PNs/VNs in the United States. These methods include document reviews, activity logs of newly licensed PNs/VNs, Subject Matter Experts knowledge, and a large-scale survey incorporating a list of LPN/LVN activities to validate current practice. Additional resources provide input such as NCSBN staff and nursing regulatory bodies or State Boards of Nursing. Data analysis followed. Based on evidence, the findings of this study were used to evaluate and validate an updated LPN/LVN test plan. "The 2024 PN Practice Analysis: Linking the NCLEX-PN® to Practice" (NCSBN, 2025) was recently published. This report will influence the next NCLEX-PN® test plan expected in 2026. The entire study is available online at https://www.ncsbn.org/public-files/24_NCLEX_PN_PA.pdf.

TEST FRAMEWORK: CLIENT NEEDS

Client needs provide an overall structure for defining nursing actions and competencies for a variety of clients across all settings and are congruent with state laws and statutes. The content of the NCLEX-PN® is divided into four client needs categories. Two of the four categories are further subdivided. The percentage of test items assigned to each category and limited examples of content are included. Additional examples of content are found in the NCLEX-PN® Examination Test Bulletin and the 2025 NCLEX® Examination Candidate Bulletin, available at https://www.nclex.com/files/2025_NCLEX_Candidate_Bulletin_English.pdf.

The categories and subcategories, based on the 2023 Test Plan are as follows:

1. Safe, Effective Care Environment
   a. Coordinated Care: 18% to 24%
      Examples: Advance directives, client rights and needs, client self-advocacy, concepts of management and supervision, confidentiality, organize and prioritize, ethical practice, legal scope of practice, information technology
   b. Safety and Infection Control: 10% to 16%
      Examples: Accident/error/injury prevention, handling hazardous and infectious materials, standard precautions/transmission-based precautions/surgical asepsis, least restrictive restraint and safety device, evaluate appropriateness of health care provider order for client
2. Health Promotion and Maintenance: 6% to 12%
   Examples: Care across the life span continuum, aging process, ante/intra/postpartum and newborn care, data collection techniques, developmental stages and transitions, high-risk behaviors, lifestyle choices, and self-care
3. Psychosocial Integrity: 9% to 15%
   Examples: Behavioral management techniques, coping mechanisms, crisis intervention, chemical and other dependencies, end-of-life concepts, mental health concepts, stress management, and therapeutic communication
4. Physiologic Integrity
   a. Basic Care and Comfort: 7% to 13%
      Examples: Assistive devices, elimination, nutrition and oral hydration, personal hygiene, and rest and sleep, postmortem care
   b. Pharmacologic Therapies: 10% to 16%
      Examples: Adverse effects/contraindications/side effects/interactions, medication administration, and pharmacologic pain management, medication safety practices
   c. Reduction of Risk Potential: 9% to 15%
      Examples: Changes/abnormalities in vital signs, diagnostic tests, laboratory values, potential for complications from surgical procedures, and health alterations
   d. Physiologic Adaptation: 7% to 13%
      Examples: Basic pathophysiology, fluid and electrolyte imbalances, medical emergencies, and unexpected response to therapies

INTEGRATION OF BODIES OF KNOWLEDGE AND NURSING CONCEPTS

Fundamental principles of clinical decision-making and critical thinking to nursing practice are applied by integrating concepts from the following bodies of knowledge (NCSBN, 2025):

- Social sciences (psychology and sociology)
- Biological sciences (anatomy, physiology, biology, and microbiology)

Concepts from the Client Needs categories and subcategories

- Caring interaction of the LPN/LVN and client in an atmosphere of mutual respect and trust
- Clinical judgment—the observed outcome of critical thinking and decision-making—observe/assess, prioritize, and generate the best possible evidence-based solutions
- Clinical problem-solving process (nursing process)—a scientific approach to client care that includes data collection, planning, implementation, and evaluation.
- Communication and documentation—verbal and nonverbal interaction between the LPN/LVN and client, as well as health care team members, written or electronic records reflecting standards of practice and accountability
- Teaching/Learning—facilitation of the acquisition of knowledge, skills, and attitudes to assist in promoting a change in behavior
- Cultural/Spiritual—interaction of the nurse and client that recognized individualized care, applicable to standards of care and legal considerations

? Critical Thinking

Client Need Categories

Provide a "real" example of a client need for each of the categories and subcategories. Where in the scheduled studies of your program do you expect to learn what is needed for each subcategory? Relate information you give in preconference to the categories and subcategories.

Try This

Categories of Client Care

Write a one-sentence example of how you might apply each of the six integrated processes of Concepts from Client Needs in planning client care.

CLINICAL JUDGMENT

Using a multistep process that uses the nurse's knowledge and ability to prioritize and generate solutions is measured by case studies or an individual stand-alone item. It will contain six items associated with the same client presentation with evolving information. The following steps are:

- Recognize cues
- Analyze cues
- Prioritize hypotheses
- Generate solutions
- Take action
- Evaluated outcomes

TYPES OF TEST QUESTIONS

The NCLEX-PN® contains items (questions) primarily at the application and analysis or higher levels of cognitive ability. This is because LPN/LVN practice requires application of knowledge, skills, abilities, and clinical judgment. These questions require prioritizing and decision-making. The two main types of test questions are multiple choice and alternate item format.

Multiple Choice

The majority of test questions are multiple choice. Each question describes a client or clinical situation. Four options are given from which to choose the correct response.

Alternate Item Format

The NCLEX-PN® also includes alternate item questions, including the following:

- *Fill in the blank*. Medicine and IV rate calculations, intake, and output totals.
- *Multiple responses*. Select **all** responses that pertain to the question, with no partial credit given. For example: Which of the following medications are antihypertensives?
- *Prioritizing* (ordered response). Options (nursing actions) are numbered as first, second, third, and so on, in order of priority, or the mouse is used to drag and drop options in the ordered priority. For example: When doing the Heimlich maneuver, which of the following actions would you do first, second, or third?
- *Figure or illustration* (hotspot). Questions are asked about a chart or figure. Either an answer is chosen from a list or the mouse is used to point and click a "hotspot" as the answer. For example: Click on the hypochondriac area.
- *Chart/exhibit questions*. A question is included with a chart or exhibit requiring use of the chart/exhibit to answer the question. For example: Which lab result is normal?

An on-screen optional calculator is available for your use during the examination. Any format item, including standard multiple-choice items, might include charts, tables, or graphic images. A tutorial is provided on the computer screen regarding the operation of the computer and how to record answers. For general information questions about the NCLEX-PN®, use the FAQs at www.ncsbn.org as a resource. You can also e-mail questions/comments to info@ncsbn.org.

Next-Generation NCLEX® (NGN)

- *Extended Multiple Response*. Same as multiple response items with more options and will use partial credit scoring.
- *Extended Drag and Drop*. Move or place response option into answer spaces. Like the current ordered response questions, not all response options may be required.
- *Cloze* (Drop–Down). Based on a case study, choose answers using drop-down lists. There may be multiple drop-down lists. Answers will be in words or phrases within a sentence, within tables and charts.
- *Enhanced Hot Spot* (Highlighting). Select answers by highlighting predefined words or phrases. A portion of a client medical record is provided; select the words or phrases to answer the item.
- *Matrix/Grid*. Select one or more answer options for each row/column. Measures multiple aspects of the clinical scenario.

Try This

What Is an Alternate Item Question?

Write an example of an alternate item format using problem solving in the geriatric setting.

OVERVIEW OF APPLICATION PROCESS

It is customary for an instructor to introduce you to the application process when it is time to apply to the state board of nursing (the Board) for a license to become an LPN or LVN.

NATIONAL COUNCIL LICENSING EXAMINATION FOR PRACTICAL NURSES PROCESS OVERVIEW[a]

Submit an application for licensure/registration to the state board of nursing/nursing regulatory body (SBON/NRB) where you wish to be licensed/registered.

1. Meet all of the eligibility requirements of the SBON/RB to take the NCLEX-PN®.
2. Register for the NCLEX-PN® with Pearson VUE.
3. Receive NCLEX-PN® Registration Acknowledgment e-mail from Pearson VUE.
4. The SBON/NRB verifies and grants eligibility in the Pearson VUE system.
5. Receive Authorization to Test or ATT via e-mail from Pearson VUE.
6. Schedule your exam with Pearson VUE online or by telephone.

For more details, see the 2025 NCLEX® Examination Candidate Bulletin and NCLEX® Frequently Asked Questions www.ncsbn.org.

REGISTRATION TIME LIMIT AND ATT

Upon completing the registration, Pearson Vue notifies the SBON/NRB, who must respond within 365 days. If you don't get an e-mail from Pearson Vue after 30 days, contact the SBON/BRN registration website and check status of your application to determine if there are any issues to resolve.

If you are not declared eligible for taking the NCLEX-PN® within the 365-day time limit, you forfeit

[a]Excerpted from National Council of State Boards of Nursing: 2025 NCLEX-PN® Examination Candidate Bulletin, 2025, https://www.ncsbn.org/public-files/2025_NCLEX_Candidate_Bulletin_English.pdf.

the Pearson Vue registration and the fee. To reapply, you must submit a new application and pay the fee again. Do not re-register for the examination until you call Pearson Vue to verify the SBON/NRB declared that you were ineligible. Registration fees are not refunded.

Once your board declares you eligible to test, you will receive an ATT from Pearson VUE via email. The ATT letter includes your authorization number, candidate identification number, and an expiration date. The ATT letter is valid for a specified time (determined by the SBON/NRB) and averages approximately 90 days. If you do not test within the specified ATT period, you must reregister and repay to take the examination with Pearson Vue.

As soon as possible after receiving the ATT, schedule a test session for the NCLEX-PN® at a Pearson Vue Center, either by phone or website. Test centers may fill up quickly. Attempting to make a last-minute testing appointment may result in missing the ATT validity deadline. You may test at any Pearson Vue Test Center in the United States and select international sites. Most test centers are open during the week except on holidays. Some are busier than other sites. If you are flexible regarding time and site location, this author's experience has been that students can generally secure an appointment within 2 weeks. Should you need to change the appointment, read the Candidate Bulletin carefully for detailed instructions.

Take the NCLEX-PN® on the scheduled day and time. You must have valid identification to be admitted to the Pearson Center. It is recommended to bring the ATT. See acceptable ID and identification requirements in more detail at www.ncsbn.org.

Validity dates for the ATT will not be extended for any reason. Once approved for testing, the candidate must take the NCLEX-PN® within the approved time frame.

Critical Thinking

Authorization to Test

Explain the significance of attaining the ATT before scheduling your appointment to take the NCLEX-PN®. What problem-solving steps will you take if you don't get your ATT within a month of registering for examination with Pearson Vue?

FEES AND OTHER IMPORTANT INFORMATION

There is a fee for the NCLEX-PN® (https://www.ncsbn.org/public-files/2025_NCLEX_Candidate_Bulletin_English.pdf). In addition, the SBON/NRB has fees where you are applying for licensure. Fees vary. There is no refund of any registration fee for any reason.

Try This

List any fees required by your state's board of nursing (or by the jurisdiction where you are applying).

HOW TO REGISTER (INTERNET OR TELEPHONE) FOR THE NCLEX-PN® EXAMINATION

Internet or telephone can be used to register. Pearson VUE will confirm receipt of registration and send an ATT to the candidate. Visit https://www.ncsbn.org/public-files/2025_NCLEX_Candidate_Bulletin_English.pdf for details.

NATIONAL COUNCIL LICENSING EXAMINATION FOR PRACTICAL NURSES ADMINISTRATION IN THE UNITED STATES AND ITS TERRITORIES

The NCLEX-PN® is given in the United States and territories including American Samoa, Guam, the Northern Mariana Islands, the Virgin Islands and other international sites to include Canada. Because the examination is the same at any location, it is possible to provide licensure by endorsement from one board of nursing to another within the United States and its territories.

Endorsement means that an LPN/LVN may apply for licensure in a different state or territory without retesting.

Try This

Practicing in Other States

Research how to apply for licensure by endorsement in another state. Start by contacting the **state board of nursing** of a state in which you may be interested in applying for a job.

THE CHECKING-IN PROCESS

The NCLEX-PN® ensures *minimal competency* to protect the public, and because of this, strict rules have been established for testing. Read and reread the current candidate bulletin, published every January before arriving to the testing center. BE PREPARED! (Excerpt from: https://www.ncsbn.org/public-files/2025_NCLEX_Candidate_Bulletin_English.pdf).

- Arrive at the testing center at least 30 minutes before the scheduled testing time. If you arrive more than 30 minutes after the scheduled appointment, you may be required to forfeit your NCLEX® appointment.
- Proper identification: Present a valid acceptable ID. NOTE: Use your first and last name in *exactly* the same form you used when applying for the NCLEX-PN®. If your legal name has changed since you applied, check the candidate bulletin for the most up-to-date document requirements.
- Additional identification: Provide a digital signature, palm vein scan, and have your photograph taken. NOTE: These items accompany the examination results sent to the board and can be used to confirm your identity.
- Attire: Hats, coats, or scarves may not be worn in the testing room or while your photo is being taken. You will be asked to remove any watches, large

jewelry, or other accessories before entering the testing room.

- Electronic devices: You will be required to place all electronic devices in a Pearson VUE–provided sealable bag to be placed in the lockable storage provided to you for the duration of the examination appointment.
- Friends, relatives, or children who accompany you to the test center are not allowed to wait in the test center while you take the examination.
- All personal belongings must be left outside of the testing room. Secure storage will be provided; however, candidates are NOT allowed to access any of the prohibited personal items at any time during the exam, including breaks. Storage space is small, so candidates should plan appropriately. Test centers assume no responsibility for candidates' personal belongings.
- The test administrator (TA) will give you a short orientation and then will escort you to a computer terminal. You must remain in your seat during the examination, except when authorized to leave by test center staff. You may not change your computer terminal unless a TA directs you to do so.
- Reference the Candidate Bulletin for Test Site Rules and Regulations for additional information on the check-in process.
- Direct observation by staff, video, and audio recording of the session occurs at all times during the examination.
- The CAT includes both a calculator and a time device that tells you how much time remains to complete the NCLEX-PN®. (Refer to your candidate bulletin for a list of other items that are not permitted in the testing room.)
- Erasable note boards are provided for use during the test and collected before you leave the room during a break or at the end of testing. Note boards cannot be taken outside the room.
- Breaks: You will have 5 hours to complete the examination, which includes a short introductory screen, two preprogrammed optional breaks (2 hours after testing and 3½ hours after testing) and any unscheduled breaks. If you decide to take a break, you must leave the testing room. It is strongly advised that you not leave the test center during breaks. When you take a break, all personal items accessed may be inspected by the test administrator. Any tampering of the electronic device bag provided will be reported. This could result in the cancellation of your examination results. You will be required to provide a palm vein scan before and after a break.
- When the exam is finished, you will complete a brief computer-delivered questionnaire about your testing experience. When finished, raise your hand to summon the TA. The TA will collect and inventory your note board.
- If you have electronic devices in a Pearson Vue–provided bag, you must take the bag to the TA to be opened and inspected. Removal of devices by the candidate will result in a case report and could lead to the cancellation of your examination result.
- The TA will dismiss you when all requirements are fulfilled.

Violation of the NCSBN Examination Candidate Rules or not following the instructions of the TA may result in examination results being withheld and/or cancelled, and your examination fee will not be refunded. NCSBN and your nursing regulatory body may take other action, up to and including license revocation and referral to law enforcement for criminal prosecution.

Try This

Security Rules

Discuss why a student cannot access their cell phone (even for an urgent call) during a break.

Examination Confidentiality Agreement (Source: https://www.nclex.com/files/NCLEX_Bulletin_English_October_%202025.pdf)

A confidentiality agreement will appear on the computer, which you must read and sign before you begin the examination. The **confidentiality agreement** includes not disclosing the contents of the examination items before, during, or after the examination. Disclosure includes, but is not limited to, discussing examination items with faculty, students, friends, family, and others. Do not send information via e-mail or discuss content verbally with anyone, including faculty. This is a confidentiality breach. Any irregular behavior can result in criminal prosecution, civil liability, and/or disciplinary action by the nursing licensing board.

DURING THE TEST (Source: https://www.ncsbn.org/candidatebulletin.htm)

You may ask for assistance with the computer at any time. Raise your hand for assistance, or if you want to change note boards, or if you need a break. Remain in your seat, until given permission to leave the room. Creating any disturbance can cause you to be dismissed from the room.

After you complete the exam, raise your hand. There will be a brief questionnaire on the computer to complete regarding the testing experience. You may also ask for a confidential comment sheet to write personal comments to the NCSBN. When all exam requirements are met, the TA will collect and inventory the note boards and dismiss you from the testing room.

REPORTING THE RESULTS OF THE EXAMINATION (Source: https://www.ncsbn.org/candidatebulletin.htm)

The Pearson VUE Center does not release final results to you directly. The official result is available only from the board approximately 1 month after testing.

The NCSBN provides an opportunity to get unofficial results in 2 business days.

A fee may be assessed. Access further information through this link: https://www.nclex.com/quick-results.page *Do not call the board, the NCLEX-PN® Candidate Services, the Pearson VUE Centers, or the NCSBN for results.* The *official* results will be sent to you by postal mail or e-mail from the state board of nursing. In addition, you can check whether a license has been issued on your state's electronic website where you initially applied for licensure.

Your state's board of nursing (not Pearson Center) notifies you of the test results. Boards are the only agencies that can release the examination results and issue a license.

? Critical Thinking

Examination Results

Explain why the state board of nursing (rather than the Pearson VUE Center) provides you with the results of the NCLEX-PN®.

? Critical Thinking

Computerized Adaptive Testing

Explain why the CAT method of testing provides a clearer picture of the candidate's competency than does the usual paper/pencil test.

A WORD ABOUT NATIONAL COUNCIL LICENSURE EXAMINATION FOR PRACTICAL NURSES REVIEW BOOKS AND NATIONAL COUNCIL LICENSURE EXAMINATION FOR PRACTICAL NURSES PREPARATION PROGRAMS

The major nursing publishing companies have developed review books based on the NCLEX-PN® format. Each review book usually includes an outline of LPN/LVN nursing content, questions with explanations and rationale, and references for the answers. Questions are intended to simulate the NCLEX-PN® format. Realize that the test questions of the NCLEX-PN® itself are highly guarded and confidential. Actual NCLEX-PN® questions are not included in any review book. Some review books provide online access with practice test questions. These resources do not simulate CAT testing, but they do provide computer experience. Silvestri's (2024) book *Comprehensive Review for the NCLEX-PN® Examination* and its companion website contain thousands of NCLEX-PN®-type questions and a comprehensive exam with a wide variety of testing formats. HESI's (2023) book *Comprehensive Review for the NCLEX-PN® Examination* and companion website include a study exam. Both resources have Next-Generation NCLEX® (NGN)-style questions.

The best preparation is to study faithfully from the beginning of the program to its conclusion, on a regular basis, until you take the NCLEX-PN®. Merely reading a review book at the end of the program without studying the nursing content throughout the program will rarely help you pass the examination. The identified outcome of a nursing program is for the graduate to learn, understand, and be able to apply basic nursing information to provide safe, quality care of clients.

Countless other vendors provide NCLEX-PN® preparation and success products, including Comprehensive Practical Nurse Predictor Examinations, which can identify your weak areas and provide an in-depth remediation plan. Most importantly, follow your school's guidelines and/or the vendor's guidelines to maximize the positive impact of the product. Purchasing the product is only the first step, integrating the product throughout your program, focusing on remediation when indicated, and avoiding "shortcuts" will prepare you very well to excel on the NCLEX-PN® and graduate as a competent practitioner. In addition, some publishers provide adaptive testing as used by the NCLEX-PN® examination. If your school's pass rates are above the state and national mean, feel confident in the products assigned and use them effectively. If NCLEX-PN® pass rates at your school are below the state and national mean, question why this is so in a professional manner and discuss what other products or strategies that your school recommends to support your NCLEX-PN® preparation. Use these experiences as additional means of preparing for your nursing licensure examination. Good luck, and keep a positive mental attitude!

Get Ready for the Next-Generation NCLEX® Examination

Key Points

- The NPA provides a foundation to guide and govern nursing practice. It exists to protect the public.
- The NPA varies from state to state, which can create some confusion regarding the LPN's scope of practice.
- It is the LPN's/LVN's responsibility to fully understand their state's NPA and educate others on the health care team if needed.
- Preparation for the NCLEX-PN® begins when the student enrolls in a nursing program.
- GPNs/GVNs (candidates) take the NCLEX-PN® to become an LPN/LVN.
- The candidate applies to the board of nursing in the state or territory where he or she wishes to be licensed.
- The candidate also must apply to the vendor (e.g., Pearson VUE) to complete the NCLEX-PN®.

- A computer administers the NCLEX-PN®, using the CAT method of testing.
- Each candidate takes a different track (path) during the CAT method of testing. The zigzag track is based on the answer to the content area and difficulty level, not the item type.
- Neither pass nor fail is related to the number of items answered by the candidate.
- The NCLEX-PN® provides all candidates ample opportunity to demonstrate minimum competency in LPN/LVN nursing knowledge, skills, and clinical judgment.
- The board of nursing to which you applied for licensure will provide results in approximately 1 month, although sometimes a LPN/LVN license posted on the SBON website within a few weeks indicates the candidate has passed the examination, even if you have not been formally notified of your examination results.
- The Next-Generation NCLEX® was implemented in 2023 and measures clinical judgment. The exam format implements different types of questions.

Additional Learning Resources

Go to your Evolve website (http://evolve.elsevier.com/Carroll/success/) for the following FREE learning resources:

- Answers to Critical Thinking Review Scenarios
- Additional learning activities
- Additional Review Questions for the NCLEX-PN® examination
- Helpful phrases for communicating in Spanish and more!

Clinical Judgment Questions

1. A group of practical/vocational nursing students are discussing how the NPA impacts their nursing practice. Which of the following statements best indicates their understanding of the NPA?

- **a.** "The Nurse Practice Act provides a foundation to guide and govern nursing practice."
- **b.** "The Nurse Practice Act provides a laundry list regarding all the tasks that an LPN is allowed to complete."
- **c.** "The Nurse Practice Act is updated every 3 years."
- **d.** "The Nurse Practice Act is the same in every state."

2. Which statement best describes how the CAT determines that a candidate has passed the NCLEX-PN®?

- **a.** The computer calculates accuracy or inaccuracy of a distracter chosen by a candidate.
- **b.** The computer subtracts the number of wrong answers from the number of right questions answers to determine the score.
- **c.** The computer makes a decision regarding minimum competency once the candidate has answered 100 questions.
- **d.** The computer continually re-estimates the candidate's ability based on previous answers and difficulty level of the question until minimal competency is determined.

3. Which statement best describes how the NCLEX-PN® is kept up to date with what LPNs/LVNs are really doing in nursing?

- **a.** Each nursing school surveys its students during the first year after graduation.
- **b.** The state board of nursing requires a work survey as a part of license renewal.
- **c.** The NCSBN sponsors a job analysis of newly licensed nurses throughout the United States.
- **d.** Each state board of nursing is required to do a work survey and submit questions.

4. A candidate attempts to access their cell phone while taking a break during the NCLEX-PN®. Which of the following is most likely to occur?

- **a.** The test center will confiscate the cell phone.
- **b.** The test administrator will ask to observe the text that was sent to ensure the candidate was not cheating.
- **c.** The test center will dismiss or cancel the testing result of the candidate.
- **d.** The candidate will return to the test area and resume testing.

5. Which of the following are required as security during the NCLEX-PN®? *(Select all that apply.)*

- **a.** Fingerprint
- **b.** Palm vein technology
- **c.** Observation
- **d.** Identification
- **e.** Signature

6. A practical/vocational nursing student has just completed the NCLEX-PN® examination. Which of the following actions are examples of this student ignoring the confidentiality statement signed prior to taking the examination? *(Select all that apply.)*

- **a.** Express relief to your family at passing the examination successfully.
- **b.** Make notes of questions you recall immediately after leaving the testing center.
- **c.** Contact your nursing program director to give her a list of questions you recall.
- **d.** Discuss the examination questions with a friend who has recently entered the PN program.
- **e.** Send examples of major content tested on the exam to current students enrolled in the nursing program.

Critical Thinking Scenarios

Scenario 1

Kar, a friend of yours in another state, is also taking a practical nursing course. You both have completed about 25% of the program. Kara has expressed concern about being prepared for the NCLEX-PN®. Kara is an average student; however, she does not see the value in completing NCLEX-type questions due to delay in taking the NCLEX-PN® for almost 1 year from now. What are you going to say to your friend?

Scenario 2

You are working for a staffing agency, and they assign you to a facility in a neighboring state. You had obtained a license 6 months ago but have never worked in this state. Describe how you will prepare for this assignment.

appendix A

Answer Key for Review Questions for the National Council Licensure Examination for Licensed Practical/Licensed Vocational Nurses (NCLEX-PN®)

CHAPTER 1

1. a
2. c
3. a
4. d
5. a, d
6. a, e

CHAPTER 2

1. d
2. b
3. a
4. a
5. d
6. b
7. a, b, c, d, e
8. a, b
9. a, d
10. Read aloud, concentrating on the words; make up "silly" rhymes or songs (mnemonic clues); listen to the words of the instructor instead of taking notes (obtain permission of the instructor and students to record the instructor).

CHAPTER 3

1. a
2. b
3. a
4. a, b, c
5. a, b, c, d, e

CHAPTER 4

1. d
2. c
3. a, b, c, d
4. b, c, d

Chapter 5

1. c
2. d
3. d
4. b
5. a, c, d, e
6. b, c, d, e

CHAPTER 6

1. c
2. a
3. a
4. b
5. a, b, d
6. True: c, e; False: a, b, d

CHAPTER 7

1. b
2. d
3. c
4. d
5. a, b, c, e
6. c, d, e
7. The nurse asked the health care provider if she could come to the unit to evaluate the client's condition. The dose was large, and the nurse repeated the order and asked if the health care provider really meant the amount stated. The health care provider became angry, insisted that the nurse immediately give the client the dosage instructed and to repeat the dose in an hour, and threatened to lodge a complaint against the nurse if she did not follow instructions.

CHAPTER 8

1. c
2. b
3. Positive Interaction: Face the resident when discussing the options for breakfast. Say, "Good morning, my name is______, I am a nursing student from_____ and I will be caring for you today." Knock on the door before entering. Not Positive Interaction: Walk in the room with great enthusiasm and say, "Hi, how are you doing?" Talk loudly in the client's left ear to be sure they hear you.
4. a, c, d
5. b, c, d

CHAPTER 9

1. d
2. b
3. c
4. a
5. a, b, c

6. Insidious on-the-job aggression: As I was talking to the health care provider, another nurse interrupted me to report on my client. I am routinely assigned the heaviest client on the unit each morning. One group of nurses is bullying the new nurse on the unit. Not insidious on-the-job aggression: When I am asked to go to lunch with someone, I explain that I am studying for my classes. A nurse is busy caring for their clients and cannot assist another nurse when requested.

CHAPTER 10

1. a
2. a
3. d
4. c
5. a, d

CHAPTER 11

1. b
2. d
3. Appropriate: Asks the client if they would like to meet with the pastoral team or their spiritual advisor. Asks the client if they would like to discuss their feelings.
   Not Appropriate: Tells the client that everything is going to be OK. Hugs the client and tells them they are safe. After the bath, stays with the client and recites a prayer that she knows.

CHAPTER 12

1. d
2. b
3. d
4. a
5. Client states they fell yesterday at home when they tripped while in the kitchen. Spouse states the client fell off a step stool in the kitchen.
   Client denies pain with movement but supports wrist gingerly, and facial grimaces are noted when attempting to move the wrist.
6. a, c, d, b, e

CHAPTER 13

1. d
2. b
3. d
4. a
5. b, a, d, c
6. a, b, c, d, e

CHAPTER 14

1. c
2. b
3. a
4. a, b, d
5. LPN/LVN: b, c, e. RN: a, b, c, d, e
6. a, b, c, d

CHAPTER 15

1. b
2. c
3. c
4. Community Health: b, c, e. Home Health: a, d
5. c, d, e
6. a, b, c, d

CHAPTER 16

1. a
2. c
3. d
4. d
5. a, c, d, e

CHAPTER 17

1. a
2. b
3. d
4. a
5. a
6. a
7. b, c, d
8. a, c, d
9. Resident B, Resident D, Resident C, Resident A

CHAPTER 18

1. c
2. c
3. a
4. a
5. a, b, c, d, e
6. a, b, c, e

CHAPTER 19

1. a
2. d
3. c
4. c
5. a, b, c, d, e
6. b, c, d, e

Glossary

A

Accountability Obligation to answer for personal actions.
Acting disinterested Showing no interest. Can be a communication block and discount the client as a person.
Active learning Taking charge of own education.
Active listener Listener who is open minded and curious and is always asking questions about content.
Active listening Hearing sounds and searching for information relevant to those sounds so the sounds may be understood.
Acute care Higher level of care required for seriously ill patients.
Adult day care center A service that provides mental stimulation, socialization, assistance with some activities of daily living (ADLs), and basic observation. Services often include transportation, meals, therapeutic activities, nursing interventions, and rehabilitation activities. The service is hospital-based or freestanding.
Advance directives Written documents to state personal wishes regarding future health care.
Affective communication Sending or receiving information through feeling tone.
Aggressive An attacking type of behavior that occurs in response to frustration and hostile feelings.
Agnostic A person who holds the belief that the existence of God can neither be proved nor disproved.
Allah Muslim name of the one supreme being; God of Islam.
Alliances New partnerships among hospitals, clinics, laboratories, health care systems, and physicians. They coordinate the delivery of care, contain costs, and attempt to provide a seamless system.
Ambulatory care facilities Primary health care services for walk-in patients. Also known as Urgent Care, Express Care, and Quick Care.
Ambulatory surgery centers One-day surgery centers that perform surgery at a scheduled date and time. Patient discharged home when recovered from surgery and is stable.
Analysis Break down complex information into its basic parts and relate it to the whole picture.
Application Use learned information in new situations.
Apps Abbreviation for applications; programs that can be stored on an electronic device.
Artificial Intelligence or AI A branch of computer science dealing with the simulation of intelligent human behaviors by computers
Assault An unjustified attempt or threat to touch someone.
Assertiveness A way of accepting responsibility for oneself by expressing thoughts and feelings directly and honestly, without blaming oneself or others.
Assigning (assignment) Allotting tasks that are in the job description of workers. Assigned tasks are the ones that workers are hired and paid to perform.
Assimilation Giving up parts of your own culture and adopting parts of the culture of the dominant group.
Assisted care Residences that provide "a home with services."
Assisting Licensed practical nurse/licensed vocational nurse (LPN/LVN) role in four phases (steps) of nursing process.
Associate degree nursing (ADN) program A 2-year community college or technical school program. The title registered nurse (RN) is used after passing the National Council Licensure Examination-Registered Nurse (NCLEX-RN®).
Atheist A person who does not believe the supernatural exists and therefore does not believe in God.
Attitude Nonverbal expression of the way a person thinks or feels.
Auditory learner Talks to himself or herself or hears sounds when thinking. Learns best by hearing.
Authorization to test (ATT) Denotes that the graduate practical/vocational nurse has met the requirements for eligibility to take the National Council Licensure Examination-Registered Nurse (NCLEX-RN®). ATT applied for and obtained from the testing center.
Authorized consent Parents cannot give informed consent for medical care of a child but can give authorized consent instead.
Autocratic leadership A purely task-centered leadership style that thrives on power.
Automatic responses Both passive and aggressive responses result from being caught by an emotional hook. These responses are not based on choice.
Autonomy Control over personal decisions.

B

Bachelor of Science in Nursing (BSN) program A 4-year college program to prepare graduates for nursing and leadership roles.
Barton, Clara Founder of the American Red Cross.
Basic client situation Patient's clinical condition is predictable. Medical and nursing orders are not changing continuously. No complex modifications of nursing care are needed.
Battery Causing acute physical harm to someone.
Belittling Mimicking or making fun of a person in some way.
Beneficence Doing good.
Beneficent paternalism Health care provider making decisions for the patient based on "I know what's best for you." Discounts patient autonomy.
Biomedicine Belief that abnormalities in structure and function of body organs are caused by pathogens, biochemical alterations, and/or environmental factors.

Blended course A course that combines face-to-face instruction with online learning.
Board and care homes Offer housing and custodial care. Also known as adult care homes or group homes.
Bodily/kinesthetic learner Learns best by touching, moving, and processing knowledge through bodily sensations.
Breach of duty One of the elements needed to prove negligence; means that the nurse did not adhere to standards of care.
Bucket theory Suggests that merely by lecturing, the teacher can transfer knowledge from the teacher's mind to the student's mind.
Buddha The enlightened one; Siddhartha Gautama, founder of Buddhism.
Bullying Negative acts perpetrated by one at a higher level.

C

Cadet Nurse Corps 1943 Bolton Act was the basis of the government subsidizing schools to teach nursing skills in 2 1/2 years. More than 150,000 nurses graduated from these programs. Discontinued in 1948.
Call number Series of letters and numbers used to identify library materials and assist in locating materials.
Candidate Graduate practical/vocational nurse who will take (or is taking) the National Council Licensure Examination-Registered Nurse (NCLEX-RN®).
Capability Ability or capacity.
Case management method Focus is on quality, service, and cost.
Case method A method of patient care in which one nurse is assigned to give total care to one patient.
Case scenarios A printed or computer patient story that brings reality to theory in the form of a clinical situation.
Centers for Medicare and Medicaid Services (CMS) Formerly Health Care Financing Administration (HCFA). Federal agency of Department of Health and Human Services. Certifies nursing homes for Medicare and Medicaid reimbursement.
Certification Certificate awarded to a registered nurse (RN) or licensed practical nurse/licensed vocational nurse (LPN/LVN) after passing a comprehensive examination in a select area of practice.
Certification in Long-Term Care (CLTC) Postgraduate course offered by the National Association of Practical Nurse Education and Service (NAPNES). Replaces previous gerontology certification. Recertification is every 5 years.
Certification in Managed Care Nursing Postgraduate course including basic knowledge of managed care, health care economics, health care management, and patient issues.
Certification in Pharmacology (NCP) Postgraduate course offered by the National Association of Practical Nurse Education and Service (NAPNES). Recertification is every 5 years.
Certified nursing assistant Minimum 75-hour course prepares nursing assistant to give bedside care. Successful completion of a national exam makes Certified Nursing Assistant (CNA) eligible for state registry.
Change-of-shift report Report on patient condition at beginning and end of shift.
Choice Act of choosing. For example, to speak assertively is to speak out of choice.
Civil action (related to individual rights) Involves the relationships between individuals and the violation of those rights.
Clark, Mildred L. Chief of Army Nurse Corps from 1963 to 1967.
Client outcomes Focus on whether patient has accomplished what was desired during treatment. Does not focus on what the nurse did.
Client-centered care Another name for patient-centered care, which is nursing care that is specific to the individual client's/patient's needs.
Client competency Relates to ability to understand and make decisions. Has both legal and clinical meaning.
Clinical judgment The process the nurse uses to decide to collect and interpret data about a client and act/not act on the interpretation. The process involves critical thinking, problem solving, and decision making.
Clinical pathway Blueprint for patient care. Includes time frame of significant events that are expected to occur each day a patient with a specific diagnosis is in the hospital.
Closed-ended questions Questions that require specific answers from a patient.
Clustering A form of mapping is a method of note-making.
Cognitive level Intellectual level of functioning.
Coinsurance Percentage of total bill paid for by insurance company once deductible is paid.
Commitment Pledge to do one's best.
Common law Judge-made law, which has its origins in the courts.
Communication blocks Stops meaningful conversation. Examples include chiding, belittling, probing, giving advice, and providing pat answers.
Community health nursing Nursing that focuses on improving the health status of communities or groups of people through public education, screening for early detection of disease, and providing services for people who need care outside the acute care setting.
Community resources Include a diverse group of people, organizations, and facilities (in-person and virtual) that assist community members in achieving their personal and professional goals. This includes social service, educational, health, workforce, and professional-related services.
Compensation Coping mechanism used to cover for real or imagined inadequacy by developing or exaggerating a desirable trait.
Complementary and alternative medicine (CAM) Focus is on assisting the body's own healing powers and restoring body balance.
Complex nursing situation Patient's clinical condition is not predictable. Medical and nursing orders are likely to involve continuous changes or complex modifications.
Comprehension Basically understand information, recall it, and identify examples of that information.
Computer simulation Learning activities on a CD-ROM or floppy disc that use an imaginary patient situation. The student uses the nursing process as he or she would in an actual clinical situation.
Computer-aided instruction An increasingly used teaching strategy in nursing education.
Computerized adaptive testing (CAT) Method by which the National Council Licensure Examination for Licensed Practical

Nurses (NCLEX-PN®) examination is administered to the candidate (a nursing graduate who has fulfilled requirements for testing).

Conditional job offer Job offer contingent on passing physical, drug screening, and/or background check.

Confidentiality Avoid sharing patient information with anyone not directly involved in care without the patient's permission.

Confidentiality agreement Before taking the National Council Licensure Examination for Licensed Practical Nurses (NCLEX-PN®) examination, read and sign agreement not to disclose contents of examination.

Conflict resolution A method of resolving differences in a peaceful way.

Constructive evaluation Critique directed toward performance and behavior; has no bearing on one's value as a person.

Continued competency The ability of a nurse to maintain, update, and demonstrate sufficient knowledge, skills, judgement, and qualifications necessary to practice safely and ethically in a designated role and setting in accordance with the scope of nursing practice

Continuing care retirement community Provides a continuum living option from independent living, assisted living, and skilled nursing home, all on one campus.

Continuous quality improvements (CQIs) Search for new ways to improve patient care, prevent errors, and identify and fix problems.

Continuum A way to look at two extremes (from least complex to most complex).

Cooperative learning Emphasis on individual accountability for learning a specific academic task while working in small groups.

Copayment Percentage of the bill that is paid by a person (subscriber) who is enrolled in a health insurance plan.

Copyright laws These laws permit a single copy of an article for personal use. Instructors may not make copies of articles, chapters, or books for distribution to each student.

Cost containment Holding costs within fixed limits.

Course outlines Up-to-date listings of what is covered in a course. Provided by the instructor.

Criminal action Involves persons and society as a whole, for example, murder.

Critical thinking Used to resolve problems and find ways to make improvements, even when no problem exists.

Cultural bias Unquestioned, unproved way of thinking.

Cultural competence The continuous attempt of licensed practical nurses/licensed vocational nurses to gain the knowledge and skills that will allow them to effectively provide care for patients of different cultures.

Cultural diversity Differences in elements of culture in groups of people.

Cultural sensitivity Learning about other cultures and being respectful of their customs, rites, and beliefs.

Culture The total of all the ideas, beliefs, values, attitudes, communication, customs, traditions, and objects that a group of people possess. Culture includes ways of doing things.

Customs Ways of doing things that are common to a group of people of the same culture.

D

Damages One of four elements needed to prove negligence. Patient must be able to show the nurse's negligent act injured the patient in some way.

Data collection Phase 1 of nursing process for practical/vocational nurses. Involves systematic gathering and reviewing of information about the patient.

Deductible Amount the subscriber must pay before health insurance begins to cover costs.

Defamation Damage to someone's reputation through false communication or communication without permission.

Delano, Jane Of the American Red Cross and who began to recruit and train nurses for overseas duty in World War I.

Delegated medical act Physician's orders given to a registered nurse (RN), licensed practical nurse (LPN), or licensed vocational nurse (LVN) by a physician, dentist, or podiatrist.

Delegating Generally, duties within the licensed practical nurse/licensed vocational nurse (LPN/LVN) job description that can be given to another worker to perform.

Denial Coping mechanism that includes rejection of events as they really are. Eliminates need for anxiety.

Dependent role The licensed practical nurse/licensed vocational nurse (LPN/LVN) functions with supervision in a dependent role to the registered nurse (RN), physician, or dentist.

Depositions Gathering information under oath. One of the steps in bringing legal action.

Desired Client Outcome Observable result. Focuses directly on what the patient will accomplish (not what the nurse will do).

Diagnosis-related group (DRG) Prospective payment system. Specifies number of days for which Medicare will pay, based on illness category.

Diploma program A 3-year nursing educational program conducted by a hospital-based school of nursing.

Direct supervision Supervisor is continuously present to coordinate, direct, or inspect nursing care. Supervisor is in building.

Directed (or focused) thinking Purposeful and outcome-oriented thinking. Focuses on particular problem to find solution.

Discrimination Rights and privileges are withheld from those of another cultural group.

Discussion buddy Another student with whom you discuss a topic to comprehend the information.

Distance learning A course in which the teacher and student are separated by physical distance, using such tools as two-way television, videotapes, audiotapes, and the Internet.

Distracters Incorrect options for multiple-choice items.

Dix, Dorothea Lynde Appointed Superintendent of Nurses during the American Civil War to organize a corps of nurses to tend to wounded soldiers.

Do-not-resuscitate (DNR) Order written by physician. Patient will not recover. Patient may have signed an advance directive regarding end-of-life care that states personal wishes.

Durable medical power of attorney Identifies who will make decisions regarding future care, extent of treatment, and kinds of treatment if the person is unable to make his or her own decisions. Written while the person is mentally competent.

Duty One of four elements needed to prove negligence. Refers to nurse's responsibility to provide care in an acceptable way. As used in the text, responsibilities directly related to nursing licensure and scope of practice. Usually not delegated to someone with less education and nursing skill.

E

Electronic device Smartphone (BlackBerry, Android, iPhone), notebook, tablet, laptop, computer.
Electronic Health Record (EHR) Computerized charting system utilized by the healthcare team across healthcare settings.
Electronic simulation Uses mannequins that are high-tech, more costly simulation models that can be programmed to set up different patient situations and allow practice of nursing procedures and data collection (assessment).
Emotional needs How people respond and deal with feelings of joy, anger, sadness, guilt, remorse, sorrow, love, etc.
Empathy Respectful, detached concern.
Enculturation Process of learning your culture: the way your group does things, resulting in a worldview.
End-of-life principles Support core principles for end-of-life care.
Endorsement Agreement among states that nurses licensed in one state may become licensed in another if they meet the state nursing board criteria.
Entitlement program Those eligible because of age, disability, or economic status are entitled by law to benefits of certain programs, namely, Social Security, Medicare, and Medicaid.
Ethics Rules or principles that govern correct conduct.
Ethnic groups Cultural groups composed of people who are members of the same race, religion, or nation, or who speak the same language.
Ethnocentrism The belief that one's own culture is best; the belief that one's way of doing things is superior/right/best.
Euthanasia Physician or other person administering lethal dose of medication to end life; illegal in the United States and Canada.
Evaluation Phase 4 of nursing process for licensed practical nurses/licensed vocational nurses (LPNs/LVNs). Compares actual patient outcomes to expected outcomes.
Evidence-based practice Nursing procedures/interventions that have been proven to be effective.
External distractions Interruptions in concentration from outside oneself, such as background sounds, lighting, peers, and so forth.

F

Facilitator Instructor who creates a learning environment by arranging for a variety of activities and experiences.
False reassurance Promising patient something you cannot deliver, such as saying, "You'll be just fine."
Feedback Response to sender's message as a part of meaningful conversation.
Fee-for-service Patient pays the physician a fee for each service provided.
Felony Serious offense, with a penalty that ranges from 1 year in prison to death.
Fidelity In nursing, to be faithful to the charge of acting in the patient's best interest when the capacity to make free choice is no longer available.
First Amendment Guarantees freedom of expression as long as it is not at the expense of harming others.
Focused questions Questions that require definitive, precise information from a patient.
Follow-up illusion Irrational belief that it is the employer's responsibility to contact applicants after an interview.
Formal education Planned, organized learning, such as the nursing course of study.
Free clinic Used by persons who cannot afford traditional health care. May have an age and income range. The clinic charges a minimal fee.
Freestanding Health facility not attached to a hospital.
Functional method A method of patient care that is task oriented and involves dividing the tasks to be done among staff members according to their abilities.

G

General hospitals Set up to treat a variety of medical/surgical problems.
General (implied) consent By entering a health facility voluntarily, a patient gives permission for treatment with noninvasive procedures. However, a patient may revoke this consent verbally and refuse to be treated.
General supervision Supervisor regularly coordinates, directs, or inspects nursing care and is within reach either in the building or by phone.
Generalization Broad, sweeping statements made about a group.
Generational personality Personality of people born around the same period of time and shaped by a common history of cultural events, images, and experiences.
Giving advice Telling someone what to do.
Goals (outcomes) Realistic, measurable, time-limited statements of resolution of a problem or need.
Good Samaritan act Stipulates that a person who provides emergency care at the scene of an accident is immune from civil liability for actions done in good faith. There is some variation of the law within states.
Goodacres, Glenna Designed and sculpted Vietnam Women's Memorial. Located on the National Mall in Washington, DC.
Goodrich, Anna Helped form the National Emergency Committee on Nursing during World War I.
Gretter, Lystra Modified the Hippocratic Oath in 1893 and named it The Nightingale Pledge.
Guest speakers Nurses or other health professionals invited to present up-to-date information on areas of expertise.

H

Hays, Colonel Anna Mae Led Army Nurse Corps during the Vietnam War. First woman to become a brigadier general and first woman in American military to attain general officer rank.
Healthcare Provider A licensed health care person, such as a physician, dentist, or nurse practitioner, whose health care services are covered by a health insurance plan.
Health Insurance Portability and Accountability Act (HIPAA) 2003 Federal law commonly called the Privacy Act.
Health maintenance organization (HMO) A comprehensive care system of medical services based on a set, prepaid fee.
Health and Medicine Division of the National Academies (HMD) A federal agency that promotes health policies.
Hidden job market Unadvertised jobs.
Higbee, Lenah S. World War I Navy nurse. Received the Navy Cross. Was the first nurse to have a warship named in her honor.

Home health nursing Provides health services supervised by a licensed professional in a patient's home. Examples include visiting nurse associations, health departments, home health agencies, etc.

Honesty To not deliberately deceive to present oneself in a better light.

Hospice care End-of-life care for the terminally ill. The philosophy is to maintain comfort as death approaches.

Howlett hierarchy Hierarchy of work motivators. Adapted from Maslow's hierarchy of needs.

Humor Communication characteristic to help "lighten up" a situation.

I

"I" messages Statements that start with the word, "I" to reduce a defensive response from others.

Idea sketches Representing a verbal concept with a picture.

Illegal questions Interview questions that do not have to be answered, such as age, marital status, number of children, and health problems, unless directly related to job.

Implementation Phase 3 of the nursing process for licensed practical nurses/licensed vocational nurses (LPNs/LVNs). Provides required nursing care to accomplish established patient goals.

Incivility Hostility among healthcare workers that risks unsafe care to clients.

Independent Function without supervision, for example, the registered nurse (RN) role in the nursing process.

Informational interview By appointment, meet with an administrator to learn about a facility. This is not a job interview, although it is treated with the same courtesy.

Informed consent Obtained by physician for invasive procedures after physician has provided patient with facts about effects, side effects, alternative treatments, prognosis, and so on. May be revoked verbally at any time up to time of procedure.

Insidious aggression Hostile behavior in the workplace that is not obvious to others.

Institute of Medicine (IOM) An independent, nonprofit organization that advises the public and decision-makers with ways to improve health.

Institutional liability Form of vicarious liability. Health setting sued for negligence of employee.

Intentional tort Intent to do a wrongful act.

Interdependent Both registered nurses (RNs) and licensed practical nurses/licensed vocational nurses (LPNs/LVNs) collaboratively carry out orders for treatments and medications written by a physician.

Interlibrary loan services Allow libraries to borrow materials from other libraries that are not a part of their holdings.

Internal distractions Interruptions in concentration from inside oneself, such as daydreaming and boredom.

Internet Physical infrastructure that allows the electronic circulation of vast amounts of information to computer users. This information is unregulated and cannot always be taken at face value.

Interpersonal learner Learns best by sharing, comparing, cooperating, and interviewing.

Interpersonal styles Four major styles: analytical type, driver type, amicable type, and expressive type.

Interstate endorsement Agreement among states that licensed nurses do not have to repeat the National Council Licensure Examination for Licensed Practical Nurses (NCLEX-PN®) examination if they meet criteria for working in the state.

Intervention Action taken to reach a patient outcome.

Intrapersonal learner Learns best by working alone, self-paced instruction, and having own space.

Intravenous Therapy Certification (IVC) Postgraduate education on intravenous therapy, offered through the National Federation of Licensed Professional Nurses (NFLPN) and National Association for Practical Nurse Education and Service (NAPNES).

Irrational thinking Based on Ellis (1994). Self-talk is often irrational thinking: Judgments are subjective and have no bearing on facts. Leads to negative emotions and stress.

ISBARR A method of clear communication between nurses and providers: I, identify; S, situation; B, background; A, assessment; R, recommendation; R, repeat back.

J

Jesus Christ Founder of Christian religion.

Judging Arriving at an opinion based on some evidence. Can be a communication block, particularly if judging is perceived as "thinking less" of the person.

Justice Giving patients their due and treating them fairly.

K

Key Correct option(s) for a multiple-choice or alternate item format question.

Kinesthetic/tactual learner Has two sub channels: movement and touch.

Kinkela-Keil, Captain Lillian Member of the Air Force Nurse Corps. Flew over 200 air evacuation missions during World War II, as well as 25 trans-Atlantic crossings. Went back to civilian flying until the Korean War. Flew several hundred more missions as a flight nurse in Korea. Numerous decorations. Inspiration for the movie *Flight Nurse*.

Knowledge Repeats information exactly as read or told. Does not imply an understanding of the information.

L

Lateral violence Between nursing colleagues. Includes both overt and covert physical, verbal, and emotional abuse by one nurse against another.

Law Nursing law is based on each state's Nurse Practice Act.

Leadership Manner in which the leader gets along with coworkers, with the goal of producing workplace changes to meet the goals of the employing agency.

Learner One who acquires knowledge and skills.

Learning Management System (LMS) Electronic platform such as Moodle, Blackboard, and Angel where resources are housed.

Learning resource center (LRC) The library.

Lecture-discussion strategy A strategy in which the instructor shares several ideas with the class and then stops to let the class discuss the ideas.

Left-brain dominant A person who is more orderly, is logical, reads and writes well, and excels at analytical thinking. Also called *linear thinkers*.

Leininger's Culture Care Theory Recognition of the link between a person's cultural background and his or her response to nursing care.
Libel Damage to someone's reputation through written communication or pictures.
Licensed Practical/Vocational Nurse (LPN/LVN) A member of the nursing team who assists the registered nurse with nursing care of clients.
Linguistic learner Learns best by saying, hearing, and seeing words.
Living will Written directive stating personal wishes regarding future health care. Not recognized as a legal document in every state or other countries.
Logical learner Learns best by using an organized method of study.
Long-term acute care Transitional medical care between critical care and rehabilitation.
Long-term care Range of medical care to assist persons with disability or chronic care needs.

M

Malpractice (professional negligence) A part of negligence that relates to lack of skill or misconduct by professional persons.
Managed care A system of controlling cost of health care by arranging health care at predetermined rates. A health maintenance organization (HMO) is an example of managed care.
Managed Care Organization (MCO) An organization that controls the costs of health care by arranging health care at predetermined rates.
Management Organizing all care required for patients in a health care setting for a specific period.
Manipulation An indirect way of dealing with issues that may be positive or negative. Negative (maladaptive) manipulation occurs if the feelings of others are disregarded or other people are treated as objects.
Mapping A form of note making in which information and its relationships are put in a visual pattern.
Maslow's human needs theory A way to look at identifying patient care priorities and responding to the patient's needs according to the patient's level of functioning.
Medicaid Financial assistance provided by the federal government for states and counties to pay for medical services for eligible poor.
Medicare Federally sponsored and supervised health insurance plan for persons 65 years of age and older and persons under 65 years who are totally and permanently disabled.
Medicare Quality Improvement Organizations (QIOs) Formerly known as peer review organizations. Under the direction of Centers for Medicare and Medicaid Services.
Melting pot The United States became known as the "melting pot" in the 19th century, when immigrants would assimilate into the dominant culture.
Mental imagery Uses the right side of the brain to generate pictures of an idea; the left side supplies the script.
Message The idea being conveyed or the question being asked.
Misdemeanor Least serious infraction of the law, except for a summary offense. Can result in a fine or up to 1 year in jail.
Mission statement A statement that defines the purpose and goals of a health care organization.
Mnemonic devices Memory aids such as rhymes or acronyms.
Mobile device PDA, smartphone (iPhone, BlackBerry), iPod Touch, e-book reader, and tablet.
Mobility program Seamless program of study from certified nursing assistant (CNA) to licensed practical nurse/licensed vocational nurse (LPN/LVN) to associate degree registered nurse (RN) to Bachelor of Science in Nursing (BSN) to Master of Science in Nursing (MSN) to Doctorate Degree in Nursing.
Morals Dealing with right and wrong behavior.
Multistate licensure (Nursing Licensure Compact) Legislation in some states that renders a nursing license obtained in that state valid for practice in other states with multistate legislation. Each state's individual regulations must still be followed.
Musical learner Learns best by humming, singing, or playing an instrument.

N

NANDA-I North American Nursing Diagnosis Association.
NAPNES National Association for Practical Nurse Education and Service, Inc.
National Certification in Gerontology Postgraduate NFLPN program leading to certification in gerontology.
National Certification in Intravenous Therapy Postgraduate course through National Association for Practical Nurse Education and Service (NAPNES).
National Patient Safety Foundation (NPSF) An organization that aims to improve safety in health care.
Naturalistic system Beliefs developed from the traditional medical practices of the ancient civilizations of China, India, and Greece.
NCLEX-PN® examination National Council Licensing Examination for Practical Nursing.
NCSBN National Council of State Boards of Nursing
NCSBN Clinical Judgment Model A framework created by the NCSBN to assist nurses in making sound clinical judgment when caring for clients.
Negligence Conduct that falls below the standard of care established by law for the protection of others.
Networking Building relationships with instructors, employers, and peers for the purposes of finding new jobs, better pay, faster promotions, and greater job satisfaction.
NFLPN National Federation of Licensed Practical Nurses
NGN Next-Generation NCLEX®
NIC Nursing Interventions Classification
Nightingale, Florence Founder of modern nursing who is known as "The Lady with the Lamp" because of her after-hours rounds with her lamp during the Crimean War.
NLN National League for Nursing.
NOC Nursing Outcomes Classification.
Nonassertive (passive) Fear-based, emotionally dishonest, self-defeating type of behavior. Gives message of "I don't count, but you count."
Nonjudgmental Taking at face value. Accepting people as they are.
Nonmaleficence First, do no harm.
Nonprofit community hospital Nonprofit hospital operated by community association or religious organization.
Nonverbal communication Sending or receiving information by facial expressions or body language.

Notes on Nursing Written by Florence Nightingale.
Nurse Practice Act Governs the practice of nursing.
Nursing Case Management Focuses on achieving client outcomes in the acute care setting by using tools, such as clinical pathways.
Nursing diagnosis Second step of the nursing process for registered nurses (RNs): Actual and high-risk problems that nurses can respond to. Exclusive responsibility of RN in nursing process.
Nursing ethics System of principles governing conduct of nurses.
Nursing Interventions Actions nurses take to assist clients in reaching their desired outcomes.
Nursing manager A registered nurse (RN) who has graduated from a baccalaureate nursing program (4-year) and is enrolled in a Master of Science in Nursing (MSN) program.
Nursing organizations Groups for nurses focused on nursing issues of importance.
Nursing process An orderly way of developing a plan of care for the individual patient. The registered nurse (RN) is responsible for developing the nursing diagnosis.
Nursing research An organized way of finding information that supports existing knowledge and develops new knowledge for clinical practice, nursing education, and nursing services.
Nursing skills lab Resource that allows student nurses to practice and develop nursing skills.
Nursing standard of care Guideline for good nursing care. Standards are based on what an ordinary, prudent nurse with similar education and nursing experience would do in a similar situation.
Nursing theories Often used as a basis for developing nursing curricula.
Nutting, Adelaide Helped form the National Emergency Committee on Nursing during World War I.

O

Objective information Data that can be observed and verified. Data obtained by seeing, hearing, touching, smelling, tasting, measuring, counting, and so on. Does not include subjective judgment.
Official (government) health care agencies Local, state, and federal health agencies supported by tax dollars.
Omnibus Reconciliation Act of 1987 (OBRA) Major federal legislation that addresses the quality of life, health, and safety of residents.
One-way communication When the sender controls a situation and offers no opportunity for feedback from the receiver; used to give a command.
Online catalog Computerized card catalog in the library.
Open-ended questions Questions that permit the patient to respond in a way most meaningful to him or her. These type of questions often begin with what, where, when.
Options Choices; for example, choices for an answer in a multiple-choice item.
Oregon Death with Dignity Act Allows terminally ill Oregonians to end their lives through voluntary self-administration of lethal medication.
Orem's Self-Care Deficit Theory This nursing theory has three subtheories: self-care, self-care deficit, and the nursing system. Nursing data collection can be used to identify the particular deficit to choose interventions that will have the desired outcomes for the patient.
Outcome Identifies the degree of progress made (or not made) by the patient toward reaching a goal.
Outpatient clinic Provides health care outside of the hospital setting. Staffed by physicians and nurses.

P

Palliative care According to the World Health Organization (WHO; www.who.int/cancer/palliative/definition/en/), an approach that improves the quality of life of patients and their families facing the problem associated with life-threatening illness, through the prevention and relief of suffering by means of early identification and impeccable assessment, and treatment of pain and other problems, physical, psychosocial, and spiritual.
Paradigm A way of thinking.
Parish nurse Works in various church settings in a health ministry.
Passive listener A person who receives sounds with little recognition or personal involvement.
Pastoral care team Members of the health team who assist nurses in meeting the spiritual needs of the patients.
Patience Willingness to put up with waiting and being okay about doing so.
Patient Self-Determination Act (PSDA) Basis for advanced directives. Federal law mandates that Medicare and Medicaid patients must be told of their right to formulate advance directives.
Peer-reviewed Information reviewed by others in a subject for accuracy, quality, and appropriateness.
Peplau's Interpersonal Relations Theory Basis for developing a therapeutic relationship with a patient (especially useful for working with adult or child psychiatric patients). The relationship has certain parameters that are a major part of the treatment. The overlapping phases are orientation, identification, exploitation, and resolution.
Perceptual learning style Refers to learning by three main sensory receivers: visual, auditory, and kinesthetic.
Performance evaluation Evaluation of clinical performance that involves input from the instructor and the student.
Periodical indexes List of periodicals by author, title, and subject.
Periodicals Magazines published weekly, monthly, and quarterly.
Personal ethics Provide personal guidelines for living.
Personal liability Holds person (nurse) responsible for own actions.
Personalistic system Belief that a deity, ghost, god, evil spirit, witch, or angry ancestor is punishing the sick person.
Physician-assisted suicide Name tagged onto "Oregon Death with Dignity Law." Physician writes prescription for medication to end life but does not administer it. Patient self-administers lethal medication.
Planning Phase 2 of the nursing process for licensed practical nurses/licensed vocational nurses (LPNs/LVNs). Involves collaborating with the registered nurse (RN) in development of the nursing diagnosis, goals, and interventions for the patient's plan of care and maintaining patient safety.
Podcast A digital audio/visual recording of information on the Internet that can be downloaded to a personal media player or a computer.

Positive mental attitude Expectation to succeed combined with hard work.

Practical/vocational nurse A person who performs, for compensation, any basic acts in the care of convalescent, subacutely, or chronically ill, injured, or infirm persons, or any act or procedure in the care of the acutely ill, injured, or infirm under the specific direction of a registered nurse, physician, podiatrist, or dentist.

Preceptor An experienced nurse who guides a newly licensed nurse or senior nursing student to adjust/learn how to "tie it all together" in the first job.

Preferred provider organizations (PPOs) Similar to health maintenance organizations (HMOs), except that physicians maintain their own practice and continue to be part of their own physician group. Part of the day is spent treating patients enrolled in a PPO.

Prejudice The opinion that a person has about something, even though facts dispute the opinion.

Premium Monthly fee a subscriber must pay for health care insurance coverage.

Preponderance Evidence that is beyond a reasonable doubt.

Primary care The point at which a person enters the health care system.

Primary Care Method RNs provide total client care without the use of supportive nursing staff.

Privacy Both a legal and ethical issue. Patient's right to choose what is done to his or her body, based on personal beliefs, feelings, and attitude.

Private health care agencies Agencies that are generally proprietary (for profit) and that charge a fee for service. The primary focus is curing illness.

Private pay The patient pays out of pocket for services received.

Probing Pushing for information beyond what is medically necessary to know.

Problem solving A series of steps used to solve problems long before the nursing process was developed.

Problem-oriented thinking Focus on a particular problem to find a solution (e.g., planning your school, work, and home schedule).

Projection A coping or mental mechanism in which an individual attributes his or her own weaknesses to others.

Proprietary hospitals (for profit) For-profit hospitals.

Prospective payment system (PPS) A system in which the federal government announces to a hospital in advance what it will pay for health care costs.

Proximate cause One of four elements needed to prove negligence. Refers to reasonable cause-and-effect relationship between omission and commission of nursing act and harm to patient.

Public Healthcare agencies Made up of official and voluntary health care agencies.

Purpose Reason.

Q

Qualitative research study Subjective study that gathers data as a narrative description of the "lived experience" of individuals.

Quantitative research study Objective study that collects numerical data that are measured using statistics. Establishes a cause–effect relationship.

R

Rationalization A coping or mental mechanism in which the individual offers a logical but untrue reason as an excuse for his or her behavior.

Receiver Person receiving the message, idea, or question.

Reference hierarchy Ranking of references from best to least by employers: current and former supervisors from work and volunteer experiences, unit managers, and teachers; workers who have seen your work; and personal references or friends.

Reference materials Includes medical and nursing dictionaries, almanacs, yearbooks, atlases, encyclopedias, handbooks, and so on. Generally cannot be checked out, but needed material can be copied.

Referral Send or direct for help.

Reflective thinking Thinking about what you are thinking about.

Registered nurse (RN) A member of the nursing team who has gone to nursing school for 2, 3, or 4 years and has passed the National Council Licensure Examination-Registered Nurse (NCLEX-RN®) to be registered. The person on the nursing team who functions independently in decision-making regarding the nursing care of patients.

Rehabilitation After acute care is completed, treatment may continue to bring person up to maximum functioning.

Reincarnation Belief in rebirth of the soul in many bodies as many times as necessary to achieve enlightenment.

Religion Attempts to give form to spiritual beliefs by adopting specific beliefs and rituals.

Religious denomination An organized group of persons with a philosophy that supports their particular concept of God.

Residency Further "training" in nursing after initial schooling and licensure.

Residential care Broadly defined as 24-hour supervision of persons, for reasons of age or impairments. Falls between skilled care and intermediate care facilities.

Resignation courtesy A 2-week notice of ending employment is considered courteous even if not part of the contract.

Respect Consideration, regard.

Restructuring Changing something that is not working out as planned.

Resume Summary of what you have accomplished; work, skills, education, experience, and sometimes personal achievements. Used to persuade an employer that you are the right person for the job. Limit to one or two pages.

Returning adult learner A learner in the age bracket of the mid-20s or older who has entered an educational program and has not experienced formal education for a period of time.

Right-brain dominant This person shows more advanced spatial relationships, recognizes negative emotions more quickly, is less verbal, adds tone and inflection to voice, and sees the total picture. Also called *global thinkers*.

Rituals Religious practices that affirm believers' connection to a higher power.

Rosenstock's health belief theory Attempts to explain why a person will or will not seek help to prevent or detect illness.

S

SBAR A method of clear communication between nurses and physicians. S, situation; B, background; A, assessment; and R, recommendation.

Scope of practice What the nurse is able to do legally.

Seacole, Mary Nurse from Jamaica, West Indies. Helped Florence Nightingale during the Crimean War. Used knowledge of tropical medicine, herbs, and natural plant medicines to treat soldiers with cholera, yellow fever, malaria, and diarrhea.

"Seamless" nursing systems Provide progressive nursing programs without the need to repeat courses as the person goes from certified nursing assistant (CNA) to licensed practical nurse/licensed vocational nurse (LPN/LVN) to associate degree registered nurse (RN) to Bachelor of Science in Nursing (BSN) to Master of Science in Nursing (MSN) to Doctorate Degree in Nursing degrees; provide ease of movement from one nursing education program to another.

Self-directed learner Takes responsibility for own learning and performance.

Self-efficacy Self-confidence, the special sense that a person can perform an action.

Self-esteem Special sense that it is okay to receive credit for something you did well.

Self-evaluation Objective look at personal performance with a plan for improvement.

Sender Person conveying an idea or asking a question.

Sensitivity Awareness of what others are feeling. Tunes in on affective and nonverbal communication.

Sexual harassment A form of assault. Abuse of power. Not about sex or passion.

Silence Avoid filling the interviewer's void of silence by providing information beyond what is needed.

Simple answers General responses. Can be a communication block and discount the patient as a person.

Simulation A learning activity that uses imaginary patient situations and mimics the reality of the clinical environment.

Sister Callista Roy's adaptation model Describes the patient as a holistic adaptive system influenced by both internal and external stimuli.

Situational leadership Varying the leadership style to meet the demands of the situation in the work environment.

Skill mix Health care staff made up of workers with different levels of education and training.

Skilled nursing facility (SNF) Patients with more serious problems need a higher level of care by skilled and well-trained staff.

Slander Damage to someone's reputation by verbalizing untrue or confidential information.

Social media Ways of using the Internet for interactive dialogue, such as Facebook, Twitter, and LinkedIn.

Social networking Gathering of individuals to share information; specifically used in this book as online communities.

Spatial learner Learns best by studying diagrams, boxes, and special lists.

Specialized hospital Offer services related to a particular disease or condition.

Spirit Life force that penetrates the person's entire body. Gives meaning to life.

Spirit of inquiry Trait of licensed practical nurses/licensed vocational nurses (LPNs/LVNs) that challenges traditional and existing practices and seeks creative approaches to problems.

Spiritual caring Recognize and support spiritual need of the patient in the health care setting.

Spiritual dimension That which gives insight into the person's meaning of life, suffering, and death.

Spiritual distress Observed in patients who are unable to practice their rituals or seen in those who experience conflict between their religious or spiritual beliefs and prescribed medical regimen.

Spiritual needs Requirements that arise out of the desire of human beings to find meaning in life, suffering, and death.

Spirituality Pertaining to the soul, one's life force.

Stacks Place in library where material that can be checked out is located.

Standards of care What a prudent nurse is expected to do.

State board of nursing Develops and enforces nurse practice act, which is the basis for nursing law. There is some variation among states.

Static simulation Simulation that uses full-size body models or models of specific parts of the body made to be realistic.

Statutory law Law developed by the legislative branch of state and federal governments.

Stem First line of a multiple-choice item.

Stereotype Casting all people in a culture as being the same in regard to thinking, feeling, and acting.

Stress management Maintenance of stress at a moderate level. The reaction to both high and low levels of stress may be overwhelming.

Student nurse Person involved in a course of study to become a nurse.

Study group Peers who are actively involved in understanding information by discussing it in a small group.

Study skills lab A place where schools provide services to assist a student with academic problems.

Subjective information Information based on a patient's opinion.

Syllabus Up-to-date course document distributed at the beginning of a course. This document usually includes a course description, course objectives, course requirements, required text, grading scale, and instructor information.

T

Taxonomy Standardized, orderly, systematic language (example, NANDA-I).

Teaching Originally thought of as lecturing to students. All responsibility was on the instructor. Current method equalizes responsibility between student and instructor and encourages a wide range of learning/teaching methods.

Teaching and research hospital Private or public hospitals that focus on treating patients; training physicians, nurses, and other health professionals; and research and development.

Team method A method of patient care in which small teams of nursing personnel are assigned to give total care to groups of patients.

Therapeutic communication Health-related, purposeful communication between the patient and the nurse. The focus is on the patient.

The Joint Commission (TJC) Sets the standards of care for hospitals and long-term care agencies. Agencies receive accreditation if they elect to be reviewed and meet standards.
Third-party coverage Health insurance.
Time management The effective use of time to meet goals.
Total client care The registered nurse (RN) is responsible for all aspects of patient care: assessing, planning, organizing, and delivering patient care. This model is often used in critical care and specialty health care settings. This model generally does not use licensed practical nurses (LPNs) to provide nursing care.
Traditional adult learner A learner who comes to an educational program directly from high school or from another program of study, usually in his or her late teens or early 20s.
Transitional practice model Helps new graduate nurses transition from their educational program to the work environment.
Trust Rely on, depend on.
Tutoring Select study group. Student arranges for special help through instructor referral or self-referral.
Two-way communication When there is feedback or discussion between the sender and receiver; the usual form of conversation.

U

Understanding Comprehension. Able to recall and provide examples.
Unit clerk Assumes responsibility for many clerical duties in the patient care area.
Unintentional torts Nurse did not intend to injure patient. Negligence and malpractice are examples.
Unit manager Has supervisor and management functions for patient units.
United Nations (UN) International organization that deals with world issues. Has representatives of many countries.
Unlicensed assistive personnel (AP) Trained by health care organizations to function in an assistive role to registered nurses (RNs) and licensed practical nurses/licensed vocational nurses (LPNs/LVNs). Also known as patient care technicians, patient care associates, nurse extenders, multiskilled workers, unlicensed assistive personnel, and direct care workers.
Unlicensed Assistive Personnel (UAP) Workers trained by healthcare organizations to assist RNs and LPNs/LVNs, as needed in the unit.
U.S. Department of Health and Human Services (HHS) A federal agency funded by taxes. Advises president on national health matters.
U.S. Public Health Service (USPHS) Division of Department of Health and Human Services. Made up of six agencies.

V

Validate information Verify data.
Values Assigned to an idea or action. Freely chosen and affected by age, experience, and maturity.
Veracity The ethical principle of telling the truth.
Verbal communication Sending or receiving communication through the spoken or written word.
Vertical violence Occurs between persons of unequal power, for example, an instructor and a student.
Vicarious liability Responsible for actions of another because of a special relationship with the other person.
Virtual clinical excursion A real clinical experience simulated on a computer, including changing physician orders.
Visual learner Generates visual images, that is, thinks primarily in pictures. Learns best by watching a demonstration first.
Visual/linguistic learner Learns best through reading and writing.
Visual/spatial learner Learns best through charts, demonstrations, videos, and other visual materials.
Voice control Be aware of how your voice sounds. A well-modulated voice makes a better impression.
Voluntary health care agencies Not-for-profit, nonofficial health care agencies that complement official health agencies and meet the needs of persons with a specific disease.

W

Wald, Lillian Began Henry Street Settlement visiting nurse service in New York in 1893 to care for indigent persons.
Watson's theory of human care Health is a harmony among body, mind, and spirit. It involves self-perception and how the self is experienced. Illness is a lack of harmony within the self and the soul.
Wellness and illness Relative terms. Have different meanings for different cultures.
Wellness center Promotes wellness. Includes nutritional counseling, exercise programs, stress reduction, and weight control programs.
World Health Organization (WHO) International health agency of the United Nations, located in Geneva.
Worldview Shared by persons with same cultural background.

References

CHAPTER 1

Appelbaum SH, Bhardwaj A, Goodyear M, Gong T, Sudha AB, Wei P: A study of generational conflicts in the workplace, *Eur J Bus Manage Res* 7(2):7–15, 2022. https://doi.org/10.24018/ejbmr.2022.7.2.1311.

Billings D, Halstead J: *Teaching in nursing: a guide for faculty*, 7th ed., St. Louis, MO, 2024, Elsevier.

Bureau of Labor Statistics, U.S. Department of Labor: *Occupational outlook handbook, licensed practical and licensed vocational nurses*, Washington, DC, 2026, U.S. Bureau of Labor Statistics. Accessed 11 February 2025. Available from. https://www.bls.gov/ooh/healthcare/licensed-practical-and-licensed-vocational-nurses.htm.

Empowerment: In *Merriam-Webster.com*, 2025. Accessed 11 November 2025. Available from: https://www.merriam-webster.com/dictionary/empowerment.

Patel D: 8 ways Generation Z will differ from millennials in the workplace, *Forbes*, 2017. Accessed 21 December 2025. Available from:. https://www.purdueglobal.edu/education-partnerships/generational-workforce-differences-infographic . Purdue Global, 2025.

Rosen M: *Understanding the generational gap and bridging it*, 2023. Accessed 12 January 2026. https://youtu.be/Z6rxzBkgvTI.

Riggs CJ: Multiple generations in the nursing workplace: part I, *J Contin Educ Nurs* 44(3):105–106, 2013.

Stewart J, Oliver E, Cravens K, Oishi S: Managing millennials: embracing generational differences, *Bus Horiz* 60:45–54, 2017.

CHAPTER 2

Barsch J: *Barsch learning style inventory*, Novato, CA, 1991, Academic Therapy Publications.

Cleveland Clinic: *What is neuroplasticity? How it works*, 2023. Accessed 3 January 2026. https://health.clevelandclinic.org/neuroplasticity.

Chall JS: *Readability: an appraisal of research and application*, Columbus, OH, 1958, The Bureau of Educational Research, Ohio State University.

Chabner DE: *The language of medicine*, 11th ed, St. Louis, 2017, Elsevier.

Ebbinghaus H: *Memory: a contribution to experimental psychology*, New York, 1885, Columbia University Teachers College.

Fleming G: *Left brain vs right brain*, 2025. Accessed 8 April 2026. Available from: https://www.thoughtco.com/left-brain-right-brain-1857174.

Gardner H, Hatch T: *Multiple intelligences go to school: educational implications of the theory of multiple intelligences [Technical Report No. 4]*, New York, 1990, Center for Technology in Education.

Gardner H: *Intelligence reframed: multiple intelligences for the 21st century*, New York: 1999, Basic Books: Perseus Books Group.

Mueller PA, Oppenheimer DM: The pen is mightier than the keyboard, *Psychol Sci* 25(6):1159–1168, 2014.

Mueller P, Oppenheimer D: Corrigendum: The Pen Is Mightier Than the Keyboard: Advantages of Longhand Over Laptop Note Taking, *Psychological Science* 29(9):1565–1568, 2018. Accessed 3 February 2026. https://www.jstor.org/stable/26957496.

National Council of State Boards of Nursing: *2023 NCLEX-PN® Test plan*, Chicago, IL, 2022, NCSBN. Accessed 11 October 2025. Available from. https://www.ncsbn.org/publications/2023-nclex-pn-test-plan.

Website Resources Cited

https://Quizlet.com
https://www.mindmup.com
https://www.ncsbn.org
https://www.thoughtco.c
https://chadd.org
https://cdc.gov
https://www.cram.com
https://docsbot.ai/article/the-11-best-free-chatgpt-alternatives

CHAPTER 3

American Nurses Association: *Social Networking Principles*, 2018. Accessed 22 October 2025. Available from: https://www.nursingworld.org/social/.

National Council of State Board Examiners (NCSBN): *A nurse's guide to the use of social media. White Paper*, 2011. https://www.ncsbn.org/public-files/Social_Media.pdf

National Council of State Board of Nursing: *A nurse's guide to the use of social media*, 2024. Available from: https://www.ncsbn.org/brochures-and-posters/nurses-guide-to-the-use-of-socialmedia.

Website Resources Cited

allnurses.com
www.napnes.org
www.nalpn.org
www.ncsbn.org
nursegroups.com
http://ajnoffthecharts.com
www.practicalclinicalskills.com
https://www.nursingworld.org/practice-policy/nursing-excellence/social-networking-Principles/
www.studentaid.gov

CHAPTER 4

Atkinson L: ANA's position paper, discussion at the ANA convention, *AORN* 4(5):15–16, 1966.

BBC News: *Mary seacole statue unveiled in London*, 2016. Accessed 20 August 2025. Available from: https://www.bbc.com/news/uk-england-london-36663206.

Berry-Caban C, Rivers F, Beltran A, Anderson L: Description of United States military nurses deployed to Afghanistan & Iraq, 2001–2015, *Open J Nurs* 8:93–101, 2018.

Bolvin J: *War on the mind, part 1: nurses deployed in Iraq and Afghanistan struggle with PTSD*, 2010. Accessed 10 November 2025. Available from: https://www.nurse.com/blog/2010/10/04/war-on-the-mind-part-1-nurses-deployed-to-iraq-and-afghanistan-struggle-with-ptsd/.

Cherry B, Jacob SR: *Contemporary nursing: issues, trends, and management*, ed 8, St. Louis, 2019, Elsevier.

Dos Santos WG: Natural history of COVID-19 and current knowledge on treatment therapeutic options, *Biomed Pharmacother*, 2020 129:110493. doi:10.1016/j.biopha.2020.110493. Available from. https://www.ncbi.nlm.nih.gov/pmc/articles/PMC7332915/.

Desch E, Doherty ME: Experiences of U.S. military nurses in Iraq and Afghanistan wars, 2003–2009, *J Nurs Sch* 42(1):3–12, 2010.

DiFilippo D: *'Blood smells the same', but for Vietnam nurses, the war never ends*, Philadelphia, 2017, WHYY. Accessed 23 March 2026. Available from. https://whyy.org/articles/vietnamnursesdd/.

Donahue P, Russac P: Nursing: the finest art, *Am J Nurs* 85(10):1080–1085, 1985.

Institute of Medicine: Future of nursing: *leading change, advancing health*, Washington, DC, 2010, The National Academies Press. Accessed 23 March 2026. Available from:. http://www.nationalacademies.org/hmd/Reports/2010/The-Future-of-Nursing-Leading-Change-Advancing-Health.aspx.

Kalish P, Kalish B: *The advance of American nursing*, ed 3, Boston, 1995, Little, Brown.

LeVasseur J: Plato, Nightingale, and contemporary nursing, IMAGE, *J Nurs Sch* 30(3):281–285, 1998.

Mosby: *Mosby dictionary of medicine, nursing & health professions*, St. Louis, MO, 2009, Elsevier.

National Black Nurse's Association: *Who we are*, 2026. Accessed 8 April 2026. Available from: https://www.nbna.org/who.

National Black Nurse's Association: *Membership benefits*, 2026. Accessed 8 April 2026. Available from: https://www.nbna.org/content.asp?contentid539.

National League for Nursing: *A vision for recognition of the role of the licensed practical/licensed vocational nurses in advancing the nation's health*, 2014. Accessed 12 November 2025. Available from: http://www.nln.org/docs/default-source/about/nln-vision-series-%28position-statements%29/nlnvision_7.pdf?sfvrsn54.

National Academies of Sciences, Engineering, and Medicine: *The future of nursing 2020–2030: charting a path to achieve health equity*, Washington, DC, 2021, The National Academies Press. Accessed 19 November 2025. Available from:. https://doi.org/10.17226/25982.

Red Cross: Jane Delano, founder of the American red cross nursing services, 2019. Accessed 19 November 2025. Available from: https://www.redcross.org/content/dam/redcross/enterprise-assets/about-us/history/nursing-history-jane-delano.pdf.

Romanoff B: Facts about Flo you may not know, *Nurse Week* 7(3):32–33, 2006.

Smiley R, Lauer P, Bienemy C, et al.: The 2017 national nursing workforce summary, *J Nurs Regul* 9(3):S1–S88, 2018.

U.S. Department of Health and Human Services Health Resources and Services Administration: *The U.S. nursing workforce: trends in supply and education*, 2013. Accessed 19 November 2025. Available from: https://bhw.hrsa.gov/sites/default/files/bhw/nchwa/projections/nursingworkforcetrendsoct2013.pdf.

Vietnam Veterans Memorial Foundation: *What innovations in medical care were introduced in Vietnam?* Echoes from the Wall. NCSS. Accessed 19 November 2025. Available from: https://www.vvmf.org/userfiles/files/VVMF%20Education%20Guide%20-%20Medical%202%20(2).pdf.

Wilson B: *Women in the Korean conflict. Women in War*, 2011. Accessed 19 November 2025. Available from: http://userpages.aug.com/captbarb/femvets6.html.

www.studentaid.org.

CHAPTER 5

Alfaro-Lefevre R: *Critical thinking and clinical judgement: a practical approach*, ed 7, Philadelphia, PA, 2020, Elsevier.

Benner P, Sutphen M, Leonard V, Day L: *Educating Nurses: A Call for Radical Transformation*, San Francisco, CA, 2009, Jossey-Bass.

Caputi L: *Think Like a Nurse: the caputi method for learning clinical judgment (USA Version)*, Rolling Meadows, IL, 2021, Windy City Publisher.

Ignatavicius D, Workman ML: *Rebar C: Medical surgical nursing*, ed 9, Philadelphia, PA, 2018, Elsevier.

Marquez J, Francis-Hew L, Humphrey N: Protective factors for resilience in adolescence: analysis of a longitudinal dataset using the residuals approach, *Child Adolesc Psychiatry Ment Health* 17(1):140, 2023. doi:10.1186/s13034-023-00687-8.

National Council of State Boards of Nursing: *Implementation of the 1999 NCLEX-PN test plan, issues*, Chicago, 1998, NCSBN.

National Council of State Boards of Nursing: *NCLEX-PN test plan—effective April 2020*, Chicago, 2019, NCSBN. Accessed 19 November 2025. Available from:. https://www.ncsbn.org/exams/exam-statistics-and-publications/exam-publications.page.

Next Generation NCLEX update. Accessed 1 November 2025. Available from: https://www.ncsbn.org/event-video-view/next-generation-nclex-ngn-forum.

NCSBN: *PN Practice Analysis: Linking the NCLEX-PN Examination to Practice*, 2024. Accessed 20 April 2025. https://www.ncsbn.org/exams-research/2024-pn-practice-analysis-linking-the-nclexpn-examination-to-practice.

NCSBN Clinical Judgment Measurement Model: NCSBN, 2019. Accessed 2 November 2025. Retrieved from: https://www.nclex.com/clinical-judgment-measurement-model.page.

Project Implicit: *Implicit association test*, 2015. Accessed 2 November 2025. Available From: https://implicit.harvard.edu/implicit/takeatest.html.

Wankier J, Beynon C: Enhancing clinical judgment in undergraduate clinical education, *Teach Learn Nurs* 20(1):32–36, 2025. Accessed 1 November 2025. https://doi.org/10.1016/j.teln.2024.08.019.

Website Resources Cited

www.ncsbn.org
www.alfaroteachsmart.com
https://implicit.harvard.edu/implicit/takeatest.html
www.nalpn.org
https://www.ncsbn.org/exams-research/2024-pn-practice-analysis-linking-the-nclexpn-examination-to-practice

CHAPTER 6

American Nurses Association: *What is veracity in nursing?* 2024. https://www.nursingworld.org/content-hub/resources/workplace/veracity-nursing/#:~:text=Veracity%2C%20also%20known%20as%20truth,%2Dmaker)%20the%20objective%20truth.

Fulham NM, Krueger KL, Cohen T: Honest feedback: Barriers to receptivity and discerning the truth in feedback, *Current Opinion in Psychology*, 101405:46, 2022. doi:10.1016/j.copsyc.2022.101405.

Miller-Keane O'Tolle: *MT: Encyclopedia and Dictionary of Medicine, Nursing, & Allied Health*, Philadelphia, PA, 2003, Elsevier.

Mosby: *Mosby dictionary of medicine, nursing & health professions*, Philadelphia, PA, 2017, Elsevier.

Potter P, Perry A, Stockert P: *Fundamentals of nursing*, 9th ed., Philadelphia, PA, 2017, Elsevier.

Seo M, Na J, Kim Y-H: Moral in whose eyes? Cross-cultural differences in moral decision making and behaviour, *International Journal of Psychology* 56(1):175–182, 2021. doi:10.1002/ijop.12681.

U.S. Bureau of Labor Statistics: *TED: The economics daily*, 2024, https://www.bls.gov/opub/ted/2024/womens-earnings-were-83-6-percent-of-mens-in-2023.htm

U.S. Bureau of Labor Statistics: *Highlights of women's earnings in 2017*, 2017, https://www.bls.gov/opub/reports/womens-earnings/2017/home.htm

U.S. Bureau of Labor Statistics: *BLS Reports*, 2014, https://www.bls.gov/opub/reports/womens-earnings/archive/highlights-of-womens-earnings-in-2013.pdf

Ulrich BT: *Leadership and Management According to Florence Nightengale*, Hoboken, N.J., 1992, Pearson.

Wheaton A: Balancing honesty and benevolence in dementia care: A commentary on therapeutic lies and codes of ethics, *Journal of Nursing Management*, 2022. doi:10.1111/jonm.13659.

Yoder-Wise P: *Leading and managing in nursing*, 8th ed, Philadelphia, PA, 2023, Elsevier.

Website Resources Cited

www.napnes.org
www.nalpn.org

CHAPTER 7

American Hospital Association: The patient care partnership, 2003. Accessed 10 January 2025. Available from: www.aha.org/advocacy-issues/communicatingpts/pt-care-partnership.shtml.

American Nurses Association & National Council State Board of Nursing: *Joint ANA and National Council of State Boards of Nursing position statement*, 2019, National Guidelines for Nursing Delegation. Accessed 10 January 2025. Available from:. https://www.ncsbn.org/public-files/NGND-PosPaper_06.pdf [new website].

ANA Center for Ethics and Human Rights: *Position statement nurses' roles and responsibilities in providing care and support at the end of Life*, 2024. Accessed 12 April 2025. https://www.nursingworld.org/practice-policy/nursing-excellence/official-position-statements/.

Byock I: A strategic path forward for hospice and palliative care: A white paper on the potential future of the field, 2025. Accessed 8 April 2026. Available from: https://pubmed.ncbi.nlm.nih.gov/40919553/, https://doi.org/10.1089/pmr.2025.0030

California Health Care Foundation: Conversation project, 2012. Accessed 10 January 2025. Available from: http://theconversationproject.org.

Chen W, Chung JOK, Lam KKW, Molassiotis A: End-of-life communication strategies for healthcare professionals: a scoping review, *Palliat Med* 37(1):61–74, 2022. https://doi.org/10.1177/02692163221133670.

Cherry B, Jacob S: *Contemporary nursing: issues, trends, and management*, St. Louis, MO, 2019, Elsevier.

Garner B: Black's Law Dictionary: Negligence. In Law books, ed 5, St. Paul MN, 2014, West Publishing Company.

Interstate Commission of Nurse Licensure Compact: *Nurse licensure compact commission annual report*, 2025. Accessed 15 March 2025. https://www.ncsbn.org/publications/2024-nlc-annual-report.

National Council of State Boards of Nursing: *Discipline – initial review of complaint*, 2022. Accessed 10 January 2025. Available from: https://www.ncsbn.org/1616.htm#6038.

National Council of State Boards of Nursing: *Board action (Disciplinary Action)*, 2022. Accessed 10 January 2025. Available from: https://www.ncsbn.org/nursing-regulation/discipline/board-action.page.

National Association for Practical Nurse Education and Service: *NAPNES Standards of practice for licensed practical/vocational nurses*, Author, MD, 2003, Silver Spring.

National Council of State Boards of Nursing: *Filing a complaint*, 2019. Accessed 8 April 2026. Available from: https://www.ncsbn.org/nursing-regulation/discipline/filing-a-complaint/filing-complaint-faq.page.

National Council of State Boards of Nursing: *A nurse's guide to the use of social media, 2018*. Accessed 10 March 2025. Available from: https://www.ncsbn.org/brochures-and-posters/nurses-guide-to-the-use-of-socialmedia.

National Council of State Boards of Nursing: *Nurse licensure compact*, 2022. Accessed 10 March 2025. Available from: www.ncsbn.org/nurse-licensure-compact.htm.

National Council of State Boards of Nursing: *The interstate commission of nurse licensure compact administrators*, 2017. Accessed 10 March 2025. Available from: https://www.ncsbn.org/eNLCFinalRulesadopted121217.pdf.

National Council of State Board of Nursing: *About U.S. Nursing regulatory bodies*, 2025. Accessed 1 April 2025. https://www.ncsbn.org/nursing-regulation/about-nursing-regulatory-bodies.page.

National Council of State Board of Nursing: *NCSBN model act*, 2021. Accessed 22 May 2025. https://www.ncsbn.org/public-files/21_Model_Act.pdf.

National Council of State Board of Nursing: *What every nurse needs to know about state and territorial boards of nursing*, 2019. Accessed 1 April 2025. https://www.ncsbn.org/public-files/What_Every_Nurse_Needs_to_Know.pdf.

National Institutes of Health: *MedlinePlus. Advanced directives*, 2021. Accessed 10 April 2026. Available from: https://medlineplus.gov/advancedirectives.html.

National League for Nursing: *A vision for recognition of the role of the licensed practical/licensed vocational nurses in advancing the nation's health*, 2014. Accessed 10 April 2026. Available from: https://www.nln.org/docs/default-source/uploadedfiles/about/nlnvision_7.pdf?sfvrsn=c7e06e45_3.

Oregon Health Authority, Public Health Division, Center for Health Statistics: *2024 oregon death with dignity act data summary*, 2025. Accessed 10 April 2026. https://www.oregon.gov/oha/PH/PROVIDERPARTNERRESOURCES/EVALUATIONRESEARCH/DEATHWITHDIGNITYACT/Documents/year27.pdf.

Relias Media: *More nurses, hospitalists being sued for malpractice, studies say*, 2016. Accessed 10 April 2026. Available from: https://www.reliasmedia.com/articles/137567-more-nurses-hospitalists-being-sued-for-malpractice-studies-say.

Rokosh C: *Legal issues in nursing: the 5 most common allegations of nursing negligence*, 2022. Accessed 10 Apr 2026. https://www.clpna.com/lpn/lpn-knowledge-hub/part-4-legal-issues-in-nursing-five-most-common-allegations-of-nursing-negligence/.

Starks H, Dudzinski D, White N: (Original text written by Braddock C, Tonelli M: [1998]) Physician aid in dying, 2013. Accessed 10 April 2026. Available from: https://depts.washington.edu/bhdept/ethics-medicine/bioethics-topics/articles/physician-aid-dying.

Teoli JD, Ghazzemzadeh S: *Patient Self Determination Act*, St Petersburg FL, 2022, Treasure Island (FL). https://www.ncbi.nlm.nih.gov/sites/books/NBK538297/.

The Joint Commission: *National patient safety goals*, 2026. Available from: https://www.jointcommission.org/standards/national-patient-safety-goals/.

The Joint Commission: *Standards of care*, 2026. Accessed 10 Apr 2026. Available from: https://www.jointcommission.org/en-us/standards/standards-manuals.

The Joint Commission: *Medication Safety – High Alert and Hazardous Medication*. 2025. 10 April 2026. Accessed 5 September 2021. Available from: https://www.jointcommission.org/en-us/knowledge-library/support-center/standards-interpretation/standards-faqs/000002226.

Watson E: Nursing malpractice: costs, trends, and issues, *J Leg Nurse Consult* 25(1):26–33, 2014.

Yoder-Wise P, Sportsman S: *Leading and managing in nursing*, 8th ed., St. Louis, MO, 2023, Elsevier.

Website Resources Cited

www.nalpn.org
www.nflpn.org
www.ncsbn.org
www.napnes.org
https://www.hhs.gov
https://www.cms.gov
www.aarp.org
https://theconversationproject.org
https://www.nahc.org
https://www.polst.org/
https://deathwithdignity.org/states/
https://safeproject.us/

CHAPTER 8

Agency for Healthcare Research and Quality: About health, 2025, https://www.ahrq.gov/health-literacy/about/index.html

Agency for Healthcare Research and Quality: *TeamSTEPPS:Team strategies and tools to enhance performance and patient safety*, (n.d.). www.ahrq.gov/teamstepps/about-teamstepps/index.html

Allen-Meares P, Lowry B, Estrella ML, Mansuri S: Health literacy barriers in the health care system: Barriers and opportunities for the profession, *Health and Social Work* 45(1):62–64, 2020. https://pubmed.ncbi.nlm.nih.gov/31993624/.

Center for Disease Control and Prevention (CDC): *What is health literacy?* 2023, www.cdc.gov/healthliteracy/learn/index.html

Cherry B, Jacob S: *Contemporary nursing: Issues, trends and management*, 9th ed, Philadelphia, PA, 2022, Elsevier.

Cuddy A: *TED Global: Your body language may shape who you are*, 2012, www.ted.com/talks/amy_cuddy_your_body_language_shapes_who_you_are?language5en

Haddeland K, Marthinsen GN, Soderhamn U, Flateland SM, Moi EM: Experiences of using the ISBAR tool after an intervention: A focus group study among critical care nurses and anesthesiologists, *Intensive and Critical Care Nursing*, 70:6, 2022. doi:10.1016/j.iccn.2021.103195.

National Council of State Boards of Nursing, Inc: *A nurse's guide to the use of social media*, 2024, www.ncsbn.org/public-files/NCSBN_SocialMedia.pdf

National League of Nursing: *Advancing care excellence for peoples with disabilities*, 2025, www.nln.org/education/teaching-resources/professional-development-programsteaching-resourcesace-all/ace-d

National Student Nurses' Association: *Code of ethics*, 2022, www.dropbox.com/scl/fi/9gclyp7hh3fcxebrfqopc/Code-of-Ethics.pdf?rlkey=kqvgudd2ykwz6z17equh714vj&e=1&dl=0

Pagana K: *The nurse's etiquette advantage*, Indianapolis, IN, 2015, Sigma.

Smith A, Schieber D, Austin T: Describing confidence: Student-identified signals of presenter confidence, *International Journal of Teaching and Learning in Higher Education* 33(3):317–327, 2022. www.isetl.org/ijtlhe/pdf/IJTLHE4039.pdf.

Tennant, K, Long A, Toney-Butler TJ: *Active listening. National Library of Medicine*, 2023, www.ncbi.nlm.nih.gov/books/NBK442015/

U.S. Department of Health and Human Services: *Healthy people 2030*, (n.d.), https://health.gov/healthypeople

U.S. Department of Health and Human Services: *Healthy people 2030: Health communication*, (n.d.), https://health.gov/healthypeople/objectives-and-data/browse-objectives/health-communication

U.S. Department of Health and Human Services: *Healthy people 2030: Health IT*, (n.d.), https://odphp.health.gov/healthypeople/objectives-and-data/browse-objectives/health-it

U.S. Department of Health and Human Services: *Healthy people 2030: Healthy People 2030*, (n.d.), https://odphp.health.gov/healthypeople

CHAPTER 9

Aloisio LD, Coughlin M, Squires JE: Individual and organizational factors of nurses' job satisfaction in long-term care: A systematic review, *International Journal of Nursing Studies*, 123:104073, 2021. doi:10.1016/j.ijnurstu.2021 November.

American Nurses Association (ANA): Healthy work environment, (n.d.), mentwww.nursingworld.org/practice-policy/work-environment

American Nurses Association (ANA): *Executive Summary: American Nurses Association health risk appraisal*, 2017, www.nursingworld.org/globalassets/practiceandpolicy/work-environment/health–safety/ana-healthriskappraisalsummary_2013-2016.pdf

Castillo B: *On April 1, California healthcare employers with no workplace violence prevention plan will be breaking the law*, 2018, www.nationalnursesunited.org/blog/april-1-california-healthcare-employers-no-workplace-violence-prevention-plan-will-be-breaking

Carroll L: *Student and faculty perceptions of respect and respectful learning environments*, 2018, ProQuest Dissertations and Theses Database.

Center of Disease Control and Prevention (CDC): *Smart framework*, 2022, www.cdc.gov/healthyyouth/yac/smart-framework.htm

Clark C: Combining cognitive rehearsal, simulation, and evidence-based scripting to address incivility, *Nurse Educator* 44(2):64–68, 2019. doi:10.1097/NNE.0000000000000563.

Clark C: *Musing of the great blue*, 2016, http://musingofthegreat-blue.blogspot.com

Congress.gov: H.R. *1195 - Workplace violence prevention for health care and social service workers act*, 2022, www.congress.gov/bill/117th-congress/house-bill/1195/all-actions?overview=closed#tabs

Cuddy A: *TED global: your body language may shape who you are, 2012*, 2012, www.ted.com/talks/amy_cuddy_your_body_language_shapes_who_you_are?language5en

Draucker CD: Responses of nurses and other healthcare workers to sexual harassment in the workplace, *The Online Journal of Issues in Nursing*, 24, 2019. doi:10.3912/OJIN.Vol24No01Man03.

Equal Employment Opportunity Commission: Sexual harassment, (n.d.), www.eeoc.gov/laws/types/sexual_harassment.cfm

Kafle S, Paudel S, Thapaliya A, Acharya R: Workplace violence against nurses: A narrative review, *Journal of Clinical and Translational Research* 8(5):421–424, 2022. https://pmc.ncbi.nlm.nih.gov/articles/PMC9536186/.

Knecht P: *Demystifying job satisfaction in long-term care: The voices of licensed practical nurses*, 2014, ProQuest Dissertations and Theses Database.

Legal Information Institute: Assault, (n.d.), www.law.cornell.edu/wex/assault

Luo Y, Zhang M, Yu S, Guan X, Zhong T, Wu Q, Li Y: The impact of psychological violence in the workplace on turnover intention of clinical nurses: The mediating role of job satisfaction, *BMC Nursing* 23:844, 2024. doi:10.1186/s12912-024-02477-9.

Merriam-Webster: *Assertive*, 2024, www.merriam-webster.com/dictionary/assertive

National Institute for Occupational Safety and Health: *Types of workplace violence*, 2024, wwwn.cdc.gov/WPVHC/Nurses/Course/Slide/Unit1_5

National League for Nurses (NLN): *NLN vision series: Creating community to build a civil and healthy academic work environment*, 2018, www.nln.org/docs/default-source/uploadedfiles/professional-development-programs/vision-statement-a-vision-for-creating-community-to-build-a-civil-and-healthy.pdf?sfvrsn=2ca7ab0d_0&pdf=VisionSeries-CreatingCommunity

National Nurses United: *Nurses applaud the introduction of federal legislation to prevent workplace violence in health care, social service settings*, 2019, www.nationalnursesunited.org/press/nurses-applaud-introduction-federal-legislation-prevent-workplace-violence-health-care-social

Occupational Safety and Health Administration (OSHA): *Guidelines for preventing workforce violence for health care and social service workers*, 2016, www.osha.gov/sites/default/files/publications/osha3148.pdf

Occupational Safety and Health Administration (OSHA): *Healthcare: Overview*, (n.d.), www.osha.gov/healthcare

Pollack R: Healthcare workplace violence prevention laws by state. ROAR, (n.d.), www.roarforgood.com/blog/healthcare-workplace-violence-prevention-laws-by-state/

Spector PE, Zhou ZE, Che XX: Nurse exposure to physical and nonphysical violence, bullying, and sexual harassment: A quantitative review, *International Journal of Nursing Studies* 51(1):72–84, 2014. doi:10.1016/j.ijnurstu.2013.01.010.

Speroni KG, Fitch T, Dawson E, Dugan L, Atherton M: Incidence and cost of nurse workplace violence perpetrated by hospital patients or patient visitors, *Journal Emergency Nursing* 40(3):218–228, 2014. doi:10.1016/j.jen.2013.05.014.

The Joint Commission: *Sentinel event alert issue 59: Physical and verbal violence against health care workers*, 2021, www.jointcommission.org/resources/sentinel-event/sentinel-event-alert-newsletters/sentinel-event-alert-59-physical-and-verbal-violence-against-health-care-workers

The Joint Commission: *Workplace violence prevention compendium of resources to support joint commission accredited hospitals implementation of new and revised standards*, (n.d.), https://www.jointcommission.org/en-us/standards/national-performance-goals/preventing-workplace-violence.

CHAPTER 10

Cherry B, Jacob S: *Contemporary nursing: Issues, trends and management*, 9th ed, Philadelphia, PA, 2022, Elsevier.

D'Avanzo C, Geissler E: *Pocket guide to cultural assessment*, St. Louis, MO, 2008, Mosby.

Giger JN, Powell-Young YM: *Transcultural nursing: Assessment and intervention*, 9th ed., Philadelphia, PA, 2025, Elsevier.

Giger JN, Davidhizar R: The Giger and Davidhizar transcultural assessment model, *Journal of Transcultural Nursing* 13(3):185–188, 2002. doi:10.1177/10459602013003004.

Jackson L: Understanding, eliciting and negotiating patients' multicultural health beliefs, *Nurse Practitioner* 18(4):37–43, 1993. https://pubmed.ncbi.nlm.nih.gov/8515898.

Jensen E, Jones N, Rabe M, Pratt B, Medina L, Orozco K, Spell L: *The chance that two people chosen at random are of different race or ethnicity groups has increased since 2010*, 2021, www.census.gov/library/stories/2021/08/2020-united-states-population-more-racially-ethnically-diverse-than-2010.html#:~:text=Prevalence%20rankings%20illustrate%20the%20percent%20of%20the%20population,non-Hispanic%20population%20was%20the%20third-

Keiser Family Foundation: 2017 *Census Bureau's American community survey*, 2019, www.kff.org/other/state-indicator/distribution-by-raceethnicity/?currentTimeframe50&selectedDistributions5two-or-more-races&sortModel5%7B%22colId%22:%22Two%20Or%20More%20Races%22,%22sort%22%22desc%22%7D

Marion L, Douglas M, Lavin MA, Barr N, Gazaway S, Thomas E, Bickford C: Implementing the new ANA Standard 8: Culturally congruent practice, *OJIN*, 22:1, 2016. doi:10.3912/OJIN.Vol22No01PPT20.

Reinhardt E: *Through the eyes of others—intercultural resource directory for health care professionals*, Hennepin County Medical Society, United Way Intercultural Awareness, 1995.

Rimmer A: Can patients use family members as non-professional interpreters in consultations? *BMJ*, 368, 2020. doi:10.1136/bmj.m447.

U.S. Census Bureau: *Demographic turning points for the United States: Population projections for 2020 to 2060*, 2020, www.census.gov/content/dam/Census/library/publications/2020/demo/p25-1144.pdf

U.S. Department of Education: *Adult literacy in the United States*, 2019, 2019, https://nces.ed.gov/pubs2019/2019179.pdf

U.S. Department of Health and Human Services: *National culturally and linguistically appropriate services standards*, (n.d.), https://thinkculturalhealth.hhs.gov/clas/standards

U.S. Department of Health and Human Services: *National CLAS standards*, (n.d.), https://thinkculturalhealth.hhs.gov/clas

World Bank Group: *Population, total*, 2025, https://data.worldbank.org/indicator/SP.POP.TOTL

Website Resources Cited

https://nccih.nih.gov/

www.dimensionsofculture.com

https://www.jointcommission.org/-/media/tjc/documents/resources/patient-safety-topics/health-equity/aroadmapforhospitalsfinalversion727pdf.pdf?db=web&hash=AC3AC4BED1D973713C2CA6B2E5ACD01B&hash=AC3AC4BED1D973713C2CA6B2E5ACD01B.

www.minoritynurse.com/about/index.html

www.napnes.org

www.nalpn.org

CHAPTER 11

Carson V: *Spiritual dimensions of nursing practice*, Philadelphia, PA, 1989, WB Saunders.

Carson V, Koenig H: *Spiritual dimensions of nursing practice*, Conshohocken, PA, 2008, Templeton Foundation Press.

Cosentino C, Harrad RA, Sulla F, Bertuol M, Sarli L, Artoli G: Nursing spiritual assessment instruments in adult patients: a narrative literature review, *Acta Biomed*, 91(12-S):e2020015, 2020. https://doi.org/10.23750/abm.v91i12-S.10998.

Herdman, Kamitsuru & Lopes: *NANDA: Nursing diagnoses definitions and classifications 2024–2026*, ed 13, 2024, 2024. Available from: www.nanda.org.

Lukovsky J, McGrath E, Sun C, Frankl D, Beauchesne MA: A Survey of hospice and palliative care nurses' and holistic nurses' perceptions of spirituality and spiritual care, *J Hosp Palliat Care Nurs* 23(1):28–37, 2021. https://doi.org/10.1097/NJH.0000000000000711.

Miller M, Addicott K, Rosa WE: Spiritual care as a core component of palliative nursing, *Am J Nurs* 123(2):54–59, 2023. https://doi.org/10.1097/01.NAJ.0000919748.95749.e5.

Murgia C, Notarnicola I, Caruso R, De Maria M, Rocco G, Stievano A: Spirituality and religious diversity in nursing: a scoping review, *Healthcare* 10:1661, 2022. https://doi.org/10.3390/healthcare10091661.

PEW Research Center: *2023–2024 U. S. religious landscape study interactive database*, 2025. https://doi.org/10.58094/3zs9-jc14.

Pulchalski C: *FICA spiritual history tool: a guide for spiritual Assessment in clinical settings* Updated 2025, Washington, D.C, 1996, The George Washington Institute for Spirituality & Health. https://gwish.smhs.gwu.edu/programs/transforming-practice-health-settings/clinical-fica-tool.

The Joint Commission: *The Joint Commission: standards FAQ details. Spiritual beliefs and preferences. Does the Joint Commission specify what needs to be included in a spiritual assessment*, 2022. https://www.jointcommission.org/standards/standard-faqs/hospital-and-hospital-clinics/provision-of-care-treatment-and-services-pc/000001669/

United States Religion Census: 2020. https://usreligioncensus.org.

World Statistics: *The largest religions in the world 2025*, 2025. https://worldstatistics.net/the-largest-religions-in-the-world-2025.

CHAPTER 12

Betts J, Muntean W, Kim D, Jorion N, Dickison P: Building a method for writing clinical judgment items for entry-level nursing exams, *Journal of Applied Testing Technology* 10(S2):21–36, 2019. www.ncsbn.org/public-files/

Building_a_Method_for_Writing_Clinical_Judgment_It.pdf.
National League for Nurses (NLN): *Vision Series: A Vision for recognition of the role of licensed practical/vocational nurses in advancing the nation's health*, 2014, www.nln.org/docs/default-source/uploadedfiles/about/nlnvision_7.pdf?sfvrsn=c7e06e45_3
National Council of States Board of Nursing (NCSBN): *Clinical judgment measurement model*, 2025, https://nclex.com/clinical-judgment-measurement-model.page
National Council of State Boards of Nursing (NCSBN): *Next generation NCLES: NCLES-PN test plan*, 2023, www.ncsbn.org/public-files/2023_PN_Test%20Plan_FINAL.pdf
National Council State Boards of Nursing (NCSBN): *Report of findings from the 2021 LPN/VN nursing knowledge survey*, 2022, https://www.ncsbn.org/public-files/21_PN_KSA_FINAL.pdf
Nightingale F: *Notes on nursing: What it is and what it is not*, New York, NY, 2009, Appleton and Company.
The Joint Commission (TJC): *Nursing assessments - Licensed Practical Nurse: Can a Licensed Practical Nurse (LPNM) perform assessments?* 2022, www.jointcommission.org/standards/standard-faqs/critical-access-hospital/provision-of-care-treatment-and-services-pc/000001666/
White A: *The use of SMART goals in nursing*, 2022, https://nursingcecentral.com/the-use-of-smart-goals-in-nursing/

CHAPTER 13

Ackley BJ, Ladwig GB, Swan BA, Tucker SJ: *Evidence-based nursing care guidelines*, St. Loius, MO, 2008, Mosby.
Billings DM, Halstead JA: *Teaching in Nursing: A Guide for Faculty*, 6th edition, Philadelphia, PA, 2019, Elsevier.
Cherry B, Jacob S: *Contemporary nursing: Issues, trends and management*, 9th ed, Philadelphia, PA, 2022, Elsevier.
Institute of Medicine: *Crossing the quality chasm: A new health system for the 21st century*, 2001, doi:10.17226/10027
Institute of Medicine: To err is human: *Building a safer health care system*, 1999, https://nap.nationalacademies.org/resource/9728/To-Err-is-Human-1999–report-brief.pdf
Intramural Research Program: *The national academy of medicine*, 2024, https://irp.nih.gov/about-us/honors/the-national-academy-of-medicine
JBI: *About JDI*, (n.d.), https://jbi.global/about-jbi
Melnyk BM, Fineout-Overholt E: *Evidence-based practice in nursing and healthcare: A guide to best practice*, 5th ed., New York, NY, 2023, Wolters Kluwer.
Polit DF, Beck CT: *Nursing research: Generating and assessing evidence for nursing practice*, 11th ed., New York, NY, 2021, Wolters Kluwer.
National League of Nursing (NLN): *Strengthening the future of the nursing workforce*, 2025, www.nln.org/education/nursing-education-competencies/core-competencies-for-academic-nurse-educators
National League for Nursing (NLN): *Practical/vocational program outcomes: Human flourishing*, 2015, www.nln.org/docs/default-source/uploadedfiles/default-document-library/human-flourishing-final.pdf
National League for Nursing (NLN): *Outcomes and competencies for graduates of practical/vocational, diploma, associate degree, baccalaureate, masters, practice doctorate, and research doctorate programs in nursing*, New York, NY, 2012, Wolters Kluwer.

Websites Resources Cited

www.cms.gov
www.nursing-theory.org
https://www.nlm.nih.gov/bsd/medline.html
https://www.cochrane.org
http://www.ahrq.gov
https://jbi.org

CHAPTER 14

American Association of Colleges of Nursing (AACN): *About the Doctor of Nursing Practice (DNP)*, 2023, www.aacnnursing.org/our-initiatives/education-practice/doctor-of-nursing-practice/about-the-dnp
American Association of Colleges of Nursing: *Academic progression in nursing: Moving together toward a highly educated nursing workforce*, (n.d.), www.aacnnursing.org/News-Information/Position-Statements-White-Papers/Academic-Progression-in-Nursing
Desir ML, Laughon D, Tao H, Green JF: The impact of a licensed practical nurse-registered nurse care delivery model on the work environment, *Nurse Leader* 22(1):95–103, 2024. www.sciencedirect.com/science/article/abs/pii/S1541461223002215.
Institute for Patient- and Family-Centered Care: *Person-and family-centered care*, (n.d.), www.ipfcc.org/about/pfcc.html
National Council of State Boards of Nursing, Inc: *2022 Study highlights*, 2024, www.ncsbn.org/research/recent-research/workforce/2022-workforce-rn.page
National League of Nursing (NLN): *Research priorities for nursing education*, 2024, www.nln.org/education/grants-scholarships/research-priorities-in-nursing-education
National League for Nursing (NLN): *Doctoral faculty collaboration in nursing education*, 2018, www.nln.org/docs/default-source/uploadedfiles/default-document-library/dnp-20183859c75c78366c709642ff00005f0421.pdf?sfvrsn=b96fab0d_0
National League for Nursing (NLN): *Graduate preparation for academic nurse educators*, 2017, www.nln.org/docs/default-source/uploadedfiles/about/nln-vision-series-position-statements/vision-graduate-preparation2.pdf
National League for Nursing (NLN): *A vision for recognition of the role of the licensed practical/licensed vocational nurses in advancing the nation's health*, 2014. www.nln.org/docs/default-source/uploadedfiles/about/nlnvision_7.pdf?sfvrsn=c7e06e45_3
National League for Nursing (NLN): *A vision for doctoral education for nurse educators*, 2013, www.nln.org/docs/default-source/uploadedfiles/about/nlnvision_6.pdf?sfvrsn=75163694_3
Nurse.org: *Complete list of common nursing certifications*, 2025, https://nurse.org/articles/nursing-certifications-credentials-list/
Nursingschool.org: *Associate's degree in nursing: Popular fast-track to a solid career*, 2024, www.nursingschool.org/

nursing-programs/program-types/associates/#context/api/listings/prefilter
Nursingschool.org: *Hospital nursing programs: Traditional diploma*, 2024, www.bls.gov/oes/current/oes291141.htm
Porat-Dahlerbruch J, Aiken LH, Lasater KB, Sloane DM, McHugh MD: Variations in nursing baccalaureate education and 30-day inpatient surgical mortality, *Nursing Outlook* 70(2):300–308, 2022. doi:10.1016/j.outlook.2021.09.009.
U.S. Bureaus of Labor Statistics: *Occupational employment and wage statistics: Licensed practical and licensed vocational nurses*, 2024, www.bls.gov/oes/2023/may/oes292061.htm
U.S. Bureau of Labor Statistics: *Occupational employment wage statistics: Registered nurses*, 2024, www.bls.gov/oes/current/oes291141.htm
U.S. Bureau of Labor Statistics: *Occupational outlook handbook: Licensed practical and licensed vocational nurses*, 2024, www.bls.gov/ooh/healthcare/licensed-practical-and-licensed-vocational-nurses.htm
U.S. Bureau of Labor Statistics: *Occupational outlook handbook: Nursing assistants and orderlies*, 2024, www.bls.gov/ooh/healthcare/nursing-assistants.htm
Tussing TE, Chipps E, Tornwall J: Generational differences in the nursing workforce: Strategies for nurse leaders, *Nurse Leader* 22(5):602–608, 2024. doi:10.1016/j.mnl.2024.03.007.
Wintemute D: *How to become a nurse anesthetist*, 2024, https://nursejournal.org/nurse-anesthetist/how-to-become-a-crna/

Website Resources Cited

www.nsna.org
https://www.nursingworld.org/practice-policy/workforce/what-is-nursing
www.nln.org
https://nam.edu

CHAPTER 15

American Hospital Association (AHA): *AHA annual survey database*, 2024, www.ahadata.com/aha-annual-survey-database.
Centers for Medicare and Medicaid Services (CMS): *Critical access hospitals (CAHs)*, 2025, www.ruralhealthinfo.org/topics/critical-access-hospitals
Centers for Medicare and Medicaid Services (CMS): *Critical care hospital*, 2021, www.hrsa.gov/sites/default/files/hrsa/opa/critical-access-hospital-factsheet.pdf
Centers for Medicare and Medicaid Services: *Palliative care versus hospice care*, (n.d.), www.cms.gov/Medicare-Medicaid-Coordination/Fraud-Prevention/Medicaid-Integrity-Education/Downloads/infograph-PalliativeCare-[June-2015].pdf
Perkari VK: *Long-term care*, (n.d.), www.drperkari.com/Services/Internal_Medicine/Long-Term_Care.html
U.S. Department of Health and Human Services: *HHS organizational charts office of secretary and divisions*, 2024, www.hhs.gov/about/agencies/orgchart/index.html
World Health Organization (WHO): *Who we are*, 2024, www.who.int/about/who-we-are

Website Resources Cited

https://www.cms.gov/Medicare-Medicaid-Coordination/Fraud-Prevention/Medicaid-Integrity-Education/Downloads/infograph-PalliativeCare-[June-2015].pdf
www.healthaffairs.org
www.medicare.gov/coverage/skilled-nursing-facility-care.html
www.cancer.org
www.diabetes.org
www.lung.org
www.heart.org
www.strokeassociation.org
www.also.org
www.easterseals.org
www.lalecheleague.org
www.na.org
www.ostomy.org
www.voa.org

CHAPTER 16

AARP International: United States, 2024, www.aarpinternational.org/initiatives/aging-readiness-competitiveness-arc/united-states
Bajwa J, Munir U, Nori A, Williams B: Artificial intelligence in healthcare: Transforming the practice of medicine, *Future Healthcare Journal*, 8(2):188-194, 2021, doi:10.7861/fhj.2021-0095
Bergman A: Great Speculations: Social security feels pinch as baby boomers check out for good, 2018, Forbes, 2018, www.forbes.com/sites/greatspeculations/2018/06/21/social-security-feels-pinch-as-baby-boomers-clock-out-for-good/#bb45f8249951
Center for Disease and Prevention (CDC): Health insurance coverage: Early release of estimates from the national health interview survey, 2023, 2024, www.cdc.gov/nchs/data/nhis/earlyrelease/insur202406.pdf
Center for Medicare Advocacy: Medicare enrollment numbers, 2023, https://medicareadvocacy.org/medicare-enrollment-numbers/
Center for Medicare and Medicaid Services: NHE fact sheet: Historical NHE, 2022, 2024, www.cms.gov/data-research/statistics-trends-and-reports/national-health-expenditure-data/nhe-fact-sheet
Cherry B, Jacob S: *Contemporary nursing: Issues, trends and management*, 9th ed, Philadelphia, PA, 2022, Elsevier.
Gunja MZ, Gumas ED, Williams RD: U.S. health care from a global perspective, 2022: Accelerating spending, worsening outcomes, 2023, www.commonwealthfund.org/publications/issue-briefs/2023/jan/us-health-care-global-perspective-2022
Hamilton C: The impact of the 2014 Medicaid expansion on the health, health care access, and financial well-being of low-income young adults, *Health Economics* 22(8):1895–1925, 2024. doi:10.1002/hec.4839.
Health and Medicine Division of the National Academies (HMD): About Health and Medicine Division: Impact, 2024, www.nationalacademies.org/hmd/about

Institute of Medicine: Report brief: To err is human: Building a safer health care system, 1999, https://nap.nationalacademies.org/resource/9728/To-Err-is-Human-1999–report-brief.pdf
Institute of Medicine: Report brief: Crossing the quality chasm: A new health system for the 21st century, 2001, doi:10.17226/10027.
Institute of Medicine: *Report brief retooling for an aging America: Building the health care workforce*, National Academy of Sciences, 2008. doi:10.17226/12089.
Keisler-Starkey K, Bunch LN: *Health insurance coverage in the United States: 2023*, U.S. Department of Commerce: U.S. Census Bureau, 2024. https://www2.census.gov/library/publications/2024/demo/p60-284.pdf.
Library of Congress: The individual mandate for health insurance coverage: In brief, 2020, www.congress.gov/crs-product/R44438
Library of Congress: H.R. 1628 - American health care act of 2017, (n.d.), www.congress.gov/bill/115th-congress/house-bill/1628
Mastrorosa I, Lepri AC, Borgo CD, Rosati S, Rueca M, Sarmati L, Mastroianni C, Fantoni M, Maggi F, Nicastri E, Girardi E, Lichtner M, Antinori A, Mazzotta V: Incidence and predictors of clinical failure after early treatment for mild-to-moderate COVID-19 in high-risk individuals, A multicentric cohort study, *Journal if Internal Medicine* 297(3):328–334, 2025. doi:10.1111/joim.20030.
Medicare.gov: Value-based care, 2025, www.cms.gov/priorities/innovation/key-concepts/value-based-care
Medicare.gov: Inpatient hospital care, (n.d.), www.medicare.gov/coverage/inpatient-hospital-care
Medicare.gov: Skilled nursing facility care, (n.d.), www.medicare.gov/coverage/skilled-nursing-facility-care
Medicare.gov: What part B covers, (n.d.), www.medicare.gov/providers-services/original-medicare/part-b
Mortada EM: Evidence-based complementary and alternative medicine in current medical practice, *Cureus* 16(1):e52041, 2024. doi:10.7759/cureus.52041.
Muller F, Abdelnour AM, Rutaremara DN, Arnet JE, Achtyes ED, Alshaarawy O, Holman HT: Association between sociodemographic factors, clinic characteristics and mental health screening rates in primary care, *PLoS ONE* 193:1–14, 2024. doi:10.1371/journal.pone.0301125.
National Academies: Sciences, Engineering, and Medicine: Future of nursing: Leading change, advancing health, (n.d.), www.nationalacademies.org/hmd/Reports/2010/The-Future-of-Nursing-Leading-Change-Advancing-Health.aspx
National Center for Health Workforce Analysis: State of the behavioral health workforce, 2024, https://bhw.hrsa.gov/sites/default/files/bureau-health-workforce/state-of-the-behavioral-health-workforce-report-2024.pdf
National Committee for Quality Assurance (NCQA): HEDIS and performance measurement, 2025, www.ncqa.org/hedis/
National Human Genome Research Institute: Personalized medicine, 2025, www.genome.gov/genetics-glossary/Personalized-Medicine
Pellegrini CA: Revisiting To Err is Human 20 year later, American College of Surgeons, 2020, www.facs.org/for-medical-professionals/news-publications/news-and-articles/bulletin/2020/02/revisiting-to-err-is-human-20-years-later/
Petrullo J: US has highest infant, maternal mortality rates despite the most health care spending, *AJMC*, 2023. www.ajmc.com/view/us-has-highest-infant-maternal-mortality-rates-despi.

CHAPTER 17

Accreditation Commission for Education in Nursing (2024): *2023 ACEN report to constituents*, 2024. Accessed 15 April 2025. Available from: https://www.acenursing.org/students-public/report-to-constituents
Bass BM: *Leadership and performance beyond expectations*, New York, NY, 1985, Free Press.
Bass BM: *The Bass handbook of leadership—theory, research and managerial applications*, New York, NY, 2008, Free Press.
Blanchard K, Oncken W, Burrows H: *The one-minute manager meets the monkey*, New York, NY, 1991, Harper Collins Publisher.
Ellis A: *Reason and emotion in psychotherapy*, New York, NY, 1994, Carol Publishing Group.
Grumet J: 2005 Effective delegation, *Nurs Manag* 36(6):50–60, 2005.
Hansten R, Jackson M: *Clinical delegation skills: a handbook for professional practice*, Burlington, MA, 2009, Jones & Bartlett Publishers.
Herzberg F, Mausner B, Snyderman B: *The motivation to work*, New York, NY, 1959, John Wiley.
Hill SS, Howett HS: *Success in practical/vocational nursing: Howlett hierarchy of work motivators*, 7th ed., St. Louis, 2013, Elsevier.
Huber P, Shubert H: Attitudes about work engagement of different generations—a cross-sectional study with nurses and supervisors, *J Nurs Manag* 27:1341–1350, 2019. Available from:. https://doi.org/10.1111/jonm.12805.
Knecht P, Sosik JJ: Transformational leadership of nurses in long-term care contexts: propositions and implications for research and practice, Nashville, TN. *Proceedings of the institute of behavioral and applied management, Publisher IBAM in Peru, NE*.
Lee A, Willis S, Tian A: *When empowering employees works, and when it doesn't*, 2018, Harvard Business Review. Available from:. https://hbr.org/2018/03/when-empowering-employees-works-and-when-it-doesnt.
National Association of Licensed Practical Nurses (former National Federation of Licensed Practical Nurses): *Nursing practice standards for the licensed practical/vocational nurse*, 2003. Accessed 10 April 2026. Available from: https://nalpn.org/standards/.
National Council State Board of Nursing & American Nurses Association: *Joint ANA and National Council of State Boards of nursing position statement. National guidelines for nursing delegation*, 2019. Accessed 10 April 2026. Available from: https://www.ncsbn.org/public-files/NCSBN_Delegation_Guidelines.pdf.

NCSBN 2024 LPN/VN Practice Analysis: 2025. Accessed 10 April 2026. Available from: https://www.ncsbn.org/public-files/24_NCLEX_PN_PA.pdf.

Nightingale F: *Notes on nursing*, New York, NY, 1859, Fall River Press.

Wong CA, Cummings GG, Ducharme L: The relationship between nursing leadership and patient outcomes: a systematic review, *J Nurs Manag* 21(5):709–724, 2013.

Website Resources Cited

http://www.jointcommission.org
http://www.cms.gov
http://www.napnes.org
http://www.nalpn.org
www.ncsbn.org
https://www.ncsbn.org/contact-bon.htm

CHAPTER 18

American Nurse Association: *Why nurses quit and leave the profession*, 2023. Accessed 15 Feb 2026. https://www.nursingworld.org/content-hub/resources/nursing-leadership/why-nurses-quit/.

Beshara T: *Acing the interview: how to ask and answer the questions that will get you the job*, New York, NY, 2008, AMACON.

Bureau of Labor Statistics: *U.S. Department of labor: occupational outlook handbook, licensed practical and licensed vocational nurses, 2024–2025 edition*, 2025. Accessed 15 February 2026. Available from: https://www.bls.gov/ooh/healthcare/licensed-practical-and-licensed-vocational-nurses.htm.

Canadian Nurses Association: Nursing statistics, 2025. Accessed 15 April 2025. https://www.cna-aiic.ca/en/nursing/regulated-nursing-in-canada/nursing-statistics.

Congressional Budget Office: *The demographic outlook: 2025 to 2055*, 2025. Accessed 15 April 2025. https://www.cbo.gov/publication/61164#_idTextAnchor001, https://vacareers.va.gov/VeteransAdministration.

Favreault, M. M., Johnson, R. W. US Department of Health and Human Services. Projections of risk of needing long-term services and support at ages 65 and older, 2021. Accessed 15 April 2025. https://aspe.hhs.gov/sites/default/files/private/pdf/265136/LTSSRisk.pdf.

Hospice Foundation of America, 2018 National Hospice and Palliative Care Organization: *Facts and figures: hospice care in America*, 2025. Accessed 15 February 2026. Available from: https://allianceforcareathome.org/2024-nhpco-facts-and-figures-report-now-available/.

Hospital Foundation of America: 2025. Accessed 15 April 2025. https://hospicefoundation.org/what-is-hospice/on.

Institute of Medicine, Committee on the Future Health Care Workforce for Older Americans: *Retooling for an aging America: building the health care workforce*, Washington, DC, 2008, The National Academies Press. Accessed 15 February 2026. Available from:. https://www.nationalacademies.org/publications/all?search=retooling%20for%20an%20aging%20america.

Institute of Medicine: *Future of nursing: leading change, advancing health*, Washington, DC, 2010, The National Academies Press. Available from:. http://www.nationalacademies.org/hmd/Reports/2010/The-Future-of-Nursing-Leading-Change-Advancing-Health.aspx.

Knecht P: *Demystifying job satisfaction in long-term care: the voices of licensed practical nurses*, 2014, Pennsylvania State University.

National Council of State Boards of Nursing: *2024 PN practical analysis: linking the NCLEX-PN to practice*, 2024. Accessed 15 February 2026. Available from: https://www.ncsbn.org/exams-research/2024-pn-practice-analysis-linking-the-nclex-pn-examination-to-practice.

National Council State Board of Nursing: *Transition to practice*, 2024. Available from: https://www.ncsbn.org/transition-to-practice.htm.

National League for Nursing: *A vision for recognition of the role of the licensed practical/licensed vocational nurses in advancing the nation's health*, 2014. Accessed 15 February 2026. Available from: https://www.nln.org/docs/default-source/uploadedfiles/about/nlnvision_7.pdf?sfvrsn=c7e06e45_3.

National Academies of Sciences, Engineering: *Medicine: The future of nursing 2020–2030: charting a path to achieve health equity*, Washington, DC, 2021, The National Academies Press. https://doi.org/10.17226/25982.

NCSBN: *2024 RN practice Analysis: linking the NCLEX-RN® examination to practice*, 2025. Accessed 15 April 2025. https://www.ncsbn.org/public-files/24_NCLEX_RN_PA.pdf.

NCSBN: *2024 PN practice analysis: linking the NCLEX-PN® examination to practice*, 2025. Accessed 15 April 2025. https://www.ncsbn.org/public-files/24_NCLEX_PN_PA.pdf.

Podcasting for Beginners: How it All Works, Easily Explained! Accessed 15 Feb 2026. Available from: https://www.thepodcasthost.com/planning/podcastingfor-beginners/

Provides guidance in their publication, a nurse's guide to the use of social media, 2024. https://www.ncsbn.org/brochures-and-posters/nurses-guide-to-the-use-of-socialmedia.

Robert Woods Johnson Campaign for Action, 2025. Accessed 15 Feb 2025. https://campaignforaction.org/

Schrager S: Tips for writing effective DVs and cover letters, *Fam Pract Manag* 28(5):4–5, 2021. Accessed 15 February 2025. Available at:. https://www.aafp.org/pubs/fpm/issues/2021/0900/p4.html.

Schrager SB: Tips for writing effective CVs and cover letters, *Fam Pract Manag* 28(5):4–5, 2021. Accessed 15 February 2025. Available at:. https://www.aafp.org/pubs/fpm/issues/2021/0900/p4.html.

Skilled Nursing Workforce: *Mission care collective*, 2025. Accessed 15 February 2026. https://www.missioncare.com/snf-workforce-report-2025.

Smiley R, Kaminski-Ozturk N, Reid M, Burwell P, Oliveira C, Shobo Y, Allgeyer R, Zhong E, O'Ohara Ch, Volk A, Martin B: The 2024 National nursing workforce survey, *K Mirs Regi* 16(1):S1–S88, 2025.

Smiley RA, Ruttinger C, Oliveira CM, et al.: The 2020 National Nursing Workforce Survey, *J Nurs Regul* 12(1):S1–S96, 2021.

Smiley R, Lauer P, Bienemy C, et al.: The 2017 national nursing workforce summary, *J Nurs Regul* 9(3):S1–S88, 2018.

Spector N, Blegen MA, Silvestre J, Barnsteiner J, Lynn MR, Ulrich B: Transition to practice in nonhospital settings, *J Nurs Regul* 6(1):4–13, 2015.

Website Resources Cited

www.napnes.org
https://nalpn.org/
www.va.gov/jobs/
www.careerbuilder.com
www.healthcarefinancenews.com
www.employmentguide.com/job-fairs/browse
www.resumehelp.com/home-1?utm_source5bing%20&utm_medium5cpc&utm_keyword5%2Bresume%20%2Btemplates
https://owl.purdue.edu/owl/purdue_owl.html
www.ncsbn.org
www.ncsbn.org/transition-to-practice.htm
www.bls.gov/oes/current/oessrcst.htm
www.bls.gov.
https://www.medscape.com
https://www.ftc.gov/about-ftc/bureaus-offices/bureau-consumer-protection/our-divisions/division-privacy-and-identity
https://owl.purdue.edu/owl/job_search_writing/resumes_and_vitas/sample_resumes/index.html
https://www.thepodcasthost.com/planning/podcasting-for-beginners/
https://www.acenursing.org/
https://www.aacnnursing.org/ccne-accreditation
https://cnea.nln.org/

CHAPTER 19

Boehning AP, Haddad LM: *Nursing practice act*, Treasure Island (FL), 2025, StatPearls Publishing. [Updated 2023 Jul 17] Accessed 15 March 2026. Available from:. https://www.ncbi.nlm.nih.gov/books/NBK559012/.

Candon M, Bergman A, Rose A, Song H, David G, Spetz J: The relationship between scope of practice laws for task delegation and nurse turnover in home health, *J Am Med Dir Assoc* 24(11):1773–1778, 2023 e2.

Corazzini KN, Anderson RA, Mueller C, Thorpe JM, McConnell ES: Licensed practical nurse scope of practice and quality of nursing home care, *Nurs Res* 62(5):315–324, 2013.

National Council of State Boards of Nursing: *Next generation NCLEX® project*. 2021. Available from: https://www.ncsbn.org/event-video-view/next-generation-nclex-update.

National Council of State Boards of Nursing: *2021 PN practical analysis: linking the NCLEX-PN to practice*, 2022. Accessed 15 April 2025. Available from: https://www.ncsbn.org/exams-research/2021-pn-practice-analysis-linking-the-nclex-pn-examination-to-practice.

National Council of State Boards of Nursing: *2023 NCLEX-PN® examination test plan for the National Council Licensure Examination for practical nurses*, Chicago, IL, 2023, NCSBN. Accessed 15 April 2025. Available from:. https://www.ncsbn.org/publications/2023-nclex-pn-test-plan.

National Council of State Boards of Nursing: 2025 NCLEX-PN® examination candidate bulletin, 2022. Accessed 15 June 2025. Available from: https://www.ncsbn.org/publications/2025-nclex-candidate-bulletin.

National Council of State Boards of Nursing: *New nurses: your license to practice*, 2015. Accessed 15 April 2025. https://www.ncsbn.org/video/new-nurses-your-license-to-practice.

National Council of State Boards of Nursing: *Quick results: how to access your "unofficial" NCLEX results*, 2025. Accessed 15 April 2025. https://www.nclex.com/quick-results.page.

National Council of State Boards of Nursing. *Nurse Practice Toolkit*. 2025. Accessed 1 April 2025. https://www.ncsbn.org/policy-gov/npa-toolkit.page.

Silvestri LA, Silvestri AE: *Saunders comprehensive review for the NCLEX-PN® examination, ed*, New York, NY, 2025, Elsevier.

Website Resources Cited

www.ncsbn.org
https://www.ncsbn.org/newnurses.htm
https://www.ncsbn.org/membership/us-members/contact-bon.page

Index

Note: Page numbers followed by "*f*" indicate figures, "*t*" indicate tables, and "*b*" indicate boxes.

F

G

H